CANCER RESEARCH FRONT OF JAPAN, 2003

Gann Monograph on Cancer Research

The "Gann Monograph on Cancer Research" series is promoted by the Japanese Cancer Association. This semiannual series of monographs was initiated in 1966 by the late Dr. Tomizo Yoshida (1903–1973) and is now published jointly by Japan Scientific Societies Press, Tokyo and S. Karger AG, Basel. Each volume consists of collected contributions on current topics in cancer problems and allied research fields. The planning for each volume is done by the Monograph Committee of the Japanese Cancer Association, with the final approval of the Board of Directors. It is hoped that the series will serve as an important source of information in the field of cancer research.

The publication of these monographs owed much to the financial support given by the late Professor Kazushige Higuchi, the Jikei University School of Medicine.

Japanese Cancer Association

JAPANESE CANCER ASSOCIATION
Gann Monograph on Cancer Research No. 52

CANCER RESEARCH FRONT OF JAPAN, 2003

SPECIAL ISSUE IN COMMEMORATION OF THE 100 th ANNIVERSARY OF THE LATE Dr. TOMIZO YOSHIDA'S BIRTH

Edited by
TAKASHI TSURUO and TOMOYUKI KITAGAWA

JAPAN SCIENTIFIC SOCIETIES PRESS
Tokyo

KARGER
Basel·Freiburg·Paris·London·New York·Bangalore
Bangkok·Singapore·Tokyo·Sydney

July 2004

Published jointly by
JAPAN SCIENTIFIC SOCIETIES PRESS
2-10 Hongo, 6-chome, Bunkyo-ku, Tokyo 113-0033, Japan
ISBN 4-7622-3031-6

and

S. KARGER AG
P.O. Box, CH-4009 Basel, Switzerland
ISBN 3-8055-7816-4

Sole distribution rights outside Japan granted to S. KARGER AG, Basel.

PREFACE

The year 2003 was the one hundredth anniversary of the late Dr. Tomizo Yoshida's birth.

Dr. T. Yoshida was an extraordinary oncologist and pathologist. He became world famous as a young scientsit for his epoch-making success, in 1932, in inducing hepatocellular carcinomas in rat liver by feeding a single chemical substance *o*-aminoazotoluene (*o*-amidoazotoluol) (Virchows Archiv 1935; 195: 175-200). This was the first experimental proof that environmental carcinogens entering the body may cause malignancies in human visceral organs. His achievement was also particularly important in cancer research because liver model systems have subsequently been widely applied for studies of cancer biochemistry, multistep carcinogenesis, carcinogen metabolism, carcinogenecity testing and risk assessment. His review book on experimented carcinogenesis entitled "Development of Cancer" (Nihon Ishoshuppan Inc., 1944) filled with his unique comments and considerations became a kind of bible for cancer researchers in Japan for a long time.

In 1943, Dr. Yoshida further discovered an ascitic tumor spontaneously developed in the peritoneal cavity of a rat bearing a small hepatoma. Since he had been actively seeking such a tumor because of his conviction that cancer cells free from stroma might provide essential clues to neoplasia , he made the most of this rare opportunity and, after a dramatic struggle, established a transplantable ascitic tumor line (later named Yoshida's sarcoma). Soon he progressed to the idea of employing the ascitic tumor line for screening for chemotherapeutic drugs. Cooperating with chemists with passion, he paved a broad path in experimental cancer chemotherapy and drug screening. In addition, with his young colleague pathologists, he produced many ascites tumor lines from azo-dye-induced rat hepatocellular carcinomas. Comparative observations of these ascitic tumors then led him to the concrete notion of individuality of cancers, regarding malignant grade, chromosomal features, genetic instability, antigenicity and, most importantly, chemosensitivity (National Cancer Institute Monograph 16, 1964). He may therefore be called the father of individualized chemotherapy, which has now become one of the most important challenges of cancer treatment in the 21st century.

As is well-known in Japan, Dr. Yoshida was not only a pioneering scientist but also remarkable philosopher, artist, idealist, organizer, mentor, husband and father. The following few examples should provide some understanding of his character traits and capabilities: 1. In 1960, when he became a member of the National Language Council, he drew on his deep thought and knowledge about Japanese culture and successfully persuaded the governmental council, hitherto biased under the influence of kanji-abolition advocates, to adopt his important proposal to officially recognize that written sentences comprised of both the Chinese characters (kanji) and the Japanese alphabet (kana) constitute the written Japanese. 2. In 1964, he ran for the presidency of the Japan Medical Association campaigning for both the government and the medical doctors to act together for providing on ideal medical system for Japan. It is of note that he did this from a sense of responsibility of a medical person, although he knew from the conservative nature of the body that he would not get more than 10% of the ballot. 3. In 1966, he acted as Chair of the organizing Committee for the 9th UICC International Cancer Congress and, bringing out the devotion of all the cancer researchers of Japan, made it the largest international congress after World War II and a springboard for subsequent remarkable progress of Japanese cancer research with the distinct increment in governmental financial aid. 4. In 1968, he organized the cancer research system of Ministry of Education, Culture and Science, Japan, implementing his novel idea to create an “invisible” National Cancer Institute comprised of many local research units throughout Japan, instead of making a single large National Institute. This system worked quite efficiently and received much praise from abroad. 5. In 1992, his eldest son Mr. Naoya Yoshida, a famous TV director and essayist, published a marvelous book entitled “Thus spoke the cancer cells”, which is widely recognized the best and most impressive record of the multiple activities and fascinating personality of his father.

It is therefore not surprising that in 2003 as many as 7 professional scientific societies, including the Japanese Cancer Association, the Japanese Society of Pathology, the Japanese Association of Medical Sciences and the Science Council of Japan, all held special symposia or a workshops in commemoration of Dr. Yoshida. In addition, two large commemorative ceremony / assemblies were held in Tokyo and in Asakawa-machi, the small town in Fukushima prefecture where he was born and in which the Yoshida-memorial Museum located.

This special volume of Gann Monograph is envisaged as another contribution to his memory. The volume is comprised of minireview articles written by current top researchers of Japan, dedicated to the late Dr. Tomizo Yoshida. To avoid disadvantages with inevitable delays in making a book composed of collected papers, most of the articles were already published in Cancer Science immediately when they were submitted.

We are very grateful to Drs. George Klein and Henry C. Pitot who kindly provided such attractive and informative Forewords for this volume.

March 2004

Tomoyuki Kitagawa

FOREWORD-I

My contacts with Professor Tomizo Yoshida started in the early 1960s. We were working with mouse ascites tumors and have greatly enjoyed reading his exciting papers about the Yoshida rat ascites sarcoma. This started a correspondence in the early 1960s and exchange of cells and information. I have also become familiar with the earlier, very important work of Tomizo Yoshida, discovering the hepatoma inducing effect of azo dyes. This was a pioneering discovery that has given rise to many experimental and also practical, prevention-related developments.

In 1965, the Cancer Section of the World Health Organization asked me to go Japan and set up a joint bank of mouse and rat ascites tumors, in collaboration with Professor Yoshida. I then met him at the first time. I stayed at the house of a young attaché at the Swedish Embassy in Tokyo (later an outstanding cabinet minister) who gave me "good advice" on the way to behave in Japan and also to negotiate an agreement with Professor Yoshida whom he has never met. His experience was largely restricted to business. His advice was to proceed very slowly, very cautiously, very indirectly, and to spend several days with polite formalities, before discussing the business part of the visit. He also advised me to avoid mentioning anything about the Second World War or, absolutely, about the atomic bomb.

Professor Yoshida did not fit any part of this stereotype. He received me with two younger professor colleagues, offered me tea and immediately asked: "What does WHO want?". When I told him he asked about the financial support for the proposed bank. Then he said: "OK. I agree. Now let us talk about more interesting things".

In the evening, my Swedish diplomat friend gave a dinner party in the honor of Professor Yoshida and some of his colleagues. During the party, Yoshida told us about many aspects of life and work in Japan. He also spoke freely, and without being specifically asked, about the war years, including the fact that he had the good fortune of leaving Nagasaki a few weeks before the atomic bomb.

This taught me two things. The stereotypes of young Swedish diplomats do not fit with the Japanese reality, at least as far as scientists are concerned. But I have also suspected, rightly, as it turned out, that Tomizo Yoshida was a scientist and thinker of great originality who would make up his own mind on all issues rather than follow an established stereotype.

During my three days visit, Professor Yoshida showed me many things in Tokyo, starting with the Korean Buddha, and has placed everything we saw into context. I particularly valued the introduction he gave me into Japanese ways of thinking. He told me that the Japanese respected the West for technological innovations, but for philosophical thinking and attitude to life and death they looked up to the Chinese.

I asked Tomizo Yoshida to give me an example of the Chinese attitude that was particularly respected by Japanese. He thought about this for a long while during which he did not speak. I already thought that I asked an impossible question. But then the answer came. The first word was in German: Wasservogel (bird of water). After some more silence, a beautiful metaphore emerged. The waterbird flies over a lake. The surface of the lake is my soul. The shadows of the bird on the water are the events.

Even though Tomizo Yoshida appeared to give the impression that this image of perfect serenity was a goal the Japanese could only strive for to attain, while the Chinese had it, he himself was the perfect image of that serenity: wise, quiet, firm and decisive.

I have learned much of him. In the field of cancer biology, he taught me the great diversity of tumors and particularly the fact that, even among tumors induced by the same agent in the same species, each tumor was an unique individual. That notion has been born out fully by the modern, molecular evidence.

I remember Professor Tomizo Yoshida as a great cancer researcher, a warm friend and a great teacher.

George Klein
Karolinska Institute
Microbiology and Tumor Biology Center
MTC

FOREWORD-II

It is a singular honor and privilege to be asked by my Japanese colleagues to write a Foreword for this distinguished volume in memory of the 100th anniversary of Dr. Tomizo Yoshida's birth. I believe that it was at the International Cancer Congress in Tokyo in 1966 that I first met Dr. Yoshida, having been introduced to him by my colleagues at the McArdle Laboratory, Drs. James and Elizabeth Miller. I had the feeling of a small boy meeting one of his distinguished heroes whom he admired and respected. I had already been teaching medical students of Dr. Yoshida's seminal contributions to cancer research in their first course in pathology.

Japanese scientists laid the foundation of our knowledge of the chemistry and pathology of chemical carcinogenesis, first discovered in animals and within the last several decades applied extensively to the human experience. It was Drs. K. Yamagiwa and K. Ichikawa who first demonstrated the carcinogenic action of the direct application of coal tar to the skin of rodents. It was their discovery that led Dr. E. L. Kennaway and his colleagues using a modification of the carcinogen bioassay applied to mouse skin to isolate a pure chemical substance from coal tar that exhibit potent epidermal carcinogenicity. This material was identified as 3,4,-benzpyrene. In the same year, 1932, Dr. Yoshida reported his epoch-making discovery that a pure chemical, *o*-aminoazotoluene, when fed to rats for extended periods induced malignant neoplasms of the liver. Perhaps the two most important ramifications of Dr. Yoshida's discovery were first, that a pure chemical when administered to rodents by feeding induced neoplasms, not of the mouth, pharynx, esophagus, or stomach, but of the liver, anatomically quite removed from these tissues that can come in direct contact with the carcinogen. I believe many scientists today do not realize the significance of this finding. Since the discovery of carcinogenesis by coal tar application to an external tissue, the skin, by Drs. Yamagiwa and Ichikawa, the concept was inherent that the carcinogenic substance must come in direct contact with the target tissue. Dr. Yoshida's findings demonstrated that such was not the case and in fact laid the foundation for later experiments demonstrating the necessity of the metabolism by the target tissue of the carcinogenic substance to its ultimate carcinogenic form. The second incisive experimental result was the demonstration that a chemical unrelated in structure to polycyclic hydrocarbons could induce neoplasia in any tissue in the living organism. This result in fact laid the foundation for our knowledge of the numerous chemicals of varied structures, organic and inorganic, that have demonstrated carcinogenic activity today.

As with many exceptional discoveries, especially in medical research, it took years, even decades for Dr. Yoshida's contributions to our basic understanding of chemical carcinogenesis to be appreciated. But Dr. Yoshida did not wait for out basic knowledge of the chemical and metabolic characteristics of chemical carcinogens to be elucidated. Rather, he continued his studies in the biology of neoplastic development, investigating the relationship between neoplastic cells and their supporting interstitial tissues. His conclusions that neoplastic cells could progress to live and proliferate without any connection with a supporting stroma in the acidic form led to his many experiments in the production of neoplasms capable of growing in liquid suspension as an ascites *in vivo* and as found later by others as a suspension in appropriate tissue culture vessels. He was able to identify individual characteristics of different strains of ascites hepatomas and proposed from these findings the individuality of malignant neoplasms. This phenomenon has been demonstrated time and again in both primary and secondary neoplasms in animals and in the human, although not appreciated at the time. His experimental findings laid the foundation for the demonstration of the major characteristics of the stage of progression in neoplastic development, that of genetic of karyotypic instability. As with most, if not all scientists who make contributions seminal to the advancement of medical science and ultimately enhanced patient care, Dr. Yoshida was concerned with and actively sought to better the medical care of his fellow countrymen. In 1964 he ran for the Presidency of the Japan Medical Association with the objective of reconciling the Japanese government and physicians to act cooperatively to develop the ideal medical system for his country. Later he developed the concepts of a number of cancer research laboratories throughout the country rather than having only a single National Cancer Institute. While working for the establishment of international cooperative cancer research programs, Dr. Tomizo Yoshida passed away on April 27, 1973 at the age of 70.

The civilized world owes an enormous debt of gratitude to Dr. Tomizo Yoshida for his basic findings on the chemical induction of neoplasia in all animals species. No one disputes that it is chemicals in out environment obtained through diet, tobacco abuse, therapeutic or self administration and inherent in the atmosphere in which we live that cause the majority of human cancers to develop. Ultimately, the goal of medical science is the complete control of cancer through prevention and therapy. When this happens, it will be in no small part the result of the life and scientific contributions of Dr. Tomizo Yoshida.

Henry C. Pitot
McARDLE Laboratory for Cancer Research
(Oncology and Pathology and Laboratory Medicine)

BIOGRAPHY of Dr. TOMIZO YOSHIDA

1903 Born on February 27th at Asakawa machi, Ishikawa-gun, Fukushima-ken, Japan

1927 Graduated from the Faculty of Medicine, the Imperial University of Tokyo and entered the Department of Pathology

1929 Research Fellow, Sasaki Institute, Tokyo

1932 Succeeded in inducing hepatomas in rat liver by feeding an azo-compound, *O*-amidoazotoluol

1935 Associate Professor of Pathology, Nagasaki Medical University
Awarded the 18th Japanese Cancer Research Society Yamagiwa Prize
Awarded the Hattori Hokokai Prize

1935–38 Overseas Researcher of the Ministry of Education at the Universität zu Berlin (Prof. Rössle)

1936 Awarded the Imperial Prize of the Imperial Academy of Japan

1938 Professor of Pathology, Nagasaki Medical University

1943 Established an ascitic tumor later known as the Yoshida Sarcoma

1944 Professor of Pathology, the Imperial University of Tohoku

1948 Elected as a member of the Science Council of Japan

1951 Science Promotion Award from the Japanese Council in Brazil

1952 Awarded the Asahi Prize
Professor of Pathology, University of Tokyo

1953 Director, Sasaki Institute, Tokyo
Awarded the Imperial Prize, Academy of Japan, for the second time, for "Pathological studies of Yoshida Sarcoma"

1954 Worked as vice president of the 6th UICC International Cancer Congress held in London

1955 Elected as an Honorary member of the American Cancer Society

1956 Awarded the Schoele Medal from the Swedish Chemical Society

1958 Dean, Faculty of Medicine, University of Tokyo
Professor of Pathology, the Institute of Infectious Diseases, University of Tokyo

1959 Awarded the Order of Cultural Merit
Member, Expert Committee, Council for Science and Technology

1960 Chair person, 7th Division, Science Council of Japan
Member, University Chartering Committee
Awarded the Honorary degree from the University of Perugia, Italy
Member, National Language Council

1961 President of Japanese Society of Pathology

1962 Worked as a principal in organizing the US-Japan Science Cooperation Program Awarded the Fujiwara Prize

1963 Retired from the University of Tokyo and became director of the Cancer Institute of the Japanese Foundation for Cancer Research (JFCR)
Vice President, Science Council of Japan
Advisor to the Minister of the Education
Awarded the Robert Koch Stiffung

1964 Ran for the Presidency of the Japan Medical Association

1965 Elected as Professor Emeritus, University of Tokyo

1966 Chair, the organizing Committee for the 9th UICC International Cancer

1968 Awarded an Honorary degree from the University of Milan
Organized the cancer research system of the Ministry of Education, Culture and Science, Japan

1969 Awarded the Maude E. Abbott Prize
Member, Tokyo Metropolitan Public Safety Commission

1972 Member, Council for Science and Technology

1973 Worked to establish the US-Japan Cooperative Cancer Research Program. Founded the Cancer Chemotherapy Center of JFCR

1973 Passed away on April 27 at Kyoundo Sasaki Institute Hospital, Tokyo
Awarded Third Grade Senior of the Court and Grand Cordon of the Order of the Rising Sun

(Arranged by Kazuyoshi Yamaguchi)

CONTENTS

PATHOLOGY

ISOLATION OF p53-TARGET GENES AND THEIR FUNCTIONAL ANALYSIS

Yusuke NAKAMURA

*Laboratory of Molecular Medicine, Human Genome Center, The Institute of Medical Science, The University of Tokyo**

Mutations of the *p53* gene are the most common genetic alterations found in human cancers, and are known to play crucial roles in tumor development and progression. The *p53* gene encodes a protein functioning as a transcription factor, and the biological functions of p53 are manifested through the activities of its downstream genes. Identification of these downstream genes involved in the p53-signaling pathway should provide more detailed insight into the molecular mechanisms that mediate tumor-suppressor activities, as well as various responses to cellular stress. We have been attempting to isolate p53-target genes by means of various approaches, including differential display, cDNA microarray analysis, and direct cloning of the p53-binding sequences from human genomic DNA. Here I review our recent work on isolation of p53-target genes and their functional analysis. The physiological functions of p53-target genes include apoptosis (GML, p53AIP1, and STAG1), DNA repair (p53R2), inhibition of angiogenesis (BAI1), re-entry into the cell cycle (p53RFP), oxidative stress (CSR), and determination of cell fate (p53RDL1).

p53 Mutations in Human Cancer

The *p53* gene is the most frequent target of genetic alteration so far identified in human cancers, and cells in which p53 is inactivated are known to have a selective growth advantage (*1*). Many studies have indicated that p53 has multiple physiological functions through transcriptional regulation of its downstream genes by binding to specific genomic sites as a tetramer. p53 was shown to bind DNA in a sequence-specific fashion (*2*) and to activate transcription of genes containing a consensus binding site; these DNA sequences are likely to function as transcriptional enhancers. Normal p53 function can be lost in a variety of ways, most commonly by loss of a chromosomal region containing one allele of the gene (or of the entire chromosome 17p) and a subtle mutation involving the other allele. This scenario fits the "two-hit" model proposed by Knudson (*3*) for the definition of what came to be known as tumor suppressor genes. Inactivation of both alleles of p53 has been documented in a large number of human cancers, including tumors arising in the colon, brain, lung,

* 4-6-1 Shirokanedai, Minato-ku, Tokyo 108-8639, Japan

This paper is dedicated to the memory of late Dr. Tomizo Yoshida on the occasion of the 100th anniversary of his birth. It was originally published in Cancer Science in January, 2004.

liver, and bladder. However, in some cases a missense mutation occurring in one allele of p53 is sufficient to inactivate p53 function, when such an event increases the proportion of hetero-tetramers that contain both mutant and wild-type p53 molecules; the chimeric complexes cannot activate transcription of target genes. This "dominant-negative" effect may be exacerbated by the increased stability (and therefore higher intracellular concentration) of the mutant protein compared with that of the wild-type p53 protein. The other mechanism for inactivation is often seen in soft-tissue sarcomas, in which amplification of MDM2 creates a similar loss of functional p53 through binding and subsequent degradation of the p53 protein (*4*).

Strategies for Identifying p53-Target Genes

Several biological functions of p53 have been described, including induction of cell cycle arrest or apoptosis after DNA damage or other cellular insults, maintenance of genomic stability, and inhibition of angiogenesis. Positive and negative feedback mechanisms by downstream genes were also reported. We have adopted three strategies to identify biologically important genes that are transcriptionally regulated by p53; two of these approaches are the differential display method and cDNA microarray analysis, with which we were able to screen genes showing different expression levels between cells with or without wild-type p53. These techniques could successfully detect p53-target genes that are expressed in relative abundance. However, identifying p53-regulated genes that are expressed less abundantly or in a tissue-specific manner has proven to be difficult. To effectively isolate such genes we applied another strategy, based on the idea that p53-target genes must contain p53-binding sites in their promoter regions or within their introns. We used for this purpose a yeast system (*Saccharomyces cerevisiae*) to identify human genomic sequences, "p53-tagged sites," that activate transcription from an adjacent reporter gene in a p53-dependent manner (*5*), and then isolated and characterized several genes including GML and BAI1 (*6, 7*).

For screening p53-target genes that are expressed in relative abundance, we established a colon-cancer cell line SW480-LOWp53-1 carrying a wild-type *p53* transgene that is inducible under the control of the lactose operon. Induction of this transgene by isopropyl-1-thio-β-D-galactoside (IPTG) arrests growth of the transfected cells (*8*). We applied a differential-display method to screen mRNAs isolated from this cell line, and looked for genes whose expression was activated or suppressed after induction of wild-type p53. Expression of seven known genes was significantly induced or suppressed by induction of wild-type p53 protein (*9*). To identify genes that are transcriptional targets of p53 by cDNA microarray analysis, we prepared an adenovirus designed to express the wild-type p53. We used cDNA-microarray slides bearing 23,000 genes and hybridized them with cDNAs reversely-transcribed from mRNAs of p53-deficient U373MG cells infected with either Ad-p53 or Ad-LacZ. Duplicate microarrays were hybridized with a mixture of Cy5-labeled cDNA probes corresponding to Ad-p53-infected cells and Cy3-labeled cDNA probes corresponding to Ad-LacZ-infected cells. Dozens of genes showed increased signal intensities of Cy5, in a time-dependent manner.

By applying a combination of these approaches, we have isolated and characterized more than a dozen genes of biological and medical importance, as summarized

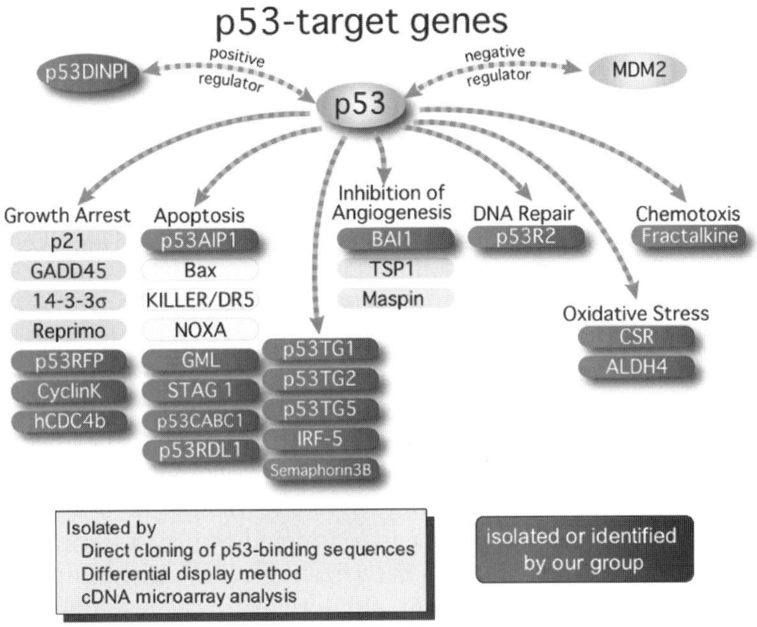

FIG. 1. p53-target genes and their physiological roles
A subset of the p53-target genes that play important biological functions, as well as genes isolated by our group, is shown.

below (Fig. 1).

DNA Repair; p53R2, a Novel Ribonucleotide Reductase

The DNA-damage checkpoint plays a critical role in preventing genomic instability by regulating the cell cycle and DNA repair. Inactivation of the checkpoint may impair the DNA-repair mechanism and increase the susceptibility of cells to genotoxic agents. The *p53R2* gene contains a p53-binding sequence in intron 1 and encodes a 351-amino-acid peptide that showed striking similarity to ribonucleotide reductase small subunit (R2). Expression of the p53R2 was induced by γ- and UV-irradiation, and also by adriamycin treatment in a wild-type p53-dependent manner, while a previously known R2, that plays an important role in DNA synthesis during cell division, was not. Induction of p53R2 expression in p53-deficient cells caused G2/M arrest and prevented cell death in response to adriamycin. Inhibition of endogenous p53R2 expression in cells with an intact p53-dependent DNA damage checkpoint reduced ribonucleotide reductase (RR) activity, DNA repair, and cell survival after exposure to various genotoxins (*10*). Thus, inactivation of p53 could directly interfere with damage-induced transcription of p53R2, enhance misincorporation of dNTPs and increase the frequency of mutations, and thereby result in genomic instability in cancers where p53 has undergone mutation. We examined the role of this p53R2-dependent pathway for DNA synthesis in a p53-regulated cell-cycle checkpoint, comparing it to R2-dependent DNA synthesis. The elevation of DNA synthesis activity through RR in response to γ-irradiation was closely correlated with the level of expression of p53R2, but not that of R2. The p53R2 product accumulated in nuclei, while the R2 levels in cytoplasm decreased. We found a point mutation of p53R2 in the cancer-cell line HCT116, which resulted in loss of RR activity, suggesting that p53R2-dependent DNA synthesis plays a pivotal role in cell survival by repairing damaged DNA in the nucleus (*11*).

We also generated and analyzed mice lacking *p53R2*. They developed normally until weaned, but thereafter displayed growth retardation and early mortality; all mice died by the age of 14 weeks from severe renal failure. Pathological examination of these mice indicated multiple organ failure in kidney, heart, liver, skeletal muscle, lymphatic organs, and nervous system. The TUNEL staining of kidneys of *p53R2−/−* mice at the age of 8 weeks showed an increase of apoptotic cells. In kidney and liver of *p53R2−/−* mice, p53 protein was activated, leading to transcriptional induction of p53-target genes including *Bax*, *Noxa*, and *p53Dinp1*, followed by apoptosis of a large number of cells and organ failure. *p53R2−/−* embryonic fibroblasts (MEFs) showed similar rates of proliferation to *p53R2+/+* MEFs, but they became immortal much earlier and were more susceptible to apoptosis induced by oxidative stress than *p53R2+/+* MEFs. dNTP pools were severely attenuated in *p53R2−/−* MEFs suffering oxidative stress. Hence, p53R2 is considered to play a pivotal role in maintaining dNTP levels for DNA repair in the arresting cells, and an impairment of this pathway may activate the p53-dependent apoptotic pathway, resulting in severe renal failure, growth retardation and early mortality *in vivo* (*12*). We speculate that p53 might function as a checkpoint for damaged cells by balancing the death and survival signals.

Apoptosis-Related Genes; p53AIP1, GML, p53ABC1L, STAG1, and Semaphorin3B

Through direct cloning of p53-binding sequences from human genomic DNA, we have isolated a novel gene, designated *p53AIP1* (p53-regulated Apoptosis Inducing Protein 1), whose expression is inducible by wild-type p53 (*13*). Ectopically expressed p53AIP1, which is localized at mitochondria, induced down-regulation of mitochondrial $\Delta\Psi m$ and release of cytochrome *c* from mitochondria in human cells. Immunoprecipitation and immunostaining experiments indicated interaction between p53AIP1 and bcl-2 proteins at mitochondria. Over-expression of bcl-2 blocked the down-regulation of mitochondrial $\Delta\Psi m$ and the pro-apoptotic activity of p53AIP1. We have also found that upon severe DNA damage, Ser46 on p53 is phosphorylated and apoptosis is induced. In addition, substitution of Ser46 inhibits the ability of p53 to induce apoptosis, and selectively blocks expression of p53AIP1. Our results suggest that p53AIP1 is likely to play an important role in mediating p53-dependent apoptosis, and phosphorylation of Ser46 regulates the transcriptional activation of this apoptosis-inducing gene. Considering the function of this gene, gene therapy involving p53AIP1 is expected to be useful for treatment of p53-resistant tumors (Fig. 2) (*14*).

Through the same approach, we isolated a *GML* (GPI-anchored molecule-like protein) gene and demonstrated an apparent correlation between its expression and the sensitivity of esophageal cancer cells to several anticancer drugs (*6*). The *GML* gene product was shown to play an important role in control of the cell cycle and/or the apoptotic pathway induced by wild-type p53 after DNA damage (*15*). Subsequently we introduced GML cDNA into TE10, an esophageal cancer cell line that

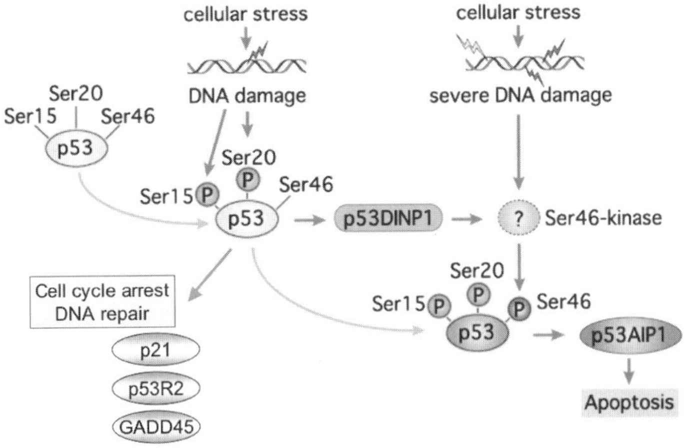

FIG. 2. Selective model for p53-target genes in cell death or survival process

When DNA damage is limited and repairable, phosphorylation of p53 occurs at certain sites (for example, Ser15 and Ser20 residues) and the modified p53 activates genes related to cell cycle arrest and DNA repair (for example, *p21*, *GADD45*, and *p53R2*). When DNA damage in cells is very severe, p53 has an additional phosphorylation at the 46th serine residue by Ser46-kinase with the cooperation of p53DINP1, and it then activates genes inducing apoptosis (for example, *p53AIP1*).

lacks endogenous GML expression. In two resulting stable cell lines which expressed GML cDNA in the absence of wild-type p53, cell death occurred within 6 h after treatment with Taxol. TE10 parent cells or TE10 cells transfected with vector alone displayed relative resistance for 36 h. Induction of GML did not by itself affect viability. Morphological analysis confirmed that the increased chemosensitivity to Taxol conferred by GML was due to apoptosis (*16*).

p53ABC1L (p53-inducible Activity of bc1 complex Like) encodes a 647-amino-acid peptide with significant sequence similarity to ABC1 (Activity of bc1 complex) in *Arabidopsis thaliana* and *Schizosaccharomyces pombe*. The *p53ABC1L* product was located in mitochondria. Inhibition of p53ABC1L expression by transfection with antisense oligonucleotide significantly reduced the apoptotic response induced by wild-type p53, suggesting that p53ABC1L plays an important role in mediating p53-inducible apoptosis through the mitochondrial pathway (*17*).

A mutant version of p53 (p53-121F), in which phenylalanine replaces the 121st serine residue, can induce apoptosis more effectively than wild-type p53 (wt-p53). The *STAG1* gene was one of the transcripts showing higher expression levels in cells infected with Ad-*p53-121F* compared to those infected with Ad-wt*p53*. The encoded product appears to contain a transmembrane domain, and binding motifs for SH3 and WW. Suppression of endogenous *STAG1* using the RNA-interference method reduced the apoptotic response, whether induced by Ad-*p53-121F* or Ad-*p53* (*18*).

Several groups have reported a possible role of *p53* in neuronal apoptosis; expression of p53 mRNA precedes neuronal apoptosis in neurons of injured brain and spinal cord and neuronal cells from p53−/− knock-out mice are resistant to apoptosis induced by neuronal injury, both *in vitro* and *in vivo*. These data indicate that p53 plays an important role in regulating neuronal apoptosis, probably through the transcriptional regulation of target gene(s). Semaphorin3A (Sema3A), a member of the same class as Semaphorin3B, was shown to induce neuronal apoptosis by binding to its receptor, neurophilin-1 (NRP1). Hence, Sema3B (a target molecule of p53) might be one of the mediators involved in p53-dependent neuronal apoptosis. The information presented here should help toward a fuller understanding of the myriad physiological functions of p53.

Angiogenesis Inhibition: BAI1

As normal cells progress toward malignancy, they must switch to an angiogenic phenotype to attract the nourishing vasculature that they depend on for their growth. This switch was found to coincide with loss of the wild-type allele of p53 and to be a result of reduced expression of thrombospondin-1 (TSP-1), a potent inhibitor of angiogenesis, in cultured fibroblasts from patients with Li-Fraumeni syndrome (*19*). p53 stimulates the endogenous *TSP-1* gene and positively regulates TSP-1 promoter sequences; therefore, wild-type p53 in fibroblasts inhibits angiogenesis through regulation of TSP-1. Furthermore, in clinical cases genetic alterations of p53 are known to be associated with neovascularization during progression of a glioma to its more malignant form, glioblastoma. A novel p53-inducible gene, named *BAI1* (brain- specific angiogenesis inhibitor 1), encodes a 1584-amino-acid product that contains five thrombospondin type 1 (TSP-type 1) repeats and is specifically expressed in the brain (*7*). We showed that a recombinant protein corresponding to the TSP-type 1 repeats present in this gene product inhibited *in vivo* neovascularization induced by bFGF in the rat cornea, and we suggested that BAI1 might play a significant role as a mediator of p53 in inhibiting angiogenesis. We also identified two novel human genes homologous to *BAI1*. Like *BAI1*, these two genes, designated *BAI2* and *BAI3*, were specifically expressed in brain, and they are likely to be expressed in the same type of cells. However, in spite of similar tissue specificity among the three *BAI* genes, only *BAI1* is transcriptionally regulated by p53 (*20*).

Oxidative Stress: CSR and ALDH4

Oxidative stress is a pathogenic condition that causes cellular damage, and in a normally functioning cell, several transcription factors respond to this threat by modulating expression of genes whose products ameliorate the altered redox status in some way. *CSR* (Cellular Stress Response) is a novel macrophage scavenger receptor-like gene, whose transcription in normal fibroblasts was significantly elevated by exposure to UV-radiation or hydrogen peroxide, but not by DNA-damaging anti-cancer reagents, in a p53-dependent manner. Pretreatment with antioxidants prevented induction of CSR. Under conditions of oxidative stress, reactive oxygen intermediates (ROIs) were significantly depleted in CSR-overexpressing cells, indicating that the CSR product protects cells by scavenging oxidative molecules or harmful products of oxidation. Investigations into the connection of p53 as transcription factor with the regulation and function of CSR should open a way to understanding the pathogenic processes caused by oxidative stress (*21*).

We also identified the aldehyde dehydrogenase 4 (*ALDH4*) gene as a direct target of p53. ALDH4 is a mitochondrial matrix NAD^+-dependent enzyme catalyzing the second step of the proline degradation pathway. The expression of *ALDH4* mRNA was induced by various cellular stresses, including hydrogen peroxide, UV-, γ-irradiation or adriamycin treatment, in a p53-dependent manner (unpublished data).

Eat-me Signal: Fractalkine and IRF5

Fractalkine, a CX3C-type chemokine that induces chemotaxis of monocytes and cytotoxic T-cells, was induced by ectopic expression of p53 (*22*). The strong induction of *fractalkine* when p53 protein was expressed by a wild-type transgene in p53-defective cells brought to light a novel role for p53; that is, potential elimination of damaged cells via the host immune-response system through transcriptional regulation of fractalkine, implying a pivotal role of p53 in immuno-surveillance to prevent cells from undergoing malignant transformation.

Expression of interferon regulatory factor 5 (*IRF5*) mRNA was also increased in the presence of exogenous p53. Expression of *IRF5* was induced in normal human dermal fibroblast (NHDF4042) cells when DNA was damaged by adriamycin or γ-irradiation, in a wild-type p53-dependent manner. Our results suggested that IRF5 might mediate the p53-dependent immune response (*23*).

Cell-Cycle Control: Cyclin K, hCDC4, and p53RFP

Cyclin K, a newly recognized member of the "transcription" cyclin family, may play a dual role by regulating CDK and transcription. We found that *cyclin K* mRNA was dramatically increased in U373MG, a glioblastoma cell line deficient in wild-type p53, by the introduction of exogenous p53 (*24*). A heterologous reporter assay revealed that p53BS (p53-binding site) in this gene possessed p53-dependent transcriptional activity. Colony-formation assays indicated that over-expression of cyclin K suppressed growth of T98G, U373MG, and SW480 cells, suggesting that cyclin K may play a role in regulating the cell cycle after being targeted for transcription by p53.

Expression of *hCDC4b*, which encodes one of the four subunits of the SCF (ubiquitin ligase) complex responsible for degradation of cyclin E, was dramatically up-regulated by infection with Ad-p53. An electrophoretic mobility-shift assay and a chromatin immunoprecipitation assay indicated that a potential p53-binding site (p53BS) present in exon 1b of the *hCDC4* gene was able to bind to p53. Expression of endogenous *hCDC4b*, but not the alternative transcript of this gene, *hCDC4a*, was induced in a p53-dependent manner in response to genotoxic stresses caused by UV-irradiation and adriamycin treatment. By negatively regulating cyclin E through induction of *hCDC4b*, p53 might stop cell-cycle progression at G0–G1 and may represent a novel mechanism for p53-dependent control of the cell cycle, in addition to the well-known $p21^{WAF1}$ machinery (*25*).

We also isolated *p53RFP* (p53-inducible RING-finger protein), whose product has E3 ubiquitin ligase activity as a transcriptional target of p53. Inhibition of p53RFP expression using antisense oligonucleotides resulted in accumulation of $p21^{WAF1}$ protein. Furthermore, over-expression of exogenous p53RFP in the HCT116 cell line followed by exposure to γ-irradiation caused a decrease in the level of $p21^{WAF1}$ protein. The $p21^{WAF1}$ gene is a direct transcriptional target of p53, and its product in-

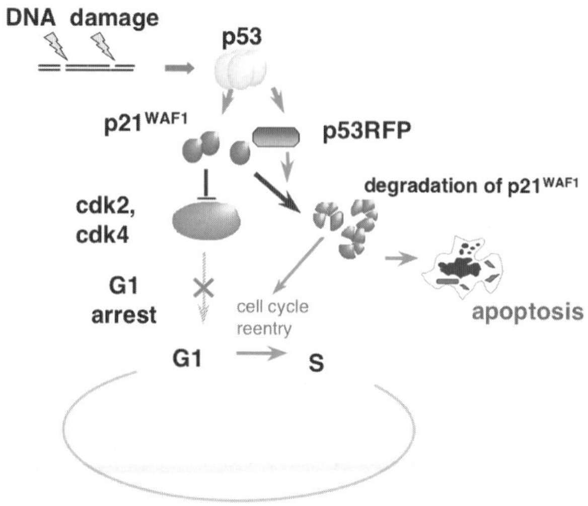

FIG. 3. Model for re-entry into the cell cycle after G1 arrest caused by $p21^{WAF1}$
p53RFP has E3 ubiquitin ligase activity and interacts with $p21^{WAF1}$ *in vitro* and *in vivo*. After cell cycle arrest and DNA repair, p53 recognizes the completion of DNA repair through an unknown mechanism and activates p53RFP for degradation of p21, resulting in re-entery of cells into the cell cycle progression. Destabilization of $p21^{WAF1}$ through transcriptional regulation of *p53RFP* represents a novel mechanism for a p53-dependent cell-cycle checkpoint.

hibits cell proliferation through direct binding to cyclin-dependent kinase (CDK) or subunits of E2F transcription factor, or by interacting with proliferating-cell nuclear antigen (PCNA) to inhibit DNA replication. In DNA-damaged cells, p53 induces $p21^{WAF1}$ to arrest cells at G1. When cells have to be released from cell-cycle arrest and undergo apoptosis, $p21^{WAF1}$ is cleaved by caspase-3 or is degraded. In mammalian cells $p21^{WAF1}$ is an unstable and short-lived protein that exhibits ubiquitination *in vivo* and proteasome-dependent turnover. In humans the $p19^{SKP1}$/$p45^{SKP2}$/CUL-1 complex is likely to function as an E3 ligase that targets $p21^{WAF1}$ for ubiquitin-dependent degradation. The $p21^{WAF1}$ protein can also be degraded by the proteasome without ubiquitin attachment; 20S proteasomes are able to mediate rapid degradation of $p21^{WAF1}$ by interacting with the C-terminus of $p21^{WAF1}$ in the absence of ubiquitin conjugation. We showed that p53RFP interacts with $p21^{WAF1}$ *in vitro* and *in vivo*. Hence, p53RFP appears to represent the second known example, the first being MDM2, of an E3 ubiquitin ligase as a p53-target. Our results suggested destabilization of $p21^{WAF1}$ through transcriptional regulation of *p53RFP*, and represent a novel mechanism for a p53-dependent cell-cycle checkpoint (Fig. 3) (*26*).

Novel Mechanism to Determine Cell Death or Survival: p53RDL1

p53RDL1 (p53-regulated Receptor for Death and Life) contains a death-domain in the cytoplasmic C-terminal region that is highly homologous to rat Unc5H2, a dependence receptor involved in apoptosis-regulation, as well as axon guidance and migration of neural cells. It mediates p53-dependent apoptosis. However, in the presence of its ligand, Netrin-1, the p53RDL1 signaling blocked p53-dependent apoptosis through its interaction with Netrin-1, suggesting that p53 might regulate both cell death and survival of damaged cells, by balancing regulation of the p53RDL1-Netrin-1 signaling for survival and cleavage of p53RDL1 for apoptosis, thereby helping to maintain the integrity of the genome. Although the mechanism still remains to be elucidated, the possibility of applying this pathway for neuronal regeneration is interesting. In neural cells whose apoptosis is regulated by p53, Netrin-1, the ligand of p53RDL1 might be a promising drug to prevent neural cell death related to injury, neurodegenerative disorders or dementias (*27*).

Positive Regulation of p53: p53DINP1

The transcription-activating function of p53 is eliminated by interaction with the *MDM2* gene product, because MDM2 promotes rapid degradation of a phosphorylated form of p53 (*4*). On the other hand, p53 activates expression of the *mdm2* gene in an auto-regulatory feedback loop. This system is well known as the negative feedback system of p53. MDM2 is amplified in 30–40% of human sarcomas; this observation indicates that inhibition of p53 function by over-expression of MDM2 plays a crucial role in development of many sarcomas.

We isolated a novel p53-inducible gene, termed *p53DINP1* (p53-dependent Damage Inducible Nuclear Protein 1), that is involved in positive regulation of the p53-apoptotic pathway (*28*). Cell death induced by DSBs, as well as Ser46-phosphorylation of p53 and induction of p53AIP1, was blocked when we inhibited expression of p53DINP1 by means of an antisense oligonucleotide. Over-expression of p53DINP1 and DNA damage by DSBs synergistically enhanced Ser46-phosphorylation of p53, induction of p53AIP1 expression, and apoptotic cell death. The protein-complex interacting with p53DINP1 was shown to have a function to phosphorylate Ser46 of p53, suggesting that p53DINP1 regulates p53-dependent apoptosis through phosphorylation of p53 at Ser46, serving as a cofactor for the putative p53-Ser46-kinase.

Conclusion

We have isolated and characterized more than a dozen novel p53-target genes. We believe that our efforts have contributed to a better understanding of the physiological roles of wild-type p53, as well as the pathological effects of p53 mutations in human carcinogenesis. However, the more new information we obtain about how p53 functions, the more mysterious the physiological roles of the p53 protein become. Indeed, we are far from a full understanding of the complicated functions of the p53 protein. Although we now have almost complete information about human genome sequences, it is clear that our knowledge of human internal processes or human carcinogenesis is still very limited.

REFERENCES

1. Hollstein M, Sidransky D, Vogelstein B, Harris CC. p53 mutation in human cancers. *Science* 1991; **253**: 49–53.
2. Kern SE, Pietenpol JA, Thiagalingam S, Seymour A, Kinzler KW, Vogelstein B. Oncogenic forms of p53 inhibit p53-regulated gene expression. *Science* 1991; **252**:

1708–11.

3. Knudson AG Jr. Hereditary cancer, oncogenes, and antioncogenes. *Cancer Res* 1985; **45**: 1437–43.
4. Kubbutat MHG, Jones SN, Vousden KH. Regulation of p53 stability by Mdm2. *Nature* 1997; **387**: 299–303.
5. Tokino T, Thiagalingam S, el-Deiry WS, Waldman T, Kinzler KW, Vogelstein B. p53 tagged sites from human genomic DNA. *Hum Mol Genet* 1994; **3**: 1537–42.
6. Furuhata T, Urano T, Tokino T, Nakamura Y. Isolation of a novel GPI-anchored gene specifically regulated by p53, and correlation between its expression and anti-cancer drug sensitivity. *Oncogene* 1996; **13**: 1965–70.
7. Nishimori H, Shiratsuchi T, Urano T, Kimura Y, Kiyono K, Tatsumi K, Yoshida S, Ono M, Kuwano M, Nakamura Y, Tokino T. A novel brain-specific p53-target gene, BAI1, containing thrombospondin type1 repeats inhibits experimental angiogenesis. *Oncogene* 1997; **15**: 2145–50.
8. Takei Y, Ishikawa S, Tokino T, Muto T, Nakamura Y. Isolation of a novel p53-target gene from a colon-cancer cell line carrying a highly-regulated wild-type p53 expression system. *Genes Chromosom Cancer* 1998; **23**: 1–9.
9. Okamura S, Ng CC, Koyama K, Takei Y, Monden M, Nakamura Y. Identification of seven genes regulated by wild-type p53 in a colon-cancer cell line carrying a well-controlled wild-type p53 expression system. *Oncol Res* 1999; **11**: 281–5.
10. Tanaka H, Arakawa H, Shiraishi K, Yamaguchi T, Takei Y, Nakamura Y. A ribonucleotide reductase gene involved in a p53 dependent DNA damage checkpoint. *Nature* 2000; **404**: 42–9.
11. Yamaguchi T, Matsuda K, Sagiya Y, Iwadate M, Fujino MA, Nakamura Y, Arakawa H. p53R2-dependent pathway for DNA synthesis in a p53-regulated cell-cycle checkpoint. *Cancer Res* 2001; **61**: 8256–62.
12. Kimura T, Takeda S, Sagiya Y, Gotoh M, Nakamura Y, Arakawa H. Impaired function of p53R2 in *Rrm2b*-null mice causes severe renal failure through attenuation of dNTP pools. *Nat Genet* 2003; **34**: 440–5.
13. Oda K, Arakawa H, Tanaka T, Matsuda K, Tanikawa C, Mori T, Nishimori H, Tamai K, Tokino T, Nakamura Y, Taya Y. Isolation of a novel gene encoding a mitochondrial protein, *p53AIP1*, a potential mediator of p53-dependent apoptosis, and its regulation by Ser46-phosphorylated p53. *Cell* 2000; **102**: 849–62.
14. Matsuda K, Yoshida K, Taya Y, Nakamura K, Nakamura Y, Arakawa H. p53AIP1 regulates the mitochondrial apoptotic pathway. *Cancer Res* 2002; **62**: 2883–9.
15. Kimura Y, Furuhata T, Urano T, Hirata K, Nakamura Y, Tokino T. Genomic structure and chromosomal localization of GML (GPI-anchored molecule-like protein), a gene induced by p53. *Genomics* 1997; **41**: 477–80.
16. Ueda K, Miyoshi Y, Tokino T, Watatani M, Nakamura Y. Induction of apoptosis in T98G glioblastoma cells by transfection of GML, a p53-target gene. *Oncol Res* 1999; **11**: 125–32.
17. Iiizumi M, Arakawa H, Mori T, Ando A, Nakamura Y. Isolation of a novel human p53-target gene encoding a mitochondrial protein, p53ABC1L, that is highly homologous to yeast activity of bc1 complex. *Cancer Res* 2002; **62**: 1246–50.
18. Anazawa Y, Arakawa H, Nakagawa H, Nakamura Y. Identification of STAG1 as a key

mediator of a p53-dependent apoptotic pathway. *Oncogene* in press.
19. Dameron KM, Volpert OV, Tainsky MA, Bouck N. Control of angiogenesis in fibroblasts by p53 regulation of thrombospondin-1. *Science* 1994; **265**: 1582–4.
20. Oda K, Shiratsuchi T, Nishimori H, Inazawa J, Yoshikawa H, Taketani Y, Nakamura Y, Tokino T. Identification of BAIAP2 (BAI-associated protein 2), a novel human homologue of hamster IRSp53, whose SH3 domain interacts with the cytoplasmic domain of BAI1. *Cytogenet Cell Genet* 1999; **84**: 75–82.
21. Han HJ, Tokino T, Nakamura Y. CSR, a scavenger receptor-like gene with a protective role from cell death caused by UV irradiation and oxidative stress. *Hum Mol Genet* 1998; **7**: 1039–46.
22. Shiraishi K, Fukuda S, Mori T, Matsuda K, Yamaguchi T, Tanikawa C, Ogawa M, Nakamura Y, Arakawa H. Identification of fractalkine, a CX3C-type chemokine, as a direct target of p53. *Cancer Res* 2000; **60**: 3722–6.
23. Mori T, Anazawa Y, Iiizumi M, Fukuda S, Nakamura Y, Arakawa H. Identification of the interferon regulatory factor 5 gene (IRF-5) as a direct target for p53. *Oncogene* 2002; **21**: 2914–8.
24. Mori T, Anazawa Y, Matsui K, Fukuda S, Nakamura Y, Arakawa H. Cyclin K as a direct transcriptional target of the p53 tumor suppressor. *Neoplasia* 2002; **4**: 268–74.
25. Kimura T, Gotoh M, Nakamura Y, Arakawa H. *hCDC4b*, a regulator of cyclin E, as a direct transcriptional target of p53. *Cancer Sci* 2003; **94**: 431–6.
26. Ng CC, Arakawa H, Fukuda S, Kondoh H, Nakamura Y. p53RFP, a p53-inducible RING-finger protein, regulates the stability of $p21^{WAF1}$. *Oncogene* 2003; **22**: 4449–58.
27. Tanikawa C, Matsuda K, Fukuda S, Nakamura Y, Arakawa H. $\textit{p53RDL1}^{UNC5B}$ as a positive and negative regulator of p53-dependent apoptosis. *Nature Cell Biol* 2003; **5**: 216–23.
28. Okamura S, Arakawa H, Tanaka T, Nakanishi H, Ng CC, Taya Y, Monden M, Nakamura Y. p53DINP1, a p53-inducible gene, regulates p53-dependent apoptosis. *Mol Cell* 2001; **8**: 85–94.

CELL ADHESION SYSTEM AND HUMAN CANCER MORPHOGENESIS

Setsuo HIROHASHI and Yae KANAI

*Pathology Division, National Cancer Center Research Institute**

Cell-cell adhesion determines the polarity of cells and participates in the maintenance of the cell societies called tissues. Cell-cell adhesiveness is generally reduced in human cancers. Reduced intercellular adhesiveness allows cancer cells to disobey the social order, resulting in destruction of histological structure, which is the morphological hallmark of malignant tumors. Reduced intercellular adhesiveness is also indispensable for cancer invasion and metastasis. A tumor-suppressor gene product, E-cadherin, and its undercoat proteins, catenins, which connect cadherins to actin filaments, are located at lateral borders, concentrating on adherens junctions, of epithelial cells and establish firm cell-cell adhesion. The E-cadherin cell adhesion system in cancer cells is inactivated by various mechanisms that reflect the morphological and biological characteristics of the tumor. Silencing of the *E-cadherin* gene by DNA hypermethylation around the promoter region occurs frequently, even in precancerous conditions. In diffuse infiltrating cancers, mutations are found in the genes for E-cadherin and α- and β-catenins. At the invading front of cancers, the E-cadherin cell adhesion system is inactivated by tyrosine phosphorylation of β-catenin; an oncogene product, c-*erb*B-2 protein, is found to associate directly with β-catenin. The E-cadherin cell adhesion system cross-talks with the Wingless/Wnt signaling pathway through β-catenin, and expression of genes, which participate in cancer morphogenesis, may be regulated in conjunction with the Wingless/Wnt signaling pathway. Dysadherin, a newly identified cancer-associated cell membrane glycoprotein, down-regulates E-cadherin and promotes cancer metastasis. In conclusion, inactivation of the E-cadherin cell adhesion system by both genetic and epigenetic mechanisms plays a significant role during multistage human carcinogenesis.

E-Cadherin Cell Adhesion System and the Wingless/Wnt Signaling Pathway

The cell-cell adherens junction is a specialized region of the plasma membrane, connected with cytoskeletal actin filaments, where cadherins act as Ca^{2+}-dependent adhesion molecules (*1, 2*). Cadherin molecules are integral membrane glycoproteins with a single transmembrane domain. The extracellular domain of E-cadherin, the major cadherin in epithelial cells, is composed of five cadherin domains (EC1 to

* 5-1-1 Tsukiji, Chuo-ku, Tokyo 104-0045, Japan

This paper is dedicated to the memory of late Dr. Tomizo Yoshida on the occasion of the 100th anniversary of his birth. It was originally published in Cancer Science in July, 2003.

EC5). Ca^{2+}-binding motifs are located between neighboring cadherin domains. Cadherins mainly interact in a homophilic manner, e.g., E-cadherin binds selectively to E-cadherin. The extracellular cadherin fragments exist in the form of stable parallel lateral dimers. The cytoplasmic undercoat proteins for cadherins have been named catenins. β-Catenin interacts with cadherins through its cytoplasmic domain, which exhibits the strongest degree of homology between different members of the cadherin family. α-Catenin connects the E-cadherin and β-catenin complex to actin filaments. Interactions between cadherins and cytoskeletal proteins through catenins confer stability on the cell-cell adherens junction.

These observations suggested the possibility that suppression of E-cadherin activity triggers the release of cancer cells from primary cancer nests. Indeed, early *in vitro* experiments using cultured cells revealed that E-cadherin has invasion-suppressing properties (*3*, *4*). In addition, a later study on a large kindred of early-onset, diffuse-type stomach cancer revealed that the *E-cadherin* gene satisfies the criteria for tumor-suppressor genes (*5*). Today, there is evidence for inactivation of the E-cadherin cell adhesion system by various mechanisms during multistage human carcinogenesis.

The structure of β-catenin is remarkably similar to that of the Armadillo protein, an important element in the Wingless/Wnt signaling pathway of the fruit fly *Drosophila* (*6*, *7*). Wingless is a cell-cell signal in *Drosophila* that triggers many key developmental processes, and Wnt is the analogous molecule in vertebrates. β-Catenin directly interacts with adenomatous polyposis coli (APC) protein through its Armadillo domain. Truncated APC protein resulting from mutation of the *APC* gene often lacks the repeats that are necessary for degradation of β-catenin by the ubiquitin-proteasome pathway. Mutations of the *β-catenin* gene in the glycogen synthase kinase-3β (GSK3β) phosphorylation site also make β-catenin itself resistant to proteolysis. As well as its involvement in cell adhesion, β-catenin acts as a transcriptional co-activator by forming a complex with T-cell factor/lymphoid enhancer factor (TCF/LEF) DNA-binding proteins (*8*). β-Catenin may participate in cross-talk between cell-cell adhesion and transcriptional regulation of cancer-related proteins.

Reduced Expression of E-Cadherin by DNA Hypermethylation

In an attempt to understand the significance of reduced expression of E-cadherin in human cancer tissues *in vivo*, we performed immunohistochemical studies with an anti-human E-cadherin monoclonal antibody (*9–11*). E-Cadherin was expressed uniformly in most cohesive stomach cancers, but was not detected in diffuse-type stomach cancers, which lack tight cell-cell adhesion (*9*, *10*). Since then, many other studies on E-cadherin protein expression in various human cancers have been reported. Generally, E-cadherin expression is strong in well-differentiated cancers, which maintain their cell-cell adhesiveness and are less invasive, but are reduced in undifferentiated cancers, which have lost their cell-cell adhesion and show a strong invasive tendency (Fig. 1). Significant correlations between abnormalities of E-cadherin expression and the clinical outcome of patients with cancers have been reported (*12*).

In order to clarify the mechanism of regulation of E-cadherin expression in cancers, we cloned and sequenced the promoter region of the human *E-cadherin* gene

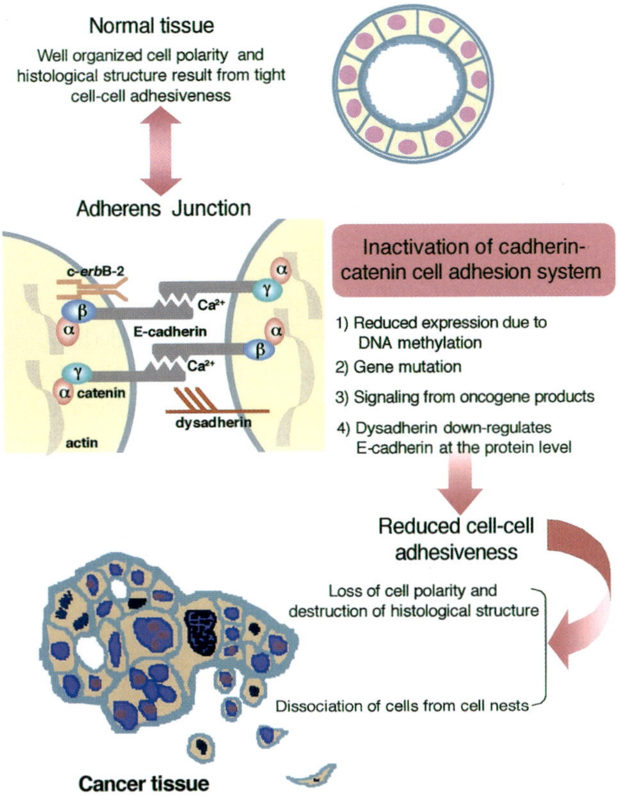

FIG. 1. Multiple mechanisms of inactivation of the E-cadherin cell adhesion system in human cancers

(*13*). We demonstrated CpG methylation around the promoter region of the *E-cadherin* gene and induction of E-cadherin expression following treatment with the DNA methyltransferase inhibitor 5-azacytidine in human cancer cell lines lacking E-cadherin expression (*13*). Thus, the *E-cadherin* gene became the third example of tumor-suppressor genes that are silenced by DNA hypermethylation, chronologically following the *RB* and *VHL* genes (Fig. 1). Today, it is widely recognized that considerable numbers of tumor-suppressor genes and tumor-related genes are silenced by DNA hypermethylation in various human cancers, and correction of DNA methylation status has gained recognition as a new anti-cancer strategy.

We assessed the DNA methylation status *in vivo* of primary hepatocellular carcinomas and their corresponding liver tissues showing chronic hepatitis or cirrhosis, which are widely considered to be precancerous conditions. DNA methylation around the promoter region of the *E-cadherin* gene was detected frequently in liver tissues showing chronic hepatitis or cirrhosis, and the incidence and the degree of DNA methylation increased as these precancerous conditions progressed to hepatocellular carcinomas (*14*). Heterogeneous E-cadherin expression in liver tissues showing chronic hepatitis or cirrhosis, which was not observed in normal liver tissues, may be due, at least in part, to DNA methylation around the promoter region of the *E-cadherin* gene. DNA methylation around the promoter region correlated significantly with reduced E-cadherin expression detected immunohistochemically in hepatocellular carcinomas (*14*). DNA methylation around the promoter region may participate in hepatocarcinogenesis, even during the early developmental stages of hepatocellular carcinomas, by reducing E-cadherin expression, resulting in loss of cell-cell adhesiveness and destruction of tissue morphology.

We also reported that α-catenin expression is frequently decreased in diffuse-type human cancers (*15, 16*). In patients with esophageal squamous cell carcinomas, reduced α-catenin expression correlated significantly with poor prognosis (*16*).

Mutations of the E-Cadherin, α-Catenin and β-Catenin Genes

The tumor cells in diffuse-type cancers are dissociated throughout the entire tumor mass. Although immunohistochemical examination revealed strong E-cadherin expression even in some diffuse-type cancers, in such cancers E-cadherin molecules failed to localize at the cell membrane but were diffusely distributed throughout the cytoplasm, suggesting that these molecules lack cell-cell adhesive properties. These findings led us to think that the E-cadherin cell adhesion system in cancer cells may also be inactivated by genetic alterations. We started to explore this hypothesis by looking for mutations, and found genetic alterations of α-catenin in a lung cancer cell line as the first evidence that our hypothesis was correct (Fig. 1) (*17, 18*). In this cell line, genetic alteration of the *α-catenin* gene may affect the RNA splicing recognition signal and result in both mRNA splicing errors and marked mRNA instability (*18*). This cell line regained its cell-cell adhesiveness when transfected with wild-type α-catenin cDNA (*19*), providing the first evidence that functional α-catenin is indispensable to the E-cadherin cell adhesion system. However, later studies showed that mutational inactivation of the *α-catenin* gene is, if anything, a rare event *in vivo* in human cancers.

Mutations of the *E-cadherin* gene itself were detected subsequently in other human cancer cell lines (*20*) and *in vivo* (*21–24*). The reported *E-cadherin* gene mutations resulted in exon skipping owing to mRNA splicing errors and/or in-frame and frame-shift deletions and insertions. Cell lines possessing *E-cadherin* gene mutations show loss of the wild-type E-cadherin allele, suggesting that E-cadherin dysfunction in such cell lines results from a two-hit mechanism, as occurs with the classical tumor-suppressor genes (*20*). Recently, a large kindred study (*5*) of early-onset, diffuse-type stomach cancers from New Zealand revealed a germ-line mutation located at the same position as the mutation that we reported in a stomach cancer cell line (*20*).

In contrast to the reduced expression of E-cadherin frequently detected in poorly differentiated carcinomas derived from various organs, mutations of the *E-cadherin* gene were restricted to certain histological types of cancers, such as signet ring cell carcinomas of the stomach and lobular carcinomas of the breast. In these cancers, cellular atypia is rather mild and their most obvious characteristic, which occurs even in intraepithelial lesions, is the complete loss of cell-cell adhesiveness. Indeed, tissue microdissection revealed that *E-cadherin* gene mutations in introns, resulting in skipping of exon 9, occurred even in the intramucosal lesions of signet ring cell carcinomas of the stomach, as well as in deeply invading areas (*23*). These findings indicate that genetic alterations of E-cadherin are involved not only in the later events of carcinogenesis, invasion and metastasis, but also during the early stages of some histological types of human cancers.

Several years before attention became focused on mutations of exon 3 of the *β-catenin* gene, which affect serine/threonine phosphorylation by GSK3β and protect the β-catenin protein from degradation through the ubiquitin-proteasome pathway, we reported genetic alterations of β-catenin that abolished cell-cell adhesiveness in two cell lines derived from a signet ring cell carcinoma of the stomach (Fig. 1) (*25*). Homozygous deletion of a part of the *β-catenin* gene caused an identical in-frame mRNA deletion in both cell lines. Although the truncated β-catenin was co-precipitated in immunoprecipitation experiments using an anti-human E-cadherin monoclonal antibody, α-catenin was not, suggesting the possibility that the interaction between α-catenin and E-cadherin is not direct, but mediated by β-catenin. This speculation was proved to be correct by later biochemical analysis (*26*).

Tyrosine Phosphorylation of β-Catenin and Its Association with the c-erbB-2 Oncogene Product

A fibroblast cell line was shown to be loosely associated, with the ability to migrate from colonies, after transfection with v-*src* (*27*). Treatment with a tyrosine kinase inhibitor restored tight cell-cell adhesion of the transformed cells, whereas a tyrosine phosphatase inhibitor inhibited cadherin-mediated aggregation (*27*). β-Catenin in these transformed cells was strongly tyrosine-phosphorylated (*27*), suggesting that tyrosine phosphorylation of β-catenin may affect the function of the cadherin cell adhesion system. Strong tyrosine phosphorylation of β-catenin was also observed in loosely adherent cancer cell lines that had no mutations and did not show reduced expression of E-cadherin or α- and β-catenins (*28*). These observations prompted a search for kinases that participate in aberrant tyrosine phosphorylation in cancers. We showed that both β-catenin and plakoglobin (γ-catenin) directly interact with the c-*erb*B-2 gene product, the first evidence for direct interaction between oncogene products and cell-cell adhesion molecules (Fig. 1) (*29, 30*). This direct interaction was mediated by the c-*erb*B-2 gene product core region, which is highly homologous with the epidermal growth factor receptor. Tyrosine phosphorylation of catenins was found to be initiated by epidermal growth factor, which can induce scattering of cancer cell lines. Another group also identified direct interaction between epidermal growth factor receptor and β-catenin (*31*).

We divided colorectal cancers into two types according to a particular macroscopic feature, the presence or absence of white streak lesions at the invasion front. The frequency of liver metastasis was significantly higher in patients with streak-type than non-streak-type tumors (*32*). The incidence of recurrent liver metastasis after curative resection was also significantly higher in patients with streak-type primary tumors than in patients with non-streak-type (*32*). The white streaks corresponded histologically to cancer cells showing focal dedifferentiation, with marked stromal fibrosis extending towards the serosa or adventitia (*33*). Western blotting analysis with an anti-phosphotyrosine monoclonal antibody after immunoprecipitation with an anti-β-catenin monoclonal antibody revealed strong tyrosine phosphorylation of β-catenin in the streaks (*34*). Tyrosine phosphorylation of β-catenin may participate in focal dedifferentiation in streak lesions, resulting in invasion and metastasis *in vivo*.

In cancer cell lines, transfection with N-terminally deleted β-catenin, which binds to c-*erb*B-2 but not to cadherin, inhibited the association between endogenous β-catenin and c-*erb*B-2 protein and suppressed the tyrosine phosphorylation of β-catenin (*35*). Cancer cells expressing N-terminally deleted β-catenin exhibited markedly reduced invasiveness *in vitro* and reduced peritoneal dissemination (*35*) and hematogenous metastases *in vivo* when inoculated into nude mice, and developed a well-differentiated epithelial morphology (Fig. 2). These results suggest that tyrosine phosphorylation of β-catenin regulated by c-*erb*B-2 protein or other receptor-type tyrosine kinases plays an important role in the invasion, metastasis and morphogenesis of cancer cells.

β-Catenin in the Wingless/Wnt Signal Transduction System

We demonstrated immunohistochemically the cytoplasmic and nuclear accumulation of β-catenin protein in adenomas and adenocarcinomas from patients with familial adenomatous polyposis (FAP) (*36*). It is known that sporadic colorectal cancers with wild-type APC harbor mutually exclusive mutations in the GSK3β phosphorylation site of β-catenin. Therefore, aberrant transactivation of a certain set of target genes by β-catenin and TCF/LEF complexes has been implicated in familial and sporadic colorectal tumorigenesis. This is supported by studies with a colorectal can-

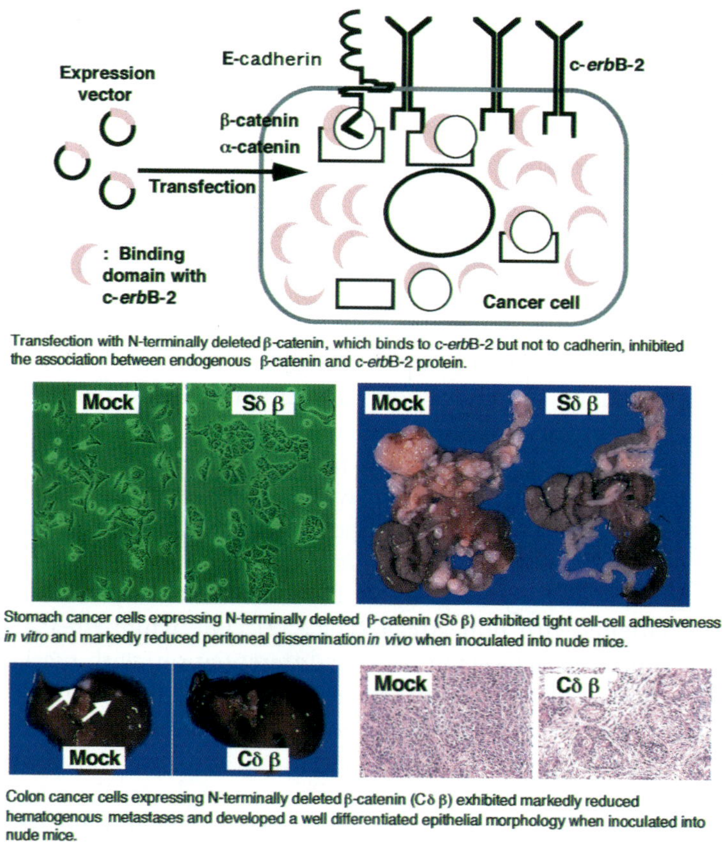

FIG. 2. Transfection of cancer cell lines with N-terminally deleted β-catenin, which binds to c-*erb*B-2, but not to cadherin

cer cell line that showed irregular multilayered growth and formed numerous dome-like polypoid loci piled-up over the surface of cell sheets (*37*). The continuous suppression of β-catenin and TCF/LEF-mediated gene transactivation by transfection of dominant-negative TCF4B reduced these piled-up foci and restored a simple monolayer of polarized columnar cells resembling normal intestinal epithelium (*37*). Reduction of contact inhibition and the loss of epithelial cell polarity may be critical events during β-catenin and TCF/LEF-mediated intestinal tumorigenesis.

However, only a limited number of genes, including c-*myc*, *cyclin D1*, *matrilysin*, *TCF1* and *peroxisome proliferator-activated receptor δ*, have so far been reported to be the direct targets of β-catenin and TCF/LEF-mediated transactivation in colorectal cancer cells. A large-scale expression profile analysis using two-color fluorescence hybridization of a cDNA microarray in dominant-negative TCF4B transfectants led to the identification of the multidrug resistance 1 (*MDR1*) gene as a target gene of β-catenin and TCF/LEF complexes (*38*). Corresponding to the accumulation of β-catenin, expression of the *MDR1* gene product was steadily up-regulated in adenomas and adenocarcinomas of patients with FAP (*38*). In combination with the cell proliferative activities of c-myc and cyclin D1, MDR1 may initiate colorectal tumorigenesis by suppressing cell death pathways programmed in intestinal epithelial cells.

We have also reported mutations of exon 3 of the *β-catenin* gene in cancers of the uterine endometrium (*39*), liver (*40*), and renal pelvis (*41*), sporadic fundic gland polyps (*42*) and craniopharyngiomas of adamantinomatous type (*43*). Synovial sarcomas without mutations of exon 3 of the *β-catenin* gene also showed cytoplasmic and nuclear accumulation of β-catenin, suggesting the possible involvement of mechanisms for β-catenin accumulation other than mutation of the *β-catenin* gene itself, such as alterations of axin, which forms a complex with GSK3β and participates in phosphorylation of β-catenin (*44*). In nodule-in-nodule type hepatocellular carcinomas, which represent the stepwise progression of hepatocarcinogenesis, early hepatocellular carcinoma components showed neither β-catenin accumulation nor mutation of the *β-catenin* gene, but progressed hepatocellular carcinoma components did show these features (*40*).

Integrin β4 in Cancer-Stromal Interactions

Immunohistochemical examination revealed that β-catenin protein frequently accumulates in the nuclei of cancer cells at the invading front of colorectal cancers. After stimulation of a stomach cancer cell line with transforming growth factor α, β-catenin concentrated at the cell membrane gradually moved into the nuclei. These findings suggested that growth factors, regionally released as a result of cancer-stromal interaction at the invading front of cancers, may activate the Wingless/Wnt signaling pathway. Gel retardation assays revealed a direct interaction between nuclear extracts of stomach cancer cells transfected with N-terminally deleted β-catenin, as described above, and DNA fragments containing the TCF/LEF responsive element. In cells transfected with N-terminally deleted β-catenin, transcriptional activity of the TCF/LEF family is persistently activated and expression of integrin β_4 subunit is increased. Consequently, we investigated the mechanism of transcriptional regulation of the *integrin* β_4 gene (*45*). The basal promoter of the *integrin* β_4 gene contains the binding sequence of the *Cdx2* homeobox gene. Transfection of the *Cdx2* gene into a colon cancer cell line has been reported to induce up-regulation of integrin β_4. We isolated the 5′-flanking region of the *Cdx2* gene and confirmed that the 5′-flanking region contains the TCF/LEF responsive element. These data suggest that integrin β_4 expression may be regulated downstream of cross-talk between the E-cadherin cell adhesion and Wingless/Wnt signaling pathways.

In a mouse inoculation model, the level of integrin β_4 subunit expression by gastric cancer cell lines was significantly negatively correlated with dissemination potential (*46*). Transfection of cancer cells showing negligible β_4 subunit expression with integrin β_4 subunit markedly suppressed peritoneal dissemination. Inhibition of endogenous integrin $\alpha_6\beta_4$ by introduction of a cytoplasmic domain-deleted β_4 subunit promoted peritoneal dissemination. The suppression of peritoneal dissemination by

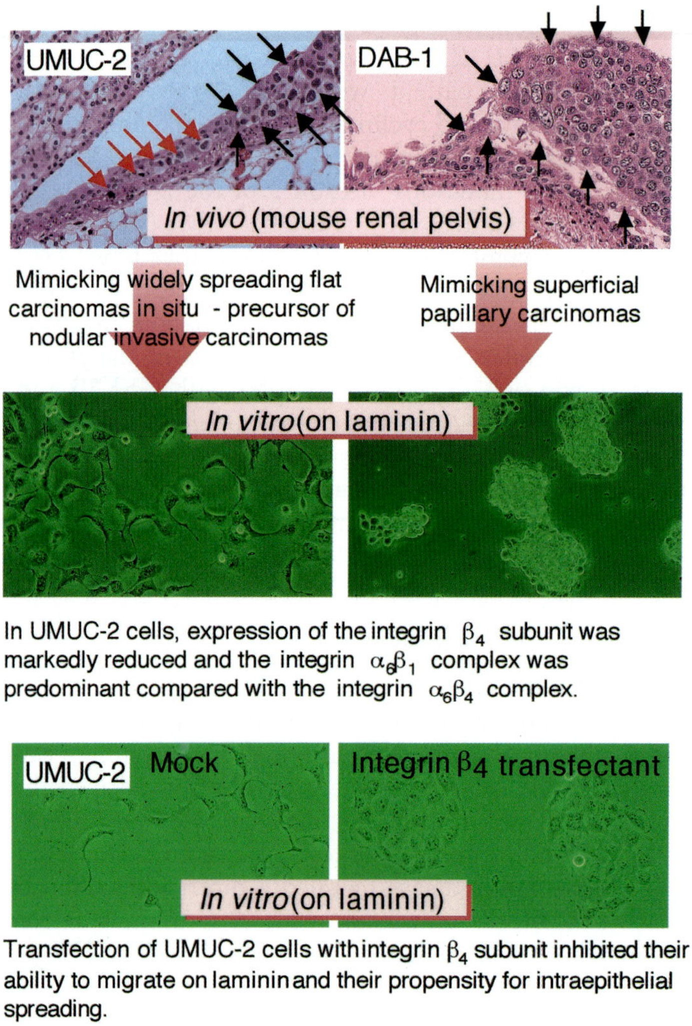

FIG. 3. Reduction of integrin β_4 and enhanced migration on laminin in association with intraepithelial spreading of urinary bladder carcinomas

UMUC-2 and DAB-1 urinary bladder carcinoma cell lines were inoculated into murine renal pelvis. Black arrows, grown tumor derived from inoculated cells; red arrows, IES of UMUC-2 cells.

integrin $\alpha_6\beta_4$ may be caused by induction of apoptosis mediated by laminin ligand (*46*). Patients with β_4 subunit-positive primary gastric cancer exhibited peritoneal dissemination only infrequently and had a better outcome (*46*).

Reduced expression of integrin β_4 also participates in the morphogenesis of urothelium-derived cancer (Fig. 3). Most nodular invasive carcinomas of the urinary bladder, which have a poor clinical outcome compared with papillary carcinomas, are believed to develop directly from widely spreading flat carcinomas *in situ*. Transitional carcinoma cell lines that showed a high propensity for intraepithelial spreading (IES) in mouse inoculation models scattered when cultured on laminin, which is a major component of the basement membrane (*47*). IES cells showed strong adhesiveness, haptotaxis and enhanced migration on laminin. In IES cells, expression of the integrin β_4 subunit was markedly reduced and the integrin $\alpha_6\beta_1$ complex was predominant compared with the integrin $\alpha_6\beta_4$ complex (*47*). Transfection of IES cells with integrin β_4 subunit inhibited their ability to migrate on laminin and their propensity for IES (*47*). In addition, expression of the integrin β_4 subunit was reduced in surgically resected specimens of widely spreading flat carcinomas *in situ* of the urinary bladder (*47*). A reduction in integrin β_4 may provide a molecular basis for IES of widely spreading flat carcinomas *in situ* through enhanced migration on laminin in the basement membrane.

Dysadherin: A Newly Identified Mechanism for Inactivation of the E-Cadherin Cell Adhesion System

We established a monoclonal antibody showing strong reactivity for a wide variety of cancer cells, but for only a limited number of normal cells, including lymphocytes, endothelial cells and basal cells of the stratified squamous epithelium (*48*). The cDNA for the antigen encodes 178 amino acids, including a putative signal sequence, an *O*-glycosylated extracellular domain, a single transmembrane domain and a short cytoplasmic tail. Transfection of a hepatocellular carcinoma cell line with the cDNA resulted in reduced cell-cell adhesiveness as indicated by the Ca^{2+}-dependent cell aggregation assay (*48*). In the transfectants, E-cadherin was markedly reduced at the protein level in inverse proportion to the expression level of the antigen. Aggregation of the antigen by antibody-coated beads triggered accumulation of actin, suggesting some interplay between this antigen and E-cadherin through actin. We named this antigen, a cell membrane glycoprotein down-regulating E-cadherin, dysadherin (*48*). After injection into mouse spleen, dysadherin transfectants formed a markedly higher number of intrahepatic metastatic nodules compared with mock transfectants, suggesting the metastasis-promoting ability of dysadherin (Fig. 4).

Colorectal carcinomas frequently showed dysadherin immunoreactivity at the cell membrane, whereas dysadherin was not expressed in normal mucosae (Fig. 4) (*49*). Increased expression of dysadherin was significantly associated with lung metastasis and had a significant impact on patients' survival (Fig. 4) (*49*). Furthermore, colorectal cancers with increased expression of dysadherin and reduced expression of E-cadherin showed the worst prognosis. Increased dysadherin expression by pancreatic ductal adenocarcinomas was also significantly correlated with an infiltrative-type growth pattern and distant metastasis (*50*). Thus, dysadherin expression may become a biological predictor of aggressiveness of tumors and poor prognosis in human can-

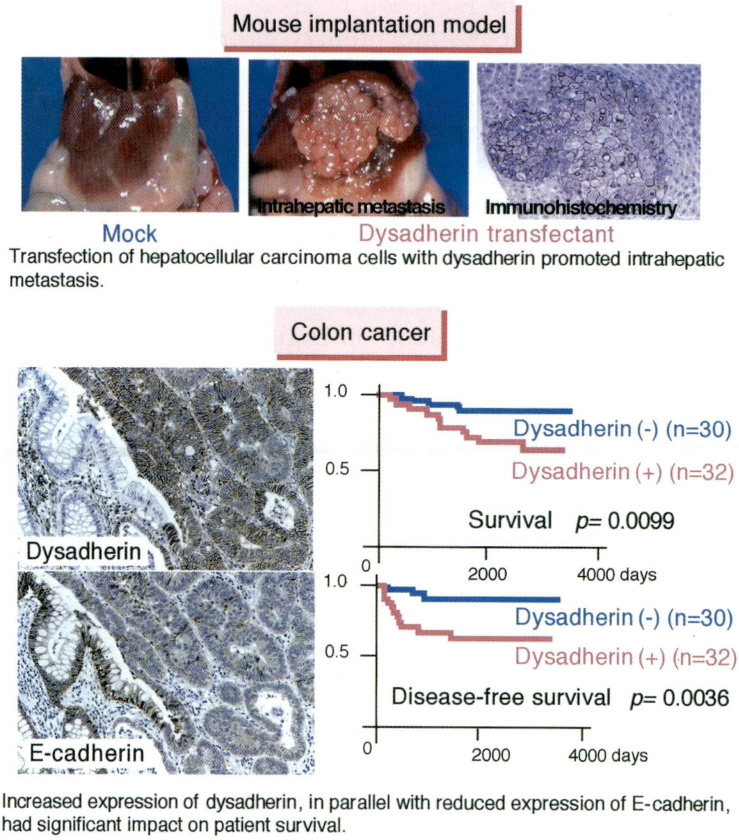

FIG. 4. Dysadherin, a newly identified cell membrane glycoprotein, promotes cancer metastasis

cers.

Perspectives

Abnormality of cell adhesion is the basis for human cancer morphogenesis and affects the biological characteristics of human cancers. Therefore, it is not unexpected that the clinicopathological parameters of various cancers are frequently and significantly associated with molecular events inactivating the cell adhesion system. Recent studies have highlighted cancer-related genes regulated by the Wingless/Wnt signaling pathway. Further understanding of genetic and epigenetic events in the E-cadherin cell adhesion system will cast further light on the mechanisms of multistage human carcinogenesis. Moreover, it is expected that molecules participating in such genetic and epigenetic changes will emerge as the targets of new strategies for prevention and therapy of multistage human carcinogenesis.

REFERENCES

1. Takeichi M. The cadherins: cell-cell adhesion molecules controlling animal morpho-

genesis. *Development* 1988; **102**: 639–55.
2. Takeichi M. Cadherin cell adhesion receptors as a morphogenetic regulator. *Science* 1991; **251**: 1451–5.
3. Behrens J, Mareel MM, van Roy FM, Birchmeier W. Dissecting tumor cell invasion: epithelial cells acquire invasive properties after the loss of uvomorulin-mediated cell-cell adhesion. *J Cell Biol* 1989; **108**: 2435–47.
4. Vleminckx K, Vakaet L Jr, Mareel M, Fiers W, van Roy F. Genetic manipulation of E-cadherin expression by epithelial tumor cells reveals an invasion suppressor role. *Cell* 1991; **66**: 107–19.
5. Guilford P, Hopkins J, Harraway J, McLeod M, McLeod N, Harawira P, Taite H, Scoular R, Miller A, Reeve AE. E-Cadherin germline mutations in familial gastric cancer. *Nature* 1998; **392**: 402–5.
6. Hinck L, Nelson WJ, Papkoff J. Wnt-1 modulates cell-cell adhesion in mammalian cells by stabilizing β-catenin binding to the cell adhesion protein cadherin. *J Cell Biol* 1994; **124**: 729–41.
7. Peifer M. Regulating cell proliferation: as easy as APC. *Science* 1996; **272**: 974–5.
8. Behrens J, von Kries JP, Kuhl M, Bruhn L, Wedlich D, Grosschedl R, Birchmeier W. Functional interaction of β-catenin with the transcription factor LEF-1. *Nature* 1996; **382**: 638–42.
9. Shimoyama Y, Hirohashi S, Hirano S, Noguchi M, Shimosato Y, Takeichi M, Abe O. Cadherin cell-adhesion molecules in human epithelial tissues and carcinomas. *Cancer Res* 1989; **49**: 2128–33.
10. Shimoyama Y, Hirohashi S. Expression of E- and P-cadherin in gastric carcinomas. *Cancer Res* 1991; **51**: 2185–92.
11. Shimoyama Y, Hirohashi S. Cadherin intercellular adhesion molecule in hepatocellular carcinomas: loss of E-cadherin expression in an undifferentiated carcinoma. *Cancer Lett* 1991; **57**: 131–5.
12. Bringuier PP, Umbas R, Schaafsma HE, Karthaus HF, Debruyne FM, Schalken JA. Decreased E-cadherin immunoreactivity correlates with poor survival in patients with bladder tumors. *Cancer Res* 1993; **53**: 3241–5.
13. Yoshiura K, Kanai Y, Ochiai A, Shimoyama Y, Sugimura T, Hirohashi S. Silencing of the E-cadherin invasion-suppressor gene by CpG methylation in human carcinomas. *Proc Natl Acad Sci USA* 1995; **92**: 7416–9.
14. Kanai Y, Ushijima S, Hui AM, Ochiai A, Tsuda H, Sakamoto M, Hirohashi S. The E-cadherin gene is silenced by CpG methylation in human hepatocellular carcinomas. *Int J Cancer* 1997; **71**: 355–9.
15. Ochiai A, Akimoto S, Shimoyama Y, Nagafuchi A, Tsukita S, Hirohashi S. Frequent loss of α catenin expression in scirrhous carcinomas with scattered cell growth. *Jpn J Cancer Res* 1994; **85**: 266–73.
16. Nakanishi Y, Ochiai A, Akimoto S, Kato H, Watanabe H, Tachimori Y, Yamamoto S, Hirohashi S. Expression of E-cadherin, α-catenin, β-catenin and plakoglobin in esophageal carcinomas and its prognostic significance: immunohistochemical analysis of 96 lesions. *Oncology* 1997; **54**: 158–65.
17. Shimoyama Y, Nagafuchi A, Fujita S, Gotoh M, Takeichi M, Tsukita S, Hirohashi S. Cadherin dysfunction in a human cancer cell line: possible involvement of loss of α-

catenin expression in reduced cell-cell adhesiveness. *Cancer Res* 1992; **52**: 5770–4.
18. Oda T, Kanai Y, Shimoyama Y, Nagafuchi A, Tsukita S, Hirohashi S. Cloning of the human α-catenin cDNA and its aberrant mRNA in a human cancer cell line. *Biochem Biophys Res Commun* 1993; **193**: 897–904.
19. Hirano S, Kimoto N, Shimoyama Y, Hirohashi S, Takeichi M. Identification of a neural α-catenin as a key regulator of cadherin function and multicellular organization. *Cell* 1992; **70**: 293–301.
20. Oda T, Kanai Y, Oyama T, Yoshiura K, Shimoyama Y, Birchmeier W, Sugimura T, Hirohashi S. E-Cadherin gene mutations in human gastric carcinoma cell lines. *Proc Natl Acad Sci USA* 1994; **91**: 1858–62.
21. Becker KF, Atkinson MJ, Reich U, Becker I, Nekarda H, Siewert JR, Hofler H. E-Cadherin gene mutations provide clues to diffuse type gastric carcinomas. *Cancer Res* 1994; **54**: 3845–52.
22. Kanai Y, Oda T, Tsuda H, Ochiai A, Hirohashi S. Point mutation of the E-cadherin gene in invasive lobular carcinoma of the breast. *Jpn J Cancer Res* 1994; **85**: 1035–9.
23. Muta H, Noguchi M, Kanai Y, Ochiai A, Nawata H, Hirohashi S. E-Cadherin gene mutations in signet ring cell carcinoma of the stomach. *Jpn J Cancer Res* 1996; **87**: 843–8.
24. Saito A, Kanai Y, Maesawa C, Ochiai A, Torii A, Hirohashi S. Disruption of E-cadherin-mediated cell adhesion systems in gastric cancers in young patients. *Jpn J Cancer Res* 1999; **90**: 993–9.
25. Oyama T, Kanai Y, Ochiai A, Akimoto S, Oda T, Yanagihara K, Nagafuchi A, Tsukita S, Shibamoto S, Ito F, Takeichi M, Matsuda H, Hirohashi S. A truncated β-catenin disrupts the interaction between E-cadherin and α-catenin: a cause of loss of intercellular adhesiveness in human cancer cell lines. *Cancer Res* 1994; **54**: 6282–7.
26. Hinck L, Nathke IS, Papkoff J, Nelson WJ. Dynamics of cadherin/catenin complex formation: novel protein interactions and pathways of complex assembly. *J Cell Biol* 1994; **125**: 1327–40.
27. Matsuyoshi N, Hamaguchi M, Taniguchi S, Nagafuchi A, Tsukita S, Takeichi M. Cadherin-mediated cell-cell adhesion is perturbed by v-src tyrosine phosphorylation in metastatic fibroblasts. *J Cell Biol* 1992; **118**: 703–14.
28. Shibata T, Gotoh M, Ochiai A, Hirohashi S. Association of plakoglobin with APC, a tumor suppressor gene product, and its regulation by tyrosine phosphorylation. *Biochem Biophys Res Commun* 1994; **203**: 519–22.
29. Ochiai A, Akimoto S, Kanai Y, Shibata T, Oyama T, Hirohashi S. c-erbB-2 gene product associates with catenins in human cancer cells. *Biochem Biophys Res Commun* 1994; **205**: 73–8.
30. Kanai Y, Ochiai A, Shibata T, Oyama T, Ushijima S, Akimoto S, Hirohashi S. c-erbB-2 gene product directly associates with β-catenin and plakoglobin. *Biochem Biophys Res Commun* 1995; **208**: 1067–72.
31. Hoschuetzky H, Aberle H, Kemler R. β-Catenin mediates the interaction of the cadherin-catenin complex with epidermal growth factor receptor. *J Cell Biol* 1994; **127**: 1375–80.
32. Inomata M, Ochiai A, Sugihara K, Moriya Y, Yamaguchi N, Adachi Y, Kitano S, Hirohashi S. Macroscopic features at the deepest site of tumor penetration predicting

liver metastases of colorectal cancer. *Jpn J Clin Oncol* 1998; **28**: 123–8.
33. Ono M, Sakamoto M, Ino Y, Moriya Y, Sugihara K, Muto T, Hirohashi S. Cancer cell morphology at the invasive front and expression of cell adhesion-related carbohydrate in the primary lesion of patients with colorectal carcinoma with liver metastasis. *Cancer* 1996; **78**: 1179–86.
34. Hirohashi S. Inactivation of the E-cadherin-mediated cell adhesion system in human cancers. *Am J Pathol* 1998; **153**: 333–9.
35. Shibata T, Ochiai A, Kanai Y, Akimoto S, Gotoh M, Yasui N, Machinami R, Hirohashi S. Dominant negative inhibition of the association between β-catenin and c-erbB-2 by N-terminally deleted β-catenin suppresses the invasion and metastasis of cancer cells. *Oncogene* 1996; **13**: 883–9.
36. Inomata M, Ochiai A, Akimoto S, Kitano S, Hirohashi S. Alteration of β-catenin expression in colonic epithelial cells of familial adenomatous polyposis patients. *Cancer Res* 1996; **56**: 2213–7.
37. Naishiro Y, Yamada T, Takaoka AS, Hayashi R, Hasegawa F, Imai K, Hirohashi S. Restoration of epithelial cell polarity in a colorectal cancer cell line by suppression of β-catenin/T-cell factor 4-mediated gene transactivation. *Cancer Res* 2001; **61**: 2751–8.
38. Yamada T, Takaoka AS, Naishiro Y, Hayashi R, Maruyama K, Maesawa C, Ochiai A, Hirohashi S. Transactivation of the multidrug resistance 1 gene by T-cell factor 4/β-catenin complex in early colorectal carcinogenesis. *Cancer Res* 2000; **60**: 4761–6.
39. Fukuchi T, Sakamoto M, Tsuda H, Maruyama K, Nozawa S, Hirohashi S. β-Catenin mutation in carcinoma of the uterine endometrium. *Cancer Res* 1998; **58**: 3526–8.
40. Kondo Y, Kanai Y, Sakamoto M, Genda T, Mizokami M, Ueda R, Hirohashi S. β-Catenin accumulation and mutation of exon 3 of the *β-catenin* gene in hepatocellular carcinoma. *Jpn J Cancer Res* 1999; **90**: 1301–9.
41. Zhu X, Kanai Y, Saito A, Kondo Y, Hirohashi S. Aberrant expression of β-catenin and mutation of exon 3 of the β-catenin gene in renal and urothelial carcinomas. *Pathol Int* 2000; **50**: 945–52.
42. Sekine S, Shibata T, Yamauchi Y, Nakanishi Y, Shimoda T, Sakamoto M, Hirohashi S. β-Catenin mutations in sporadic fundic gland polyps. *Virchows Arch* 2002; **440**: 381–6.
43. Sekine S, Shibata T, Kokubu A, Morishita Y, Noguchi M, Nakanishi Y, Sakamoto M, Hirohashi S. Craniopharyngiomas of adamantinomatous type harbor β-catenin gene mutations. *Am J Pathol* 2002; **161**: 1997–2001.
44. Sato H, Hasegawa T, Kanai Y, Tsutsumi Y, Osamura Y, Abe Y, Sakai H, Hirohashi S. Expression of cadherins and their undercoat proteins (α-, β-, and γ-catenins and p120) and accumulation of β-catenin with no gene mutations in synovial sarcoma. *Virchows Arch* 2001; **438**: 23–30.
45. Takaoka AS, Yamada T, Gotoh M, Kanai Y, Imai K, Hirohashi S. Cloning and characterization of the human β4-integrin gene promoter and enhancers. *J Biol Chem* 1998; **273**: 33848–55.
46. Ishii Y, Ochiai A, Yamada T, Akimoto S, Yanagihara K, Kitajima M, Hirohashi S. Integrin α6β4 as a suppressor and a predictive marker for peritoneal dissemination in human gastric cancer. *Gastroenterology* 2000; **118**: 497–506.
47. Harabayashi T, Kanai Y, Yamada T, Sakamoto M, Ochiai A, Kakizoe T, Koyanagi T, Hirohashi S. Reduction of integrin β4 and enhanced migration on laminin in associa-

tion with intraepithelial spreading of urinary bladder carcinomas. *J Urol* 1999; **161**: 1364–71.

48. Ino Y, Gotoh M, Sakamoto M, Tsukagoshi K, Hirohashi S. Dysadherin, a cancer-associated cell membrane glycoprotein, down-regulates E-cadherin and promotes metastasis. *Proc Natl Acad Sci USA* 2002; **99**: 365–70.
49. Aoki S, Shimamura T, Shibata T, Nakanishi Y, Moriya Y, Sato Y, Kitajima M, Sakamoto M, Hirohashi S. Prognostic significance of dysadherin expression in advanced colorectal carcinoma. *Br J Cancer* 2003; **88**: 726–32.
50. Shimamura T, Sakamoto M, Ino Y, Sato Y, Shimada K, Kosuge T, Sekihara H, Hirohashi S. Dysadherin overexpression in pancreatic ductal adenocarcinoma reflects tumor aggressiveness: relationship to E-cadherin expression. *J Clin Oncol* 2003; **21**: 659–67.

GASTROINTESTINAL STROMAL TUMORS (GIST): A MODEL FOR MOLECULE-BASED DIAGNOSIS AND TREATMENT OF SOLID TUMORS

Yukihiko KITAMURA[*1], Seiichi HIROTA[*1] and Toshirou NISHIDA[*2]

*Departments of [*1]Pathology and [*2]Surgery, Medical School/Graduate School of Frontier Biosicence, Osaka University*

Gastrointestinal stromal tumor (GIST) is the most common mesenchymal tumor of the human gastrointestinal (GI) tract. The c-kit receptor tyrosine kinase (KIT) is expressed by practically all GISTs, and gain-of-function mutations of KIT are present in most GISTs. Interstitial cells of Cajal (ICC) are the pacemaker of the peristaltic movement of the GI tract. Since signals through KIT are essential for development of ICC and since multiple GISTs develop from the hyperplastic lesion of ICCs in familial GIST patients with germline mutations of KIT, GISTs are considered to originate from ICC. Imatinib mesylate, which was developed for treatment of chronic myeloid leukemia (CML), was found to be useful for treatment of GISTs. Imatinib mesylate inhibits BCR-ABL fused tyrosine kinase that causes CML. Imatinib mesylate also inhibits the mutated KIT observed in most GISTs, and this explains the effectiveness of Imatinib mesylate on GISTs. GISTs appear to serve as a model for molecule-based diagnosis and treatment of solid tumors.

The gastrointestinal stromal tumor (GIST) is the most common mesenchymal tumor of the human gastrointestinal (GI) tract (*1*, *2*). GIST used to be a collective term referring to primary mesenchymal tumors of the GI tract (*2*, *3*), but now it is considered to be a particular tumor that originates from an interstitial cell of Cajal (ICC) or its precursor (*1*, *4*). ICC is a pacemaker of the peristaltic movement of the GI tract (*5*). In 1998, we found the expression of c-kit receptor tyrosine kinase (KIT) in practically all GISTs, and the presence of gain-of-function mutations of KIT in most GISTs (*1*). Metastatic GISTs had been resistant to all available chemotherapy (*6*). However, soon after our report, Imatinib mesylate (STI-571), which was developed for the treatment of chronic myeloid leukemia (CML), was found to be useful for the treatment of metastatic GISTs as well (*7*). Imatinib mesylate inhibits BCR-ABL fused tyrosine kinase and thereby kills CML cells (*8*). Imatinib mesylate also inhibits normal KIT (*9*) as well as the mutated KIT found in most GISTs (*10*). GISTs appear to serve as a good model for molecule-based diagnosis and treatment

[*1, *2] 2-2 Yamada-oka, Suita, Osaka 565-0871, Japan

This paper is dedicated to the memory of late Dr. Tomizo Yoshida on the occasion of the 100th anniversary of his birth. It was originally published in Cancer Science in April, 2003.

of solid tumors. In the present review, we describe the remarkable progress that has occurred recently in the diagnosis and treatment of GISTs.

KIT and Its Loss-of-Function Mutations

Our story about GISTs does not start from the classical histopathology of GI tumors, but from mutant mice that lack mast cells (*11*, *12*). Through these mutant mice, we became familiar with KIT (*13*), then ICC (*14*) and finally arrived at GISTs (*1*). The c-kit is the cellular homologue of the oncogene v-kit of HZ4 feline sarcoma virus, and encodes a receptor tyrosine kinase that is structurally similar to the receptors for macrophage colony-stimulating factor (M-CSF) and platelet-derived growth factor (PDGF) (*15*). These receptor tyrosine kinases have unique features: an extracellular (EC) domain made up of five immunoglobulin-like repeats, and a tyrosine kinase (TK) domain that is split into two domains by an insert sequence of variable length. The structure and amino acid sequence of KIT are well preserved in humans, mice and rats. For many years after the discovery of v-kit gene, it remained unclear whether KIT played any role in the development of human neoplasms.

The W locus of mice was demonstrated to encode KIT (*16*, *17*). Many types of loss-of-function mutants have been reported at the W locus. Among them, double heterozygous mice of W/W^v genotype are most frequently used. The W mutant allele encodes a truncated KIT without the transmembane domain; as a result, the extracellular domain is not expressed on the cell surface (*18*, *19*). The W^v mutant allele is a point mutation at the TK domain, resulting in a remarkable decrease in the TK activity (*18*). W/W^v mice show five abnormalities due to the loss of KIT function: 1) anemia due to hypoproduction of erythrocytes, 2) white coat color due to the lack of melanocytes, 3) sterility due to depletion of germ cells, 4) depletion of mast cells (*11*), 5) depletion of ICCs (*20*). Abnormalities 1 to 3 have been known for a long time. We found the depletion of mast cells in 1978 (*11*), and Maeda *et al.* (*20*) found the depletion of ICCs in 1992.

The ligand of KIT was identified and named stem cell factor (SCF) (*21*). Since SCF is encoded by the Sl locus, homozygous or double heterozygous mutant mice at the W or Sl locus have the same phenotype. The most frequently used mutant mice of the Sl locus are of Sl/Sl^d genotype. Sl/Sl^d mice show anemia, white coat color, sterility, depletion of mast cells and depletion of ICCs.

We found spontaneous development of forestomach papillomas (*22*) and antral ulcers (*23*) in W/W^v and Sl/Sl^d mutant mice at around the same time when we discovered depletion of mast cells in these mice (*11*, *12*). We identified bile reflux from duodenum to stomach as a cause of the stomach lesions (*24*). However, the mechanism of the bile reflux remained unclear. Since the depletion of ICCs was identified as the fifth abnormality of W/W^v and Sl/Sl^d mice (*20*, *25*, *26*) and since ICCs regulate the peristaltic movement of the GI tract (*5*), the bile reflux is now attributed to the depletion of ICCs.

Gain-of-Function Mutation of KIT as a Cause of Mast Cell Neoplasms

Binding of dimerized SCF induces the dimerization of KIT (*27*). This leads to autophosphorylation of KIT on tyrosine and to association of KIT with substrates such as phophatidylinositol 3-kinase (PI3K) (*27*). In human mast cell leukemia cell line HMC-1, KIT was constitutively phosphorylated on tyrosine, activated, and then could associate with PI3K without the addition of SCF. Furitsu *et al.* (*28*) found that KIT gene of HMC-1 cells was composed of normal, wild-type allele and mutant allele with point mutations resulting in substitution of Val-560 to Gly in the juxtamembrane (JM) domain and Asp-816 to Val in the tyrosine kinase-II (TK-II) domain. Amino acid sequences in the region of the two mutations are completely conserved in mouse, rat and human KIT.

In order to determine the causal role of these mutations in the constitutive activation, mutant KIT gene with Val-560 to Gly mutation in the JM domain or with Asp-816 to Val mutation in the TK-II domain was constructed and expressed in a human embryonic kidney cell line, 293T (*28*). In the transfected cells, KIT with either mutation was abundantly phosphorylated on tyrosine and activated in the immune complex kinase reaction without the addition of SCF. Tsujimura *et al.* (*29, 30*) found the mutation corresponding to Asp-816 to Val of the human HMC-1 cell line in the P-815 mouse mastocytoma cell line (Asp-817 to Tyr) and the RBL-2H3 rat mast cell leukemia cell line (Asp-814 to Tyr). Both P-815 and RBL-2H3 cells showed constitutive activation of KIT without SCF. These KIT mutations were considered to induce the transformation of mast cells. In fact, the Asp-816 to Val mutation has been found in various types of mast cell neoplasms of human patients (Fig. 1) (*31, 32*). Moreover, in some dog mastocytomas, internal tandem duplication has been found in the JM domain of KIT (*33*). Mast cell neoplasms are very rare in humans, but they are the most common malignant tumors in dogs. In some human germ cell tumors, Asp-816 to His mutation has been reported (*34*).

To examine the transformation potential of the KIT activation mutation, we used the murine inerleukin-3 (IL-3)-dependent IC-2 mast cell line as a transfectant (*35*). The IC-2 cells that had been established by Koyasu *et al.* (*36*) from murine cultured mast cells did not express KIT on the surface. The Asp-814 to Val or Val-559 to Gly murine type mutant KIT cDNA was introduced into IC-2 cells using a retrovirus vector. The mutant KIT expressed in IC-2 cells was constitutively phosphorylated on tyrosine and demonstrated kinase activity in the absence of SCF. IC-2 cells expressing mutant KIT showed factor-independent growth in suspension culture and produced tumors in nude athymic mice (*35*). Introduction of the mutant KIT cDNAs also resulted in the transformation of the IL-3-dependent Ba/F3 murine pro-B

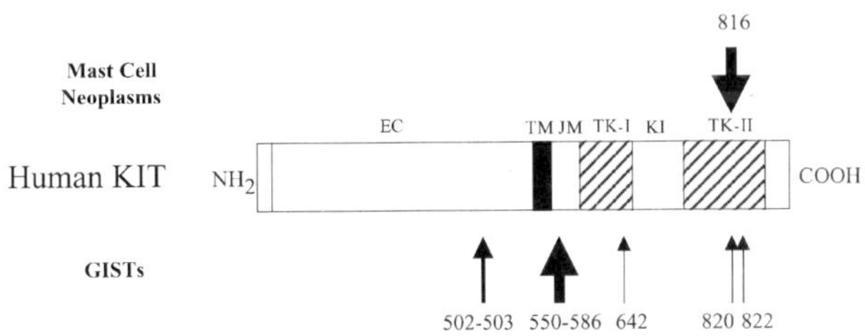

FIG. 1. KIT mutations reported in human mast cell neoplasms and GISTs
EC, extracellular domain; TM, transmembrane domain, JM, juxtamembrane domain; TK-I, tyrosine kinase-I domain; KI, kinase insert; TK-II, tyrosine kinase-II domain. Sizes of arrows roughly parallel the proportion of cases with each mutation. The mutation of the TK-II domain at position 820 has been reported only in a family with familial GISTs.

cells (*37*).

The mechanisms of constitutive activation were different in the cases of Val-559 to Gly JM mutation and Asp-814 to Val TK-II (*37*). This was shown by chemical cross-linking analysis. A substantial fraction of phosphorylated KIT with Val-559 to Gly mutation dimerized, whereas phosphorylated KIT with Asp-814 to Val mutation did not. Tsujimura *et al.* (*38*) found another gain-of-function mutation at the JM domain of the FMA3 murine mastocytoma cell line. The KIT cDNA of FMA3 cells carried an in-frame deletion of 21 base pairs (bp). The FMA3-type KIT cDNA was introduced into IC-2 cells. The FMA3-type KIT was constitutively phosphorylated on tyrosine and activated. IC-2 cells expressing FMA3-type KIT grew in suspension culture without IL-3 and SCF, and became leukemic in nude athymic mice. Although the Val-559 to Gly mutation and the FMA3-type mutation with 21-bp deletion were different in nature, their biological effects were comparable (*37*, *38*).

Sporadic GISTs

Loss-of-function mutation of KIT resulted in depletion of mast cells (*11*), while gain-of-function mutation resulted in mast cell neoplasms (*28*, *31*, *32*, *35*, *38*). Since loss-of-function mutation of KIT caused depletion of ICCs (*20*, *25*), it seems reasonable that gain-of-function mutation might induce neoplasms of ICCs. However, when we started examining this possibility, the existence of ICC-derived tumors was not known. Therefore, we examined whether any mesenchymal tumors in the human GI tract express KIT, by using immunohistochemistry (*1*) (Fig. 2). Authentic leiomyomas and schwannomas did not express KIT, but most tumors designated as GISTs did express it (*1*). This suggested that GISTs originated from ICCs. Soon after the publication of our paper, Kindblom *et al.* (*4*) independently reported a similar result. Practically all gastric and intestinal tumors that were previously classified as leiomyomas and leiomyosarcomas express KIT, and consequently they are currently considered to be GISTs (*39*).

The whole coding region of KIT was obtained from six GISTs and sequenced.

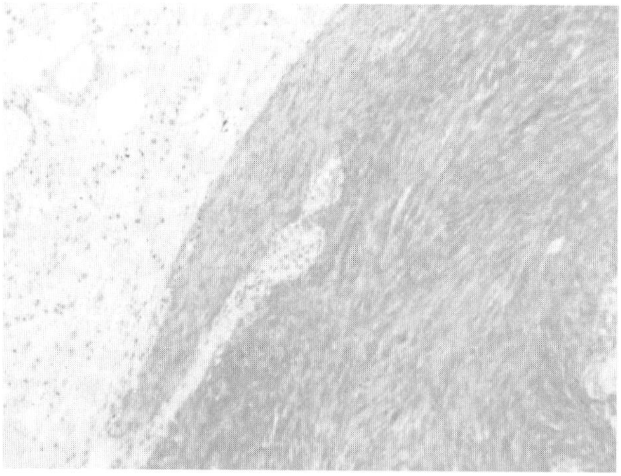

FIG. 2. Expression of KIT in a GIST revealed by immunohistochemistry

Mutations were observed in 5 out of 6 GISTs (Fig. 1) (*1*). All mutations were detected in the JM domain, but not at identical sites. We next examined whether the KIT mutations found in the GISTs resulted in constitutive activation, by means of transient introduction of mutant KIT cDNAs into 293T human embryonic kidney cell line. The KIT mutants found in GISTs showed constitutive tyrosine phosphorylation in 293T cells without SCF (*1*). The KIT mutants also exhibited constitutive kinase activation in *in vitro* kinase assay. To investigate the biological consequences of mutant KIT, we introduced the KIT mutations found in GISTs into mouse KIT cDNA and then stably transfected it into the IL-3-dependent Ba/F3 murine pro-B cell line. Ba/F3 cells with the mutated murine KIT grew autonomously in nude mice (*1*).

Mutations in the JM domain were most common in GISTs (~80%), and therefore were firstly found. Mutations in other domains were found thereafter; duplication of two particular amino acids in the EC domain (~5%) (*40–42*), a point mutation at the TK-I domain (~3%) (*40, 41*), and a point mutation at the TK-II domain (~2%) (Fig. 3) (*43*). The site of this TK-II mutation was different from that of the Asp-816 to Val mutation, which is found in human mast cell neoplasms (Fig. 1) (*31, 32*). In approximately 10% of GISTs, no KIT mutations were found even when the whole coding region was examined using fresh materials (*40, 42*).

Recently Heinlich *et al.* (*44*) investigated the cause of GISTs without KIT mutations and found gain-of-function mutations of PDGF receptor α in about one-third of GISTs without KIT mutations. We independently obtained a similar result (Hirota *et al.*, unpublished data). Mutated PDGF receptor α activated not only itself, but also wild-type KIT. Since the signal transduction pathway of PDGF receptor α is similar to that of KIT (*27*), gain-of-function mutation of PDGF receptor α by itself may cause transformation of ICCs. Another possibility is that the mutated PDGF receptor α may affect ICCs through activation of the wild-type KIT. These two possibilities are not mutually exclusive (Hirota *et al.*, unpublished data).

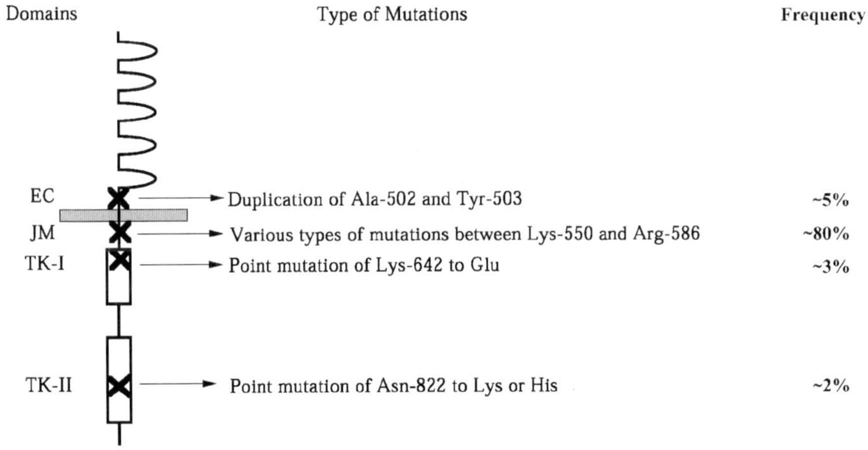

FIG. 3. KIT mutations in sporadic GISTs
KIT mutations were detected in ~90% of GISTs, but not in ~10% of them. The frequency of each mutation in sporadic GISTs is shown. EC, extracellular; JM, juxtamembrane; TK-I, tyrosine kinase-I; TK-II, tyrosine kinase-II.

Allander *et al.* (*45*) examined the gene expression profile of KIT mutation-positive GISTs by cDNA microarray and found a remarkably distinct and uniform expression profile. This homogeneity suggests that the molecular pathogenesis of GIST involves expansion of a clone that has acquired an activating mutation in KIT without the extreme genetic instability found in the common epithelial cancers. This is consistent with the results of Corless *et al.* (*46*), who found mutated KIT in very small GISTs that were incidentally found at the time of surgical operations for other purposes.

The presence of KIT mutation has been correlated with survival of GIST patients (*47*). We extracted DNA samples from paraffin sections of 124 GIST cases (*47*). Exon 11 encoding the JM domain and exon 17 encoding the TK-II domain were amplified by PCR and sequenced. Survival was better in patients without KIT mutation than in patients with KIT mutation (*47*). However, the mutation rate was rather low (57%) in this study. When the whole KIT coding region was sequenced in fresh materials, the observed mutation rate increased to ~90% (*42*). In such studies, the presence of KIT mutation did not significantly correlate with survival.

There is a tendency that GISTs that are small (<2 cm in diameter) and show low mitotic activity (<5/50 high-power fields) have a good prognosis. However, a few GISTs apparently lacking mitotic activity may metastasize (*39*). It is difficult to clearly divide GISTs to benign and malignant classes. Therefore, GISTs are practically classified into low-risk, intermediate-risk and high-risk groups (*48*). Even when GISTs do metastasize, the sites of metastasis are limited to the liver and peritoneal cavity.

Familial GISTs

Most GISTs are sporadic, but we found three families with germline mutation of KIT and development of multiple GISTs (*49–51*). Firstly, we found multiple GISTs in 60-year-old Japanese woman who received two surgical operations due to intestinal obstruction (*49*). A nephew of this woman also suffered from multiple GISTs. Analysis of the family pedigree revealed that many family members suffered from intestinal obstruction that may be attributable to multiple GISTs. Although the GISTs of the 60-year-old woman and her nephew were benign, a niece of the woman died of malignant GISTs that disseminated to the peritoneal cavity. DNA was extracted from GISTs and leukocytes of the woman and the nephew. An identical mutation was found in the JM domain of KIT, while this mutation was not detected in leukocytes obtained from other family members in whom GISTs were not observed (*49*).

The second family was originally reported by O'Brien *et al.* (*52*) under the diagnosis of multiple familial gastrointestinal autonomic nerve tumors (GANTs). Multiple GANTs were observed in a mother and a daughter, and at least one GANT metastasized to the liver of the daughter. O'Brien *et al.* kindly made available to us the paraffin blocks of the GANTs and surrounding tissues. An identical JM mutation of KIT was found in both GANTs and the normal surrounding tissues of the mother and the daughter (*50*). This showed that the multiple familial GANTs were identical to familial GISTs. Since sporadic GANTs also showed JM mutations of KIT, GANTs in general are now considered to be a subtype of GISTs with particular histological characteristics (*48*).

The third family showed a unique symptom. The family members with multiple GISTs claimed dysphagia, a difficulty in swallowing (*51*). However, no mechanical obstruction was found, and the esophagus was not remarkably dilated. Endoscopic ultrasonography at the esophagocardiac junction showed a thickened hyperechoic layer between the circular and longitudinal muscle layers, suggesting hyperplasia of ICCs at the myenteric plexus layer. Manometry showed low resting lower esophageal sphincter pressure and abnormal simultaneous contractions of the esophagus without normal peristalsis. These findings indicate that the dysphagia of this family is different from typical achalasia (*51*). The family members with dysphagia showed germline gain-of-function mutation of KIT at the TK-II domain (Asp-820 to Tyr), which is different from the Asp-816 to Val mutation found in mast cell neoplasms (Fig. 1). Although this family is the first case of familial GISTs with the TK-II domain mutation, it was not clear whether the presence of dysphagia was related to this type of KIT mutation.

In addition to the above-mentioned three families, other three families with multiple GISTs and gain-of-function mutation of KIT have been described (*53–55*). Two families possessed KIT mutation at the JM domain (*54*, *55*), and the remaining one family, at the TK-I domain (*53*).

In addition to multiple GISTs, hyperpigmentation of the skin (*49*, *54*, *55*) and/or mast cell tumors (*55*) were reported in some families. Most family members with multiple GISTs survive and can have offspring, and moreover, various KIT mutations cause the familiar GISTs. Therefore, this disease entity may be a more common cancer syndrome than is presently supposed.

In familial GISTs, remarkable hyperplasia of ICCs was observed in the small and large intestines (*50*, *51*, *53*, *55*). ICCs constitute only one or two cell layers in the normal intestine, whereas hyperplasia with 10 to 20 cell layers was observed in familial GIST patients (Fig. 4). Multiple GISTs developed from the hyperplasia. We examined the clonality of the hyperplastic lesions and GISTs in patients with familial GISTs (*56*). To examine the clonality of human samples, random inactivation of one of two female X chromosomes is commonly used. Currently, the polymorphism of the human androgen receptor (HUMARA) locus, which is located on the X chromosome, is most frequently used as it has a highly polymorphic tandem repeat. Samples obtained with a laser capture microdissection system were used. The hyperplastic le-

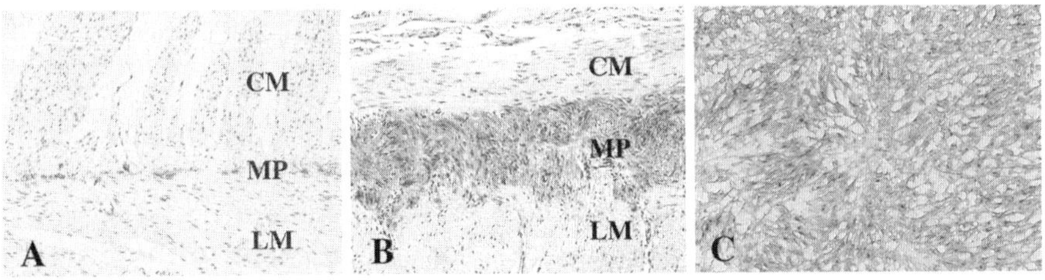

FIG. 4. Hyperplasia of ICCs in a familial GIST patient
A, ICCs in the small intestine of a normal subject. ICC hyperplasia (B) and a GIST (C) in a familial GIST patient with germline mutation of the c-kit gene. Each monoclonal GIST develops from a polyclonal hyperplastic lesion of ICCs. KIT expression is demonstrated by immunohistochemistry. CM, circular muscle layer; MP, myenteric plexus layer; LM, longitudinal muscle layer.

sion was polyclonal and each GIST derived from the hyperplastic lesion was monoclonal. This clearly indicated that each GIST was derived from an ICC (*56*).

Molecular Target Therapy of GISTs

Treatment of GISTs has changed dramatically since the introduction of Imatinib mesylate. Since GISTs were not routinely distinguished from other mesenchymal tumors of the peritoneal cavity, it is difficult to determine accurately the response rate of GISTs to conventional chemotherapeutic agents. However, it appears to be less than 10% (*6*).

Imatinib mesylate was initially developed at Ciba-Geigy (now Novartis) as a specific inhibitor of the PDGF receptor (*57*). However, it was found to be a potent and selective inhibitor of ABL TKs, including BCR-ABL. BCR-ABL is a fusion protein produced by balanced translocation between chromosomes 9 and 22. BCR-ABL has uncontrolled TK activity, which leads to constitutive intracellular signaling and induces the development of CML. Druker and scientists at Novartis showed that Imatinib mesylate selectively blocked BCR-ABL and killed CML cells *in vitro* (*8*). They also examined the utility of this finding by means of a clinical trial. Data from the clinical trial were published in early 2001 (*58*). The US Food and Drug Administration approved Imatinib mesylate as a safe and effective therapy for CML patients in May 2001. The efficacy of Imatinib mesylate is striking, with greater than a 90% complete response rate in chronic-phase CML (*58*).

As already mentioned, we reported gain-of-function mutations of KIT in GISTs, in 1998 (*1*). We speculated that the constitutive activation of KIT functioned as a critical step in the development of GISTs. In addition to the inhibitory effect of Imatinib mesylate on the PDGF receptor and ABL, Buchdunger *et al.* (*9*) found an inhibitory effect on wild-type KIT. Some reports showed that Imatinib mesylate also inhibited various types of mutated KIT found in GISTs (*10*, *59*). Before the publication of these data, the treatment of the first GIST patient with Imatinib mesylate started in Finland. The patient's tumor expressed KIT and contained a JM mutation of KIT. The patient had progressive, widely metastatic disease after failure of previous extensive therapy, including multiple surgical procedures, chemotherapy, and even investigational antiangiogenic therapy (*6*, *7*). Within a few weeks of starting daily oral administration of Imatinib mesylate, the patient exhibited an objective clinical response that was maintained for more than 18 months. This encouraging result was published in 2001 (*7*). A multicenter trial on advanced GISTs was done and reported in 2002 (*60*). The US Food and Drug Administration has approved Imatinib mesylate as effective therapy for advanced GIST patients, and the role of Imatinib mesylate in adjuvant therapy is now being evaluated.

The position of KIT mutation appears to be related to the effectiveness of Imatinib mesylate. Since JM domain mutations of KIT are found in 80% of all GISTs (*40*, *42*), the therapeutic effect of Imatinib mesylate on such GISTs with JM mutations is definitive. In contrast, effectiveness is not so apparent in the case of GISTs without KIT mutations (*6*). The proportions of EC, TK-I or TK-II mutations are small, and therefore it is rather difficult to evaluate the effectiveness of Imatinib mesylate against such GISTs with EC, TK-I or TK-II mutation. The Asp-816 to Val TK-II mutation has not been observed in GISTs, but it was frequently found in human mast cell neoplasms (*31, 32*). Imatinib mesylate did not inhibit the growth of COS cells, into which KIT cDNA with the Asp-816 to Val mutation had been introduced (*61*).

Remaining Problems

The definition of GISTs as tumors of ICC origin was established after our findings that most GISTs express KIT and that most GISTs have gain-of-function mutations of KIT (*1*). In the 4 years after those findings, the treatment of GISTs has changed dramatically. The primary cause of such rapid progress was the prior existence of Imatinib mesylate as a molecular target drug for CML (*6*). GIST and CML appear to have similar pathogenic mechanisms, each being driven by a single dominant stimulus (*6*). On the other hand, most human carcinomas are caused by more complicated mechanisms. If carcinomas can be divided into certain types with definitely identifiable molecular changes, a specific molecule-based therapy might be possible for each type.

In spite of the remarkable progress, there are many problems remaining to be clarified in the pathogenesis and therapy of GISTs. The KIT mutation appears to be an early event in the development of a GIST (*46*). Although polyclonal hyperplasia of ICCs was observed throughout the GI tract of familial GIST patients, benign monoclonal GISTs developed within the hyperplasia (*56*). In addition to the KIT mutation, other factors appear to be necessary for development of even benign GISTs. Such factors should be identified.

The signal transduction pathways from KIT should be clarified. Frequent development of GISTs in neurofibromatosis (NF)-1 patients is known (*62*). Loss-of-function mutation of the NF-1 gene, which causes neurofibromatosis (*62*), may be involved in the development of GISTs. The NF-1 protein negatively regulates the signal transduction of RAS (*62*). Interaction of the KIT signal with RAS may play an important role. Further investigation of GISTs, which developed in NF-1 patients, may clarify the mechanisms of interaction among KIT, RAS and NF-1.

Although multiple benign GISTs develop in persons with germline mutation of KIT (*49–51, 53–55*), most benign GISTs do not become malignant. More than half of such persons with germ-line mutation of KIT survive to rather old age without development of malignant GISTs. This suggests that KIT mutation alone does not cause malignant transformation of GISTs. This is consistent with data on the prognosis of patients with sporadic GISTs. The proportion of GISTs with KIT mutation reached ~90% when the whole coding region of the KIT gene obtained from fresh materials was sequenced (*40, 42*). When prognosis was compared between GISTs with KIT mutation and those without KIT mutation, no significant difference was found (*6*). Factors causing the transformation of benign GISTs to malignant GISTs should be examined. If such factors are identified, the selection of patients for adjuvant therapy with Imatinib mesylate will become much easier.

REFERENCES

1. Hirota S, Isozaki K, Moriyama Y, Hashimoto K, Nishida T, Ishiguro S, Kawano K, Hanada M, Kurata A, Takeda M, Tunio GM, Matsuzawa Y, Kanakura Y, Shinomura

Y, Kitamura Y. Gain-of-function mutations of c-kit in human gastrointestinal stromal tumors. *Science* 1998; **279**: 577–80.

2. O'Leary T, Berman JJ. Gastrointestinal stromal tumors: answers and questions. *Hum Pathol* 2002; **33**: 456–8.
3. Heinrich MC, Rubin BP, Longley BJ, Fletcher JA. Biology and genetic aspects of gastrointestinal stromal tumors: KIT activation and cytogenetic alterations. *Hum Pathol* 2002; **33**: 484–95.
4. Kindblom LG, Remotti HE, Aldenborg F, Meis-Kindblom JM. Gastrointestinal pacemaker cell tumor (GIPACT): gastrointestinal stromal tumors show phenotypic characteristics of the interstitial cells of Cajal. *Am J Pathol* 1998; **152**: 1259–69.
5. Thomsen L, Robinson TL, Lee JC, Farraway LA, Hughes MJ, Andrews DW, Huizinga JD. Interstitial cells of Cajal generate a rhythmic pacemaker current. *Nat Med* 1998; **4**: 848–51.
6. Dematteo RP, Heinrich MC, El-Rifai WM, Demetri G. Clinical management of gastrointestinal stromal tumors: before and after STI-571. *Hum Pathol* 2002; **33**: 466–77.
7. Joensuu H, Roberts PJ, Sarlomo-Rikala M, Andersson LC, Tervahartiala P, Tuveson D, Silberman S, Capdeville R, Dimitrijevic S, Druker B, Demetri GD. Effect of the tyrosine kinase inhibitor STI571 in a patient with a metastatic gastrointestinal stromal tumor. *N Engl J Med* 2001; **344**: 1052–6.
8. Druker BJ, Tamura S, Buchdunger E, Ohno S, Segal GM, Fanning S, Zimmermann J, Lydon NB. Effects of a selective inhibitor of the Abl tyrosine kinase on the growth of Bcr-Abl positive cells. *Nat Med* 1996; **2**: 561–6.
9. Buchdunger E, Cioffi CL, Law N, Stover D, Ohno-Jones S, Druker BJ, Lydon NB. Abl protein-tyrosine kinase inhibitor STI571 inhibits *in vitro* signal transduction mediated by c-kit and platelet-derived growth factor receptors. *J Pharmacol Exp Ther* 2000; **295**: 139–45.
10. Tuveson DA, Willis NA, Jacks T, Griffin JD, Singer S, Fletcher CD, Fletcher JA, Demetri GD. STI571 inactivation of the gastrointestinal stromal tumor c-KIT oncoprotein: biological and clinical implications. *Oncogene* 2001; **20**: 5054–8.
11. Kitamura Y, Go S, Hatanaka K. Decrease of mast cells in W/W^v mice and their increase by bone marrow transplantation. *Blood* 1978; **52**: 447–52.
12. Kitamura Y, Go S. Decreased production of mast cells in Sl/Sl^d anemic mice. *Blood* 1979; **53**: 492–7.
13. Tsujimura T, Koshimizu U, Katoh H, Isozaki K, Kanakura Y, Tono T, Adachi S, Kasugai T, Tei H, Nishimune Y, Nomura S, Kitamura Y. Mast cell number in the skin of heterozygotes reflects molecular nature of c-kit mutation. *Blood* 1993; **81**: 2530–8.
14. Isozaki K, Hirota S, Nakama A, Miyagawa J-I, Shinomura Y, Xu Z, Nomura S, Kitamura Y. Disturbed intestinal movement, bile reflux to the stomach, and deficiency of c-kit-expressing cells in Ws/Ws mutant rats. *Gastroenterology* 1995; **109**: 456–64.
15. Yarden Y, Kuang WJ, Yang-Feng T, Coussens L, Munemitsu S, Dull TJ, Chen E, Schlessinger J, Francke U, Ullrich A. Human proto-oncogene c-kit: a new cell surface receptor tyrosine kinase for an unidentified ligand. *EMBO J* 1987; **6**: 3341–51.
16. Chabot B, Stephenson DA, Chapman VM, Besmer P, Bernstein A. The proto-oncogene c-kit encoding a transmembrane tyrosine kinase receptor maps to the mouse W locus. *Nature* 1988; **335**: 88–9.

17. Geissler EN, Ryan MA, Housman DE. The dominant-white spotting (W) locus of the mouse encodes the c-kit proto-oncogene. *Cell* 1988; **55**: 185–92.
18. Nocka K, Tan JC, Chiu E, Chu TY, Ray P, Traktman P, Besmer P. Molecular bases of dominant negative and loss of function mutation at the murine c-kit/white spotting locus: W^{37}, W^{v}, W^{41} and W. *EMBO J* 1990; **9**: 1805–13.
19. Hayashi S, Kunisada T, Ogawa M, Yamaguchi K, Nishikawa S. Exon skipping by mutation of an authentic splice site of c-kit gene in W/W mouse. *Nucleic Acids Res* 1991; **19**: 1267–71.
20. Maeda H, Yamagata A, Nishikawa S, Yoshinaga K, Kobayashi S, Nishi K, Nishikawa S-I. Requirement of c-kit for development of intestinal pacemaker system. *Development* 1992; **116**: 369–75.
21. Witte ON. Steel locus defines new multipotent growth factor. *Cell* 1990; **63**: 5–6.
22. Kitamura Y, Yokoyama M, Matsuda H, Shimada M. Coincidental development of forestomach papilloma and prepyloric ulcer in nontreated mutant mice of W/W^{v} and Sl/Sl^{d} genotypes. *Cancer Res* 1980; **40**: 3392–7.
23. Shimada M, Kitamura Y, Yokoyama M, Miyano Y, Maeyama K, Yamatodani A, Takahashi Y, Tatsuta M. Spontaneous stomach ulcer in genetically mast cell depleted W/W^{v} mice. *Nature* 1980; **293**: 662–4.
24. Yokoyama M, Tatsuta M, Baba M, Kitamura Y. Bile reflux: a possible cause of stomach ulcer in nontreated mutant mice of W/W^{v} genotype. *Gastroenterology* 1982; **82**: 857–63.
25. Huizinga JD, Thuneberg L, Kluppel M, Malysz J, Mikkelsen HB, Bernstein A. W/kit gene required for interstitial cells of Cajal and for intestinal pacemaker activity. *Nature* 1995; **373**: 347–9.
26. Ward SM, Burns AJ, Torihashi S, Harney SC, Sanders KM. Impaired development of interstitial cells and intestinal electrical rhythmicity in steel mutants. *Am J Physiol* 1995; **269**: 1577–85.
27. Ullrich A, Schlessinger J. Signal transduction by receptors with tyrosine kinase activity. *Cell* 1990; **61**: 203–12.
28. Furitsu T, Tsujimura T, Tono T, Ikeda H, Kitayama H, Koshimizu U, Sugahara H, Butterfield JH, Ashman LK, Kanayama Y, Matsuzawa Y, Kitamura Y, Kanakura Y. Identification of mutations in the coding sequence of the proto-oncogene c-kit in a human mast cell leukemia cell line causing ligand-independent activation of c-kit product. *J Clin Invest* 1993; **92**: 1736–44.
29. Tsujimura T, Furitsu T, Morimoto M, Isozaki K, Nomura S, Matsuzawa Y, Kitamura Y, Kanakura Y. Ligand-independent activation of c-kit receptor tyrosine kinase in a murine mastocytoma cell line P-815 generated by a point mutation. *Blood* 1994; **83**: 2619–26.
30. Tsujimura T, Furitsu T, Morimoto M, Kanayama Y, Nomura S, Matsuzawa Y, Kitamura Y, Kanakura Y. Substitution of an aspartic acid results in constitutive activation of c-kit receptor tyrosine kinase in a rat tumor mast cell line RBL-2H3. *Int Arch Allergy Immunol* 1995; **106**: 377–85.
31. Nagata H, Worobec AS, Oh CK, Chowdhury BA, Tannenbaum S, Suzuki Y, Metcalfe DD. Identification of a point mutation in the catalytic domain of the protooncogene c-kit in peripheral blood mononuclear cells of patients who have mastocytosis with an as-

sociated hematologic disorder. *Proc Natl Acad Sci USA* 1995; **92**: 10560–4.

32. Longley BJ, Tyrrell L, Lu S-Z, Ma Y-S, Langley K, Ding T-G, Duffy T, Jacobs P, Tang LH, Modlin I. Somatic c-kit activating mutation in urticaria pigmentosa and aggressive mastocytosis: establishment of clonality in a human mast cell neoplasm. *Nat Genet* 1996; **12**: 312–4.
33. London CA, Galli SJ, Yuuki T, Hu ZQ, Helfand SC, Geissler EN. Spontaneous canine mast cell tumors express tandem duplications in the proto-oncogene c-kit. *Exp Hematol* 1999; **27**: 689–97.
34. Tian Q, Frierson HF Jr, Krystal GW, Moskaluk CA. Activating c-kit gene mutations in human germ cell tumors. *Am J Pathol* 1999; **154**: 1643–7.
35. Hashimoto K, Tsujimura T, Moriyama Y, Yamatodani A, Kimura M, Tohya K, Morimoto M, Kitayama H, Kanakura Y, Kitamura Y. Transforming and differentiation-inducing potentials of constitutively activated c-kit mutant genes in the IC-2 murine interleukin-3-dependent mast cell line. *Am J Pathol* 1996; **148**: 189–200.
36. Koyasu S, Nakauchi H, Kitamura K, Yonehara S, Okumura K, Tada T, Yahara I. Production of interleukin 3 and gamma-interferon by an antigen-specific mouse suppressor T cell clone. *J Immunol* 1985; **134**: 3130–6.
37. Kitayama H, Kanakura Y, Furitsu T, Tsujimura T, Oritani K, Ikeda H, Sugahara H, Mitsui H, Kanayama Y, Kitamura Y, Matsuzawa Y. Constitutively activating mutations of c-kit receptor tyrosine kinase confer factor-independent growth and tumorigenicity of factor-dependent hematopoietic cell lines. *Blood* 1995; **85**: 790–8.
38. Tsujimura T, Morimoto M, Hashimoto K, Moriyama Y, Kitayama H, Matsuzawa Y, Kitamura Y, Kanakura Y. Constitutive activation of c-kit in FMA3 murine mastocytoma cells caused by deletion of seven amino acids at the juxtamembrane domain. *Blood* 1996; **87**: 273–83.
39. Miettinen M, El-Rifai W, H L Sobin L, Lasota J. Evaluation of malignancy and prognosis of gastrointestinal stromal tumors: a review. *Hum Pathol* 2002; **33**: 478–83.
40. Lux ML, Rubin BP, Biase TL, Chen C-J, Maclure T, Demetri G, Xiao S, Singer S, Fletcher CDM, Fletcher JA. KIT extracellular and kinase domain mutations in gastrointestinal stromal tumors. *Am J Pathol* 2000; **156**: 791–5.
41. Lasota J, Wozniak A, Sarlomo-Rikala M, Rys J, Kordek R, Nassar A, Sobin LH, Miettinen M. Mutations in exons 9 and 13 of *KIT* gene are rare events in gastrointestinal stromal tumors. *Am J Pathol* 2000; **157**: 1091–5.
42. Hirota S, Nishida T, Isozaki K, Taniguchi M, Nakamura J, Okazaki T, Kitamura Y. Gain-of-function mutation at the extracellular domain of KIT in gastrointestinal stromal tumours. *J Pathol* 2001; **193**: 505–10.
43. Rubin BP, Singer S, Tsao C, Duensing A, Lux ML, Ruiz R, Hibbard MK, Chen CJ, Xiao S, Tuveson DA, Demetri GD, Fletcher CD, Fletcher JA. KIT activation is a ubiquitous feature of gastrointestinal stromal tumors. *Cancer Res* 2001; **61**: 8118–21.
44. Heinrich MC, Corless CL, Duensing A, McGreevey L, Chen CJ, Joseph N, Singer S, Griffith DJ, Haley A, Town A, Demetri GD, Fletcher CD, Fletcher JA. PDGFRA activating mutations in gastrointestinal stromal tumors. *Science* 2003; **299**: 708–10.
45. Allander SV, Nupponen NN, Ringner M, Hostetter G, Maher GW, Goldberger N, Chen Y, Carpten J, Elkahloun AG, Meltzer PS. Gastrointestinal stromal tumors with KIT mutations exhibit a remarkably homogenous gene expression profile. *Cancer Res*

2001; **61**: 8624–8.
46. Corless CL, McGreevey L, Haley A, Town A, Heinrich MC. KIT mutations are common in incidental gastrointestinal stromal tumors one centimeter or less in size. *Am J Pathol* 2002; **160**: 1567–72.
47. Taniguchi M, Nishida T, Hirota S, Isozaki K, Ito T, Nomura T, Matsuda H, Kitmura Y. Effect of c-*kit* mutation on prognosis of gastrointestinal stromal tumors. *Cancer Res* 1999; **59**: 4297–300.
48. Fletcher CD, Berman JJ, Corless C, Gorstein F, Lasota J, Longley BJ, Miettinen M, O'Leary TJ, Remotti H, Rubin BP, Shmookler B, Sobin LH, Weiss SW. Diagnosis of gastrointestinal stromal tumors: a consensus approach. *Hum Pathol* 2002; **33**: 459–65.
49. Nishida T, Hirota S, Taniguchi M, Hashimoto K, Isozaki K, Nakamura H, Kanakura Y, Tanaka T, Takabayashi A, Matsuda H, Kitamura Y. Familial gastrointestinal stromal tumours with germline mutation of the KIT gene. *Nat Genet* 1998; **19**: 323–4.
50. Hirota S, Okazaki T, Kitamura Y, O'Brien P, Kapusta L, Dardick I. Cause of familial and multiple gastrointestinal autonomic nerve tumors with hyperplasia of interstitial cells of Cajal is germline mutation of the c-*kit* gene. *Am J Surg Pathol* 2000; **24**: 326–7.
51. Hirota S, Nishida T, Isozaki K, Taniguchi M, Nishikawa K, Ohashi A, Takabayashi A, Obayashi T, Okuno T, Kinoshita K, Chen H, Shinomura Y, Kitamura Y. Familial gastrointestinal stromal tumors associated with dysphagia and novel type germline mutation of KIT gene. *Gastroenterology* 2002; **122**: 1493–9.
52. O'Brien P, Kapusta L, Dardick I, Axler J, Gnidec A. Multiple familial gastrointestinal autonomic nerve tumors and small intestinal neuronal dysplasia. *Am J Surg Pathol* 1999; **23**: 198–204.
53. Isozaki K, Terris B, Belghiti J, Schiffmann S, Hirota S, Vanderwinden J-M. Germline-activating mutation in the kinase domain of *KIT* gene in familial gastrointestinal stromal tumors. *Am J Pathol* 2000; **157**: 1581–5.
54. Maeyama H, Hidaka E, Ota H, Minami S, Kajiyama M, Kuraishi A, Mori H, Matsuda Y, Wada S, Sodeyama H, Nakata S, Kawamura N, Hata S, Watanabe M, Iijima Y, Katsuyama T. Familial gastrointestinal stromal tumor with hyperpigmentation: association with a germline mutation of the c-*kit* gene. *Gastroenterology* 2001; **120**: 210–5.
55. Beghini A, Tibiletti MG, Roversi G, Chiaravalli AM, Serio G, Capella C, Larizza L. Germline mutation in the juxtamembrane domain of the kit gene in a family with gastrointestinal stromal tumors and urticaria pigmentosa. *Cancer* 2001; **92**: 657–62.
56. Chen H, Hirota S, Isozaki K, Sun H, Ohashi A, Kinoshita K, O'Brien P, Kapusta L, Dardick I, Obayashi T, Okazaki T, Shinomura Y, Matsuzawa Y, Kitamura Y. Polyclonal nature of diffuse proliferation of interstitial cells of Cajal in patients with familial and multiple gastrointestinal stromal tumours. *Gut* 2002; **51**: 793–6.
57. Mauro MJ, Druker BJ. STI571: targeting BCR-ABL as therapy for CML. *Oncologist* 2001; **6**: 233–8.
58. Druker BJ, Talpaz M, Resta DJ, Peng B, Buchdunger E, Ford JM, Lydon NB, Kantarjian H, Capdeville R, Ohno-Jones S, Sawyers CL. Efficacy and safety of a specific inhibitor of the BCR-ABL tyrosine kinase in chronic myeloid leukemia. *N Engl J Med* 2001; **344**: 1031–7.
59. Chen H, Isozaki K, Kinoshita K, Ohashi A, Shinomura Y, Matsuzawa Y, Kitamura Y, Hirota S. Imatinib inhibits various types of activating mutant KIT found in gastrointestinal stromal tumors. *Int J Cancer* 2003; **105**: 130–5.

60. Demetri GD, von Mehren M, Blanke CD, Van den Abbeele AD, Eisenberg B, Roberts PJ, Heinrich MC, Tuveson DA, Singer S, Janicek M, Fletcher JA, Silverman SG, Silberman SL, Capdeville R, Kiese B, Peng B, Dimitrijevic S, Druker BJ, Corless C, Fletcher CD, Joensuu H. Efficacy and safety of imatinib mesylate in advanced gastrointestinal stromal tumors. *N Engl J Med* 2002; **347**: 472–80.
61. Ma Y, Zeng S, Metcalfe DD, Akin C, Dimitrijevic S, Butterfield JH, McMahon G, Longley BJ. The c-KIT mutation causing human mastocytosis is resistant to STI571 and other KIT kinase inhibitors; kinases with enzymatic site mutations show different inhibitor sensitivity profiles than wild-type kinases and those with regulatory-type mutations. *Blood* 2002; **99**: 1741–4.
62. Fuller CE, Williams GT. Gastrointestinal manifestations of type 1 neurifibromatosis (von Recklinghausen's disease). *Histopathology* 1991; **19**: 1–11.

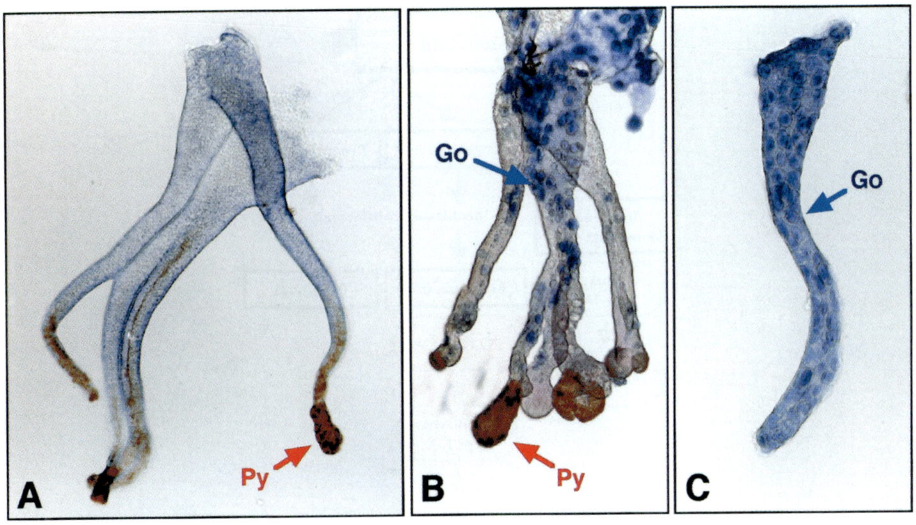

FIG. 3. Morphological and mucin histochemical classification of isolated pyloric glands from human stomach

(A) G type glands consisting of surface mucous cells in the upper part and pyloric gland cells (Py) at the bottom. (B) Glands with GI mixed IM still preserving pyloric gland cells with emergence of goblet cells (Go). (C) I type IM glands losing pyloric glands but with many goblet cells appeared. Goblet cells are shown in blue with Alcian blue staining and pyloric gland cells containing class III mucins are stained brown using DAB utilizing paradoxical concanavalin A staining.

testinal absorptive cells with or without Paneth cells (Fig. 3C). In the GI mixed type, on the other hand, gastric phenotype cells are found sharing the same metaplastic glands with intestinal phenotype cells in various combinations (Fig. 3B). All of the subtypes of GI mixed type IM and a subtype of the I type without Paneth cells belong to the incomplete IM category while the subtype of I type with Paneth cells corresponds to complete type IM. In many cases of the GI mixed type, atrophied pyloric glands are present under the intestinalized cells.

A mixture of gastric and intestinal phenotypes occurs at the cellular level as well as at the glandular level, involving cells of gastric phenotype together with those of intestinal phenotype as mentioned above in GI mixed type IM. Intestinal metaplastic glands are easily found with hematoxylin and eosin (H&E) staining by the presence of goblet cells and brush border lining the apical side of the epithelium (Fig. 1E). Goblet cells are confirmed to exhibit intestinal phenotype, as shown with MUC2 immunostaining (Fig. 1G), which is not present in gastric epithelium (Fig. 1C). Brush border is positive for villin, as is normal intestinal epithelium (Fig. 1H). However, gastric mucin sometimes remains in both goblet and absorptive cells as revealed with MUC5AC immunohistochemistry (Fig. 1F, red arrowhead), villin expression being weaker in such a gland (Fig. 1H, red arrowhead) compared to ones without MUC5AC expression (Fig. 1, F and H, blue arrowheads). The intestinal metaplastic gland still preserving gastric mucin is also considered to be GI mixed type IM at the cellular level, whereas the others are considered to be I types, indicating the presence in the gland of a phenotypic shift from gastric toward intestinal. Thus, IM subtypes may be considered as not independent entities, but rather a sequence of pathological states with a gradual change from stomach to intestinal character. Experimentally, a

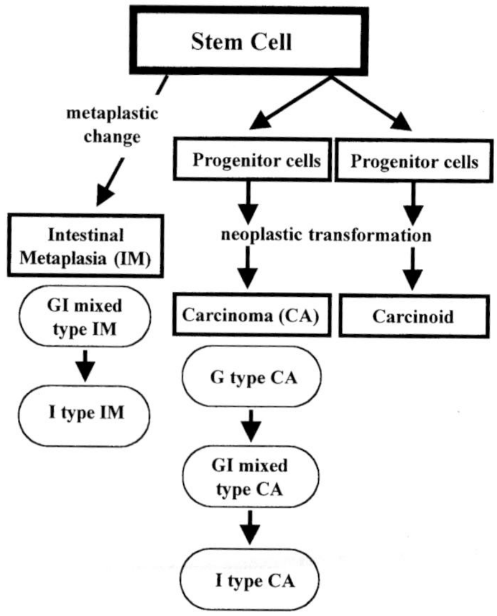

FIG. 4. Schematic illustration of the hypothesis for pathways of intestinal metaplasia and intestinalization of gastric carcinoma based on the pathological findings of human materials and experimental results with rodent models

Intestinalization progresses from GI mixed type toward I type in non-cancerous (left flow) and cancerous (middle flow) tissue independently. GI mixed type IM, gastric and intestinal mixed type intestinal metaplasia; I type IM, solely intestinal type intestinal metaplasia; G type CA, gastric epithelial cell type carcinoma; GI mixed type CA, mixed gastric and intestinal epithelial cell type carcinoma; I type CA, intestinal epithelial cell type carcinoma.

phenotypic shift from GI mixed type to an I type IM could be clearly observed on sequential observation of rat stomach treated with X-rays (*6*). GI mixed type IM may be composed of a mixture of cells with various degrees of intestinal phenotypic shift rather than just a random mixture of gastric and intestinal type cells. This allows us to introduce the notion that IM might be due to abnormal stem cell differentiation still obeying a certain order (Fig. 4, left flow).

It is believed that stem cells (multipotent progenitor cells) are present in the proliferative cell zone in the isthmus region of the gastric glands, giving rise to all the various cell types by differentiation, so that consequently gastric glands are monoclonal in the adult stage (*30, 31*). In the environment of a normal gastric gland, cells derived from stem cells undergo complex bipolar migration from the isthmus either upward or downward. In pyloric mucosa, surface mucous cells move upward, while pyloric gland cells migrate downward (*32*). In the crypts of the small intestine, on the other hand, stem cells would be expected to be present in the proliferative cell zone at the bottom of the crypts. In the normal intestinal gland, cells that will become absorptive and goblet cells move up, and only these differentiating into Paneth cells migrate lower from the proliferative cell zone. In GI mixed IM, gastric surface mucous cells, intestinal absorptive cells and goblet cells are found in the upper glandular portions from the proliferative zone and pyloric gland cells and Paneth cells are found in the lower glandular portions from the proliferative zone (Fig. 5, A and B) (*14*). GI mixed type IM might be the consequence of abnormal differentiation of stem cells that can produce both gastric and intestinal type cells, with the normal cell migration

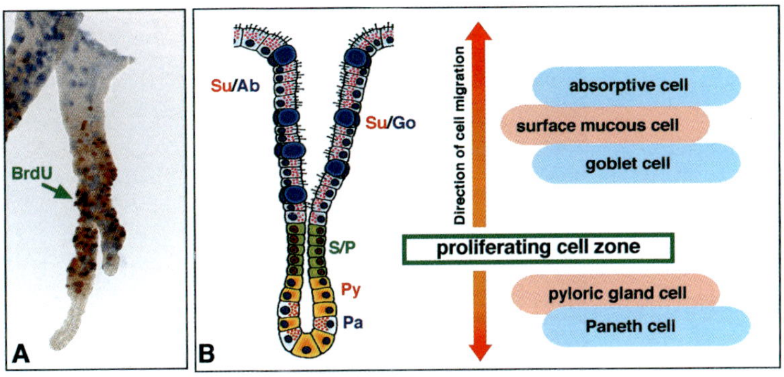

FIG. 5. Direction of cell migration and differentiation of gastric and intestinal phenotypic cells in GI mixed IM

(A) Isolated GI mixed intestinal metaplastic glands are incubated in the presence of 10 mg/ml bromodeoxyuridine (BrdU) for 2 h. Proliferating cells are visualized with BrdU immunohistochemistry. Goblet cells are visualized with Alcian blue. Original magnification, ×100. (B) Schematic view of the cell differentiation (left panel) and direction of cell migration in GI mixed intestinal metaplastic glands consisting of both gastric (highlighted red) and intestinal (highlighted blue) phenotypic cells (right panel). Su, surface mucous cells; Ab, absorptive cells; Go, goblet cells; Su/Ab, absorptive cells retaining mucin of surface mucous cells; Su/Go, goblet cells containing both gastric and intestinal mucin; S/P, stem cells and proliferating cells; Py, pyloric gland cells; Pa, Paneth cells.

pattern preserved. Since epithelial cell differentiation and migration of gastric glands are thought to be closely linked, it is not clear why only the former is disturbed. Recently, epithelial-mesenchymal interactions have attracted attention due to their alteration under miscellaneous conditions, as well as interest in their role in organogenesis (*33*). It clearly warrants further study whether the organization of intestinal metaplastic lesions might be influenced by interstitial cells.

Expression of Homeobox Genes in Intestinal Metaplasia

Caudal genes are necessary for determination of anteroposterior polarity during early *Drosophila* development (*34*) and caudal-type homeobox (*Cdx*) 1 and *Cdx2* are mammalian members of the caudal-related homeobox gene family (*35*). In the adult mouse and in humans, expression is strictly confined to the gut, from the duodenum to the rectum. Silberg *et al.* (*36*) previously reported the presence of *Cdx1* protein in intestinal metaplastic lesions of the human stomach. Mizoshita *et al* (*37*). demonstrated the expression of *Cdx1* and *Cdx2* in both the small and large intestine and in intestinal metaplastic mucosa of the human stomach. On the other hand, *in situ* analysis of the chicken *cSox2* gene, a member of the transcription factor family containing an *Sry*-like high-mobility group box, demonstrated localized expression in the embryonic endoderm. Transcripts of *cSox2* appear before commencement of morphogenesis and cytodifferentiation in the rostral gut epithelium from the pharynx to the stomach. The caudal limit of *cSox2* expression coincides with that of the region competent for proventricular differentiation and to the rostral limit of the domain of *CdxA*, a homologue of *Drosophila* caudal (*38*). In the human digestive tract, *Sox2* expression is found in stomach epithelium but is very low in intestine, as observed in the chicken. However, in IM, *Sox2* transcripts begin to decrease and gradually disappear as IM progresses from GI mixed type to I type (Fig. 6). The expression patterns

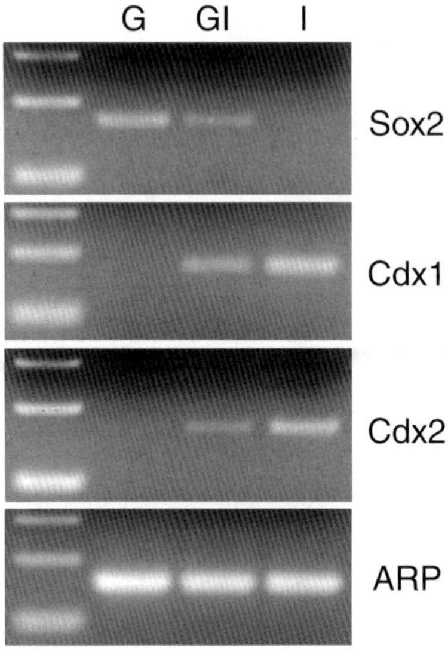

FIG. 6. Semi-quantitative reverse transcription-polymerase chain reaction of *Sox2*, *Cdx1*, and *Cdx2* transcripts in isolated stomach glands

G type (lane G), GI mixed type (lane GI), and I type glands (lane I). *Sox2* is expressed in gastric epithelium, is down-regulated when IM starts, and finally disappears in I type glands. On the other hand, *Cdx* genes are ectopically transcribed in intestinal metaplastic glands of both GI mixed and I types, being upregulated with the progression towards the I type. Acidic ribosomal phosphoprotein PO (ARP) is shown as an internal control. Left lane, DNA molecular weight markers corresponding to 100, 200, and 300 base pairs from the bottom.

of *Sox2* and *Cdx1/Cdx2* are inversely related and down-regulation of *Sox2* could be an important mechanism in IM in addition to ectopic expression of *Cdx1/Cdx2* (*39*).

Gastric and Intestinal Phenotypic Expression of Gastric Cancer Cells

It is widely believed that the phenotypic expression of tumor cells tends to be the same as that of the tissue of origin of the cells. Histologically, human gastric carcinomas have been classified into two major groups, the "intestinal" and "diffuse" types of Lauren (*1*), which respectively nearly correspond to the "differentiated" and "undifferentiated" types of Nakamura *et al.* (*40*) and Sugano *et al.* (*41*) in Japan. Using several gastric and intestinal cellular differentiation markers as mentioned above, phenotypic expression of human and rat gastric cancer cells of each histologic type can be clearly classified into a gastric epithelial cell type (G type), including pyloric gland cells and surface mucous cells and an intestinal epithelial cell type (I type) including goblet cells and intestinal absorptive cells (*3–5*). Based on findings for monoclonal growth of gastric cancers (*2*), it is assumed that individual lesions are derived from a single cell with intrinsic potential to differentiate into G type and I type cancer cells. Although Lauren's classification (*1*) has been widely used, it is inadequate for studies of histogenesis of gastric cancers and phenotypic expression at the cellular level, because it confuses I type cancer cells with "diffuse" structure and G types with the "intestinal" type of Lauren.

Sugihara *et al.* (*42*) and Fujimori *et al.* (*43*) have revealed an organoid differentiation of intramucosal signet ring cell carcinomas. The upper and lower layers of the typical intramucosal laminated structure consist of carcinoma cells containing surface mucous cell and pyloric gland cell type mucins, respectively, whereas the middle layer is occupied by immature carcinoma cells. Such a structure appears to simulate cellular differentiation occurring in normal mucosa. Similar organoid differentiation, mimicking pyloric gland mucosa, with GI type IM and I type IM, is often found within differentiated adenocarcinomas (*44*).

Phenotypic Change from G to I Type Cancer Cells in Gastric Cancers

Focusing on the histogenesis of gastric cancer, we have compared the frequency of IM in the surrounding mucosa in the two types to clarify whether "intestinal" type carcinomas arose in intestinalized mucosa and "diffuse" type carcinomas in the gastric mucosa proper. Phenotypic expression of gastric cancers originating from IM should be of the I type. Even if the phenotypic expression of I type cells of gastric cancer is unstable, the incidence of I type cells in small gastric cancers should be higher than that in large gastric cancers, although in fact it appears to be stable (*45*). Sequential and quantitative analysis of the appearance of IM and I type tumor cells in gastric tumors during gastric carcinogenesis induced by a chemical carcinogen in rats clearly demonstrated the following (Fig. 4, middle flow) (*3*). (i) Adenomatous hyperplasia totally consisting of G type cells appears first. (ii) All adenocarcinomas mainly consist of G type cancer cells and in more than 50% of cases they are composed entirely of cells of G type. No tumors consisting only of I type cells were found. (iii) The incidence of I type tumor cells increased significantly in gastric lesions with progression from adenomatous hyperplasia through small well-differentiated adenocarcinomas to large well-differentiated adenocarcinomas. (iv) Tumor cells of G and I types may be present in the same acini in adenocarcinomas. (v) Adenocarcinomas with I type cells occasionally develop in pyloric mucosa in the absence of IM, and tumors without I type tumor cells sometimes occur in pyloric mucosa with IM. Therefore we earlier proposed that IM may not be a preneoplastic change in gastric carcinoma, but rather that cells of the I type may appear independently in the gastric mucosa in IM or in gastric cancers.

Recently, a similar phenomenon was also observed in human gastric cancers. Gastric cancers consisting of G type cancer cells in gastric mucosa with IM and the presence of gastric cancers consisting of I type cancer cells in ordinary mucosa suggest phenotypic expression of gastric cancer cells is independent of phenotypic changes in the surrounding gastric mucosa (*44*, *46*). Yamachika *et al.* (*46*) and Bamba *et al.* (*47*) found signet ring cell carcinomas at early stages to consist mainly of G type cancer cells, with a phenotypic shift from G type to I type expression accompanying increasing depth of invasion. In addition, Yoshikawa *et al.* (*44*) revealed over 40% of early stage Lauren's "intestinal" type carcinomas to consist mainly of G type cancer cells, and again a phenotypic shift from G to I type expression was evident with progression.

Expression of Homeobox Genes in Gastric Carcinomas

Intestinalization of gastric cancer cells differs from the non-systematic deregulation of a single gene that is often seen during carcinogenesis. For intestinalization, changes in the expression of various genes determining cell structures and functions may be involved. Intestinalization of gastric cancer cells may represent a kind of homeotic transformation. In the course of human ontogenesis, homeobox genes play a key role in developmental processes. Fetal stomach, which develops from the foregut, displays areas of "intestinal type mucosa" with goblet cells and epithelial cells with striated borders in the antrum and cardia (*48*). Intestinalization of gastric cancer cells may thus indicate a loss of ability to inhibit the primitive intestinal phenotype, which was present in the fetal tissue but is normally inhibited in adult cells. Initiation of carcinogenesis may lead to a less differentiated appearance or the capacity to differentiate in both gastric and intestinal directions, perhaps with deregulation of homeobox gene expression. Recent evidence suggests roles for several homeobox genes in processes leading to malignancy. Silberg *et al.* (*36*) and Bai *et al.* (*49*) have shown that *Cdx1* is sometimes expressed in adenocarcinomas of the stomach. Mizoshita *et al.* (*50*) suggested *Cdx1* to be linked with I type cancer cells in both "intestinal" and "diffuse" type lesions of Lauren's histological classification. Ectopic expression of Cdx may be related to I type phenotypic expression of cancer cells. As mentioned regarding GI mixed IM, investigation of *Sox2* expression could provide essential clues to understanding G type and GI mixed type cancer. Disturbance of regulation of *Sox2* and *Cdx1/2* within cancer originating from single cells with multipotential for differentiation might play important roles in determining phenotypic expression of gastric neoplastic cells and in the biological behavior of gastric cancers.

Acknowledgments

This work was supported in part by a Research Grant from the Princess Takamatsu Cancer Research Fund (00-23207), a Grant-in-Aid for the 2nd Term Comprehensive 10-Year Strategy for Cancer Control and a Grant-in-Aid for Cancer Research from the Ministry of Health, Labour and Welfare, Japan, and a Grant-in-Aid from the Ministry of Education, Culture, Sports, Science and Technology of Japan.

REFERENCES

1. Lauren P. The two histological main types of gastric carcinoma: diffuse and so-called intestinal-type carcinoma: an attempt at a histo-clinical classification. *Acta Pathol Microbiol Scand* 1965; **64**: 31–49.
2. Tatematsu M, Fukami H, Yamamoto M, Nakanishi H, Masui T, Kusakabe N, Sakakura T. Clonal analysis of glandular stomach carcinogenesis in C3H/HeN↔BALB/c chimeric mice treated with N-methyl-N-nitrosourea. *Cancer Lett* 1994; **83**: 37–42.
3. Tatematsu M, Furihata C, Katsuyama T, Hasegawa R, Nakanowatari J, Saito D, Takahashi M, Matsushima T, Ito N. Independent induction of intestinal metaplasia and gastric cancer in rats treated with N-methyl-N′-nitro-N-nitrosoguanidine. *Cancer Res* 1983; **43**: 1335–41.
4. Tatematsu M, Furihata C, Katsuyama T, Miki K, Honda H, Konishi Y, Ito N. Gastric and intestinal phenotypic expressions of human signet ring cell carcinomas revealed by their biochemistry, mucin histochemistry, and ultrastructure. *Cancer Res* 1986; **46**:

4866–72.
5. Tatematsu M, Ichinose M, Miki K, Hasegawa R, Kato T, Ito N. Gastric and intestinal phenotypic expression of human stomach cancers as revealed by pepsinogen immunohistochemistry and mucin histochemistry. *Acta Pathol Jpn* 1990; **40**: 494–504.
6. Yuasa H, Inada K, Watanabe H, Tatematsu M. A phenotypic shift from gastric-intestinal to solely intestinal cell types in intestinal metaplasia in rat stomach following treatment with X-rays. *J Toxicol Pathol* 2002; **15**: 85–93.
7. Katsuyama T, Spicer SS. Histochemical differentiation of complex carbohydrates with variants of the concanavalin A-horseradish peroxidase method. *J Histochem Cytochem* 1978; **26**: 233–50.
8. Tatematsu M, Katsuyama T, Fukushima S, Takahashi M, Shirai T, Ito N, Nasu T. Mucin histochemistry by paradoxical concanavalin A staining in experimental gastric cancers induced in Wistar rats by N-methyl-N-nitro-N-nitrosoguanidine or 4-nitroquinoline 1-oxide. *J Natl Cancer Inst* 1980; **64**: 835–43.
9. Furihata C, Tatematsu M, Miki K, Katsuyama T, Sudo K, Miyagi N, Kubota T, Jin SS, Kodama K, Ito N, Konishi Y, Suzuki K, Matsushima T. Gastric- and intestinal-type properties of human gastric cancers transplanted into nude mice. *Cancer Res* 1984; **44**: 727–33.
10. Tatematsu M, Furihata C, Katsuyama T, Mera Y, Inoue T, Matsushima T, Ito N. Immunohistochemical demonstration of pyloric gland-type cells with low-pepsinogen isozyme 1 in preneoplastic and neoplastic tissues of rat stomachs treated with N-methyl-N′-nitro-N-nitrosoguanidine. *J Natl Cancer Inst* 1987; **78**: 771–7.
11. Tatematsu M, Katsuyama T, Furihata C, Fukushima S, Shirai T, Kato T, Ito N. Cellular differentiation and histogenesis of rat glandular stomach cancers. *Jpn J Cancer Res* 1990; **81**: 760–7.
12. Iwata H, Itzkowitz SH, Werther JL, Hayashi K, Nakamura H, Ichinose M, Miki K, Tatematsu M. Expression of sialosyl-Tn in intestinal type cancer cells of human gastric cancers. *Acta Pathol Jpn* 1993; **43**: 646–53.
13. Inada K, Nakanishi H, Fujimitsu Y, Shimizu N, Ichinose M, Miki K, Nakamura S, Tatematsu M. Gastric and intestinal mixed and solely intestinal types of intestinal metaplasia in the human stomach. *Pathol Int* 1997; **47**: 831–41.
14. Inada K, Tanaka H, Nakanishi H, Tsukamoto T, Ikehara Y, Tatematsu K, Nakamura S, Porter EM, Tatematsu M. Identification of Paneth cells in pyloric glands associated with gastric and intestinal mixed-type intestinal metaplasia of the human stomach. *Virchows Arch* 2001; **439**: 14–20.
15. Tajima Y, Shimoda T, Nakanishi Y, Yokoyama N, Tanaka T, Shimizu K, Saito T, Kawamura M, Kusano M, Kumagai K. Gastric and intestinal phenotypic marker expression in gastric carcinomas and its prognostic significance: immunohistochemical analysis of 136 lesions. *Oncology* 2001; **61**: 212–20.
16. Fialkow PJ. Clonal origin of human tumors. *Biochim Biophys Acta* 1976; **458**: 283–321.
17. Kakizoe T, Tanooka H, Tanaka K, Sugimura T. Single-cell origin of bladder cancer induced by N-butyl-N-(4-hydroxybutyl) nitrosamine in mice with cellular mosaicism. *Gann* 1983; **74**: 462–5.
18. Nomura S, Esumi H, Job C, Tan SS. Lineage and clonal development of gastric glands. *Dev Biol* 1998; **204**: 124–35.

19. Kusakabe M, Yokoyama M, Sakakura T, Nomura T, Hosick HL, Nishizuka Y. A novel methodology for analysis of cell distribution in chimeric mouse organs using a strain specific antibody. *J Cell Biol* 1988; **107**: 257–65.
20. Tatematsu M, Masui T, Fukami H, Yamamoto M, Nakanishi H, Inada K, Kusakabe M, Sakakura T. Primary monoclonal and secondary polyclonal growth of colon neoplastic lesions in C3H/HeN↔BALB/c chimeric mice treated with 1,2-dimethylhydrazine immunohistochemical detection of C3H strain-specific antigen and simple sequence length polymorphism analysis of DNA. *Int J Cancer* 1996; **66**: 234–8.
21. Stemmermann GN, Hayashi T. Intestinal metaplasia of the gastric mucosa: a gross and microscopic study of its distribution in various disease states. *J Natl Cancer Inst* 1968; **41**: 627–34.
22. Morson BC. Carcinoma arising from areas of intestinal metaplasia in the gastric mucosa. *Br J Cancer* 1955; **9**: 377–85.
23. Correa P. Human gastric carcinogenesis: a multistep and multifactorial process—First American Cancer Society Award Lecture on Cancer Epidemiology and Prevention. *Cancer Res* 1992; **52**: 6735–40.
24. You WC, Blot WJ, Li JY, Chang YS, Jin ML, Kneller R, Zhang L, Han ZX, Zeng XR, Liu WD, Zhao L, Correa P, Fraumeni JJF, Xu GW. Precancerous gastric lesions in a population at high risk of stomach cancer. *Cancer Res* 1993; **53**: 1317–21.
25. Kawachi T, Kogure K, Tanaka N, Tokunaga A, Sugimura T. Studies of intestinal metaplasia in the gastric mucosa by detection of disaccharidases with "Tes-Tape." *J Natl Cancer Inst* 1974; **53**: 19–30.
26. Matsukura N, Suzuki K, Kawachi T, Aoyagi M, Sugimura T, Kitaoka H, Numajiri H, Shirota A, Itabashi M, Hirota T. Distribution of marker enzymes and mucin in intestinal metaplasia in human stomach and relation to complete and incomplete types of intestinal metaplasia to minute gastric carcinomas. *J Natl Cancer Inst* 1980; **65**: 231–40.
27. Teglbjaerg PS, Nielsen HO. "Small intestinal type" and "colonic type" intestinal metaplasia of the human stomach, and their relationship to the histogenetic types of gastric adenocarcinoma. *Acta Pathol Microbiol Scand [A]* 1978; **86A**: 351–5.
28. Segura DI, Montero C. Histochemical characterization of different types of intestinal metaplasia in gastric mucosa. *Cancer* 1983; **52**: 498–503.
29. Jass JR, Filipe MI. A variant of intestinal metaplasia associated with gastric carcinoma: a histochemical study. *Histopathology* 1979; **3**: 191–9.
30. Karam SM, Leblond CP. Dynamics of epithelial cells in the corpus of the mouse stomach. I. Identification of proliferative cell types and pinpointing of the stem cell. *Anat Rec* 1993; **236**: 259–79.
31. Ponder BA, Schmidt GH, Wilkinson MM, Wood MJ, Monk M, Reid A. Derivation of mouse intestinal crypts from single progenitor cells. *Nature* 1985; **313**: 689–91.
32. Hattori T, Fujita S. Tritiated thymidine autoradiographic study of cell migration and renewal in the pyloric mucosa of golden hamsters. *Cell Tissue Res* 1976; **175**: 49–57.
33. Ichinose M, Tsukada S, Fujimitsu Y, Tatematsu M, Matsubara Y, Yahagi N, Oka M, Suzuki T, Shimizu Y, Yonezawa S, Kageyama T, Miki K, Fukamachi H. Proliferation, differentiation and morphogenesis of fetal rat glandular stomach transplanted under the kidney capsule of syngeneic hosts. *Dev Growth Differ* 1997; **39**: 635–42.
34. Macdonald PM, Struhl G. A molecular gradient in early *Drosophila* embryos and its

role in specifying the body pattern. *Nature* 1986; **324**: 537–45.

35. Mallo GV, Rechreche H, Frigerio JM, Rocha D, Zweibaum A, Lacasa M, Jordan BR, Dusetti NJ, Dagorn JC, Iovanna JL. Molecular cloning, sequencing and expression of the mRNA encoding human Cdx1 and Cdx2 homeobox. Down-regulation of Cdx1 and Cdx2 mRNA expression during colorectal carcinogenesis. *Int J Cancer* 1997; **74**: 35–44.
36. Silberg DG, Furth EE, Taylor JK, Schuck T, Chiou T, Traber PG. CDX1 protein expression in normal, metaplastic, and neoplastic human alimentary tract epithelium. *Gastroenterology* 1997; **113**: 478–86.
37. Mizoshita T, Inada K, Tsukamoto T, Kodera Y, Yamamura Y, Hirai T, Kato T, Joh T, Itoh M, Tatematsu M. Expression of Cdx1 and Cdx2 mRNAs and relevance of this expression to differentiation in human gastrointestinal mucosa—with special emphasis on participation in intestinal metaplasia of the human stomach. *Gastric Cancer* 2001; **4**: 185–91.
38. Ishii Y, Rex M, Scotting PJ, Yasugi S. Region-specific expression of chicken Sox2 in the developing gut and lung epithelium: regulation by epithelial-mesenchymal interactions. *Dev Dyn* 1998; **213**: 464–75.
39. Tsukamoto T, Inada K, Tanaka H, Mizoshita T, Mihara M, Ushijima T, Yamamura Y, Nakamura S, Tatematsu M. Down-regulation of a gastric transcription factor, Sox2 and ectopic expression of intestinal homeobox genes Cdx1 and Cdx2: inverse correlation during progression from gastric/intestinal-mixed to complete intestinal metaplasia. *J Cancer Res Clin Oncol* 2004; **130**: 135–45.
40. Nakamura K, Sugano H, Takagi K. Carcinoma of the stomach in incipient phase: its histogenesis and histological appearances. *Gann* 1968; **59**: 251–8.
41. Sugano H, Nakamura K, Kato Y. Pathological studies of human gastric cancer. *Acta Pathol Jpn* 1982; **32** Suppl 2: 329–47.
42. Sugihara H, Hattori T, Fukuda M, Fujita S. Cell proliferation and differentiation in intramucosal and advanced signet ring cell carcinomas of the human stomach. *Virchows Arch A Pathol Anat Histopathol* 1987; **411**: 117–27.
43. Fujimori Y, Akamatsu T, Ota H, Katsuyama T. Proliferative markers in gastric carcinoma and organoid differentiation. *Hum Pathol* 1995; **26**: 725–34.
44. Yoshikawa A, Inada Ki K, Yamachika T, Shimizu N, Kaminishi M, Tatematsu M. Phenotypic shift in human differentiated gastric cancers from gastric to intestinal epithelial cell type during disease progression. *Gastric Cancer* 1998; **1**: 134–41.
45. Tatematsu M, Katsuyama T, Furihata C, Tsuda H, Ito N. Stable intestinal phenotypic expression of gastric and small intestinal tumor cells induced by N-methyl-N′-nitro-N-nitrosoguanidine or methylnitrosourea in rats. *Gann* 1984; **75**: 957–65.
46. Yamachika T, Inada K, Fujimitsu Y, Nakamura S, Yamamura Y, Kitou T, Itzkowitz SH, Werther JL, Miki K, Tatematsu M. Intestinalization of gastric signet ring cell carcinomas with progression. *Virchows Arch* 1997; **431**: 103–10.
47. Bamba M, Sugihara H, Kushima R, Okada K, Tsukashita S, Horinouchi M, Hattori T. Time-dependent expression of intestinal phenotype in signet ring cell carcinomas of the human stomach. *Virchows Arch* 2001; **438**: 49–56.
48. Salenius P. On the ontogenesis of the human gastric epithelial cells: a histologic and histochemical study. *Acta Anat* 1962; **50** Suppl 46: 1–76.
49. Bai YQ, Yamamoto H, Akiyama Y, Tanaka H, Takizawa T, Koike M, Kenji Yagi O, Saitoh K, Takeshita K, Iwai T, Yuasa Y. Ectopic expression of homeodomain protein

CDX2 in intestinal metaplasia and carcinomas of the stomach. *Cancer Lett* 2002; **176**: 47–55.

50. Mizoshita T, Inada K, Tsukamoto T, Nozaki K, Joh T, Itoh M, Yamamura Y, Ushijima T, Nakamura S, Tatematsu M. Expression of the intestine-specific transcription factors, Cdx1 and Cdx2, correlates shift to an intestinal phenotype in gastric cancer cells. *J Cancer Res Clin Oncol* 2004; **130**: 29–36.

CARCINOGENESIS

RENAL CARCINOGENESIS: GENOTYPE, PHENOTYPE AND DRAMATYPE

Okio HINO[*1, *2], Toshiyuki KOBAYASHI[*1], Shuji MOMOSE[*1], Yasushi KIKUCHI[*1], Hiroyuki ADACHI[*1] and Kazuo OKIMOTO[*1]

*Department of Experimental Pathology, Cancer Institute, Japanese Foundation for Cancer Research[*1] and Department of Pathology, Juntendo University School of Medicine[*2]*

Cancer is a heritable disorder of somatic cells. Environment and heredity are both important in the carcinogenic process. The Eker rat model of hereditary renal carcinoma (RC) is an example of a Mendelian dominantly inherited predisposition to a specific cancer in an experimental animal. Forty years after the discovery of the Eker rat in Oslo, we and Knudson's group independently identified a germline retrotransposon insertion in the rat homologue of the human tuberous sclerosis (*TSC2*) gene. To our knowledge, this was the first isolation of a Mendelian dominantly predisposing cancer gene in a naturally occurring animal model. Recently, we discovered a new hereditary renal carcinoma in the rat. This rat was named the "Nihon" rat and its predisposing (*Nihon*) gene could be a novel renal tumor suppressor gene. This article will review the utility of these unique models for the study of problems in carcinogenesis; e.g., species-specific differences in tumorigenesis, cell stage and tissue/cell-type specific tumorigenesis, multistep carcinogenesis, modifier gene(s) in renal carcinogenesis, cancer prevention and the development of therapeutic treatments which can be translated to human patients, as well as how environmental factors interact with cancer susceptibility gene(s).

History of the Eker Rat

A naturally occurring hereditary cancer in rat was described by Reidar Eker in Oslo in 1954 (*1*). After 1971, Alfred G. Knudson (Fox Chase Cancer Center, Philadelphia, PA) was looking for an animal model of "two-hit carcinogenesis" that might parallel hereditary retinoblastoma in humans (*2*), and found it in the Eker rat. In 1983, Eker sent some Eker rats to Knudson in Philadelphia. I (O.H.) went to Knudson's laboratory from 1989 to 1991, and began to isolate rat genetic markers (*3*). Unfortunately, these initial linkage studies were negative. When I returned to the Cancer Institute in Tokyo, Knudson sent some Eker rats to me and they have been bred on a normal Long-Evans (LE) strain background at the Animal Facility of the Cancer Institute since 1991. I (O.H.) have since continued investigating them in To-

[*1] 1-37-1 Kami-Ikebukuro, Toshima-ku, Tokyo 170-8455, Japan
[*2] 2-1-1 Hongo, Bunkyo-ku, Tokyo 113-8421, Japan
This paper is dedicated to the memory of late Dr. Tomizo Yoshida on the occasion of the 100th anniversary of his birth. It was originally published in Cancer Science in February, 2003.

kyo. Thus, Eker rat research is being continued by a third generation of investigators (Oslo→Philadelphia→Tokyo).

Identification of the Predisposing Gene of the Eker Rat

The predisposing gene of the Eker rat was mapped to the proximal part of rat chromosome 10 (*4, 5*). We then established a method for early detection of Eker gene carrier rats as early as 2 weeks of age by transplacental administration of N-ethyl-N-nitrosourea (ENU) (*6*), and this dramatically sped up the linkage analysis. Shortly thereafter, we used the conserved linkage between parts of rat chromosome 10q and human chromosome 16p to show that the Eker mutation is tightly linked to the tuberous sclerosis (*Tsc2*) gene (*7*). Finally, we and Knudson's group independently identified a germline retrotransposon insertion in the rat homologue of the human tuberous sclerosis (*TSC2*) gene (*8, 9*).

Then, we constructed transgenic Eker rats with a wild-type *Tsc2* gene and ascertained that germline suppression of the Eker phenotype is possible for both embryonic lethality of the homozygote and tumor predisposition in the heterozygote (gene therapy or prevention), thus confirming that tumor predisposition in the Eker rat is caused by the *Tsc2* germline mutation (*10*).

Phenotype of the Tsc2 Gene Mutant (Eker) Rat

We found that the homozygous mutant condition is lethal at around the 13th day of fetal life (*11*). In heterozygotes, renal carcinomas develop from early preneoplastic lesions (phenotypically altered renal tubules, which begin to appear at 2 months of age) to adenomas around the age of 1 year, penetrance for this RC (*Tsc2*) gene is virtually complete.

Investigation of extra-renal primary tumors revealed hemangiomas/hemangiosarcomas of the spleen, leiomyomas/leiomyosarcomas of the uterus (*12*) and pituitary adenomas (*13–15*). The Eker rat thus bears a single gene mutation with a dominant predisposition to four different tumors, although predisposition for extra-renal tumors is not as complete as with RCs (*16*). Recently brain lesions in the Eker rat, such as subependymal and subcortical hamartomas, were also reported (*17*). In the Eker rat cerebrum, we identified two novel lesions, a cortical tuber and anaplastic ganglioglioma, in addition to the two types of hamartomas described above (*18*). The presence of a cortical tuber is important, as tubers are epileptogenic, and likely to be associated with autism and other neurological symptoms of human TSC.

Species-Specific Difference in Tumorigenesis

Human tuberous sclerosis is an autosomal dominant multisystem disorder caused by a mutation in either the *TSC1* or the *TSC2* gene, characterized by phacomatosis with manifestations that include mental retardation and seizures. The phenotype in human differs from that in the Eker rat, except for the occurrence of RCs (in human, angiomyolipomas are more common), although subependymal, subcortical hamartomas and cortical tuber in the Eker rat were recently reported (*17, 18*). Thus, the same gene shows diverse phenotypes between species, although we do not have any good explanation for this difference. Similar phenomena have been observed in knock-out mice for a number of tumor suppressor genes.

To elicit insights into species-specific tumorigenesis caused by *Tsc2* gene inactivation, we generated a *Tsc2* knock-out mouse (*19*). Mice heterozygous for *Tsc2* mutation developed RCs but no angiomyolipoma, with a complete penetrance as seen in the Eker rat, although there is still a species-specific difference between rat and mouse (liver hemangiomas are observed only in mouse) (*19*). Recently, we also prepared a *Tsc1* knock-out mouse. The phenotype was similar to that of *Tsc2* knock-out mouse. However, it is noteworthy that renal carcinogenesis is slower and milder than that of *Tsc2* mutants (*20*).

Cell Stage and Cell/Tissue-Type Specific Tumorigenesis in Tsc2 Gene Mutants

ENU-induced transplacental renal carcinogenesis in the rat results primarily in Wilms' tumors, not RCs, apparently because primitive nephroblasts are the preferred target. To examine further this specificity of tumor type, we undertook transplacental carcinogenesis in the Eker rat, which is heterozygous for a mutation that predisposes to RC with high penetrance, but not to Wilms' tumor (*6*). Surprisingly, RCs but no Wilms' tumors began to appear from as early as 1 week after birth (*6*). Thus, the Eker rat is highly susceptible to induction of RCs (but not Wilms' tumors) by transplacental administration of ENU. The inheritance of the Eker mutation reduces the required number of carcinogenic events, as evidenced by the finding of renal lesions under conditions where ENU produces no tumors in controls, and determines the specificity of tumor histology even with *in utero* carcinogenesis, where nephroblasts are the preferred target. Nephroblasts might be the targets for development of both kinds of tumor in ENU-induced transplacental renal carcinogenesis.

Our data thus support the hypothesis that the Wilms' tumor gene may control differentiation of nephroblasts (metanephric stem cells) into renal tubular stem cells, while the Eker (*Tsc2*) gene may control terminal differentiation of these stem cells, but permit differentiation of nephroblasts to renal cells (*6*).

Qualitative Differences in the Second Hit of Tsc2 Gene among Mutagens—Spontaneous vs. Chemicals vs. Radiation

We previously reported that in spontaneous RCs of Eker rats, 60% (6 of 10) showed loss of heterozygosity (LOH) covering over 30 cM and, in contrast, 0% (0 of 9) did so in ENU-induced RCs using several DNA markers located on rat chromosome 10 (*14*). We characterized the second hit (intragenic mutations including point mutation) in LOH-negative lesions at the DNA-sequencing level of the predisposing *Tsc2* gene using polymerase chain reaction-single strand conformations. We showed that a qualitative difference in the second hit exists between spontaneous and ENU-induced mutations (e.g., deletion or duplication versus point mutation) (*21*). Quite recently, we investigated the second hit of radiation-induced RCs in Eker rat and compared the results with other findings (*22*).

We further detected loss of heterozygosity in 4 of 11 uterine leiomyosarcomas (36%) and 11 of 31 pituitary adenomas (35%) from Eker rats, but in none of 9 pituitary adenomas from non-carrier rats, suggesting that inactivation of the *Tsc2* gene is also a critical event in the pathogenesis of these extra-renal tumors (*15*). Our data indicate that there might be different pathways for tumorigenesis of pituitary adenomas between Eker and non-carrier rats (*15*).

Structure and Function(s) of Tsc2 Gene

We described the entire cDNA (5375 bp without exons 25 and 31) of the rat *Tsc2* gene, and the genomic structure of the rat *Tsc2* gene (*23*). There are 41 coding exons with relatively small-sized introns, and the length covering all the exons is ~35 kb, although there is a noncoding exon(s) in the 5′ upstream region (*24*). Two alternative splicing events [involving exons 25 (129 bp) and 31 (69 bp)] make for complex diversity of the Tsc2 product. The deduced amino acid sequence (1743 amino acids) shows 92% identity to the human counterpart. The determination of the *Tsc2* gene and establishment of strong conservation between rat and man provided clues to the gene functions.

As a next step, we checked the effect of wild-type *Tsc2* gene expression in Eker RC cells using a tetracycline-responsive promoter system. Transfection and expression of an exogenous *Tsc2* gene affect both cell morphology and growth rate (*25*), as well as anchorage independence *in vitro* and tumorigenicity *in vivo* (*26*). This provides direct support for the classification of *Tsc2* as a tumor suppressor gene.

TSC Signalling Pathway—AKT-mTOR-S6K (Fig. 1)

As patients having *TSC1* and *TSC2* mutations show similar symptoms, involvement of tuberin (TSC2 product) and hamartin (TSC1 product) in a common pathway has been suggested (*27*). Phenotypic resemblance between *Tsc1* and *Tsc2* knockout mice and between *Drosophila Tsc1* and *Tsc2* mutants supports this hypothesis, although the possibility of independent functions of each molecule should not be excluded (*19, 20*). Tuberin and hamartin form a complex and are thought to stabilize each other (*28*). *In vivo*, in accordance with the reciprocal stabilization found *in vitro*, homozygous *Tsc2* mutant rat embryos show a reduced level of hamartin protein ex-

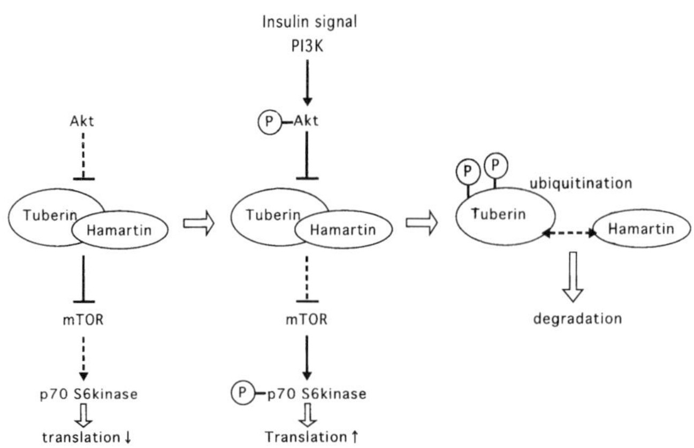

FIG. 1. TSC signalling pathway

pression (*29*). Phosphorylation of tuberin at tyrosine and serine/threonine residues modulates its binding activity with hamartin (*30*). One of the kinases that phosphorylates serine/threonine residues in tuberin is Akt. After the phosphorylation of Akt, binding of tuberin to hamartin is inhibited. Hamartin is also phosphorylated, although the significance of this for functional activities is not clear.

Genetic studies of *Drosophila* revealed that tuberin and hamartin regulate the insulin-signaling pathway (*31*). Initially, both fly *Tsc1* and *Tsc2* homologues were cloned as causative genes for mutants that exhibit common phenotypes such as enlarged cell size and aberrant expression of cell cycle regulators such as cyclins and Cdks (*32*). The appearance of large cell phenotype may be relevant to that found in tuberous sclerosis lesions. In *Drosophila*, one of the pathways regulating cell size is insulin-signaling through PI3-kinase, Akt and p70 S6 kinase (*33*). Subsequent genetic crossing experiments in the fly suggested that hamartin and tuberin function between Akt and S6 kinase.

Interestingly, we observed the specific development of hepatocellular adenomas (enlarged hepatocytes) only in Eker rats, although we observed no difference in the number of preneoplastic "traditional" GST-P-positive foci (small hepatocytes) between Eker and non-Eker rats (*34*). The *Tsc2* gene mutation might influence the phenotype of preneoplastic initiated hepatocytes.

Biochemical studies with mammalian cells further demonstrated a functional link between tuberin/hamartin complex and Akt-S6 kinase signaling (*35*). Phosphorylation of 4E-BP1 and S6 kinase and its downstream target, ribosomal protein S6 subunit, are up-regulated in cells lacking functional *Tsc1* or *Tsc2*, or by RNAi-mediated down-regulation of hamartin and tuberin expression. Inactivation of 4E-BP1 and activation of S6 kinase by phosphorylation result in increased translation. Forced expression of both hamartin and tuberin significantly suppresses basal and insulin- or nutrient-induced S6 kinase activity. Tuberin has several serine/threonine residues in the consensus sequence for phosphorylation by Akt (*36*). Two of these residues (Ser 939 and Thr 1462) appeared to be main phosphorylation sites by Akt. Mutations that introduce acidic residues in these sites abolish tuberin function against S6 kinase activity (*37*). Upon phosphorylation by Akt, hamartin/tuberin complex is destabilized and degraded, probably via the ubiquitin-proteasome pathway (*28*).

Rapamycin—Molecular Targeted Therapy

In terms of the regulation of S6 kinase activity, one candidate for the direct downstream targets of hamartin/tuberin complex is the mammalian target of rapamycin (mTOR) (*35*). Physical association of mTOR with hamartin and tuberin has been found and phosphorylation (Ser 2448) of mTOR is inhibited by hamartin/tuberin expression (*35*). However, the dependency of hamartin/tuberin-mediated suppression of S6 kinase on mTOR inhibition is still unclear (*37*). Recent reports suggested that 14-3-3 family proteins bind to tuberin and modulate the Akt-S6 kinase pathway (*37*).

The relationship of the hamartin/tuberin complex and the insulin-signaling pathway is not fully understood so far, and involvement of S6 kinase activation in the pathogenesis of tuberous sclerosis remains to be determined.

Functional Domain(s) Responsible for Eker Phenotypes (RC and Embryonic Lethality) (Fig. 2)

Our transgenic rescue system using various deletion mutants of the *Tsc2* gene will be useful for the analysis of functional *TSC2/Tsc2* domains (*10, 29*). Therefore, to elucidate the functional domain(s) of tuberin *in vivo*, we generated transgenic Eker rats carrying deletion mutants of the *Tsc2* gene (*29*) (Fig. 2).

Tsc2-DCT55-flag, which lacks only exon 41, completely suppressed ENU-induced RCs of the Eker rat. A Tg coding the C-terminal region (amino acids 1425–1755: TSC2-RGH) suppressed renal carcinogenesis in the Eker rat, and interestingly the degree of this suppression correlated with the level of expression of the Tg. However, Tsc2-DRG, which lacks the region corresponding to Tsc2-RGH, has no tumor suppressor activity. These results prove that the crucial region for the tumor suppressor in *Tsc2* gene is located in Tsc2-RGH (Fig. 2).

Notably, the product of this Tg lacks the ability to bind to the Tsc1 product (hamartin) (*29*). Thus, tuberin could function as a tumor suppressor without binding

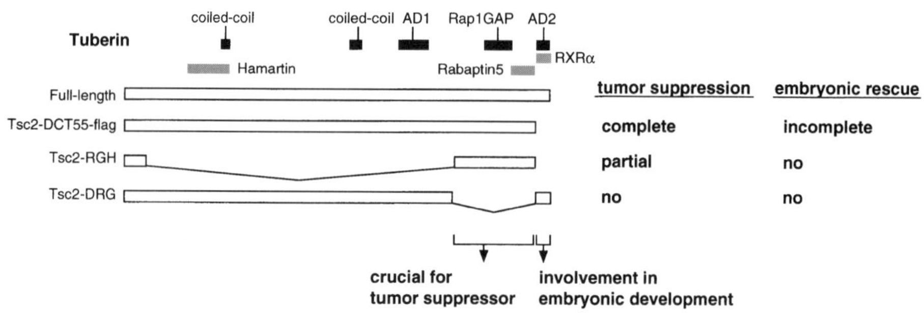

FIG. 2. Protein structure of tuberin (*29*)

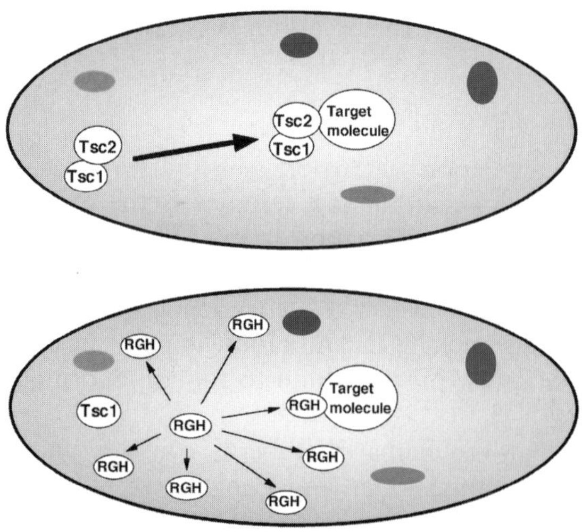

FIG. 3. A model for the behavior of Tsc2-RGH

to hamartin (Fig. 3). As the suppression of renal tumor development by Tsc2-RGH was not complete, the N-terminal two-thirds of tuberin including the hamartin-binding domain would be necessary for the complete tumor suppressor function *in vivo* (Fig. 3).

The reason why the Tg expression-dependent tumor suppression observed in Tsc2-RGH between two independent lines (no. 15 and no. 26) occurred is not yet known. However, one possibility may be the following: From an observation that the increased expression amount of Tsc2-RGH reflects stronger tumor suppression, it was suggested that a high concentration of Tsc2-RGH resulted in increased accessibility of tuberin to the target molecule by diffusion (Fig. 3). In other words, binding of the N-terminal region of tuberin to hamartin might bring tuberin to the appropriate localization efficiently.

We also investigated which Tg would rescue homozygous mutants from embryonic lethality. Though Tsc2-DRG and Tsc2-RGH were not effective, surprisingly, Tsc2-DCT55-ins.flag was partially effective (*38*) (Fig. 2). Therefore, the requirements of the functional domain(s) of tuberin might differ for prevention of embryonic lethality and for suppression of renal carcinogenesis. We are investigating whether there are any characteristic phenotypes in these rescued homozygous mutants.

Role of Association of Tuberin and Hamartin

The *in vivo* association of tuberin and hamartin remained to be elucidated. As expected from the previous reports, hamartin bound with endogenous, Tsc2-DCT55-flag-derived and Tsc2-DRG-derived tuberin, but not with Tsc2-RGH-derived one. In the case of Tsc2-DRG, though the Tg expression was much higher than endogenous tuberin, the amount of Tg-product binding to hamartin was smaller than that of endogenous tuberin. Therefore, it is suggested that the ability to bind to hamartin or the stability of the complex depends on the integrity of tuberin (*29*).

The effect of Tg-derived product on the level of expression of hamartin was also examined. The protein expression of hamartin gradually decreased with deletion of the C-terminal region of tuberin. Furthermore, the hamartin expression in a homozygous mutant embryo carrying Tsc2-RGH seemed to be equal to that in a homozygous mutant embryo (*29*). These results suggested that the hamartin expression depends on the integrity of tuberin, and its expression was regulated at the translational or post-translational level (*29*).

Multistep Renal Carcinogenesis in the Tsc2 Gene Mutant Rat

Successive stages in the development of RCs were observed, beginning with isolated phenotypically altered renal tubule. These foci of atypical tubules were seen in all kidneys exhibiting tumors and are presumed to give rise to the smaller, rounded early adenomas as well as to the later, larger carcinomas; they were not observed in normal rats. Microscopic invasion of perirenal tissue was detected infrequently.

Using laser microscopic dissection, we detected LOH of the wild-type allele even in the earliest preneoplastic lesions, e.g., phenotypically altered renal tubules (*39*), supporting the hypothesis that a second, somatic mutation (second hit) might be a rate-limiting step for renal carcinogenesis in the Eker rat model of dominantly inherited cancer, as well as indicating a tumor-suppressor function for the *Tsc2* gene (*25*). Although the initial event that triggers Eker rat renal cancer is a somatic mutation of the *Tsc2* wild-type allele, other genetic or epigenetic modifications may also contribute to tumor progression in multistep renal carcinogenesis.

Secondary Changes in Gene Expression in Multistep Carcinogenesis

Carcinogenesis can be considered as resembling an opened Japanese fan, because initiated cells grow in several directions, and clinical studies of tumors suggest the edge of the fan contains many gene abnormalities (*40*) (Figs. 4 and 5). To search for such alterations, we identified genes that were expressed more abundantly in Eker rat RC cells than in the normal kidney by representational difference analysis (*40*, *41*).

We identified the highly expressed genes in Eker RCs as *C3* gene encoding the third component of complement, *annexin II* gene encoding the calpactine 1 heavy-chain, *Erc* (expressed in renal carcinoma) gene and *fra-1* gene encoding a transcriptional factor activator protein 1 (AP-1) (*42*). We also found that other members of the AP-1 transcriptional factor family were involved in renal carcinogenesis in the Eker rat model (*43*). Interestingly, AP-1 proteins were highly expressed even in the earlist preneoplastic lesions (e.g., phenotypically altered tubules) as suggested by im-

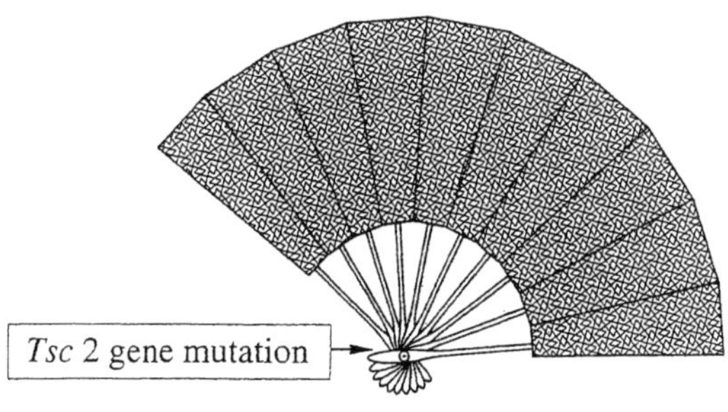

FIG. 4. Fan model of renal carcinogenesis (*40*)
Carcinogenesis looks like an opened Japanese fan. Primal force is "two hits" of the predisposing *Tsc2* gene. Initiated cells grow into many directions and culminate in diverse clinical cancers at the periphery. The edge of the fan corresponds to clinical tumors.

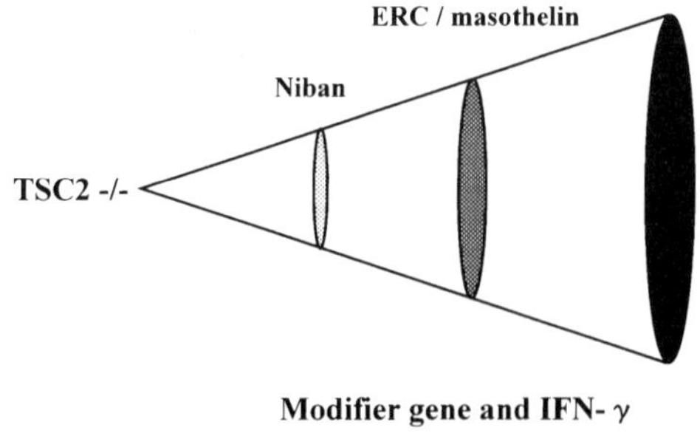

FIG. 5. Multistep renal carcinogenesis in Eker (*Tsc2* mutant) rat

munohistochemistry. Moreover, we transfected antisense oligonucleotides targeting *AP-1* genes into RC cells and demonstrated that cell growth was strongly inhibited (*43*). Thus, the data suggest that expession of *AP-1* genes might play a crucial role in renal carcinogenesis in the Eker rat model.

We also elucidated the underlying regulatory mechanisms of the *Tsc2* gene expression via two Ets-transcription factor binding sites (EBSs) in opposite directions and found that Ets family proteins were highly expressed in the RCs. These observations might be helpful to search the downstream molecular targets and gene network of the *Tsc2* gene.

Erc Gene/MPF/Mesothelin

After we determined the complete primary strucure of rat *Erc* cDNA, we showed that the putative rat Erc product has 56.1% identity to human MPF/mesothelin (*44*). Rat *Erc* and its human homologue were localized in chromosomes 10q12-21 and 16p13.3, respectively, both of which coincide with the locus of the *Tsc2/TSC2* gene (*44*). As mesothelin is a cell surface protein, it may function as a cell adhesion molecule. Our transfection data also suggest a role of the Erc product in cell adhesion and/or cell shape dynamics (*44*). *Erc* may be related to carcinogenesis in the Eker rat model (Fig. 5). Recently, we prepared *Erc* knock-out mice and we are currently mating them with *Tsc1* and *Tsc2* knock-out mice.

In addition, we found the Erc product was cleaved and secreted into the culture medium (unpublished results). We are now establishing an ELISA assay system for serum diagnosis.

A Novel Gene, Niban

Recently, we also isolated a novel gene, using the cDNA-amplifed fragment length polymorphisms approach, and named it "*Niban*," meaning the second in Japanese, because it is the second new gene to be found after *Erc* in our laboratory (*45*). The *Niban* gene consists of 14 exons and is located on RNO13, MMU1 and HSA1. The expression of *Niban* was upregulated even in early preneoplastic lesions (phenotypically altered renal tubules) in the renal carcinogenesis models (unpublished results). *Niban* might be a candidate marker for early-stage renal carcinogenesis and its molecular analysis should provide new insights into multistep carcinogenesis in the kidney (Fig. 5).

Loss of Rat Chromosome 5 in Late Stage of Renal Carcinogenesis

Microsatellite instability was not observed in 26 Eker rat tumors (*46*). Nonrandom loss of rat chromosome 5 in RC-derived cell lines is sometimes associated with homologous deletion of the interferon gene loci at rat chromosome bands 5q31-33 (*11*). Homozygous deletion of the *Ink4* homologue on rat chromosome 5q was observed in 14 of 24 (58%) RC-derived cell lines, *Ifn*α gene in five of 24 cases (21%) and the *Ifn*β gene in one of 24 cases (4%), so the order of the genes may be *Ink4-Ifn*α*-Ifn*β (*46*). Since this locus is not linked with the predisposing inherited *Tsc2* gene in the Eker rat, it probably represents a second tumor suppressor gene involved in late events in tumor progression.

Additional Event(s) for Metastatic RC

Although inactivation of *Tsc2* results in development of renal tumors, it is not sufficient for metastatic RCs in the Eker rat. Their transformation to carcinomas may require additional rate-limiting events. To investigate the additional genetic event(s) necessary for cancer metastasis, we established highly metastatic cell lines from a non-metastatic RC cell line (*48*). They should be useful experimental tools to investigate metastasis-promoting events in renal carcinogenesis.

Tsc Gene Mutations in Chemically Induced Renal Carcinogenesis

We searched for mutations of the *Tsc2* gene in chemically induced non-Eker rat RCs by SSCP analysis (*49, 50*). We simultaneously searched for mutation in the *Vhl* gene, a rat homologue of von Hippel-Lindau disease (*VHL*). Mutations in the *VHL* gene were not detected in any spontaneous RCs of the Eker rat model, or in chemically induced non-Eker rat tumors. In contrast, *Tsc2* gene mutations were detected at a high frequency in N-ethyl-N-hydroxyethylnitrosamine (EHEN)- and diethylnitrosamine (DEN)-induced non-Eker rat primary RCs. We infrequently found mutations of the *Tsc1* gene, a rat homologue of the *TSC1* gene, in chemically induced rat RCs (*51*). These findings call attention to possible *TSC1* and *TSC2* gene mutation in human RCs, especially of the non-clear cell type, which are not related to the *VHL* gene. Up to now, mutations of the *TSC1*/*TSC2* genes in human RCs have not been extensively examined. Interestingly, we recently found LOH of the *TSC2*/*ERC* gene locus in human lung carcinomas (*52*).

Presence of Modifier Gene(s) in Renal Carcinogenesis

It is well known that tuberous sclerosis shows a variety of phenotypes even within the same family. There are effects of genetic background on renal carcinogenesis in the Eker rat model. Interestingly, there is a difference of tumor development between the original Eker rats (LE/LE) and hybrid Eker rat (LE/BN) F1 hybrids. These data indicate there is a modifier gene(s) in the BN rat genome that suppresses the growth of tumors. The identification of such a modifier gene(s) might help us to understand diverse phenotypes of tuberous sclerosis in humans. We subsequently succeeded in mapping a new modifier locus on the rat chromosome (*53*).

Prevention of Renal Carcinogenesis in Tsc Genes Knock-Out Mice: Manipulatable Phenotype (Dramatype)

We reported that tumor buds repeatedly appeared and disappeared in Eker rats on a high-fat diet, and indicated that carcinogenesis does not proceed only in a forward direction (*54*).

In comparison with the rat system, one of the advantages of the mouse system is the availability of various genetically modified lines for genetic cross experiments. Nothing is known about prevention of tumorigenesis of human tuberous sclerosis, and animal models have great potential in that regard. We will describe here an example of disease prevention.

We mated the *IFN-γ* transgenic mice with *Tsc2* gene knock-out mice. Surprisingly, renal carcinogenesis was dramatically suppressed in *Tsc2* gene knockout mice, both macro- and microscopically (*55*). These transgenic mice specifically expressed IFN-γ in the liver, because of the link to liver-specific serum amyloid P component gene promoter, and developed chronic hepatitis (*56–58*). Values of circulating IFN-γ in these transgenic mice were more than 100 pg/ml, while in non-transgenic mice IFN-γ could not be detected. IFN-γ is a pleotrophic cytokine and suppression of tumor development has been reported using several systems. Various mechanisms have been considered, including immunity and non-immunity such as cell arrest and apoptosis. Previously, we reported that the capacity to stimulate allogeneic and antigen-specific T lymphocytes, as well as the ability to produce IL-12 and to process soluble protein antigens, was significantly higher in dendritic cells from *IFN-γ* transgenic mice compared to normal mice. It should be noted that lymphoid infiltration was lacking in the kidneys of these *IFN-γ* transgenic mice. Long-term application of IFN-γ is feasible, because chronic systemic administration of low-dose IFN-γ is already being given to mycosis fungoides (cutaneous T cell lymphoma) patients.

As mentioned before, recent studies have implicated a possible relationship of *TSC* genes to the PI3 kinase-Akt/PKB-S6K signaling pathway. Our findings might be helpful in understanding the mechanisms of disease, as well as in the development of new therapeutic treatments for TSC patients (*59*).

From Eker Rat to Nihon Rat

Recently, we discovered a new hereditary RC in the rat. This rat was named the "Nihon" rat (*60, 61*), and its predisposing (*Nihon*) gene is a novel renal tumor suppressor gene (*62*).

Acknowledgments

This work was supported in part by Grants-in-Aid for Cancer Research from the Ministry of Education, Culture, Sports, Science and Technology of Japan, the Ministry of Health, Labour and Welfare of Japan, and the Organization for Pharmaceutical Safety and Research (OPSR). We thank Drs. H. Sugano, T. Kitagawa and A. Knudson for encouragement throughout this work.

REFERENCES

1. Eker R, Mossige J. A dominant gene for renal adenomas in the rats. *Nature* 1961; **189**: 858–9.
2. Knudson AG. Mutation and cancer: statistical study of retinoblastoma. *Proc Natl Acad Sci USA* 1971; **68**: 820–3.
3. Hino O, Testa J, Buetow K, Taguch T, Zhou JY, Bremer M, Bruzel A, Yeung R, Levan G, Knudson AG, Tartof KD. Universal mapping probes and origin of human chromsome 3. *Proc Natl Acad Sci USA* 1993; **90**: 730–4.
4. Yeung RS, Buetow KH, Testa JR, Knudson AG. Susceptibility to renal carcinoma in

the Eker rat involves a tumor suppressor gene on chromosome 10. *Proc Natl Acad Sci USA* 1993; **90**: 8038–42.

5. Hino O, Mitani H, Nishizawa M, Katsuyama H, Kobayashi E, Hirayama Y. A novel renal cell carcinoma susceptibility gene maps on chromosome 10 in the Eker rat. *Jpn J Cancer Res* 1993; **84**: 1106–9.
6. Hino O, Mitani H, Knudson AG. Genetic predisposition to transplacentally induced renal cell carcinomas in the Eker rat. *Cancer Res* 1993; **53**: 5856–8.
7. Hino O, Kobayashi T, Tsuchiya H, Kikuchi Y, Kobayashi E, Mitani H, Hirayama Y. The predisposing gene of the Eker rat inherited cancer syndrome is tightly linked to the tuberous sclerosis (Tsc2) gene. *Biochem Biophys Res Commun* 1994; **203**: 1302–8.
8. Kobayashi T, Hirayama Y, Kobayashi E, Kubo Y, Hino O. A germline insertion in the tuberous sclerosis (Tsc2) gene gives rise to the Eker rat model of dominantly inherited cancer. *Nat Genet* 1995; **9**: 70–4.
9. Yeung RC, Xiao GH, Jin F, Lee W-C, Testa JR, Knudson AG. Predisposition to renal carcinoma in the Eker rat is determined by germ-line mutation of the tuberous sclerosis 2 (TSC2) gene. *Proc Natl Acad Sci USA* 1994; **91**: 11413–6.
10. Kobayashi T, Mitani H, Takahashi R, Hirabayashi M, Ueda M, Tamura H, Hino O. Transgenic rescue from embryonic lethality and renal carcinogenesis in the Eker rat model by introduction of a wild-type *Tsc2* gene. *Proc Natl Acad Sci USA* 1997; **94**: 3990–3.
11. Hino O, Klein-Szanto AJP, Freed JJ, Testa JR, Brown DQ, Vilensky M, Yeung RS, Tartof KD, Knudson AG. Spontaneous and radiation-induced renal tumors in the Eker rat model of dominantly inherited cancer. *Proc Natl Acad Sci USA* 1993; **90**: 327–31.
12. Everitt JI, Goldsworthy TL, Wolf DS, Walker CL. Hereditary renal cell carcinoma in the Eker rat: a rodent familial cancer syndrome. *J Urol* 1992; **148**: 1932–6.
13. Hino O, Mitani H, Katsuyama H, Kubo Y. A novel cancer predispostion syndrome in the Eker rat model. *Cancer Lett* 1994; **83**: 117–21.
14. Kubo Y, Mitani H, Hino O. Allelic loss at the predisposing gene locus in spontaneous and chemically induced renal cell carcinomas in Eker rat. *Cancer Res* 1994; **54**: 2633–5.
15. Kubo Y, Kikuchi Y, Mitani H, Kobayashi E, Kobayashi T, Hino O. Allelic loss at the tuberous sclerosis (*Tsc2*) gene locus in spontaneous uterine leiomyosarcomas and pituitary adenomas in the Eker rat model. *Jpn J Cancer Res* 1995; **86**: 828–32.
16. Hino O, Kobayashi T, Mitani H, Kubo H, Tsuchiya Y, Kikuchi Y, Nishizawa M, Hirayama Y. The Eker rat, a model of dominantly inherited cancer syndrome. *Transplant Proc* 1995; **27**: 1529–31.
17. Yeung RS, Katsetos CD, Klein-Szanto A. Subependymal astrocytic hamartomas in the Eker rat model of tuberous sclerosis. *Am J Pathol* 1997; **151**: 1477–86.
18. Mizuguchi M, Takahashi S, Yamanouchi H, Nakazato Y, Mitani H, Hino O. Novel cerebral lesions in the Eker rat model of tuberous sclerosis: cortical tuber and anaplastic ganglioglioma. *J. Neuropathol Exp Neurol* 2000; **59**: 188–96.
19. Kobayashi T, Minowa O, Kuno J, Mitani H, Hino O, Noda T. Renal carcinogenesis, hepatic hemangiomatosis, and embryonic lethality caused by a germ-line *Tsc2* mutation in mice. *Cancer Res* 1999; **59**: 1206–11.
20. Kobayashi T, Minowa O, Sugitani Y, Takai S, Mitani H, Kobayashi E, Noda T, Hino O. A germ-line *Tsc1* mutation causes tumor development and embryonic lethality that

are similar, but not identical to, those caused by Tsc2 mutation in mice. *Proc Natl Acad Sci USA* 2001; **98**: 8762–7.

21. Kobayashi T, Urakami S, Hirayama Y, Yamamoto T, Nishizawa M, Takahara T, Kubo Y, Hino O. Intragenic *Tsc2* somatic mutations as Knudson's second hit in spontaneous and chemically induced renal carcinomas in the Eker rat model. *Jpn J Cancer Res* 1997; **88**: 254–61.
22. Hino O, Mitani H, Sakurai J. "Second hit" of Tsc2 gene in radiation induced renal tumors of Eker rat model. *Int Congr Ser* 2002; **1236**: 163–74.
23. Kobayashi T, Nishizawa M, Hirayama Y, Kobayashi E, Hino O. cDNA structure, alternative splicing and exon-intron organization of the predisposing tuberous sclerosis (*Tsc2*) gene of the Eker rat model. *Nucleic Acids Res* 1995; **23**: 2608–13.
24. Kobayashi T, Urakami S, Cheadle JP, Aspinwall R, Harris P, Sampson JR, Hino O. Identification of a leader exon and a core promoter for the rat tuberous sclerosis 2 (Tsc2) gene and structural comparison with the human homologue. *Mamm Genome* 1997; **8**: 554–8.
25. Orimoto K, Tsuchiya H, Kobayashi T, Matsuda T, Hino O. Suppression of the neoplastic phenotype by replacement of the Tsc2 gene in Eker rat renal carcinoma cells. *Biochem Biophys Res Commun* 1996; **219**: 70–5.
26. Jin F, Wienecke R, Xiao GH, Maize JC Jr, DeClue JE, Yeung RS. Suppression of tumorigenicity by the wild-type tuberous sclerosis 2 (*Tsc2*) gene and its C-terminal region. *Proc Natl Acad Sci USA* 1996; **93**: 9154–9.
27. van Slegtenhorst M, Nellist M, Nagelkerken B, Cheadle J, Snell R, van der Ouweland A, Reuser A, Sampson J, Halley D, van der Sluijs P. Interaction between hamartin and tuberin, the *TSC1* and *TSC2* products. *Hum Mol Genet* 1998; **7**: 1053–7.
28. Benvenuto G, Li S, Brown SJ, Braverman R, Vass WC, Cheadle JP, Halley DJJ, Sampson JR, Wienecke R, DeClue JE. The tuberous sclerosis-1 (*TSC1*) gene product hamartin suppresses cell growth and augments the expression of the *TSC2* gene product tuberin by inhibiting its ubiquitination. *Oncogene* 2000; **19**: 6306–16.
29. Momose S, Kobayashi T, Mitani H, Hirabayashi M, Ito K, Ueda M, Nabeshima Y, Hino O. Identification of the coding sequences responsible for Tsc2-mediated tumor suppression using a transgenic rat system. *Hum Mol Genet* 2002; **11**: 2997–3006.
30. Nellist M, Verhaaf B, Goedbloed MA, Reuser AJJ, van der Ouweland AMW, Halley DJJ. *TSC2* missense mutations inhibit tuberin hosphorylation and prevent formation of the tuberin-hamartin complex. *Hum Mol Genet* 2001; **10**: 2889–98.
31. Gao X, Pan D. *TSC1* and *TSC2* tumor suppressors antagonize insulin signaling in cell growth. *Genes Dev* 2001; **15**: 1383–92.
32. Ito N, Rubin GM. *gigas*, a *Drosophila* homolog of tuberous sclerosis gene product-2, regulates the cell cycle. *Cell* 1999; **96**: 529–39.
33. Stocker H, Hafen E. Genetic control of cell size. *Curr Opin Genet Dev* 2000; **10**: 529–35.
34. Fukuda T, Mitani H, Tsutsumi M, Konishi Y, Hino O. Specific induction of hepatocellular adenomas by transplacental administration of ENU in the Tsc2 gene mutant (Eker) rat. *Int J Oncol* 1998; **13**: 957–61.
35. Gao X, Zhang Y, Arrazola P, Hino O, Kobayashi T, Yeung RS, Ru B, Pan D. Tsc tumor suppressor proteins antagonize amino-acid-TOR signalling. *Nat Cell Biol* 2002; **4**:

699–704.

36. Scheid MP, Woodgett JR. PKB/AKT: functional insights from genetic models. *Nat Rev Mol Cell Biol* 2001; **2**: 760–8.
37. Nellist M, Goedbloed MA, de Winter C, Verhaaf B, Jankie A, Reuser AJJ, van den Ouweland AMW, van der Sluijs P, Halley DJJ. Identification and characterization of the interaction between tuberin and 14-3-3 z. *J Biol Chem* 2002; **277**: 39417–24.
38. Tsuchiya H, Orimoto K, Kobayashi T, Hino O. Presence of potent transcriptional activation domains in the predisposing tuberous sclerosis (*Tsc2*) gene product of the Eker rat model. *Cancer Res* 1996; **56**: 429–33.
39. Kubo Y, Klimek F, Kikuchi Y, Bannasch P, Hino O. Early detection of Knudson's two-hits in preneoplastic renal cells of the Eker rat model by the laser microdissection procedure. *Cancer Res* 1995; **55**: 989–90.
40. Hino O, Majima S, Kobayashi T, Honda S, Momose S, Kikuchi Y, Mitani H. Multistep renal carcinogenesis as gene expression disease in tumor suppressor *TSC2* gene mutant model—genotype, phenotype and environment. *Mutat Res* 2001; **477**: 155–64.
41. Tsuchiya H, Tsuchiya Y, Kobayashi T, Kikuchi Y, Hino O. Isolation of genes differentially expressed between the Yoshida sarcoma and Long-survival Yoshida sarcoma variants: origin of Yoshida sarcoma revisited. *Jpn J Cancer Res* 1994; **85**: 1099–104.
42. Hino O, Kobayashi E, Nishizawa M, Kubo Y, Kobayashi T, Hirayama Y, Takai S, Kikuchi Y, Tsuchiya H, Orimoto K, Kajino K, Takahara T, Mitani H. Renal carcinogenesis in the Eker rat. *J Cancer Res Clin Oncol* 1995; **121**: 602–5.
43. Urakami S, Tsuchiya H, Orimoto K, Kobayashi T, Igawa M, Hino O. Overexpression of members of the AP-1 transcriptional factor family from an early stage of renal carcinogenesis and inhibition of cell growth by AP-1 gene antisense oligonucleotides in the Tsc2 gene mutant (Eker) rat model. *Biochem Biophys Res Commun* 1997; **241**: 24–30.
44. Yamashita Y, Yokoyama M, Kobayashi E, Takai S, Hino O. Mapping and determination of the cDNA sequence of the Erc gene preferentially expressed in renal cell carcinoma in the *Tsc2* gene mutant (Eker) rat model. *Biochem Biophys Res Commun* 2000; **75**: 134–40.
45. Majima S, Kajino K, Fukuda T, Otsuka F, Hino O. A novel gene "Niban" upregulated in renal carcinogenesis: cloning by the cDNA-amplified fragment length polymorphism approach. *Jpn J Cancer Res* 2000; **91**: 869–74.
46. Adachi H, Majima S, Kon S, Kobayashi T, Kajino K, Mitani H, Shiina H, Igawa M, Hino O. The Niban gene is commonly expressed in renal tumors: a new candidate marker for renal carcinogenesis. *Oncogene* 2004; **23**: 3495–500.
47. Hino O, Kobayashi E, Hirayama Y, Kobayashi T, Kubo Y, Tsuchiya H, Kikuchi Y, Mitani H. Molecular genetic basis of renal carcinogenesis in the Eker rat model of tuberous sclerosis (Tsc2). *Mol Carcinog* 1995; **14**: 23–27.
48. Fukuda T, Hirayama Y, Mitani H, Maeda H, Tsutsumi M, Konishi Y, Hino O. Generation of metastatic variants of Eker renal carcinoma cell lines for experimental investigation of renal cancer metastasis. *Jpn J Cancer Res* 1998; **89**: 1104–8.
49. Urakami S, Tokuzen R, Tsuda H, Igawa M, Hino O. Somatic mutation of the tuberous sclerosis (Tsc2) tumor suppressor gene in chemically induced rat renal carcinoma cell. *J Urol* 1997; **158**: 275–8.

50. Satake N, Urakami S, Hirayama Y, Izumi K, Hino O. Biallelic mutations of the *Tsc2* gene in chemically induced rat renal carcinoma. *Int J Cancer* 1998; **77**: 895–900.
51. Satake N, Kobayashi T, Kobayashi E, Izumi K, Hino O. Isolation and characterization of a rat homologue of the human tuberous sclerosis 1 gene (Tsc1) and analysis of its mutations in rat. *Cancer Res* 1999; **59**: 849–55.
52. Kajino K, Yakurai J, Hirayama Y, Takahara T, Fukui I, Ishikawa Y, Hino O. LOH of tumor suppressor TSC2 gene locus in human renal cell carcinomas and lung carcinomas. *Proc Jpn Cancer Assoc* 1997: 279.
53. Kikuchi Y, Sudo A, Mitani H, Hino O. Presence of a modifier gene(s) affecting early renal carcinogenesis in the Tsc2 mutant (Eker) rat model. *Int J Oncol* 2004; **24**: 75–80.
54. Miki S, Miki Y, Mitani H, Sato B, Yamamoto M, Hino O. Hyperlipidemia enhancement of renal preneoplasia but not tumor formation is due to elevated apoptosis in the Eker rat. *Cancer Res* 1997; **57**: 4673–6.
55. Hino O, Kobayashi T, Mitani H. Prevention of hereditary carcinogenesis. *Proc Japan Acad* 2002; **78B**: 31–3.
56. Toyonaga T, Hino O, Sugai S, Wakasugi S, Abe K, Shichiri M, Yamamura K. Chronic active hepatitis in transgenic mice expressing interferon-γ in the liver. *Proc Natl Acad Sci USA* 1994; **91**: 614–8.
57. Okamoto T, Furuya M, Yamakawa T, Yamamura K, Hino O. TNF-alpha gene expression in the liver of the IFN-gamma transgenic mouse with chronic active hepatitis. *Biochem Biophys Res Commun* 1996; **226**: 762–8.
58. Akbar SMF, Kajino K, Tanimoto K, Yamamura K, Onji M, Hino O. Unique features of dendritic cells in IFN-γ transgenic mice: relevance to cancer development and therapeutic implications. *Biochem Biophys Res Commun* 1999; **259**: 294–9.
59. Kobayashi T, Adachi H, Mitani H, Hirayama Y, Hino O. Toward chemotherapy for Tsc2-mutant renal tumor. *Proc Japan Acad* 2003; **79B**: 22–5.
60. Okimoto K, Kouchi M, Kikawa E, Toyosawa K, Koujitani T, Tanaka K, Matsuoka N, Sakurai J, Hino O. A novel "Nihon" rat model of a Mendelian dominantly inherited renal cell carcinoma. *Jpn J Cancer Res* 2000; **91**: 1096–9.
61. Hino O, Okimoto K, Kouchi M, Sakurai J. A novel renal carcinoma predisposing gene of the Nihon rat maps on chromosome 10. *Jpn J Cancer Res* 2001; **92**: 1147–9.
62. Okimoto K, Sakurai J, Kobayashi T, Mitani H, Hirayama Y, Nickerson ML, Warren MB, Zbar B, Schmidt LS, Hino O. A germ-line insersion in the Birt-Hogg-Dubé (BHD) gene gives rise to the Nihon rat model of inherited renal cancer. *Proc Natl Acad Sci USA* 2004; **101**: 2023–7.

HETEROCYCLIC AMINES: MUTAGENS/CARCINOGENS PRODUCED DURING COOKING OF MEAT AND FISH

Takashi SUGIMURA, Keiji WAKABAYASHI, Hitoshi NAKAGAMA and Minako NAGAO

*National Cancer Center**

Research leading to the discovery of a series of mutagenic and carcinogenic heterocyclic amines (HCAs) was inspired by the idea that smoke produced during cooking of food, especially meat or fish, might be carcinogenic. More than ten kinds of HCAs, actually produced by cooking or heating of meat or fish, have now been isolated and their structures determined, most being previously unregistered compounds. They are highly mutagenic towards *Salmonella typhimurium* in the presence of S9 mix and are also mutagenic *in vitro* and *in vivo* toward mammalian cells. HCAs have now been chemically synthesized in quantity and subjected to long-term animal testing. When HCAs were fed in the diet, rodents developed cancers in many organs, including the colon, breast and prostate, and one HCA produced hepatomas in monkeys. The lesions exhibited alteration in genes including *Apc*, *β-catenin* and Ha-*ras*, and these changes provide clues to the induction mechanisms. The HCAs are oxidized to hydroxyamino derivatives by cytochrome P450s, and further converted to ester forms by acetyltransferase and sulfotransferase. Eventually, they produce DNA adducts through the formation of N-C bonds at guanine bases. There are HCA-sensitive and resistant strains of rodents and a search for the responsible genes is now under way. While the content of HCAs in dishes consumed in ordinary life is low and not sufficient in itself to explain human cancer, the coexistence of many other mutagens/carcinogens of either autobiotic or xenobiotic type and the possibility that HCAs induce genomic instability and heightened sensitivity to tumor promoters suggest that avoidance of exposure to HCAs or reduction of HCAs' biological effects as far as possible are to be highly recommended. Usage of microwave ovens for cooking and supplementation of the diet, for example with soy-isoflavones, which have been found to suppress the occurrence of HCA-induced breast cancers, should be encouraged. Advice to the general public about how to reduce the carcinogenic load imposed by HCAs would be an important contribution to cancer prevention.

Importance of Analysis of Causative Factors for Human Carcinogenesis

Much is now known concerning the mechanisms of carcinogenesis, and genetic

* 5-1-1 Tsukiji, Chuo-ku, Tokyo 104-0045, Japan

This paper is dedicated to the memory of late Dr. Tomizo Yoshida on the occasion of the 100th anniversary of his birth. It was originally published in Cancer Science in April, 2004.

alterations and epigenetic changes of crucial genes related to cancer phenotypes have been well elucidated. Knowledge on qualitative and quantitative changes of gene products during carcinogenesis has also been accumulated, and the dissection and integration of information on changes in signal transduction pathways should eventually reveal the details of the molecular mechanisms underlying malignant cancer phenotypes, namely escape from cell cycle regulation, cellular and structural atypia, and cellular behaviors such as infiltration and metastasis. Scientific research has focused on DNA modification and its repair processes relevant to genetic alterations, and much progress has been made over the past decades. For prevention of cancer, however, further information and analysis of causative factors of both genetic and epigenetic changes are required.

Early Ideas on Cancer Causation

Soon after the discovery of radium, it was noted by Furth and Lorenz that ionizing radiation was a carcinogenic hazard (*1*). Prior to this, Sir Percival Pott had described chimney sweeps in London developing scrotal skin tumors (*2*), and urinary bladder cancers in workers in the aniline dye industry were reported in 1895 (*3*), pointing to environmental influences. Lung cancers frequently occur among miners (*4*) and liver tumors with special histological features, hemangioendothelial sarcomas, develop in workers occupationally exposed to vinyl chloride monomer (*5*), removing any doubt that human cancers can be caused by heavy exposure to environmental xenobiotic carcinogens, mostly related to occupational or iatrogenic events or industrial accidents. Currently, autobiotic oxidative carcinogens are attracting much attention.

Meanwhile, scientists working on the genetic background of cancer development have provided us with important evidence about the roles of specific genes from studies of hereditary cancers, such as childhood retinoblastoma (*Rb*) (*6*), adenomatous polyposis associated malignancies of the colon (*APC*) (*7*), familial breast cancers (*BRCA-1* and *-2*) (*8*, *9*) and familial gastric cancers (*E-cadherin*) (*10*). However, heavy exposure to environmental xenobiotic carcinogens and clearly definable genetic alterations can explain only a relatively small proportion of the total cancer burden.

Most neoplasms occurring in the general population, our relatives and friends, are due to both environmental factors and genetic influences. Exposure to individual xenobiotics may be minute, so that the impact of one agent may be small, but the presence of many kinds of environmental factors that can act in concert must be considered. Among the common cancers, the contribution and penetrance of single genetic factors may similarly be low, but multiple genetic factors can interact to play major roles. Of particular interest, studies using identical twins have provided very reasonable guesses as to the relative contributions of environmental and genetic factors. For instance, Lichtenstein *et al.* indicated that genetic factors account for 42%, 35% and 27% of the risk for prostate, colon and breast cancers, respectively (*11*). The remaining contributions come from the environment.

It is generally believed that about one-fourth to one-third of all cancers are produced by smoking, dietary factors and inflammation/infection (*12*, *13*). Dietary factors for carcinogenesis include two categories, namely cancer-producing and cancer-preventing agents. Since most occupational human and experimental carcinogens have been found to show mutagenic activity toward prokaryotes (*14–17*), it is rational to expect mutagens in the diet to be carcinogenic. As proven mutagenic substances in the diet, we can point to mycotoxins, including aflatoxin B_1, which is carcinogenic to humans, rodents and fish (*18*). However, the presence of aflatoxin B_1 up to certain levels in foodstuffs such as peanut butter is accepted in many developed nations, since it is almost impossible to completely eliminate it (*19*). Various plant alkaloids are also illustrative. For example, cycasin, a β-D-glucoside of methylazoxymethanol, exerts carcinogenic activity in the intestines of rodents and is neurotoxic in man (*20*). Bracken fern containing mutagenic ptaquiloside/aquilide A induces tumors in rodents, and also causes urinary bladder-bleeding in cows (*21*, *22*). Bracken fern is nevertheless accepted as an edible plant by most Asian nations.

Based on the colorful history of environmental carcinogenesis, we initiated studies on genotoxic substances in food in 1970 and by coincidence, AF-2 [2-(2-furyl)-3-(5-nitro-2-furyl)acrylamide], which had been used as a food preservative for several years in Japan, was revealed to be mutagenic toward *Escherichia coli* (*23–25*). Based on this, intensive tests were carried out on rodents, demonstrating positive carcinogenicity (*26*, *27*) and the use of AF-2 was banned by the Ministry of Health and Welfare, Japan in 1974.

A Serendipitous Scenario for the Discovery of Heterocyclic Amines (HCAs) in Cooked Meat

One of the authors (T.S.) was inspired by an experience on holiday that has now lead to a major new research area in environmental carcinogenesis. His wife was broiling fish in the kitchen, and the smoke caught his attention. If cigarette smoke contains many mutagens, why not also smoke produced by broiling fish? On the basis of this speculation, it was soon confirmed in the laboratory that smoke produced by broiling fish, collected on glass-fiber filters and dissolved in dimethyl sulfoxide, showed strong mutagenicity to *Salmonella typhimurium* TA98 (*28*, *29*). This was a memorable day, initiating three-decade worldwide investigations of mutagens derived from broiled proteinaceous foods. These data were first introduced in a milestone symposium entitled “The Origins of Human Cancer” held in Cold Spring Harbor in 1976, and the proceedings of the meeting were published in 1977 (*28*). Commoner *et al.* also reported in 1978 that cooking of meat results in the formation of mutagens (*30*).

From pyrolysates of amino acids and proteins, Trp-P-1, Trp-P-2, Glu-P-1, Glu-P-2, AαC and MeAαC were isolated and identified (*31–33*), some being also contained in cooked meat. In collaboration with us, Spingarn *et al.* succeeded in isolating mutagenic compounds from beef extract (*34*). We subsequently isolated large quantities of mutagens and identified IQ, MeIQ and MeIQx as mutagenic principles in cooked (broiled) meat and fish (*35–38*). PhIP was added by Felton *et al.* in the USA to this series of compounds (*39*), all belonging to the heterocyclic amine (HCA) class of chemicals. The structures, chemical names and common abbreviations for these newly identified mutagens are listed in Fig. 1 and Table I. HCAs are divided in two groups. On 2 m*M* nitrite treatment, Group I HCAs, such as Trp-P-1, Trp-P-2, Aαc, MeAαC, Glu-P-1 and Glu-P-2, lose their mutagenicity through conversion of amino to hydroxyl groups, while the amino group of Group II HCAs, such as IQ, MeIQ, MeIQx, DiMeIQx and 7,8-DiMeIQx, is not changed (*40*). For the formation of Group II HCAs, creatine or creatinine in muscles serves as a precursor of imidazo moieties, as reported by Jägerstad (*41*). The concentrations of Group II HCAs are generally much higher than those of Group I HCAs in cooked meat, as described below. Various ways to prevent formation of heterocyclic amines (HCAs) are available (*42*).

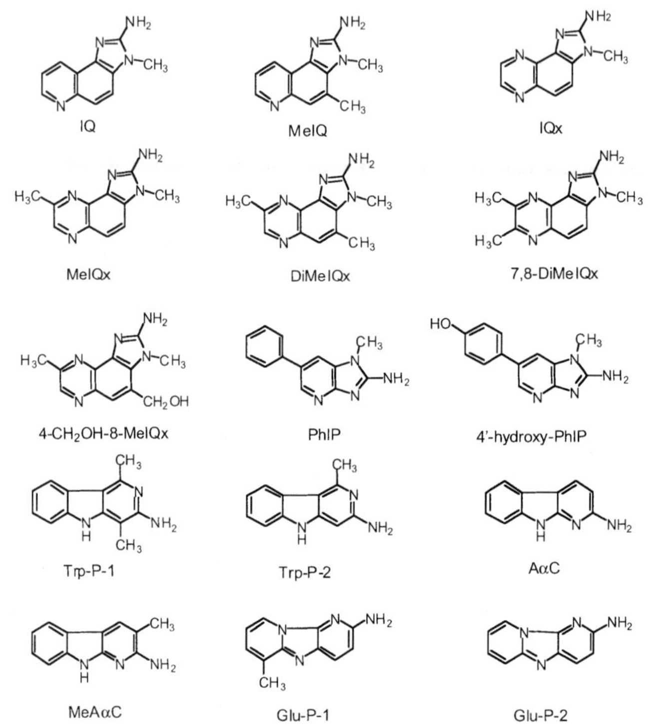

FIG. 1. Structures of HCAs.

TABLE I. Full names and common abbreviations of HCAs

Common abbreviation	Full name
IQ	2-amino-3-methylimidazo[4,5-*f*]quinoline
MeIQ	2-amino-3,4-dimethylimidazo[4,5-*f*]quinoline
IQx	2-amino-3-methylimidazo[4,5-*f*]quinoxaline
MeIQx	2-amino-3,8-dimethylimidazo[4,5-*f*]quinoxaline
DiMeIQx	2-amino-3,4,8-trimethylimidazo[4,5-*f*]quinoxaline
7,8-DiMeIQx	2-amino-3,7,8-trimethylimidazo[4,5-*f*]quinoxaline
4-CH_2OH-8-MeIQx	2-amino-4-hydroxymethyl-3,8-dimethylimidazo[4,5-*f*]quinoxaline
PhIP	2-amino-1-methyl-6-phenylimidazo[4,5-*b*]pyridine
4′-hydroxy-PhIP	2-amino-6-(4-hydroxyphenyl)-1-methylimidazo[4,5-*b*]pyridine
Trp-P-1	3-amino-1,4-dimethyl-5*H*-pyrido[4,3-*b*]indole
Trp-P-2	3-amino-1-methyl-5*H*-pyrido[4,3-*b*]indole
AαC	2-amino-9*H*-pyrido[2,3-*b*]indole
MeAαC	2-amino-3-methyl-9*H*-pyrido[2,3-*b*]indole
Glu-P-1	2-amino-6-methyldipyrido[1,2-*a*:3′,2′-*d*]imidazole
Glu-P-2	2-aminodipyrido[1,2-*a*:3′,2′-*d*]imidazole

Mutagenicity of HCAs

All HCAs listed in Table I and shown in Fig. 1 are mutagenic toward *Salmonella typhimurium*, with a range of mutagenic potential of the order of 10^3, as shown in Table II (*43*). *Salmonella typhimurium* TA98, detecting frameshift-type mutagens, shows more susceptibility to HCAs than TA100, which detects base-pair change-type mutagens. The specific mutagenicities of HCAs toward mammalian cell lines

TABLE II. Mutagenicity of HCAs in *S. typhimurium* TA98 and TA100 with S9 mix

HCA	Revertants/μg	
	TA98	TA100
MeIQ	661,000	30,000
IQ	433,000	7000
DiMeIQx	183,000	8000
7,8-DiMeIQx	163,000	9900
MeIQx	145,000	14,000
Trp-P-2	104,200	1800
4-CH_2OH-8-MeIQx	99,000	3000
IQx	75,400	1500
Glu-P-1	49,000	3200
Trp-P-1	39,000	1700
Glu-P-2	1900	1200
PhIP	1800	120
AαC	300	20
MeAαC	200	120
4′-hydroxy-PhIP	2	no data available

TABLE III. Mutational spectra of MeIQ and PhIP in mammalian cells *in vitro* and *in vivo* (*46–51*)

HCA		Target gene	Tissue	No. of total mutations detected/ analyzed	Characteristic mutation type[a] (%)	Characteristic mutation and its frequency[a] (%)
MeIQ	Rat	H-*ras*	Zymbal gland tumor	11/14	G:C to T:A, 10 (91)	G to T at 5′-GC-3′, 9 (82)
	Mouse	H-*ras*	Forestomach tumor	22/64	G:C to T:A, 22 (100)	G to T at 5′-GC-3′, 22 (100)
	Mouse	*lacI*	Colon mucosa	92/92	G:C to T:A, 50 (54)	G to T at 5′-GC-3′, 38 (41)
PhIP	Rat	*Apc*	Colon tumor	5/8	G:C deletion, 5 (100)	G deletion from 5′-GGGA-3′, 5 (100)
	Rat	*lacI*	Colon mucosa	227/227	G:C deletion, 82 (36)	G deletion from 5′-GGGA-3′, 23 (10)
	Rat	*lacI*	Mammary gland	149/149	G:C deletion, 31 (21)	G deletion from 5′-GGGA-3′, 9 (6)
	Mouse	*lacI*	Colon mucosa	115/115	G:C deletion, 30 (26)	G deletion from 5′-GGGA-3′, 8 (7)
	Mouse	*lacZ*	Colon mucosa	40/40	G:C deletion, 8 (20)	G deletion from 5′-GGGA-3′, 2 (5)
	Human fibroblast	*supF*		172/172	G:C deletion, 7 (4)	G deletion from 5′-GGGA-3′, 5 (3)
	Chinese hamster fibroblast	*Hprt*		40/40	G:C deletion, 5 (12.5)	G deletion from 5′-GGGA-3′, 4 (10)

[a] No. of the same type of mutations among total mutations detected.

using the *Hprt* gene or the *Ef-2* gene as a reporter were almost the same range among various HCAs as in *Salmonella typhimurium* (*44*, *45*). Mutation spectra *in vivo* have been reported for some HCAs, as shown in Table III (*46–51*), but these are not sufficiently specific to identify causative agents of mutations found in tissues.

Carcinogenicity of HCAs

Carcinogenicity studies of HCAs in mice and rats have mainly been carried out in Japan (Fig. 2). The sites of tumors observed in long-term standard animal tests are listed in Table IV with references. Matsukura, Ohgaki, Takayama, Ito, and Shirai are among the main contributors (*52–69*). It is noteworthy that some HCAs can produce tumors in the colon, mammary glands, and prostate, which are common sites of neoplasms in Western countries and for which rates are increasing in Japan with westernization of dietary habits. Macroscopic and histological features of some HCA-induced tumors are shown in Fig. 3 and Fig. 4. In addition to the lungs, liver, ear ducts, skin and clitoral gland are targets of HCAs. Moreover, Weisburger's group reported that intragastric intubation of IQ resulted in development of tumors in the mammary glands, liver and ear ducts of SD rats (*70*). Adamson *et al.* also demonstrated that hepatocellular carcinomas were induced in cynomolgus monkeys (*Macaca fascicularis*) after administration of IQ by gavage (*71*).

Metabolism of HCAs

HCAs are mainly metabolized first by cytochrome P450 (CYP) 1A2 in rodents as well as humans. Other P450 molecular species including CYP1A1, 1B1 and 3A4

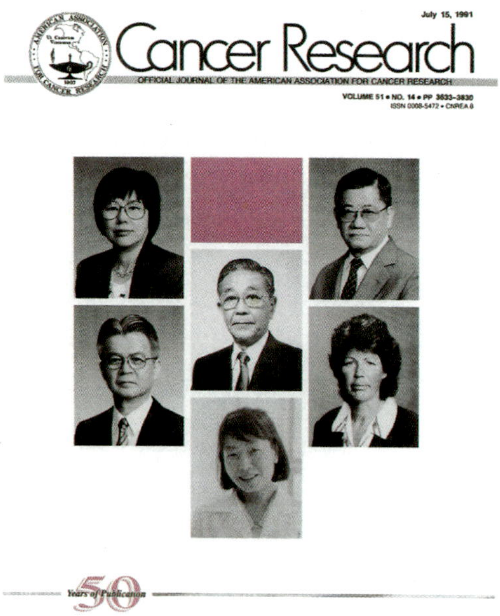

FIG. 2. Cover of Cancer Res, July 15, 1991, introducing the researchers working HCAs.

TABLE IV. Carcinogenicity of HCAs in rats and mice

HCA	Animal	Strain	Concentration in diet (ppm)	Experimental peroid (weeks)	Target organs	Reference
Trp-P-1	Rat	F344	150	52	Liver	59
	Mouse	CDF_1	200	89	Liver	52
Trp-P-2	Rat	F344	100	112	Liver, Urinary bladder	60
	Mouse	CDF_1	200	89	Liver	52
Glu-P-1	Rat	F344	500	64	Liver, Small and large intestine, Zymbal gland, Clitoral gland	61
	Mouse	CDF_1	500	57	Liver, Blood vessels	53
Glu-P-2	Rat	F344	500	104	Liver, Small and large intestine, Zymbal gland, Clitoral gland	61
	Mouse	CDF_1	500	84	Liver, Blood vessels	54
AαC	Rat	F344	800	104	No tumors	69
	Mouse	CDF_1	800	98	Liver, Blood vessels	53
MeAαC	Rat	F344	100	100	Liver	62
	Mouse	CDF_1	800	84	Liver, Blood vessels	53
IQ	Rat	F344	300	55–72	Liver, Small and large intestine, Zymbal gland, Clitoral gland, Skin	63
	Mouse	CDF_1	300	96	Liver, Forestomach, Lung	54
MeIQ	Rat	F344	300	40	Large intestine, Zymbal gland, Skin, Oral cavity, Mammary gland	64
	Mouse	CDF_1	400, 100	91	Liver, Forestomach	55
		C57BL/6	300		Liver, Large intestine	57
MeIQx	Rat	F344	400	61	Liver, Zymbal gland,Clitoral gland, Skin	65
	Mouse	CDF_1	600	84	Liver, Lung, Hematopoietic system	56
PhIP	Rat	F344	400	52	Large intestine, Mammary gland, Prostate, Lymphoid tissue	66, 67
	Mouse	CDF_1	400	82	Lymphoid tissue	58
		C57BL/6N	300	70–95	Small intestine, Lymphoid tissue	68

are also responsible, to some extent, for oxidation of the exocyclic primary amino group to a hydroxyamino group (*72–74*). Recombinant human CYP1A2 shows a much lower K_m for PhIP and a higher activity for MeIQx than rat CYP1A2, and has a low activity for detoxification by hydroxylation at the 4′ position of PhIP (*75*). The hydroxyamino group is further metabolized by *N(O)*-acetyltransferase (NAT), of which there are two isozymes, NAT1 and NAT2, in rats and humans. NAT1 is expressed mainly in extrahepatic tissues and NAT2 in the liver and intestinal epithelium (*76*). *N*-Hydroxyl metabolites of most HCAs, including PhIP, IQ and MeIQx, are poor substrates of human NAT1. However, human NAT2 catalyzes *O*-acetylation of *N*-hydroxyl derivatives of IQ, MeIQ, and PhIP (*77, 78*). There are at least two and ten polymorphic genotypes of human NAT1 and NAT2, respectively. The NAT2 fast acetylator trait (*NAT2*4* wild allele) has often, but not consistently, been associated with an increased risk of colorectal cancers (*79, 80*).

N-Acetoxy metabolites of HCAs are spontaneously converted to arylnitrenium ions (R-NH^+) and react with DNA to form adducts at the 8-position carbon of guanine bases. IQ and MeIQx also form adducts by binding to the N^2 position in guanine. Adduct structures clarified by Snyderwine and others (*81–83*) are illustrated in Fig. 5.

It would be interesting to examine the change in the cytochrome P450 molecu-

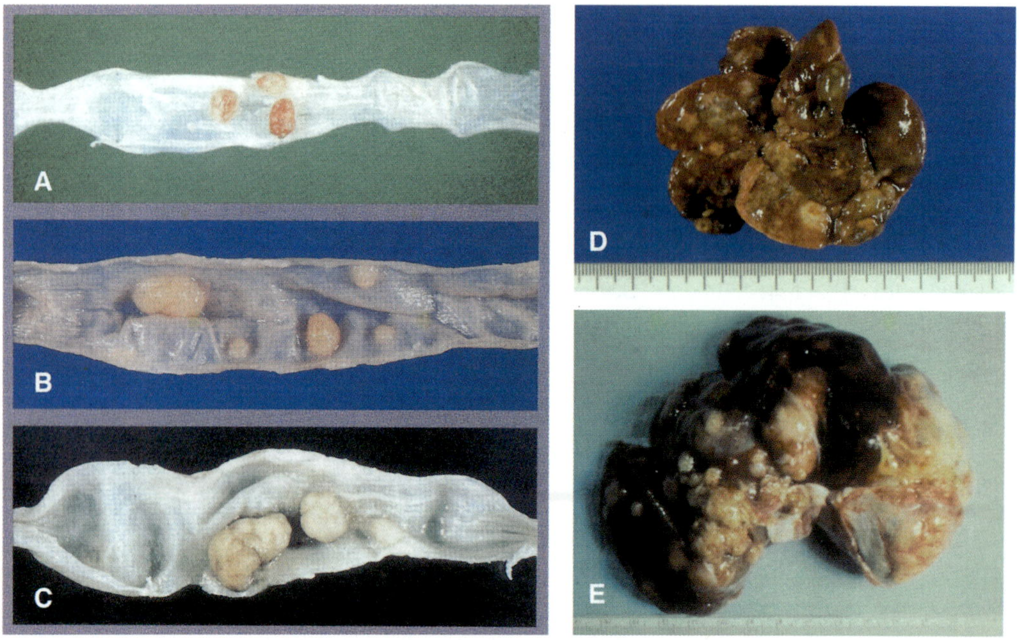

FIG. 3. Macroscopic features of HCA-induced cancers in experimental animals
A–C: Rat colon cancers induced by IQ. A: PhIP (B) and Glu-P-1. C: respectively. D and E: Liver cancers induced by MeIQx in rat (D) and by IQ in monkey.

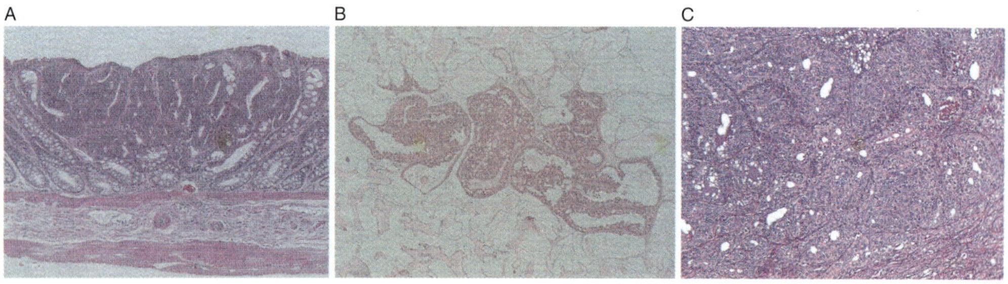

FIG. 4. Histological features of PhIP-induced colon, prostate and mammary gland cancers in rats
A: Colon cancer. B: prostate cancer. C: mammary cancer. The picture for prostate cancer was kindly provided by Dr. Tomoyuki Shirai, Nagoya City University Medical School.

lar species leading to more efficient activation in atrophic gastritis with intestinal metaplasia than in the normal stomach (*85*). It is apparent that intestinalized lesions of the stomach are produced by *Helicobacter pylori* infection, and gastric cancer often arises in areas with intestinalization.

Measurement of HCAs in Foods and HCA Adducts in DNA and Protein in the Human Body

Various convenient methods for quantification of HCAs are now being used worldwide. The simplest approach is to employ blue cotton absorption from crude homogenates and to subject the eluates to HPLC and LC/MS. However, several so-

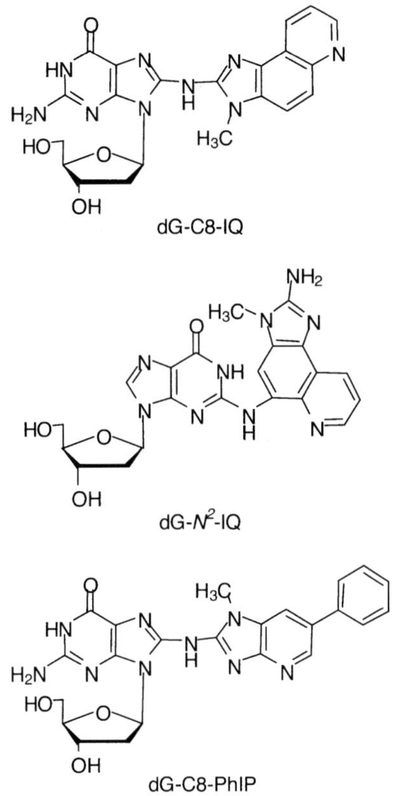

FIG. 5. Structures of major DNA adducts of IQ and PhIP
Major adducts of IQ were identified as *N*-(deoxyguanosin-8-yl)-IQ and 5-(deoxyguanosin-N^2-yl)-IQ (*81*, *83*), and of PhIP as *N*-(deoxyguanosin-8-yl)-PhIP (*82*). The *anti* form is preferred for the dG-N^2 adduct of IQ, while the *syn* form is preferred for dG-C8-IQ. In the case of PhIP, the major structure for the dG-C8-PhIP adduct is the *syn* form (*84*).

TABLE V. Amounts of HCAs in cooked foods

Food	Cooking method	HCA (ng/100 g)								Reference
		PhIP		MeIQx		4,8-DiMeIQx		7,8-DiMeIQx		
		Flesh	Skin	Flesh	Skin	Flesh	Skin	Flesh	Skin	
Salmon	Grilled	29	593	10	59	0	0	0	414	88
Salted fish	Grilled	37	700	8	59	0	9	0	446	88
Bacon	Fried	30–450		nd–2370		20–140		nd		42
Pork	Barbecued	420		40		10		nd		42
Chicken breast	Grilled	2700–4800		nd–900		nd–200		nd		42
London broiled steak		18,200		300		nd		nd		89

nd: not detected.

phisticated and sensitive methods are also available (*86*). One method currently being developed allows *N*-dimethylaminomethylene derivatives of HCAs to be analyzed by gas chromatography with nitrogen-phosphorus-selective detection (*87*). Table V summarizes data on HCA contents in various foods. MeIQx and PhIP have also been

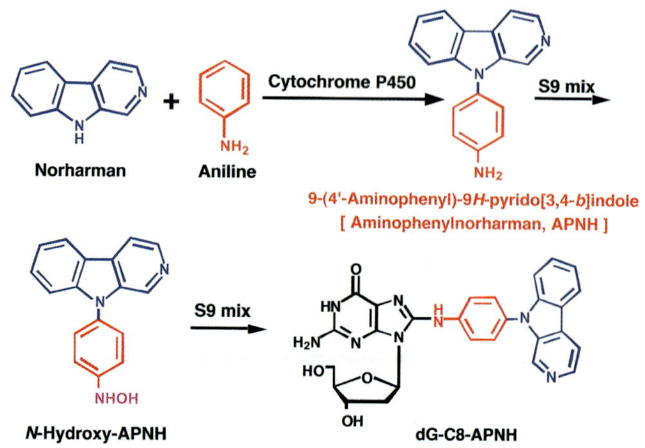

FIG. 6. Structures of aminophenylnorharman (APNH) and its DNA adduct, *N*-(Deoxyguanosin-8-yl)-APNH

The comutagens, norharman and aniline, are converted to APNH through the action of cytochrome P450, and APNH is further metabolized to a proximate form, *N*-hydroxy-APNH and then *N*-acetoxy-APNH (*99*). It is considered that the latter form is spontaneously degraded to the arylnitrenium ion, which reacts with DNA.

detected in commercial pet foods (*90*). The presence of HCAs, including MeIQx, PhIP, Trp-P-1 and Trp-P-2, in urine samples from healthy volunteers eating a normal diet, but not from in-patients receiving parenteral alimentation, has been reported (*91*) and PhIP has been detected in the milk of healthy women (*92*).

The presence of DNA adducts with HCAs in humans further points to appreciable exposure (*93*). DNA adduct levels in experimental animals after chronic administration of carcinogenic doses of HCAs reach plateau levels of around several adducts per 10^7 nucleotides (*67*, *94*). Surprisingly, similar levels of PhIP adducts were detected in mammary epithelial cells obtained from some human milk samples (*93*). HCAs also produce adducts with proteins (*95*, *96*) but most of them are not stable. Magagnotti *et al.* reported a good correlation between PhIP doses (0.1–10 mg/kg) and PhIP adduct levels (of the order of fmol/mg protein) in rat serum albumin and hemoglobin (*97*).

The Issue of Comutagenicity: Endogenous Formation of Heterocyclic Amines

During studies of purification of mutagens, including HCAs from tryptophan pyrolysate, a sudden loss of mutagenicity was observed in certain fractionation steps. Remixing of the fractions restored the original mutagenic activity. Further study demonstrated the occurrence of comutagenicity (*98*). Non-mutagenic aniline and non-mutagenic norharman (β-carboline) yield aminophenylnorharman in the presence of S9 mix of rat liver (*99*), a type of HCA which, when further activated by S9 mix to hydroxyaminophenylnorharman and finally converted to an acetoxy derivative, produces DNA adducts and induces mutations, as shown in Fig. 6 (*100*). In rodents, *in vivo* formation of aminophenylnorharman from aniline and norharman has been proven (*101*) and, as expected from the mutagenicity, carcinogenicity was observed in rats.

TABLE VI. TD_{50} of major HCAs in mice and rats

	TD_{50} (mg/kg/day)	
	Rats	Mice
PhIP	2.2	64.6
MeIQx	0.7	11
IQ	0.7	14.7
MeIQ	0.1	8.4
AαC	—	15.8
MeAαC	6.4	5.8

TABLE VII. Daily intake of HCAs

Study	Subject number		Amount		Reference
European Prospective Investigation into Cancer and Nutrition		344	Median	103 ng/day	104
Japanese Public Health Center	Man	18,290	Mean for men	66 ng/day	106
	Woman	20,745	Mean for women	58 ng/day	
USA, Case (colorectal cancer) control study in Arkansas	Case	155	Mean for cases	364 ng/day	105
	Control	380	Mean for controls	261 ng/day	

Comutagenicity can also be observed with aromatic amines other than aniline, such as *o*-toluidine and diphenylamine (*102*), and thus naturally occurring compounds or drugs and their metabolites might present a risk.

Risk of HCAs for Development of Human Cancer: Comparison of Human Dietary Intake with Carcinogenic Doses in Animals

Doses of individual HCAs that produce tumors in 50% of animals under standard experimental conditions are listed in Table VI (*103*). Reliable data on the concentrations of HCAs in cooked foods and the daily intake of HCAs by humans are given in Table VII (*104–106*). Comparison of the carcinogenic dose in rodents and the actual human daily intake suggests that the latter is definitely too low for cancer production to be explicable in terms of HCAs alone.

In animal experiments, however, simultaneous co-administration of different kinds of carcinogens can result in additive or synergistic effects (*107*). Moreover, the carcinogenic potency of HCAs is markedly enhanced in the presence of tumor promoters and agents that cause cell proliferation. When a limited amount of Trp-P-2 was painted on the skin of the back of mice, skin tumors only developed after subsequent painting of 12-*O*-tetradecanoylphorbol-13-acetate (TPA) (*108*). While it is still unlikely that the group of HCA compounds present in food account for a major proportion of cancers in human beings, considering their high metabolic activation capacity, and the finding of very high levels of PhIP-DNA adducts in epithelial cells from human milk, further extensive studies are needed before definitive conclusions can be drawn regarding the importance of HCAs in human carcinogenesis.

Carcinogenic potency could easily be modulated by other dietary factors, making risk estimation difficult. In addition, there are genotoxic substances other than HCAs that enter the human body through food intake and/or by alternative routes and cause mutations. *Apc* and *β-catenin* mutations are frequently observed in HCA-induced colon cancers, but, in contrast, *p53* and K-*ras* mutations are rarely observed (*51*, *109*, *110*). Squamous cell tumors induced by MeIQ and IQ (*109*) and mammary gland cancers induced by PhIP (*111*) are frequently associated with Ha-*ras* mutations. De-regulation of the cyclin D1/Cdk4 retinoblastoma pathway was recently reported to play a central role in PhIP mammary carcinogenesis (*112*). Mutations in genes related to repair of DNA damage would be expected to result in genomic instability, with more rapid accumulation of mutations in somatic cells. Of course, precancerous cells, in which numbers of mutations relevant to carcinogenesis have already been accumulated, would be more susceptible to transformation to cancer by further induction of mutations by HCAs. Genomic instability was observed in the rat mammary adenocarcinomas induced by PhIP (*113*, *114*).

Other mutagenic compounds include arylhydrocarbons, *N*-nitrosamines, plant alkaloids, mycotoxins, and nitroarenes, as well as oxidative agents (such as peroxides of fatty acids), metals and naturally occurring radioactive molecules such as radon and potassium.

Modulation of Carcinogenic Activity

Carcinogenic activity of HCAs can be enhanced or suppressed by various dietary factors. For example, a high-fat diet efficiently enhanced colon carcinogenesis when administered with a relatively small amount of PhIP to F344 male rats (*115*). Similarly, PhIP induced mammary tumors at a high incidence in female SD rats fed a high-fat diet (*116*). On the other hand, docosahexaenoic acid (DHA), a polyunsaturated ω3 fatty acid in fish oil, significantly reduced PhIP-induced aberrant crypt focus (ACF) formation in the colon of rats (*117*), possibly by decreasing levels of prostaglandin E_2. Conjugated linoleic acids (CLA), present in several foods, can also suppress IQ-induced ACF development in the rat colon (*118*). Epidemiologically, it has been demonstrated that frequent *miso* soup and isoflavone consumption is associated with a reduced risk of breast cancer (*119*). Consistent with these data, an isoflavone mixture (genistein:daidzein=4:1) clearly suppressed PhIP-induced rat mammary carcinogenesis (*120*). Moreover, it is reported that green tea catechins inhibit PhIP-induced mammary carcinogenesis and Glu-P-1-induced hepatocarcinogenesis in rats (*121*, *122*). Indole-3-carbinol, which is present in cruciferous vegetables, was shown to suppress ACF development in rats given PhIP or IQ (*123–125*), and its modification of the metabolic activation pathway of HCAs is probably associated with its beneficial effects. CYP1A2 plays a major role in metabolic activation of HCAs and administration of caffeine at 500 and 1000 ppm in drinking water for 2 weeks significantly increased levels of this enzyme. Concurrent administration of caffeine and PhIP resulted in a significant increase of ACF formation in the rat colon (*126*). In addition, lyophilized cultures of *Bifidobacterium longum* in yogurt have been found to inhibit colon, mammary and liver carcinogenesis by IQ (*127*).

Chlorophyllin is a stable and soluble derivative of chlorophyll, and this has been demonstrated to suppress IQ and PhIP-induced carcinogenesis in rats (*128*, *129*). Here, the mechanisms involve reduced absorption of HCAs from the intestine, probably due to interactions between these two types of planar molecules, and passage of unmetabolized HCAs in the feces.

Genetic Determinants for HCA-induced Carcinogenesis

As is now widely recognized, genetic backgrounds of individuals have a substantial impact on the development of cancers in response to exposure to various environmental carcinogens. The history of our research seeking genetic determinants of chemical-induced carcinogenesis started almost 20 years ago (*130*, *131*). Focusing on colon cancers, Demant's group in the Netherlands determined several quantitative trait loci (QTLs), including *Scc1* on mouse chromosome 2, using a DMH-induced model in mice (*132*), and *Scc1* was recently identified as *protein tyrosine phosphatase receptor type J (Ptprj)* (*133*). The secretory phospholipase A2 (*Pla2g2a*) gene has also been shown to serve as a modifier of the development of intestinal tumors in the *Apc*$^{Min/+}$ mice (*134*, *135*). Furthermore, we have observed differential susceptibility to the development of ACFs, precancerous lesions of the colon, and colon cancers due to PhIP among various rat strains (*136*). The Buffalo strain is highly sensitive to PhIP, while the Fischer 344, Brown-Norway and Wistar strains are moderately susceptible, and ACI is resistant. QTL analysis using 290 backcross progeny of (F344×ACI)F_1×ACI revealed the presence of a susceptibility locus on rat chromosome 16 (*137*). A long-term carcinogenesis experiment also demonstrated higher susceptibility of F344 rats as compared to the ACI strain. Resistant traits were also identified on several chromosomes and identification of candidate genes for these, which is currently on-going in our laboratory, should benefit us from a prophylactic point of view, namely for population-based cancer prevention of neoplasia induced by environmental HCAs.

Ways to Lessen the Intake of HCAs

Various easy and efficient ways to prevent the production of HCAs are available. Their generation mainly depends on an increase in temperature and heating time, and on dehydration of the meat (*138–140*). Therefore, prolonged cooking and broiling of meat, and direct exposure to a naked flame should be avoided. Flipping hamburgers every minute for 7 min results in less than one-tenth the level of HCA contained after flipping once with a cooking time of 8.9 min (*141*, *142*). Usage of microwave ovens can be recommended (*42*).

The formation of HCAs is inhibited by green tea extract, EGCG, β-carotene and γ-tocopherol (*143*, *144*), but this is not practical in the human situation. It is more realistic to avoid consuming charred parts produced on meat surfaces. For instance, charred black material on barbecued meat can be removed with a knife and the surface or skin of dried fish after broiling can be discarded by, for example, skilled use of chopsticks (*35*).

Proposals for Cancer Prevention Based on the Science of HCAs

Armitage and Doll had already emphasized in 1954 that cancers of the lungs, intestine and breasts are established by several events, from analyses of age-occurrence curves (*145*). In addition to the three main causes of human cancers, cigarette smoking, food components and inflammation/infection (*12*, *13*), air and water pollution, pesticides and insecticide residues, iatrogenic exposure to medicines, and food additives are claimed to make minor contributions. As food-related matters, over-eating and obesity may be particularly important factors for cancer causation. Avoidance of or quitting the smoking habit, appropriate diet intake in qualitative and quantitative terms, and establishment of hygienic conditions free from infections of *Helicobacter pylori*, hepatitis viruses and human papilloma viruses are effective cancer preventive measures. Cancer prevention should be the outcome of the integration of efforts to suppress multiple steps of carcinogenesis, involving multiple exposures to multiple carcinogenic factors, that are either environmental/xenobiotic or endogeneous/autobiotic. Thus, the holistic approach, namely life-style improvement seems important. This is the reason why we proposed twelve points for cancer prevention, and these recommendations were distributed in brochures all over Japan (*146*, *147*). In the case of HCAs, exposure levels are low, but they should still be reduced as far as possible, even though complete avoidance would be impossible.

IARC has rated many chemicals into the categories of human carcinogen, possible human carcinogen, and non-human carcinogen, based on information regarding chemical nature and pharmacobiology, as well as animal experimental and epidemiological data. IQ is in Group 2A "probably carcinogenic to humans" and MeIQ, MeIQx, PhIP are in Group 2B, "possibly carcinogenic to humans (*148*)." Accidents or other unusual occasions of exposure of humans to chemicals are sometimes important for evaluation, for instance, following factory explosions. Fortunately, there have been no industrial accidents associated with synthesis of HCAs so far, but if one occurred it would likely lead to their upgrading as human carcinogens. People tend to over-look the presence of HCAs in their daily routine lifestyle with the present ratings by the IARC. We would like to draw attention to this danger and the need for improvement. If we assume an intake of 10 μg of HCAs/day, life-time exposure could easily reach around 300 mg. Awareness of the fact that humans could be exposed to such a large dose during an ordinary life-span may indeed have a significant psychological impact, and contribute substantially to the realization that HCAs are important as environmental carcinogens.

Epidemiology and HCA Risk

Early epidemiological studies indicated a positive relation between stomach cancer and intake of broiled fish (*149*). More precise epidemiological studies have demonstrated a higher intake of HCAs among American people than Europeans or Japanese, as shown in Table VII, and a positive correlation between PhIP exposure and mammary cancer incidence was demonstrated among Americans. Correlations between MeIQx or DiMeIQx intake and colon cancer incidence were also demonstrated in studies conducted in the USA (*79*, *105*, *150*). Currently, red meat intake is being claimed to be one factor responsible for a high incidence of colon cancer (*151*). On the other hand, an European study found no relation among the type of cooking of meat, frequency of meat intake and cancer occurrence (*152*). Precise quantification of HCA intake is, however, difficult, although there has been remarkable progress in methodology. Further well-planned cohort studies are on-going in the United States and other countries, and should be assisted by establishment of surrogate markers such as HCA adducts in DNA and protein in tissue, body fluid and urine.

Concluding Comments

HCAs are readily produced by cooking meat in the kitchen and most people are exposed to appreciable, although very small, amounts of these unequivocal carcinogens (*153*). A comparable situation was noted a couple of years ago, in that acrylamide was produced by frying potatoes and flour and roasting coffee (*154*). Acrylamide induced chromosomal aberrations in mammalian cells *in vitro*, and tumors in rats in a long-term carcinogenicity test (*155*). Heavy exposure to acrylamide on the occasion of strengthening a tunnel structure occurred among workers in the south of Sweden (*156*) and this has prompted more exhaustive risk analyses of the effects of the compound and the hazard to man. To reduce the formation and intake of acrylamide to zero is impossible, just as in the case of HCAs. Common points are that they are both produced in daily life. Regulatory agencies cannot proscribe events going on in the home, and complete avoidance is clearly not possible. Therefore, it is essential to limit the formation and exposure in everyday life by increasing the public's awareness.

We would like to close this review by mentioning that organic solvent extracts of broiled horse meat induced tumors in mammary glands when repeatedly painted on the backs of mice, as reported by Widmark in Lund University, Sweden, in 1939 (*157*). This was communicated personally to one of the authors (T.S.) by Prof. B. Holmstedt of the Karolinska Institute, many years after HCAs had been isolated and their carcinogenicity demonstrated. Original scientific achievements and important information are sometimes hidden by a stream of trendy science.

REFERENCES

1. Furth J, Lorenz E. Carcinogenesis by ionizing radiations. In: Hollaender A, editor. Radiation Biology. vol 1. New York: McGraw-Hill; 1954. p. 1145.
2. Pott P. Chirurgical observations relative to the cataract, the polyps of the nose, the cancer of the scrotum, the different kinds of ruptures, and the mortification of the toes and feet. London: Hawes, Clarke and Collins; 1775.
3. Rehn L. Biasengeschwülste bei Fuchsin-Arbeitern. *Arch Klin Chir* 1895; **50**: 588–600.
4. Härting GH, Hesse W. Der Lungenkrebs, die Bergkrankheit in den Schneeberger Gruben. *Vrtijschr gerlichtl Med* 1879; **30**: 296–309 and **31**: 102–32.
5. Spirtas R, Kaminski R. Angiosarcoma of the liver in vinyl chloride/polyvinyl chloride workers. Update of the NIOSH Register. *J Occup Med* 1977; **20**: 427–9.
6. Friend SH, Bernards R, Rogeij S, Weinberg RA, Rapaport JM, Albert DM, Dryja TP. A human DNA segment with properties of the gene that predisposes to retinoblastoma and osteosarcoma. *Nature* 1986; **323**: 643–6.
7. Nishisho I, Nakamura Y, Miyoshi Y, Miki Y, Ando H, Horii A, Koyama K, Utsunomiya J, Baba S, Hedge P. Mutations of chromosome 5q21 genes in FAP and colorectal cancer patients. *Science* 1991; **253**: 665–9.
8. Miki Y, Swensen J, Shattuck-Eidens D, Futreal PA, Harshman K, Tavtigian S, Liu Q,

Cochran C, Bennett LM, Ding W *et al.* A strong candidate for the breast and ovarian cancer susceptibility gene BRCA1. *Science* 1994; **266**: 66–71.
9. Wooster R, Bignell G, Lancaster J, Swift S, Seal S, Mangion J, Collins N, Gregory S, Gumbs C, Micklem G. Identification of the breast cancer susceptibility gene BRCA2. *Nature* 1995; **378**: 762–3.
10. Guilford P, Hopkins J, Harraway J, McLeod M, McLeod N, Harawira P, Taite H, Scoular R, Miller A, Reeve AE. E-Cadherin germline mutations in familial gastric cancer. *Nature* 1998; **26**: 402–5.
11. Lichtenstein P, Holm NV, Verkasalo PK, Iliadou A, Kaprio J, Koskenvuo M, Pukkala E, Skytthe A, Hemminki K. Environmental and heritable factors in the causation of cancer—analyses of cohorts of twins from Sweden, Denmark, and Finland. *N Engl J Med* 2000; **343**: 78–85.
12. Doll R, Peto R. The causes of cancer: quantitative estimates of avoidable risks of cancer in the United States today. *J Natl Cancer Inst* 1981; **66**: 1191–308.
13. Parkin DM. Global cancer statistics in the year 2000. *Lancet Oncol* 2001; **2**: 533–43.
14. McCann J, Ames BN. Detection of carcinogens as mutagens in the *Salmonella/* microsome test: assay of 300 chemicals: discussion. *Proc Natl Acad Sci USA* 1976; **73**: 950–4.
15. Sugimura T, Sato S, Nagao M, Yahagi T, Matsushima T, Seino Y, Takeuchi M, Kawachi T. Overlapping of carcinogens and mutagens. In: Magee PN, Takayama S, Sugimura T, Matushima T, editors. Fundamentals in cancer prevention. Tokyo: Univ Tokyo Press/Baltimore: Univ Park Press; 1976. p. 191–215.
16. Nagao M, Sugimura T, Matsushima T. Environmental mutagens and carcinogens. *Annu Rev Genet* 1978; **12**: 117–59.
17. Zeiger E, Anderson B, Haworth S, Lawlor T, Mortelmans K. *Salmonella* mutagenicity tests. V. Results from the testing of 311 chemicals. *Environ Mol Mutagen* 1992; **19** Suppl 21: 2–141.
18. IARC monographs on the evaluation of carcinogenic risks to humans. Overall evaluations of carcinogenicity: An updating of IARC monographs volumes 1 to 42. IARC monographs supplement 7. Lyon: IARC; 1987. p. 83–7.
19. van Egmond HP, Dekker WH. Worldwide regulations for mycotoxins and phycotoxins in Rome, Italy. 1996 (May 27–31). The 9th IUPAC International Symposium on Mycotoxins and Phycotoxins.
20. Laqueur GL. Carcinogenic effects of cycad meal and cycasin, methyl-azoxymethanol glycoside, in rats and effects of cycasin in germ free rats. *Fed Proc* 1964; **23**: 1386–8.
21. Evans IA, Mason J. Carcinogenic activity of bracken. *Nature* 1965; **208**: 913–4.
22. van der Hoven JC, Aquilide A. A new mutagenic compound isolated from bracken fern (*Pteridium aquilinum* (L.) Kuhn). *Carcinogenesis* 1983; **4**: 1587–90.
23. Kondo S, Ichikawa-Ryo H. Testing and classification of mutagenicity of furylfuramide in *Escherichi coli*. *Jpn J Genet* 1973; **48**: 295–300.
24. Kada T. *Escherichia coli* mutagenicity of furylfuramide, *Jpn J Genet* 1973; **48**: 301–5.
25. Yahagi T, Matsushima T, Nagao M, Seino Y, Sugimura T, Bryan GT. Mutagenicity of nitrofuran derivatives on a bacterial tester strain with an R factor plasmid. *Mutat Res* 1976; **40**: 9–14.
26. Ikeda Y, Horiuchi S, Furuya T, Uchida O, Suzuki K, Azegami J. Induction of gastric

tumors in mice by feeding of furylfuramide. Food Sanitation Study Council 1974; Ministry of Health and Welfare, Japan.

27. Sano T, Kawachi T, Matsukura N, Sasajima K, Sugimura T. Carcinogenicity of food additive, AF-2, in hamsters and mice. *Z Krebsforsch* 1977; **89**: 61–8.
28. Sugimura T, Nagao M, Kawachi T, Honda M, Yahagi T, Seino Y, Sato S, Matsukura N, Matsushima T, Shirai A, Sawamura M, Matsumoto H. Mutagen-carcinogens in foods with special reference to highly mutagenic pyrolytic products in broiled foods. In: Hiatt HH, Watson JD, Winsten JA, editors. Origins of human cancer. New York: Cold Spring Harbor; 1977. p. 1561–77.
29. Nagao M, Honda M, Seino Y, Yahagi T, Sugimura T. Mutagenicities of smoke condensates and the charred surface of fish and meat. *Cancer Lett* 1977; **2**: 221–6.
30. Commoner B, Vithayathil AJ, Dolora P, Nair S, Madyastha P, Cuca GC. Formation of mutagens in beef and beef extract during cooking. *Science* 1978; **201**: 913–6.
31. Sugimura T, Kawachi T, Nagao M, Yahagi T, Seino Y, Okamoto T, Shudo K, Kosuge T, Wakabayashi K, Iitaka T, Itai A. Mutagenic principle(s) in tryptophan and phenylalanine pyrolysis products. *Proc Jpn Acad* 1977; **53**: 58–61.
32. Yamamoto T, Tsuji K, Kosuge T, Okamoto T, Shudo K, Takeda K, Iitaka K, Yamaguchi K, Seino Y, Yahagi T, Nagao M, Sugimura T. Isolation and structure determination of mutagenic substances in L-glutamic acid pyrolysate. *Proc Jpn Acad* 1978; **54B**: 248–50.
33. Yoshida D, Matsumoto T, Yoshimura R, Matsuzaki T. Mutagencity of amino-α-carboline in pyrolysis products of soybean globulin. *Biochem Biophys Res Commun* 1978; **83**: 915–20.
34. Spingarn NE, Kasai H, Vuolo LL, Nishimura S, Yamaizumi Z, Sugimura T, Matsushima T, Weisburger JH. Formation of mutagens in cooked foods. III. Isolation of potent mutagens from beef. *Cancer Lett* 1980; **9**: 177–83.
35. Wakabayashi K, Nagao M, Esumi H, Sugimura T. Food-derived mutagens and carcinogens. *Cancer Res* 1992; **52** Suppl: 2092s–8s.
36. Kasai H, Yamaizumi Z, Wakabayashi K, Nagao M, Sugimura T, Tokoyama S, Miyazawa T, Spingrn NE, Weisburger JH, Nishimura S. Potent novel mutagens produced by broiling fish under normal conditions. *Proc Jpn Acad* 1980; **56B**: 278–83.
37. Kasai H, Yamaizumi Z, Wakabayashi K, Nagao M, Sugimura T, Yokoyama S, Miyazawa T, Nishimura T. Structure and chemical synthesis of MeIQ, a potent mutagen isolated from broiled fish. *Chem Lett* 1980; 1391–4.
38. Kasai H, Yamaizumi Z, Shiomi T, Yokoyama S, Miyazawa T, Wakabayashi K, Nagao M, Sugimura T, Nishimura S. Structure of a potent mutagen isolated from fried beef. *Chem Lett* 1981; 485–8.
39. Felton JS, Knize MG, Shen NH, Lewis PR, Andresen BD, Happe J, Hatch FT. The isolation and identification of a new mutagen from fried ground beef: 2-amino-1-methyl-6-phenylimidazo[4,5-*b*]pyridine (PhIP) *Carcinogenesis* 1986; **7**: 1081–6.
40. Tsuda M, Negishi C, Makino R, Sato S, Yamaizumi Z, Hirayama T, SugimuraT. Use of nitrite and hypochlorite treatments in determination of the contributions of IQ-type and non-IQ-type heterocyclic amines to the mutagenicities in crude pyrolyzed materials, *Mutat Res* 1985; **147**: 335–41.
41. Jägerstad M, Lase Reutersward A, Olsson R, Grivas S, Nyhammar T, Olsson K,

Dahlqvist A. Creatin(in)e and Maillard reaction products as precursors of mutagenic compounds: effects of various amino acids. *Food Chem* 1983; **12**: 239–44.
42. Felton JS, Jägerstad M, Knize MG, Skog K, Wakabayashi K. Contents in foods, beverages and tobacco. In: Nagao M, Sugimura T, editors. Food borne carcinogens: Heterocyclic amines. Chichester: John Wiley & Sons Ltd; 2000. p. 31–71.
43. Nagao M. Mutagenicity. In: Nagao M, Sugimura T, editors. Food borne carcinogens: Heterocyclic amines. Chichester: John Wiley & Sons Ltd; 2000. p. 163–95.
44. Terada M, Nagao M, Nakayasu M, Sakamoto H, Nakasato F, Sugimura T. Mutagenic activities of herterocyclic amines in Chinese hamster lung cells in culture. *Environ Health Perspect* 1986; **67**: 117–9.
45. Thompson LH, Tucker JD, Stewart SA, Christense ML, Salazar EP, Carrano AV, Felton JS. Genotoxicity of compounds from cooked beef in repair-deficient CHO cells versus *Salmonella* mutagenicity. *Mutagenesis* 1987; **2**: 483–7.
46. Nagao M. A new approach to risk estimation of food-borne carcinogens-heterocyclic amines-based on molecular information. *Mutat Res* 1999; **431**: 3–12.
47. Okochi E, Watanabe N, Shimada Y, Takahashi S, Wakazono K, Shirai T, Sugimura T, Nagao M, Ushijima T. Preferential induction of guanine deletion at 5′-GGGA-3′ in rat mammary glands by 2-amino-1-methyl-6-phenylimidazo[4,5-*b*]pyridine. *Carcinogenesis* 1999; **20**: 1933–8.
48. Okonogi H, Ushijima T, Zhang XB, Heddle JA, Suzuki T, Sofuni T, Felton JS, Ticker JD, Sugimura T, Nagao M. Agreement of mutational characteristics of heterocyclic amines in lacI of the Big Blue® mouse with those in tumor related genes in rodents. *Carcinogenesis* 1997; **18**: 745–8.
49. Nagao M, Ushijma T, Toyota M, Inoue R, Sugimura T. Genetic changes induced by heterocyclic amines. *Mutat Res* 1997; **376**: 161–7.
50. Burnouf DY, Miturski R, Nagao M, Nakagama H, Nothisen M, Wagner J, Fuchs RPP. Early detection of 2-amino-1-methyl-6-phenylimidazo[4,5-b]pyridine (PhIP)-induced mutations within the *Apc* gene of rat colon. *Carcinogenesis* 2001; **22**: 329–35.
51. Nagao M. A new approach to risk estimation of food-borne carcinogens—heterocyclic amines—based on molecular information. *Mutat Res* 1999; **431**: 3–12.
52. Matsukura N, Kawachi T, Morino K, Ohgaki H, Sugimura T, Takayama S. Carcinogenicity in mice of mutagenic compounds from a tryptophan pyrolysate. *Science* 1981; **213**: 346–7.
53. Ohgaki H, Matsukura N, Morino K, Kawachi T, Sugimura T, Takayama S. Carcinogenicity in mice of mutagenic compounds from glutamic acid and soybean globulin pyrolysates. *Carcinogenesis* 1984; **5**: 815–9.
54. Ohgaki H, Kusama K, Matsukura N, Morino K, Hasegawa H, Sato S, Takayama S, Sugimura T. Carcinogenicity in mice of a mutagenic compound, 2-amino-3-methylimidazo[4,5-*f*]quinoline, from broiled sardine, cooked beef and beef extract. *Carcinogenesis* 1984; **5**: 921–4.
55. Ohgaki H, Hasegawa H, Suenaga M, Sato S, Takayama S, Sugimura T. Induction of hepatocellular carcinoma and highly metastatic squamous cell carcinomas in the forestomach of mice by feeding 2-amino-3,8-dimethylimidazo[4,5-*f*]quinoline. *Carcinogenesis* 1986; **7**: 1889–93.
56. Ohgaki H, Hasegawa H, Suenaga M, Sato S, Takayama S, Sugimura T.

Carcinogenicity in mice of a mutagenic compound, 2-amino-3,8-dimethylimidazo[4,5-*f*]quinoxaline (MeIQx) from cooked foods. *Carcinogenesis* 1987; **8**: 665–8.
57. Fujita H, Nagano K, Ochiai M, Ushijima T, Sugimura T, Nagao M, Matsushima T. Difference in target organs in carcinogenesis with a heterocyclic amine, 2-amino-3,4-dimethylimido[4,5-*f*]quinoline, in different strains of mice. *Jpn J Cancer Res* 1999; **90**: 1203–6.
58. Esumi H, Ohgaki H, Kohzen E, Takayama S, Sugimura T. Induction of lymphoma in CDF_1 mice by the food mutagen, 2-amino-1-methyl-6-phenylimidazo[4,5-*b*]pyridine. *Jpn J Cancer Res* 1989; **80**: 1176–8.
59. Takayama S, Nakatsuru Y, Ohagaki H, Sato S, Sugimura T. Carcinogenicity in rats of a mutagenic compound, 3-amino-1,4-dimethyl-5*H*-pyrido[4,3-*b*]indole from tryptophan pyrolsate. *Jpn J Cancer Res* 1985; **76**: 815–7.
60. Takahashi M, Toyoda K, Aze Y, Furuta K, Mitsumori K, Hayashi Y. The rat urinary bladder as a new target of heterocyclic amine carcinogenicity: tumor induction by 3-amino-1-methyl-5*H*-pyrido[4,3-*b*]indole acetate. *Jpn J cancer Res* 1993; **84**: 852–8.
61. Takayama S, Masuda M, Mogami M, Ohgaki H, Sato S, Sugimura T. Induction of cancers in the intestine, liver and various other organs of rats by feeding mutagens from glutamic acid pyrolysate. *Gann* 1984; **75**: 207–13.
62. Tamano S, Hasegawa R, Hagiwara A, Nagao M, Sugimura T, Ito N. Carcinogenicity of a mutagenic compound from food, 2-amino-3-methyl-9H-pyrido[2,3-*b*]indole (MeAαC), in male F344 rats. *Carcinogenesis* 1994; **15**: 2009–15.
63. Takayama S, Nakatsuru Y, Masuda M, Ohgaki H, Sato S, Sugimura T. Demonstration of carcinogenicity in F344 rats of 2-amino-3-methylimidazo[4,5-*f*]quinoline from broiled sardine, fried beef and beef extract. *Gann* 1984; **75**: 467–70.
64. Kato T, Migita H, Ohgaki H, Sato S, Takayama S, Sugimura T. Induction of tumors in the Zymbal gland, oral cavity, colon, skin and mammary gland of F344 rats by a mutagenic compound, 2-amino-3,4-dimethylimidazo[4,5-*f*]quinoline. *Carcinogenesis* 1989; **10**: 601–3.
65. Kato T, Ohgaki H, Hasegawa H, Sato S, Takayama S, Sugimura T. Carcinogenicity in rats of a mutagenic compound, 2-amino-3,8-dimethylimidazo[4,5-*f*]quinoxaline. *Carcinogenesis* 1988; **9**: 71–3.
66. Ito N, Hasegawa R, Sano M, Tamano S, Esumi H, Takayama S, Sugimura T. A new colon and mammary carcinogen in cooked food, 2-amino-1-methyl-6-phenylimidazo[4,5-*b*]pyridine (PhIP). *Carcinogenesis* 1991; **12**: 1503–6.
67. Shirai T, Sano M, Tamano S, Takahashi S, Hirose M, Futakuchi M, Hasegawa R, Imaida K, Matsumoto K, Wakabayashi K, Sugimura T, Ito N. The prostate: a target for carcinogenicity of 2-amino-1-methyl-6-phenylimidazo[4,5-*b*]pyridine (PhIP) derived from cooked foods. *Cancer Res* 1997; **57**: 195–8.
68. Ochiai M, Imai H, Sugimura T, Nagao M, Nakagama H. Induction of intestinal tumors and lymphomas in C57BL/6N mice by a food-borne carcinogen, 2-amino-1-methyl-6-phenylimidazo[4,5-*b*]pyridine. *Jpn J Cancer Res* 2002; **93**: 478–83.
69. Takayama S, Nakatsuru Y, Ohgaki H, Sato S, Sugimura T. Atrophy of salivary glands and pancreas of rats fed on diet with amino-methyl-α-carboline. *Proc Jpn Acad* 1985; **61** Ser B: 277–80.
70. Tanaka T, Barnes WS, Williams GM, Weisburger JH. Multipotential carcinogenicity

of the fried food mutagen 2-amino-3-methylimidazo[4,5-*f*]quinoline in rats. *Gann* 1985; **76**: 570–6.

71. Adamson RH, Thorgeirsson UP, Snyderwine EG, Thorgeirsson SS, Reeves J, Dalgard DW, Takayama S, Sugimura T. Carcinogenicity of 2-amino-3-methylimidazo[4,5-*f*]quinoline in nonhuman primates: induction of tumors in three macaques. *Jpn J Cancer Res* 1990; **81**: 10–4.
72. Yamazoe Y, Shimada M, Kamataki T, Kato R. Microsomal activation of 2-amino-3-methylimidazo[4,5-*f*]quinoline, a pyrolysate of sardine and beef extracts, to a mutagenic intermediate. *Cancer Res* 1983; **43**: 5768–74.
73. Shimada T, Guengerich FP. Activation of amino-α-carboline, 2-amino-1-methyl-6-phenyimidazo[4,5-*b*]pyridine, and a copper phthalocyanine cellulose extract of cigarette smoke condensate by cytochrome P-450 enzymes in rat and human liver microsomes. *Cancer Res* 1991; **56**: 2979–84.
74. Hammons GJ, Miton D, Stepps K, Guengerrich FP, Tukey RH, Kadlubar FF. Metabolism of carcinogenic heterocyclic and aromatic amines by recombinant human cytochrome P450 enzymes. *Carcinogenesis* 1997; **18**: 851–4.
75. Turesky R, Constable A, Fay LB, Guengerich FP. Interspecies differences in metabolism of heterocyclic amines by rat and human P450 1A2. *Cancer Lett* 1999; **143**: 109–12.
76. Hickman D, Pope J, Patil S, Fakis G, Smelt V, Stanley L, Payton M, Unadkat J, Sim E. Expression of arylamine *N*-acetyltransferase in human intestine. *Gut* 1998; **42**: 402–9.
77. Hein DW, Doll MA, Rustan TD, Gray K, Feng Y, Ferguson RJ, Grant DM. Metabolic activation and deactivation of arylamine carcinogens by recombinant human NAT1 and polymorphic NAT2 acetyltransferases. *Carcinogenesis* 1993; **14**: 1633–8.
78. Minchin RF, Reeves PT, Teitel CH, McManus ME, Mojarrabi B, Illett KF, Kadlubar FF. *N*- and *O*-acetylation of aromatic and HCA carcinogens by human monomorphic and polymorphic acetyltransferases expressed in COS-1 cells. *Biochem Biophys Res Commun* 1992; **185**: 839–44.
79. LeMarchand L, Hankin JH, Pierce LM, Sinha R, Nerurkar PV, Franke AA, Wilkens LR, Kolonel LN, Donlon T, Seifried A, Custer LJ, Lum-Jones A, Chang W. Well-done red meat, metabolic phenotypes and colorectal cancer in Hawaii. *Mutat Res* 2002; **506-507**: 205–214.
80. Ishibe N, Sinha R, Hein DW, Kulldorff M, Strickland P, Fretland AJ, Chow WH, Kadlubar FF, Lang NP, Rothman N. Genetic polymorphisms in heterocyclic amine metabolism and risk of colorectal adenomas. *Pharmacogenetics* 2002; **12**: 145–50.
81. Snyderwine EG, Roller PP, Adamson RH, Sato S, Thorgeirsson SS. Reaction of N-hydroxylamine and N-acetoxy derivatives of 2-amino-3-methylimidazo[4,5-*f*]quinoline with DNA. Synthesis and identification of *N*-(deoxyguanosin-8-yl)-IQ. *Carcinogenesis* 1988; **9**: 1061–5.
82. Nagaoka H, Wakabayashi K, Kim S-B, Kim I-S, Tanaka Y, Ochiai M, Tada A, Nukaya H, Sugimura T, Nagao M. Adduct formation at C-8 of guanine on *in vitro* reaction of the ultimate form of 2-amino-1-methyl-6-phenylimidazo[4,5-*b*]pyridine with 2′-deoxyguanosine and its phosphate esters. *Jpn J Cancer Res* 1992; **83**: 1025–9.
83. Turesky RJ, Rossi SC, Welti D, Lay JO Jr, Kadlubar FF. Characterization of DNA ad-

ducts formed *in vitro* by reaction of *N*-hydroxy-2-amino-3-methylimidazo[4,5-*f*]quinoline and *N*-hydroxy-2-amino-3,8-dimethylimidazo[4,5-*f*]quinoxaline at C-8 and N^2 atoms of guanine. *Chem Res Toxicol* 1992; **5**: 479–90.
84. Brown K, Hingerty BE, Guenther EA, Krishnan VV, Broyde S, Turteltaub KW, Cosman M. Solution structure of the 2-amino-1-methyl-6-phenylimidazo[4,5-*b*]pyridine C8-deoxyguanosine adduct in duplex DNA. *Proc Natl Acad Sci USA* 2001; **98**: 8507–12.
85. Tatemachi M, Nomura S, Ogura T, Sone H, Nagata H, Esumi H. Mutagenic activation of environmental carcinogens by microsomes of gastric mucosa with intestinal metaplasia. *Cancer Res* 1999; **15**: 3893–8.
86. Guy PA, Gremaud E, Richoz J, Turesky RJ. Quantitative analysis of mutagenic heterocyclic aromatic amines in cooked meat using liquid chromatography-atmospheric pressure chemical ionization tandem mass spectrometry. *J Chromatogr A* 2000; **883**: 89–102.
87. Kataoka H, Kajima KK. Analysis of heterocyclic amines as their *N*-dimethylaminomethylene derivatives by gas chromatography with nitrogen-phophorus selective detection. *J Chromatogr A* 1997; **767**: 187–94.
88. Kataoka H, Nishioka S, Kobayashi M, Hanaoka T, Tsugane S. Analysis of mutagenic heterocyclic amines in cooked food samples by gas chromatography with nitrogen-phosphorus detector. *Bull Environ Contam Toxicol* 2002; **69**: 682–9.
89. Felton JS, Knize MG, Salmon CP, Malfatti MA, Kulp KS. Human exposure to heterocyclic amine food mutagens/carcinogens: relevance to breast cancer. *Environ Mol Mutagen* 2002; **39**: 112–8.
90. Knize MG, Salmon CP, Felton JS. Mutagenic activity and heterocyclic amine carcinogens in commercial pet foods. *Mutat Res* 2003; **539**: 195–201.
91. Ushiyama H, Wakabayashi K, Hirose M, Ito H, Sugimura T, Nagao M. Presence of carcinogenic heterocyclic amines in urine of healthy volunteers eating normal diet, but not of inpatients receiving parenteral alimentation. *Carcinogenesis* 1991; **12**: 1417–22.
92. DeBruin LS, Martos PA, Josephy PD. Detection of PhIP (2-amino-1-methyl-6-phenylimidazo[4,5-*b*]pyridine) in the milk of healthy women. *Chem Res Toxicol* 2001; **14**: 1523–8.
93. Gorlewska-Roberts K, Green B, Fares M, Ambrosone CB, Kadlbar FF. Carcinogen-DNA adducts in human breast epithelial cells. *Environ Mol Mutagen* 2002; **39**: 184–92.
94. Takayama K, Yamashita K, Wakabayashi K, Sugimura T, Nagao M. DNA modification by 2-amino-1-methyl-6-phenylimidazo[4,5-*b*]pyridine in rats. *Jpn J Cancer Res* 1989; **80**: 1145–8.
95. Skipper PL, Tannenbaum SR. Protein adducts in the molecular dosimetry of chemical carcinogens. *Carcinogenesis* 1990; **11**: 507–18.
96. Umemoto A, Monden Y, Tsuda M, Grivas S, Sugimura T. Oxidation of the 2-hydroxyamino derivative of 2-amino-6-methyldipyrido[1,2-*a*:3′,2′-*d*]imidazole (Glu-P-1) to its 2-nitroso form, an ultimate form reacting with hemoglobin thiol groups. *Biochem Biophys Res Commun* 1988; **151**: 1326–31.
97. Magagnotti C, Orsi F, Bagnati R, Celli N, Rotilio D, Fanelli R, Airoldi L. Effect of diet on serum albumin and hemoglobin adducts of 2-amino-1-methyl-6-phenylimi-

dazo[4,5-*b*]pyridine (PhIP) in humans. *Int J Cancer* 2000; **88**: 1–6.
98. Nagao M, Yahagi T, Honda M, Seino Y, Matsushima T, Sugimura T. Demonstration of mutagenicity of aniline and *o*-toluidine by norharman. *Proc Jpn Acad* 1977: **53**: 34–7.
99. Totsuka Y, Hada N, Matsumoto K, Kawahara N, Murakami Y, Yokoyama Y, Sugimura T, Wakabayashi K. Structure determination of a mutagenic aminophenylnorharman produced by the co-mutagen norharman with aniline. *Carcinogenesis* 1998; **19**: 1995–2000.
100. Totsuka Y, Kataoka H, Takamura-Enya T, Kawahara N, Nishigaki R, Sugimura T. Wakabayashi K. Structure of DNA adduct formed with aminophenylnorharman, being responsible for the comutagenic action of norharman with aniline. *Chem Res Toxicol* 2002; **15**: 1288–94.
101. Totsuka Y, Kataoka H, Takamura-Enya T, Sugimura T, Wakabayashi K. *In vitro* and *in vivo* formation of aminophenylnorharman from norharman and aniline. *Mutat Res* 2002; **506-507**: 49–54.
102. Sugimura T. A new concept of co-mutagenicity from a phenomenon forgotten for the past two decades: is it more important than previously expected? *Environ Health Perspect* 1998; **106**: A522–3.
103. Sugimura T, Nagao M, Wakabayashi K. Complex factors pertinent to human hazard risk. In: Nagao M, Sugimura T, editors. Food borne carcinogens: Heterocyclic amines. Chichester: John Wiley & Sons Ltd; 2000. p. 349–59.
104. Rohrmann S, Becker N. Development of a short questionnaire to assess the dietary intake of heterocyclic aromatic amines. *Public Health Nutr* 2002; **5**: 699–705.
105. Nowell S, Coles B, Sinha R, Macleod S, Ratnasinghe DL, Stotts C, Kadlubar FF, Ambrosone CB, Lang NP. Analysis of total meat intake and exposure to individual heterocyclic amines in a case-control study of colorectal cancer: contribution of metabolic variation to risk. *Mutat Res* 2002; **506-507**: 175–85.
106. Kobayashi M, Hanaoka T, Nishioka S, Kataoka H, Tsugane S. Estimation of dietary HCA intakes in a large-scale population-based prospective study in Japan. *Mutat Res* 2002; **506-507**: 233–41.
107. Hasegawa R, Tanaka H, Tamano S, Shirai T, Nagao M, Sugimura T, Ito N. Synergistic enhancement of small and large intestinal carcinogenesis by combined treatment of rats with five heterocyclic amines in a medium-term multi-organ bioassay. *Carcinogenesis* 1994; **15**: 2567–73.
108. Takahashi M, Furukawa F, Miyakawa Y, Sato H, Hasegawa R, Hayashi Y. 3-Amino-1-methyl-5*H*-pyrido[4,3-*b*]indole initiates two-stage carcinogenesis in mouse skin but is not a complete carcinogen. *Jpn J Cancer Res* 1986; **77**: 509–13.
109. Nagao M, Ushijima T, Toyota M, Inoue R, Sugimura T. Genetic changes induced by heterocyclic amines. *Mutat Res* 1997; **376**: 161–7.
110. Dashwood RH, Suzui M, Nakagama H, Sugimura T, Nagao M. High frequency of *β-catenin* (*Ctnnb1*) mutations in the colon tumors induced by two heterocyclic amines in the F344 rat. *Cancer Res* 1998; **58**: 1127–9.
111. Yu M, Snyderwine EG. H-*ras* oncogene mutations during development of 2-amino-1-methyl-6-phenylimidazo[4,5-*b*]pyridine (PhIP)-induced rat mammary gland cancer. *Carcinogenesis* 2002; **23**: 2123–8.
112. Qiu C, Shan L, Yu M, Snyderwine EG. Deregulation of the cyclin D1/Cdk4 retino-

blastoma pathway in rat mammary gland carcinomas induced by the food-derived carcinogen 2-amino-1-methyl-6-phenylimidazo[4,5-*b*]pyridine. *Cancer Res* 2003; **63**: 5674–8.

113.Watanabe N, Okochi E, Hirayama Y, Shimada Y, Yanagihara K, Yoshida MC, Takahashi S, Mochizuki M, Sugimura T, Nagao M, Ushijima T. Single nucleotide instability without microsatellite instability in rat mammary carcinomas. *Cancer Res* 2001; **61**: 2632–40.

114.Okochi E, Watanabe N, Sugimura T, Ushijima T. Single nucleotide instability: a wide involvement in human and rat mammary carcinogenesis? Single nucleotide instability without microsatellite instability in rat mammary carcinomas. *Mutat Res* 2002; **506-507**: 101–11.

115.Ubagai T, Ochiai M, Kawamori T, Imai H, Sugimura T, Nagao M, Nakagama H. Efficient induction of rat large intestinal tumors with a new spectrum of mutations by intermittent administration of 2-amino-1-methyl-6-phenylimidazo[4,5-*b*]pyridine in combination with a high fat diet. *Carcinogenesis* 2002; **23**: 197–200.

116.Ghoshal A, Preisegger KH, Takayama S, Thorgeirsson SS, Snyderwine EG. Induction of mammary tumors in female Sprague-Dawley rats by the food-derived carcinogen 2-amino-1-methyl-6-phenylimidazo[4,5-*b*]pyridine and effect of dietary fat. *Carcinogenesis* 1994; **15**: 2429–33.

117.Takahashi M, Totsuka Y, Masuda M, Fukuda K, Oguri A, Yazawa K, Sugimura T, Wakabayashi K. Reduction in formation of 2-amino-1-methyl-6-phenylimidazo[4,5-*b*]pyridine (PhIP)-induced aberrant crypt foci in the rat colon by docosahexaenoic acid (DHA). *Carcinogenesis* 1997; **18**: 1937–41.

118.Liew C, Schut HAJ, Chin SF, Pariza MW, Dashwood RH. Protection of conjugated linoleic acids against 2-amino-3-methylimidazo[4,5-*f*]quinoline-induced colon carcinogenesis in the F344 rats: a study of inhibitory mechanisms. *Carcinogenesis* 1995; **16**: 3037–43.

119.Yamamoto S, Sobue T, Kobayashi M, Sasaki S, Tsugane S. Soy, isoflavones, and breast cancer risk in Japan. *J Natl Cancer Inst* 2003; **95**: 906–13.

120.Ohta T, Nakatsugi S, Watanabe K, Kawamori T, Ishikawa F, Morotomi M, Sugie S, Toda T, Sugimura T, Wakabayashi K. Inhibitory effects of *Bifidobacterium*-fermented soy milk on 2-amino-1-methyl-6-phenylimidazo[4,5-*b*]pyridine-induced rat mammary carcinogenesis, with a partial contribution of its component isoflavones. *Carcinogenesis* 2000; **21**: 937–41.

121.Hirose M, Hasegawa R, Kimura J, Akagi K, Yoshida Y, Tanaka H, Miki T, Satoh T, Wakabayashi K, Ito N, Shirai T. Inhibitory effects of 1-*O*-hexyl-2,3,5-trimethylhydroquinone (HTHQ), green tea catechins and other antioxidants on 2-amino-6-methyldipyrido[1,2-a;3′,2′-*d*]imidazole (Glu-P-1)-induced rat hepatocarcinogenesis and dose-dependent inhibition by HTHQ of lesion induction by Glu-P-1 or 2-amino-3,8-dimethylimidazo[4,5-*f*]quinoxaline (MeIQx). *Carcinogenesis* 1995; **16**: 3049–55.

122.Hirose M, Akagi K, Hasegawa R, Yaono M, Satoh T, Hara Y, Wakabayashi K, Ito N. Chemoprevention of 2-amino-1-methyl-6-phenylimidazo[4,5-*b*]pyridine (PhIP)-induced mammary gland carcinogenesis by antioxidants in F344 female rats. *Carcinogenesis* 1995; **16**: 217–21.

123.Guo D, Schut HAJ, Davis CD, Snyderwine EG, Bailey GS, Dashwood RH.

Protection by chlorophyllin and indole-3-carbinol against 2-amino-1-methyl-6-phenylimidazo[4,5-*b*]pyridine (PhIP)-induced DNA adducts and colonic aberrant crypts in the F344 rats. *Carcinogenesis* 1995; **16**: 2931–7.

124.Xu M, Bailey AC, Hernaez JF, Taoka CR, Schut HAJ, Dashwood RH. Protection by green tea, black tea, and indole-3-carbinol against 2-amino-3-methylimidazo[4,5-*f*]quinoline-induced DNA adducts and colonic aberrant crypts in the F344 rat. *Carcinogenesis* 1996; **17**: 1429–34.

125.Dashwood RH. Modulation of heterocyclic amine-induced mutagenicity and carcinogenicity: an 'A-to-Z' guide to chemopreventive agents, promoters, and transgenic models. *Mutat Res* 2002; **11**: 89–112.

126.Tsuda H, Sekine K, Uehara N, Takasuka N, Moore MA, Konno Y, Nakashita K, Degawa M. Heterocyclic amine mixture carcinogenesis and its enhancement by caffeine in F344 rats. *Cancer Lett* 1999; **143**: 229–34.

127.Reddy BS, Rivenson A. Inhibitory effect of *Bifidobacterium longum* on colon, mammary, and liver carcinogenesis induced by 2-amino-3-methylimidazo[4,5-*f*]quinoline, a food mutagen. *Cancer Res* 1993; **53**: 3914–8.

128.Guo D, Horio DT, Grove JS, Dashwood RH. Inhibition by chlorophyllin of 2-amino-3-methylimidazo[4,5-*f*]quinoline-induced tumorigenesis in the male F344 rat. *Cancer Lett* 1995; **95**: 161–5.

129.Hasegawa R, Hirose M, Kato T, Hagiwara A, Boonyaphiphat P, Nagao M, Ito N, Shirai T. Inhibitory effect of chlorophyllin on PhIP-induced mammary carcinogenesis in female F344 rats. *Carcinogenesis* 1995; **16**: 2243–6.

130.Ohgaki H, Kawachi T, Matsukura N, Morino K, Miyamoto M, Sugimura T. Genetic control of susceptibility of rats to gastric carcinoma. *Cancer Res* 1983; **43**: 3663–7.

131.Ushijima T, Yamamoto M, Suzui M, Kuramoto T, Yoshida Y, Nomoto T, Tatematsu M, Sugimura T, Nagao M. Chromosomal mapping of genes controlling development, histological grade, depth of invasion, and size of rat stomach carcinomas. *Cancer Res* 2000; **60**: 1092–6.

132.Demant P. Cancer susceptibility in the mouse: genetics, biology and implications for human cancer. *Nat Rev* 2003; **4**: 721–34.

133.Ruivenkamp CAL, van Wezel T, Zanon C, Stassen APM, Vlek C, Csikos T, Klous AM, Tripodis N, Perrakis A, Boerrigter L, Groot PC, Lindeman J, Mooi SK, Meijjer GA, Scholten G, Dauwerse H, Paces V, van Zandwijk N, van Ommen GJB, Demant P. *Ptprj is* a candidate for the mouse colon-cancer susceptibility locus *Scc1* and is frequently deleted in human cancers. *Nat Genet* 2002; **31**: 295–300.

134.Dietrich WF, Lander ES, Smith JS, Moser AR, Gould KA, Luongo C, Borenstein N, Dove W. Genetic identification of Mom-1, a major modifier locus affecting Min-induced intestinal neoplasia in the mouse. *Cell* 1993; **75**: 631–9.

135.MacPhee M, Chepenik KP, Liddell RA, Nelson KK, Siracusa LD, Buchberg AM. The secretory phospholipase A2 gene is a candidate for the Mom1 locus, a major modifier of ApcMin-induced intestinal neoplasia. *Cell* 1995; **81**: 957–66.

136.Ishiguro Y, Ochiai M, Sugimura T, Nagao M, Nakagama H. Strain differences of rats in the susceptibility to aberrant crypt foci formation by 2-amino-1-methyl-6-phenylimidazo[4,5-*b*]pyridine: no implication of *Apc* and *Pla2g2a* genetic polymorphisms in differential susceptibility. *Carcinogenesis* 1999; **20**: 1063–8.

137.Nakagama H, Souda K, Ochiai M, Ishiguro Y, Sugimura T, Nagao M. Genetic analysis of the susceptibility in rats to aberrant crypt foci formation by 2-amino-1-methyl-6-phenylimidazo[4,5-*b*]pyridine, PhIP. *Cancer Lett* 1999; **143**: 205–9.

138.Knize MG, Kulp KS, Salmon CP, Keating GA, Felton JS. Factors affecting human heterocyclic amine intake and the metabolism of PhIP. *Mutat Res* 2002; **506-507**, 153–62.

139.Persson E, Sjoholm I, Skog K. Effect of high water-holding capacity on the formation of heterocyclic amines in fried beefburgers. *J Agric Food Chem* 2003; **51**: 4472–7.

140.Underwood A, Springen K, Davis A. Cancer & diet. *Newsweek* 1998; **Nov 30**: 42–8.

141.Salmon CP, Kinze MG, Panteleakos FN, Wu RW, Nelson DO, Felton JS. Minimization of heterocyclic amines and thermal inactivation of *Escherichia coli* in fried ground beef. *J Natl Cancer Inst* 2000; **92**: 1773–8.

142.O'Neil. Hamburger safety may be partly in the flip. *The New York Times* 2000; **Dec 5**.

143.Johansson M, Jägerstad M. Influence of edible oils and fatty acids on the formation of heterocyclic amines in a model system. *Food Chem* 1996; **56**: 69–75.

144.Oguri A, Suda M, Totsuka Y, Sugimura T, Wakabayashi K. Inhibitory effects of antioxidants on formation of heterocyclic amines. *Mutat Res* 1998; **402**: 237–45.

145.Armitage P, Doll R. The age distribution of cancer and a multistage theory of carcinogenesis. *Br J Cancer* 1954; **8**: 1–12.

146.Sugimura T. Studies on environmental chemical carcinogenesis in Japan. *Science* 1986; **233**: 312–8.

147.Sugimura T, Nagao M, Wakabayashi K. How we should deal with unavoidable exposure of man to environmental mutagens: cooked food mutagen discovery, facts and lessons for cancer prevention. *Mutat Res* 2000; **447**: 15–25.

148.IARC. Some naturally occurring substances: food items and constituents, heterocyclic aromatic amines and mycotoxins. *IARC Monograph on the Evaluation of Carcinogenic Risks to Humans* 1992; **56**: 169–242.

149.Ikeda M, Yoshimoto K, Yoshimura T, Kono S, Kato H, Kuratsune M. A cohort study on the possible association between broiled fish intake and cancer. *Gann* 1983; **74**: 640–8.

150.Butler LM, Sinha R, Millikan RC, Martin CF, Newman B, Gammon MD, Ammerman AS, Sandler RS. Heterocyclic amines, meat intake, and association with colon cancer in a population-based study. *Am J Epidemiol* 2003; **157**: 434–45.

151.Le Marchand L, Donlon T, Seifried A, Wilkens LR. Red meat intake, CYP2E1 genetic polymorphisms, and colorectal cancer risk. *Cancer Epidemiol Biomarkers Prev* 2002; **11**: 1019–24.

152.Augustsson K, Skog K, Jagerstad M, Dickman PW, Steineck G. Dietary heterocyclic amines and cancer of the colon, rectum, bladder, and kidney: a population-based study. *Lancet* 1999; **353**: 703–7.

153.Roberts L. In: Thomas L, editor. Cancer today: Origins, prevention, and treatment. Washington: Institute of Medicine/National Academy Press; 1984. p. 68–9.

154.The National Food Administration, Sweden. Acrylamide in heat-processed foods. Report of The National Food Administration. 2002-06-06. (http://www.slv.se/engdefault.asp?FrameLocation=/templatesSLV/SLV_DocumentList____4089.asp)

155.IARC. Some industrial chemicals-acrylamide. *IARC Monographs on the Evaluation of*

Carcinogenic Risks to Humans 1994; **60**: 389–433.

156.Hagmar L, Tornqvist M, Nordander C, Rosen I, Bruze F, Kautianinen A, Magnusson A-L, Malmberg B, Aprea P, Ranath F, Axmon A. Health effects of occupational exposure to acrylamide using hemoglobin adducts as biomarkers of internal dose. *Scand J Work Environ Health* 2001; **27**: 219–26.

157.Widmark EMP. Presence of cancer-producing substances in roasted food. *Nature* 1939; **143**: 984.

A MEDIUM-TERM RAT LIVER BIOASSAY FOR RAPID *IN VIVO* DETECTION OF CARCINOGENIC POTENTIAL OF CHEMICALS

Nobuyuki ITO*1, Seiko TAMANO*2 and Tomoyuki SHIRAI*3

*Nagoya City University*1, Daiyukai Institute of Medical Science*2 and Departments of Experimental Pathology and Tumor Biology, Nagoya City University Postgraduate School of Medical Sciences*3*

A reliable medium-term bioassay system for rapid detection of carcinogenic potential of chemicals in the human environment has been developed. The 8-week-protocol consists of 2 stages; male F344 rats are given a single intraperitoneal injection of diethylnitrosamine (200 mg/kg) for initiation of liver carcinogenesis, followed by a 6-week test chemical treatment starting 2 weeks thereafter. Test chemicals are usually given in the diet or the drinking water and in the 2nd week of test chemical treatment, all rats are subjected to two-thirds partial hepatectomy in order to induce regenerative cell replication. The end-point marker is the glutathione S-transferase placental form (GST-P)-positive hepatic focus, the numbers and sizes of which are analyzed using an image-analyzer and expressed as values per unit liver section (1 cm^2). When the yield of GST-P-positive foci is significantly enhanced ($P<0.05$) over the control value, a chemical is judged to possess carcinogenic or promotion potential for the liver. Among 313 chemicals already tested in this system in our laboratory, 30/31 (97%) mutagenic hepatocarcinogens and 29/33 (88%) non-mutagenic hepatocarcinogens gave positive results. Ten out of 43 (23%) agents known to be carcinogenic in organs other than the liver were also positive. It is particularly important that only one of 48 non-carcinogens gave a very weak positive result, so that the system has a very low false-positivity rate. It is now well documented that the assay system is highly effective for detecting hepatocarcinogens, bridging the gap between traditional long-term carcinogenicity tests and short-term screening assays. At the Fourth International Conference on Harmonization, our medium-term liver bioassay based on an initiation and promotion protocol was recommended in the guidelines as an acceptable alternative to the long-term rodent carcinogenicity test.

Reduction of chemical agents with carcinogenic potential in the environment is of prime importance to reduce cancer risk in human beings. Lifetime assays for detection of carcinogenicity in experimental animals, together with data on related toxic

---

*1, *3 1 Kawasumi, Mizuho-ku, Nagoya 467-8601, Japan

*2 Ichinomiya, Japan

This paper is dedicated to the memory of late Dr. Tomizo Yoshida on the occasion of the 100th anniversary of his birth. It was originally published in Cancer Science in January, 2003.

effects on a variety of organisms, have been the foundation for prediction of carcinogenic hazard to human beings. The standard requirements are lifetime carcinogenicity testing in two rodent species, rats and mice, at 3 different doses of test compound with a control for each sex. This is very expensive in terms of financial and human resources, and time-consuming. Good animal facilities with experts in toxicology and toxicological pathology are essential for performance of the assays. These fundamentals make it practically impossible to evaluate the carcinogenic potential of the vast variety of chemicals present in our environment. Accordingly, alternative short-term screening assays have been developed which are very rapid and economical, though their validity is limited by substantial rates of false-negative and false-positive determinations and by their inability to determine target organ-specificity (*1*).

It has become clear that mutagenicity does not always correlate with carcinogenicity and there are a variety of chemical agents that are non-genotoxic but carcinogenic. It is likely that an *in vivo* system using a whole body approach is the only method applicable to non-genotoxic carcinogens, because these tend to have restricted organ-specificity. Recent questions concerning the contribution of mouse bioassay results to assessment of human hazard emphasize the necessity for an optimized approach (*2–4*). The proposed guideline of International Conference on Harmonization (ICH) recommends reducing long-term protocols, and utilizing any one species with additional of an alternative bioassay (*5*).

For the past 25 years, our laboratory has focused on development of *in vivo* medium-term bioassay systems employing the rat liver. A total of 313 chemicals have already been tested and an extremely good correlation between positive results and carcinogenicity in 2-year long-term studies has been obtained. The efficacy of the medium-term rat liver bioassay for detection of carcinogenicity is now well established, particularly for agents targeting the liver, as extensively discussed at a special meeting at the International Agency for Research on Cancer in 1997 (*6*). The most recent edition of "Casarett and Doull's TOXICOLOGY" introduces our medium-term protocol as an alternative bioassay (*7*). In the present review, the outline and characteristics of the system are briefly described, current issues underlying the system are discussed, and practical applications for other purposes are also briefly covered.

Medium-term Liver Bioassay Protocol

In 1976, with long experience of experimental research into rodent hepatocarcinogenesis, Solt and Farber were able to develop a protocol by which altered liver cell foci could be induced in rats within 4 weeks (*8*). Their protocol was based on a selective growth theory that utilized suppression of growth of normal cells by a hepatotoxic chemical and selective growth of carcinogen-initiated hepatotoxin-resistant altered liver cells by forced regenerative stimulation. However, the primary aim of their model was to study mechanisms of hepatocarcinogenesis rather than to utilize it as an assay system for carcinogens. At about the same time, Peraino and associates reported a two-stage model in which hepatic tumor formation was enhanced by chemicals such as phenobarbital given after initiation with 2-acetylaminofluorene (*9–11*). Their data suggested that this two-stage approach could be utilized for detection of carcinogenic responses of a given chemical. Based on this concept, we gradually established a new assay system in which carcinogenic potential of chemicals can be detected by measurement of altered liver foci as an end-point marker within a relatively short period (*12*). The preneoplastic nature of altered hepatic foci and the usefulness of such lesions as early indicators for hepatocarcinogenicity are now well accepted and the validity of foci in assays for detection of carcinogenic agents has been emphasized (*13*, *14*). Their phenotypic characteristics have been extensively studied using enzyme histochemical and immunohistochemical approaches, and glutathione *S*-transferase placental form (GST-P) was found to be an optimal marker for clear visualization of even very small lesions (*15*).

Fig. 1 shows the protocol employed in our laboratory as a medium-term liver bioassay. Male F344 male rats, 5 weeks old, are divided into three groups consisting of 15–20 animals each; group 1 is given a single intraperitoneal injection of diethylnitrosamine (DEN, 200 mg/kg body weight) dissolved in saline to initiate hepatocarcinogenesis and after a 2-week recovery period, receives a test compound in the basal diet, drinking water, or by repeated intraperitoneal, subcutaneous or intravenous injections. The rats are subjected to two-thirds partial hepatectomy (PH) at week 3. Group 2 is given DEN and PH in the same manner as for group 1 without administration of any test compound. Group 3 rats are injected with saline instead of DEN solution and then subjected to administration of test compound and PH. All animals are sacrificed at week 8, and 3–4 slices of their livers are fixed in ice-cold acetone for subsequent immunohistochemical demonstration of GST-P-positive foci (Fig. 2).

Numbers and areas of GST-P-positive foci more than 0.2 mm in diameter are measured using an image processor, and the results are assessed by comparing the values between group 1 (DEN-test compounds) and group 2 (DEN alone). Group 3 serves to assay the potential of the test chemicals to induce GST-P-positive foci without prior DEN exposure.

Until finalization of the protocol of this system, the following were extensively investigated in order to maximize the predictive potential of the model: 1. What is the best initiator for the liver carcinogenesis? 2. What dose of initiator is most suitable? 3. Which strain of rats is most suitable? 4. What is the minimum period for the test compound to be administered? 5. Which time point is the most efficient for PH

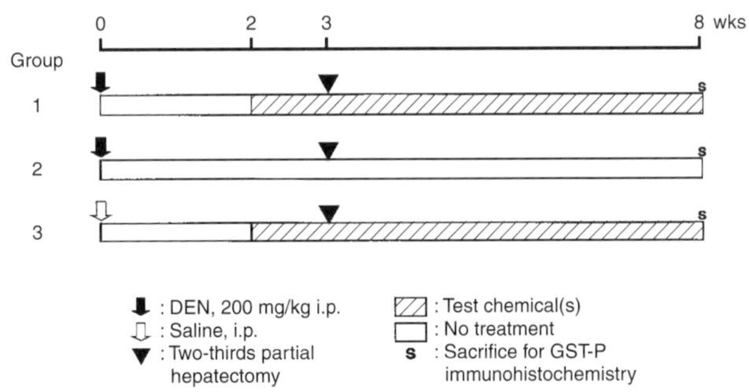

FIG. 1. Standard protocol of the medium-term liver bioassay
Animals are male F344 rats aged 5 weeks. Each group is composed 15 to 20 animals. Partial hepatectomy is performed under light ether anesthesia and all surgical operations are finished within 1 to 2 h in the morning to avoid circadian variation.

to boost the appearance of liver foci? 6. What is the best end-point surrogate marker to detect liver foci? Answers to these questions have been precisely reported in previous papers and also were mentioned in previous review papers (*6*, *16–19*).

Statistical analysis of differences between means is carried out using the Student's or Welch's *t* tests after application of the preliminary *F* test for equal variance, and scoring of carcinogenicity, promotion or inhibition, is made on the basis of differences in *P* values between groups; positive=increase at $P<0.05$ in either number or area of foci.

Results for 313 Compounds

So far, using this system, we have examined a total of 313 substances classified into 4 categories (Table I): (1) chemicals which are carcinogenic to the liver; (2) chemicals which are carcinogenic to organs other than the liver; (3) chemicals for which long-term carcinogenicity tests have been conducted in both rats and mice and

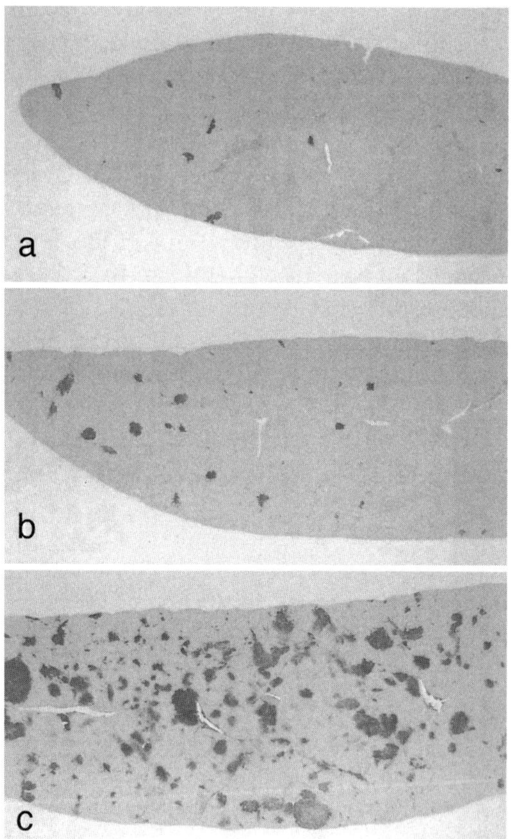

FIG. 2. Appearances of GST-P-positive foci in a rat given basal diet as a control (a), phenobarbital (b) and MeIQx (c), respectively after DEN-initiation

Note that the numbers and area of GST-P$^+$ in rats given carcinogen were increased compared with those of the control. A strong hepatocarcinogen (MeIQx) induced much more foci than did a weak carcinogen (phenobarbital).

carcinogenicity has not been proven; and (4) chemicals whose carcinogenicity had not previously been appropriately evaluated (unknowns). Chemicals for which no carcinogenicity has been proven but which had been tested only in one animal species are categorized as of unknown carcinogenicity, and those for which no carcinogenicity has been reported only in one species or which are supposed not to be carcinogenic based on their chemical structure or properties are categorized as non-carcinogens. Similarly, the compounds were divided into 3 groups according to their reported mutagenicity in the Ames' test; mutagenic compounds, non-mutagenic compounds and unknowns. Comparisons of the summarized results with reported *Salmonella*/ microsome and long-term carcinogenicity test findings are shown in Table I. The detailed results for 277 and 291 compounds have already been documented in our review papers (*18*, *19*). Newly investigated compounds since 1997 are 2 hepatocarcinogens (vinclozolin and diethylstilbesterol), one non-hepatocarcinogen (dichrolovos), 3 non-carcinogens (troglitazone, fenbendazole styrene monomer, bisphenol A) and 17 chemicals for which carcinogenicity is unknown (rutin, hesperidin, melatonin, Sho-siko-tou, Saiko-keishi-tou, Hochu-ekki-tou, purple sweet potato color, red cabbage color, protocatechuic acid, phloroglucin carbonic acid, rhEGF, nonylphenol, styrene dimmer, styrene timer dimethylarsinic acid, Ju-myo protein and proohyra tenera). Vinclozolin used to be categorized as a non-carcinogen, but we came across the report by Mellert *et al.* who found that vinclozolin induced hepatocellular carcinomas in rats when given for 24 months at a dose of 4500 ppm in a diet (*20*). Therefore, for the purpose of this review, we categorized vinclozolin as a hepatocarcinogen.

As emphasized in previous review papers, use of this assay has generated an extremely good outcome in terms of predictability of carcinogenicity. It is especially noteworthy that 60 of 65 (92%) liver carcinogens gave positive results, irrespective of their mutagenicity, leaving only 4 false-negatives; 30 out of 31 (97%) mutagenic, and 29 out of 33 (88%) non-mutagenic hepatocarcinogens gave positive results. Tamoxifen was negative in our previous assay but as shown in a study by Kim *et al.* with this assay (*21*), an increase of the dose of tamoxifen resulted in a positive finding. Three out of 4 non-mutagenic carcinogens that gave false-negative results were carcinogenic

TABLE I. Positive Rates in the Medium-Term Liver Bioassay for 313 Compounds

Carcinogenicity of test chemicals	Positive rates			
	Mutagenicity (Ames test)			Total
	Positive	Negative	Unknown	
Hepatocarcinogens	30/31 (97)[a]	29/33 (88)[b]	1/1 (100)	60/65 (92)
Non-hepatocarcinogens	7/26 (27)	2/15 (13)	1/2 (50)	10/43 (23)[d]
Non-carcinogens	0/6 (0)	1/40 (3)[c]	0/2 (0)	1/48 (2)[d]
Unknowns	4/14 (29)	30/86 (36)	14/57 (24)	48/157 (32)
Total	41/77 (53)	62/174 (36)	16/62 (25)	119/313 (38)

The numbers in parentheses represent percentages.

[a] Negative: 4,4′-diaminodiphenylmethane.

[b] Negative: clofibrate, di(2-ethylhexyl)adipate (mouse), di(2-ethylhexyl)phthalate, trichloroacetic acid (mouse).

[c] Positive: malathione.

[d] A total of 11 chemicals were positive in this model, although hepatocarcinogenicity is not proven.

peroxisome proliferators, known to suppress GST-P expression. Trichloroacetic acid is a mouse hepatocarcinogen and this chemical has also been demonstrated to possess peroxisome proliferation activity (*22*). Since the lesions associated with their hepatocarcinogenicity are not positive for GST-P as a marker enzyme (*23*), use of another end-point marker is necessary. At present only morphological appearance can be reliably applied, because no other enzyme marker has yet been found. With peroxisome proliferators, we must therefore take care and use hematoxylin and eosin stained slides for quantitative measurement of hepatic foci.

Among 43 carcinogens targeting organs other than the liver, 10 compounds gave positive results (23%), and 1 pesticide (malathion) among 43 compounds reported as not carcinogenic demonstrated positivity (3%) (*24*). Since the present system uses hepatic preneoplastic lesions as an indicator of carcinogenicity, the positive results for these 11 chemicals, as well as for 48 out of 157 chemicals of unknown carcinogenicity, suggest that they are weak hepatocarcinogens or liver tumor promoters.

Table II shows the validity of the assay system based on correlations with hepatocarcinogenicity data obtained from long-term carcinogenicity testing. The evaluation was calculated using the formula for validity of carcinogen screening tests described by Cooper *et al.* (*25*) Five categories, sensitivity, specificity, predictive value (positive predictivity), false-positive rate and false-negative rate were calculated and all demonstrated excellent values. Although carcinogenic potential of chemicals that are peroxisome proliferators cannot be accurately detected, even when they were included, the sensitivity, specificity, positive predictivity and negative predictivity were found to be 92.3%, 97.9%, 98.4% and 90.4%, respectively. When the 4 peroxisome proliferators were excluded, specificity rose to 97.9%. It is noteworthy that the false-positive and false-negative rates so far are 2.1% and 1.6%, respectively, clearly demonstrating that this medium-term liver bioassay is excellent for detection of liver carcinogens. A particular advantage of the system is that the majority of non-genotoxic carcinogens are accurately predictable. Table II also demonstrates the validity of this system for non-genotoxic hepatocarcinogens; the sensitivity, specificity, positive predictivity and negative predictivity are all more than 96.7%, when the 4 peroxisome proliferators are excluded.

Among chemicals tested in this system, seventeen are carcinogenic only in mouse: 14 target the liver and 3, other organs. Eighty-six percent (12/14) of the former were positive and 1 of the latter. These data for mouse carcinogens are impor-

TABLE II. Validity of the Medium-Term Liver Bioassay for Hepatocarcinogens

	Carcinogenic compounds[a]		Non-mutagenic carcinogens	
	Including peroxisome proliferators	Excluding peroxisome proliferators	Including peroxisome proliferators	Excluding peroxisome proliferators
Sensitivity	60/65 (92.3)	60/61 (98.4)	29/33 (87.9)	29/29 (100)
Specificity	47/48 (97.9)	47/48 (97.9)	39/40 (97.5)	39/40 (97.5)
Positive predictivity	60/61 (98.4)	60/61 (98.4)	29/30 (96.7)	29/30 (96.7)
Negative predictivity	47/52 (90.4)	47/48 (97.9)	39/43 (90.7)	39/39 (100)
False-positive rate	1/48 (2.1)	1/48 (2.1)	1/40 (2.5)	1/40 (2.5)
False-negative rate	5/65 (7.7)	1/61 (1.6)	4/33 (12.1)	0/29 (—)

All data are for hepatocarcinogens (see Table I). The numbers in parentheses represent percentages.
[a] Carcinogenic compounds include non-mutagenic and mutagenic.

TABLE III. Footnote for TABLE II

Test outcome	Carcinogenicity		Total
	Yes	No	
Positive	*a*	*b*	*a*+*b*
Negative	*c*	*d*	*c*+*d*
Total	*a*+*c*	*b*+*d*	*a*+*b*+*c*+*d*

Sensitivity: $a/(a+c)$.
Specificity: $d/(b+d)$.
Positive predictivity: $a/(a+b)$.
Negative predictivity: $d/(c+d)$.
False-positive: $b/(b+d)$.
False-negative: $c/(a+c)$.

tant since there is a recommendation to use rats for the long-term carcinogenicity test with an additional alternative animal model in the ICH.

Significance of PH as a Stimulator of Hepatocyte Proliferation

The actual protocol of the medium-term liver bioassay model is simple and there are no major practical difficulties involved in its performance. It is necessary to be familiar with the surgical procedure for PH, but basically it is not a difficult operation. Since it was introduced by Higgins and Anderson in 1931 (*26*), it has been extensively employed for investigation of cell proliferation and regeneration and as a very efficient tool to stimulate a wave of hepatocyte division. The rodent liver has been repeatedly demonstrated to become quickly restored through vigorous regeneration after two-thirds partial hepatectomy. The liver weight recovers almost to preoperative levels within 1 week with peak DNA synthesis at about 24 h. There is some concern with PH in terms of animal rights and therefore we have explored alternatives. By using a hepatotoxin such as carbon tetrachloride or β-galactosamine, so-called chemical hepatectomy can be performed. However, neither of these agents gave cell proliferative effects equivalent to PH in our system (data not shown), presumably because of the effects of the initiator used (DEN) and also the test compound. These hepatotoxins induce compensatory cell proliferation to restore cell numbers. Cell toxicity depends on hepatic enzyme activities, which can be modified by a test compound, and in some cases, test compounds themselves are toxic. Therefore, the required cell toxicity to provoke cell regeneration is not constant. Furthermore, the presence of tissue necrosis induced by hepatotoxins is not favorable condition for analysis of GST-P-positive foci. Cell mitogens active in the liver, such as lead nitrate do not work either (*27*), because after cell replication, the excess cell population is eliminated by apoptosis, a phenomenon which is not desirable for the medium-term bioassay.

Utilization of the Medium-term Liver Bioassay to Identify Chemopreventors, and to Assess Interactions among Multiple Chemicals, Dose-response Effects of Carcinogens and Physical Factors

Since GST-P-positive foci are very sensitive end-points, the present system can also provide information concerning anticancer properties of compounds, as empha-

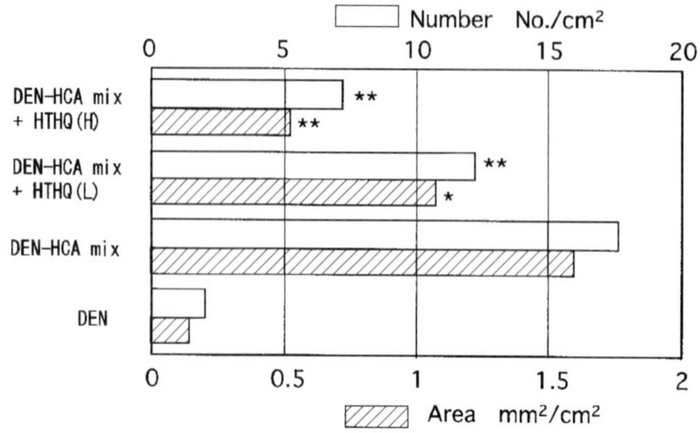

FIG. 3. Chemopreventive effects of HTHQ on HCA-hepatocarcinogenesis using the medium-term liver bioassay

Application of the system for detection of chemopreventive activity. This figure is from Table IV of ref. 28. HCAs: a mixture of 5 hepatocarcinogenic heterocyclic amines, 2-amino-6-methyldipyrido[1,2-*a*:3′,2′-*d*]imidazole (Glu-P-1), 3-amino-1,4-dimethyl-5-*H*-pyrido[4,3-*b*]indole (Trp-P-1), 2-amino-3-methyl-9*H*-pyrido[2,3-*b*]indole (MeAaC), 2-amino-3-methylimidazo[4,5-*f*]quinoline (IQ) and 2-amino-3,8-dimethylimidazo[4,5-*f*]quinoxaline (MeIQx). All were incorporated into the diet. HTHQ (a synthetic antioxidant, 1-*O*-hexyl-2,3,5-trimethylhydroquinone) was mixed in the diet at a dose of 0.125% (L) or 0.5% (H). Each group was composed of 15 male F344 rats. * $P<0.01$, ** $P<0.001$ vs. the respective DEN-HCAs group values. The numbers and area of GST-P-positive foci were suppressed in a dose-dependent manner by the simultaneous treatment with HTHQ.

sized in a review paper (*18*). Thus, the system can provide a rapid screening tool for chemopreventors (*28, 29*). As an example, Fig. 3 graphically demonstrates the chemopreventive effect of an antioxidant, 1-*O*-hexyl-2,3,5-trimethylhydroxyquinoline (HTHQ) on 2-amino-3,8-dimethylimidazo[4,5-*f*]quinoxaline (MeIQx)-induced hepatocarcinogenesis using the medium-term liver bioassay (see ref. 28). The issue of summation and synergism in response to multiple chemicals and co-carcinogenic factors in our environment is very important and needs to be clarified. The complexity inherent in looking at many factors precludes the use of long-term protocols, but our medium-term test can be applied. For example, combined effects of 20 pesticides and five heterocyclic amines have been examined and the data provided very important information (*30–32*). Carcinogen dose-dependence is of essential significance to risk assessment. Fukushima's group has been approaching this issue using the medium-term bioassay system (*33*). Since the required time is short and the quantitative measurement of GST-P-positive foci is very sensitive, it is relatively easy to conduct studies with many different doses of chemical.

The present medium-term bioassay can also be applied for assessment of physical factors for tumor-promoting potential. For example, risk with near-field electronic magnetic fields (EMF) used for cellular phones has been evaluated (*34, 35*), and the data demonstrated a lack of tumor-promoting potential in two separate experiments with different frequencies.

Other Rapid in vivo Systems

Since the medium-term liver bioassay naturally targets hepatocarcinogens, the validity for chemicals that are carcinogenic to organs other than the liver is not optimal. In order to overcome this disadvantage, we also developed whole-body system models using wide-spectrum initiation by sequential treatment with three to five potent carcinogens having different target organ spectra. Preliminary results with these medium-term multi-organ models have indicated that most carcinogens can be detected because of increased development of lesions in target organs within 24 or 36 weeks, as presented in several reviews (*6*, *18*). This approach was also intensively discussed at a special meeting at the International Agency for Research on Cancer in 1997 (*6*).

Several systems using transgenic and newborn animals have been proposed as candidate alternative whole body bioassays. The utility of genetically altered mouse models such as p53+/−, rasH2 and Tg.AC for identifying carcinogens has been extensively discussed (*36–38*) and the usefulness of those models has been validated world-wide under ILSI's collaborative evaluation program (*39*). Although there may be many advantages in terms of detection of carcinogenicity in a relatively short period, it is likely that organ-specificity is not always demonstrated and it can be argued that there seem to be undefined areas regarding mechanistic points in these genetically engineered models. In the ILSI/HESI workshop in 2000, a panel discussion concluded that such animal models have utility as screening bioassays for identification of potential human carcinogens, but it was recognized that there are limitations in organ/tissue specificity and sensitivity, and that further characterization and clarification are needed (*40–42*).

Conclusions

The medium-term liver bioassay described here is a reliable and practical tool for prediction of carcinogenic potential of chemicals and physical factors in a short period. The system is now internationally well recognized and recommended as an alternative carcinogenicity test.

Acknowledgments

This work was supported in part by Grants-in-Aid for Cancer Research from the Ministry of Education, Culture, Sports, Science and Technology and the Ministry of Health, Labour and Welfare, a Grant-in-Aid from the Ministry of Health, Labour and Welfare for the 2nd Term Comprehensive 10-Year Strategy for Cancer Control, and grants from the Society for Promotion of Pathology of Nagoya and the Experimental Pathological Research Association, Nagoya, Japan. We would like to thank the following researchers for their contributions to the establishment of the medium-term liver bioassay; Shoji Fukushima, Hiroyuki Tsuda, Masae Tatematsu, Masao Hirose, Ryohei Hasegawa, Katsumi Imaida, Akihiro Hagiwara, Masashi Sano, Mayumi Kawabe, Satoru Takahashi, Makoto Asamoto, Toshio Kato, Tadashi Ogiso, Koji Kato, Kumiko Ogawa, Mitsuru Futakuchi, Masato Ohshima, Keisuke Nakanishi, Witaya Thamavit, Ross Cameron, Joao L. de Camargo, Ricardo Cabral, Dae Joong Kim and Malcolm A. Moore.

REFERENCES

1. Ashby J, Tennant RW. Definitive relationship among chemical structure, carcinogenic-

ity and mutagenicity for 301 chemicals tested by the U.S. NTP. *Mutat Res* 1991; **257**: 229–306.

2. Huff J, Bucher J, Yang R. Carcinogenesis studies in rodents for evaluating risks associated with chemical carcinogens in aquatic food animals. *Environ Health Perspect* 1991; **90**: 127–32.
3. Huff J, Haseman J. Long-term chemical carcinogenesis experiments for identifying potential human cancer hazards: collective database of the National Cancer Institute and National Toxicology Program (1976–1991). *Environ Health Perspect* 1991; **96**: 23–31.
4. Alden CL, Smith PF, Piper CE, Brej L. A critical appraisal of the value of the mouse cancer bioassay in safety assessment. *Toxicol Pathol* 1996; **24**: 722–5.
5. International Conference on Harmonization of Technical Requirements for the Registration of Pharmaceuticals for Human Use. *Testing for Carcinogenic Activity* 1995.
6. Shirai T, Hirose M, Ito N. Medium-term bioassays in rats for rapid detection of the carcinogenic potential of chemicals. In: McGregor DB, Rice JM, editors. The use of short- and medium-term tests for carcinogens and data on genetic effects in carcinogenic hazard evaluation. Lyon: International Agency for Research on Cancer; 1999. p. 251–72.
7. Pitot H, Dragan Y. Chemical carcinogenesis. In: Klaassen CD, editor. Casertt & Doul's TOXICOLOGY: The basic science of poisons. 6th ed. McGraw-Hill; 2001. p. 241–319.
8. Solt D, Farber E. New principle for the analysis of chemical carcinogenesis. *Nature* 1976; **263**: 701–3.
9. Peraino C, Fry RJ, Staffeldt E, Christopher JP. Comparative enhancing effects of phenobarbital, amobarbital, diphenylhydantoin, and dichlorodiphenyltrichloroethane on 2-acetylaminofluorene-induced hepatic tumorigenesis in the rat. *Cancer Res* 1975; **35**: 2884–90.
10. Peraino C, Fry RJ, Staffeldt E, Christopher JP. Enhancing effects of phenobarbitone and butylated hydroxytoluene on 2-acetylaminofluorene-induced hepatic tumorigenesis in the rat. *Food Cosmet Toxicol* 1977; **15**: 93–6.
11. Peraino C, Staffeldt EF, Haugen DA, Lombard LS, Stevens FJ, Fry RJ. Effects of varying the dietary concentration of phenobarbital on its enhancement of 2-acetylaminofluorene-induced hepatic tumorigenesis. *Cancer Res* 1980; **40**: 3268–73.
12. Tatematsu M, Shirai T, Tsuda H, Miyata Y, Shinohara Y, Ito N. Rapid production of hyperplastic liver nodules in rats treated with carcinogenic chemicals: a new approach for an *in vivo* short-term screening test for hepatocarcinogens. *Gann* 1977; **68**: 499–507.
13. Bannasch P. Preneoplastic lesions as end points in carcinogenicity testing. I. Hepatic neoplasia. *Carcinogenesis* 1986; **7**: 689–95.
14. Oesterle D, Deml E. Detection of chemical carcinogens by means of the rat liver bioassay. *Exp Pathol* 1990; **39**: 197–206.
15. Ogiso T, Tatematsu M, Tamano S, Tsuda H, Ito N. Comparative effects of carcinogens on the induction of placental glutathione S-transferase-positive liver nodules in a short-term assay and of hepatocellular carcinomas in a long-term assay. *Toxicol Pathol* 1985; **13**: 257–63.
16. Ito N, Shirai T, Hasegawa R. Medium-term bioassay for carcinogens. In: Vainio H,

Magee P, editors. Mechanisms of carcinogenesis in risk assessment. Lyon: IARC; 1992. p. 345–80.

17. Hasegawa R, Ito N. Liver medium-term bioassay in rats for screening of carcinogens and modifying factors in hepatocarcinogenesis. *Food Chem Toxicol* 1992; **30**: 979–92.
18. Ito N, Hasegawa R, Imaida K, Hirose M, Shirai T, Tamano S, Hagiwara A. Medium-term rat liver bioassay for rapid detection of hepatocarcinogenic substances. *J Toxicol Pathol* 1997: 1–11.
19. Shirai T. A medium-term rat liver bioassay as a rapid *in vivo* test for carcinogenic potential: a historical review of model development and summary of results from 291 tests. *Toxicol Pathol* 1997; **25**: 453–60.
20. Evaluations 1995 Part II—Toxicological and environmental. Joint FAO/WHO Meeting on Pesticide Residues. In: IPCS editor. WHO; 1995. p. 375–404.
21. Kim DJ, Han BS, Ahn B, Lee KK, Kang JS, Tsuda H. Promotion potential of tamoxifen on hepatocarcinogenesis in female SD or F344 rats initiated with diethylnitrosamine. *Cancer Lett* 1996; **104**: 13–9.
22. Moody DE, Reddy JK, Lake BK, Popp JA, Reese DH. Symposium overview: peroxisome proliferation and nongenotoxic carcinogenesis: commentary on a symposium. *Fundam Appl Toxicol* 1991; **16**: 233–48.
23. Bentley P, Calder I, Elcombe C, Grasso P, Stringer D, Wiegand H. Hepatic peroxisome proliferation in rodents and its significance for humans. *Food Chem Toxicol* 1993; **31**: 857–907.
24. Hoshiya T, Hasegawa R, Hakoi K, Cui L, Ogiso T, Cabral R, Ito N. Enhancement by non-mutagenic pesticides of GST-P positive hepatic foci development initiated with diethylnitrosamine in the rat. *Cancer Lett* 1993; **72**: 59–64.
25. Cooper JAI, Saracci R, Cole P. Describing the validity of carcinogen screening tests. *Br J Cancer* 1979; **39**: 87–9.
26. Higginson GH, Anderson RM. Experimental pathology of the liver. 1. Restoration of the liver of the white rat following partial surgical removal. *Arch Pathol* 1931; **12**: 186–202.
27. Columbano A, Ledda-Columbano GM, Lee G, Rajalakshmi S, Sarma DS. Inability of mitogen-induced liver hyperplasia to support the induction of enzyme-altered islands induced by liver carcinogens. *Cancer Res* 1987; **47**: 5557–9.
28. Hirose M, Futakuchi M, Tanaka H, Orita S, Ito T, Miki T, Shirai T. Prevention by antioxidants of heterocyclic amine-induced carcinogenesis in a rat medium-term liver bioassay: results of extended and combination treatment experiments. *Eur J Cancer Prev* 1998; **7**: 61–7.
29. Hirose M, Ito T, Takahashi S, Ozaki M, Ogiso T, Nihro Y, Miki T, Shirai T. Prevention by synthetic phenolic antioxidants of 2-amino-3,8-dimethylimidazo[4,5-*f*]quinoxaline (MeIQx)- or activated MeIQx-induced mutagenesis and MeIQx-induced rat hepatocarcinogenesis, and role of antioxidant activity in the prevention of carcinogenesis. *Eur J Cancer Prev* 1998; **7**: 233–41.
30. Ito N, Hasegawa R, Shirai T, Fukushima S, Hakoi K, Takaba K, Iwasaki S, Wakabayashi K, Nagao M, Sugimura T. Enhancement of GST-P positive liver cell foci development by combined treatment of rats with five heterocyclic amines at low doses. *Carcinogenesis* 1991; **12**: 767–72.

31. Hasegawa R, Shirai T, Hakoi K, Takaba K, Iwasaki S, Hoshiya T, Ito N, Nagao M, Sugimura T. Synergistic enhancement of glutathione *S*-transferase placental form-positive hepatic foci development in diethylnitrosamine-treated rats by combined administration of five heterocyclic amines at low doses. *Jpn J Cancer Res* 1991; **82**: 1378–84.
32. Ito N, Imaida K, Hagiwara A, Tamano S, Shirai T. Effects of ingesting a combination of 20 or 40 pesticides at ADI levels on carcinogenesis in rats. In: Hodgson E, editor. Reviews in toxicology. The Netherlands: IOS Press; 1998. p. 85–92.
33. Kitano M, Ichihara T, Matsuda T, Wanibuchi H, Tamano S, Hagiwara A, Imaoka S, Funae Y, Shirai T, Fukushima S. Presence of a threshold for promoting effects of phenobarbital on diethylnitrosamine-induced hepatic foci in the rat. *Carcinogenesis* 1998; **19**: 1475–80.
34. Imaida K, Taki M, Watanabe S, Kamimura Y, Ito T, Yamaguchi T, Ito N, Shirai T. The 1.5 GHz electromagnetic near-field used for cellular phones does not promote rat liver carcinogenesis in a medium-term liver bioassay. *Jpn J Cancer Res* 1998; **89**: 995–1002.
35. Imaida K, Taki M, Yamaguchi T, Ito T, Watanabe S, Wake K, Aimoto A, Kamimura Y, Ito N, Shirai T. Lack of promoting effects of the electromagnetic near-field used for cellular phones (929.2 MHz) on rat liver carcinogenesis in a medium-term liver bioassay. *Carcinogenesis* 1998; **19**: 311–4.
36. Tennant RW, Stasiewicz S, Mennear J, French JE, Spalding JW. Genetically altered mouse models for identifying carcinogens. In: McGregor DB, Rice JM, editors. The use of short- and medium-term tests for carcinogens and data on genetic effects in carcinogenic hazard evaluation. Lyon: IARC; 1999.
37. Gonzalez FJ. Use of transgenic animals in carcinogenesis studies. *Mol Carcinog* 1996; **16**: 63–7.
38. Pitot HC. Animal models of neoplastic development. *Dev Biol* 2001; **106**: 53–7; discussion 7–9, 143–60.
39. Robinson DE, MacDonald JS. Background and framework for ILSI's collaborative evaluation program on alternatve models for carcinogenicity assessment. *Toxicol Pathol* 2001; **29** (Suppl.): 13–9.
40. Cohen S. Alternative models for carcinogenicity testing: weight of evidence evaluations across models. *Toxicol Pathol* 2001; **29** (Suppl.): 183–90.
41. Goodman J. A perspective on current and future uses of alternative models for carcinogenicity testing. *Toxicol Pathol* 2001; **29** (Suppl.): 183–90.
42. Ashby J. Expectations for transgenic rodent cancer bioassay models. *Toxicol Pathol* 2001; **29** (Suppl.): 177–82.

METABOLIC ACTIVATION OF POLYCYCLIC AROMATIC HYDROCARBONS TO CARCINOGENS BY CYTOCHROMES P450 1A1 AND 1B1

Tsutomu SHIMADA[*1,2] and Yoshiaki FUJII-KURIYAMA[*3,4]

Osaka Prefectural Institute of Public Health[*1]*, Department of Biochemistry and Center in Molecular Toxicology*[*2]*, The Vanderbilt University School of Medicine, Center for Tsukuba Advanced Research Alliance, University of Tsukuba*[*3]*, Core Research for Evolutional Science and Technology (CREST) Japan, Science and Technology Corporation*[*4]

Polycyclic aromatic hydrocarbons (PAHs) are ubiquitously distributed environmental chemicals. PAHs aquire carcinogenicity only after they have been activated by xenbiotic-metabolizing enzymes to highly reactive metabolites capable of attacking cellular DNA. Cytochrome P450 (CYP) enzymes are central to the metabolic activation of these PAHs to epoxide intermediates and ultimately, with the aid of epoxide hydrolase to ultimate carcinogenic diol-epoxides. Historically, CYP1A1 was believed to be the only enzyme that catalyzes activation of these procarcinogenic PAHs. However, recent studies have established that CYP1B1, a newly identified member of the CYP1 family, plays a very important role in the metabolic activation of PAHs. In *CYP1B1* gene-knock mice treated with 7, 12-dimethylbenz[*a*]anthracene and dibenzo[*a*, *l*]pyrene, decreased rates of tumor formation were observed, when compared to wild-type mice. Significantly, gene expression of CYP1A1 and 1B1 is induced by PAHs and polyhalogenated hydrocarbons such as 2, 3, 7, 8-tetrachlorodibenzo-*p*-dioxin through the arylhydrocarbon receptor. Differences in susceptibilities of individuals to the adverse action of PAHs may, in part, be due to the levels of expression of CYP1A1 and 1B1 and to genetic variations in the *CYP1A1* and *1B1* genes.

Most of the chemical carcinogens in the environment are chemically inert in themselves and require metabolic activation by cytochrome P450 (CYP) enzymes to more reactive metabolites to exhibit their carcinogenicities in experimental animals and humans (*1*, *2*). Of the 17 families of human CYPs identified to date, the CYP1, 2, and 3 family members play major roles in the metabolic activation of a variety of environmental carcinogens. It has been suggested that CYP1A1 and CYP1B1 are responsible for the activation of most of the carcinogenic polycyclic aromatic hydrocar-

[*1] 3-69 Nakamichi 1-chome, Higashinari-ku, Osaka 537-0025, Japan
[*2] Nashville, Tennessee 37232-0146, U.S.A.
[*3] 1-1-1 Tennoudai, Tsukuba 305-8577, Japan
[*4] Kawaguchi 322-0012, Japan

This paper is dedicated to the memory of late Dr. Tomizo Yoshida on the occasion of the 100th anniversary of his birth.
The essential part of this article was originally published in Cancer Science in January, 2004.

bons (PAHs) to epoxide intermediates and further to more reactive diol-epoxides with the aid of epoxide hydrolase (*1, 3*). CYP1A2 converts aryl- and heterocyclic amines to *N*-hydroxylated metabolites that are subsequently modified by phase II enzymes, such as acetyltransferase and sulfotransferase, to ultimate carcinogens (*4, 5*). CYP2A6 is a key contributor to the activation of *N*-diethylnitrosamine and other tobacco-related nitrosamines, such as 4-(methylnitrosamino)-1-(3-pyridyl)-1-butanone and *N*-nitrosonornicotine (*6, 7*). CYP2E1 activates *N*-dimethylnitrosamine and other low-molecular weight procarcinogens such as ethyl carbamate and vinyl carbamate (*8*). CYP3A4, 5 and 7 activate aflatoxin B_1, aflatoxin G_1, and sterigmatocystin by forming their respective highly reactive epoxides (*5, 9*). Other human P450 members including CYP2B6, 2C8, 2C9, 2C18, 2C19, and 2D6 are known to play relatively minor roles in the metabolic activation of procarcinogens and promutagens (*2*). Of the CYP4 family enzymes identified so far, CYP4B1 catalyzes activation of urinary bladder carcinogens, such as benzidine and 2-naphthylamine (*10*).

PAHs are ubiquitouly distributed carcinogens in the environment and their carcinogenic potentials have been extensively studied in experimental animal models (*1, 11, 12*). Historically, CYP1A1 had been thought to be the sole enzyme responsible for the metabolic activation of most of the carcinogenic PAHs to reactive electrophiles in mice, rats, and rabbits (*1*). However, recent studies have established that CYP1B1 also activates PAHs to reactive metabolites at rates similar to or even higher than CYP1A1 in experimental animals and humans. As a further cause for concern, human CYP1B1 has also been shown to metabolize 17β-estradiol to a 4-hydroxylated product, a chemical considered to cause breast cancers in women (*13*). Both CYP1A1 and 1B1 are expressed mainly in extrahepatic organs and thus make major contribution to the incidence of cancers in these organs, when PAHs and other carcinogens are ingested into the animal's body (*3, 14–16*). PAHs and polyhalogenated hydrocarbons such as TCDD induce several xenobiotic-metabolizing enzymes including CYP1A1 and 1B1 through the arylhydrocarbon receptor (AhR) and the increased synthesis of these enzymes as well as genetic variations in *CYP1A1* and *1B1* genes may determine the different susceptibilities of individuals to carcinogenesis caused by PAHs. In this review, we summarize recent progress in the investigation of the roles of CYP1A1 and 1B1 in the metabolic activation of PAHs and their relevance to the occurrence of cancers in humans.

Metabolic Activation of PAHs by P450 and Epoxide Hydrolase

A great number of studies have demonstrated that most carcinogenic PAHs are activated by the combined actions of CYPs and epoxide hydrolase to highly reactive diol-epoxides that initiate cell transformation (*1, 17*). Metabolic activation of the prototype carcinogen B[*a*]P (benzo[*a*]pyrene) for example, was extensively studied by the research groups of Jerina and Conney in the middle 1970's (*1*). Historically speaking, the so-called K-region epoxide B[*a*]P-4, 5-epoxide formed from metabolism of B[*a*]P by CYPs was thought to be the ultimate carcinogenic metabolite (*11, 17, 18*). However, the B[*a*]P-4, 5-epoxide was found to be readily hydrolyzed by epoxide hydrolase to an inactive B[*a*]P-4, 5-diol metabolite and was finally concluded not to play a major role in carcinogenesis by B[*a*]P (*1, 19*). Subsequent examination of several B[*a*]P metabolites revealed that (+)- and (−)-B[*a*]P-7, 8-diol-9, 10-epoxides, commonly refered to as bay region epoxides, were highly reactive towards DNA and, thus, were the ultimate carcinogenic metabolites of B[*a*]P (*1, 17*). The pathways leading to the formation of B[*a*]P bay region epoxides were extensively investigated in rat liver microsomes or reconstituted systems containing purified rat CYP and epoxide hydrolase (Fig. 1) (*1, 17*). B[*a*]P is first oxidized by liver microsomes of MC-treated rats to (+)- and (−)-B[*a*]P-7, 8 oxides with the conversion rate of the (+) enantiomer being much higher than the (−) form. Subsequently, microsomal epoxide hydrolase rapidly hydrolyzes these oxides to produce (−)- and (+)-B[*a*]P-7, 8-diol (*1, 17, 20*). And then, the resultant (−)- and (+)-B[*a*]P-7, 8-diols are finally activated by CYPs to highly reactive bay region epoxides, namely (−)-B[*a*]P-7, 8-diol-9, 10-epoxide-1, (+)- B[*a*]P-7, 8-diol-9, 10-epoxide-2, (+)-B[*a*]P-7, 8-diol-9, 10-epoxide-1 and (−)-B[*a*]P-7, 8-diol-9, 10-epoxide-2 (*1, 12, 21*). Although these four diol-epoxides were all highly mutagenic when assessed in Ames Salmonella tester strains and Chinese hamster V-79 cells, the (+)-B[*a*]P-7, 8-diol-9, 10-epoxide-2 was identified as the most reactive in producing tumors in newborn mice (*1, 20, 22*). Since (+)-B[*a*]P-7, 8-diol-9, 10-epoxide-2 had almost the same level of carcinogenicity as B[*a*]P itself or (−)-B[*a*]P-7, 8-diol, this diol epoxide is considered to be the ultimate carcinogenic metabolite of B[*a*]P (*1, 23, 24*).

The bay region theory has also been applied to other PAHs to explain their carcinogenic activation by CYPs and epoxide hydrolase (*1, 11, 25*). For example, DB[*a*, *l*]P and 7, 12-DMBA (7, 12-dimethylbenz[*a*]anthracene) are converted to their proximate carcinogenic metabolites, namely DB[*a*, *l*]P-11, 12-epoxide and 7, 12-DMBA-3, 4-oxide, respectively, by CYPs (Fig. 2). These epoxides are hydrolyzed by epoxide hydrolase to form DB[*a*, *l*]P(dibenzo[*a*, *l*]pyrene)-11, 12-diol and 7, 12-DMBA-3, 4-diol, which are finally oxidized again by CYPs to the ultimate carcinogenic metabolites, DB[*a*, *l*]P-11, 12-diol-13, 14-epoxide and 7, 12-DMBA-3, 4-diol-1, 2-epoxide, respectively (Fig. 2) (*1, 26, 27*).

Other typical PAH compounds considered to be activated in accordance with the bay region theory include benz[*a*]anthracene, benzo[*b*]fluoranthene, benzo[*c*]phenanthrene, benzo[*g*]chrysene, chrysene, 5, 6-dimethylchrysene and 5-

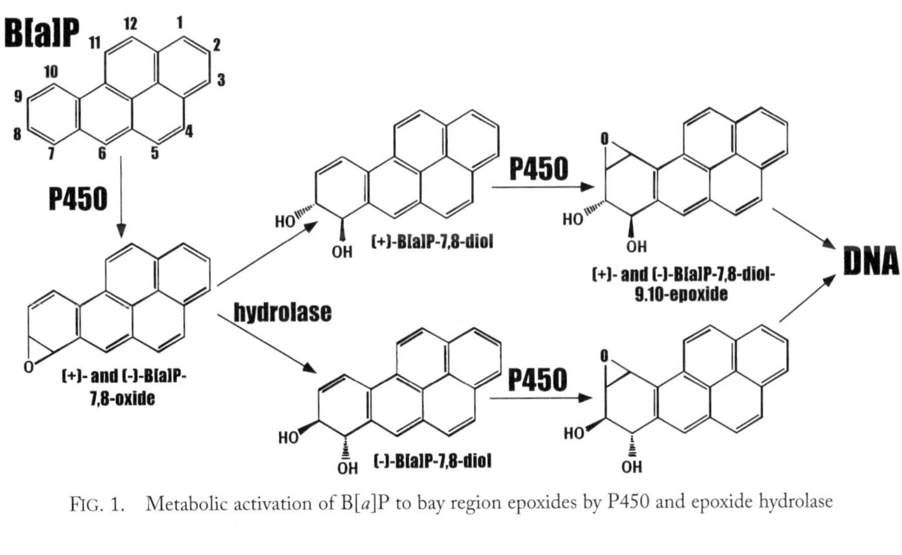

FIG. 1. Metabolic activation of B[*a*]P to bay region epoxides by P450 and epoxide hydrolase

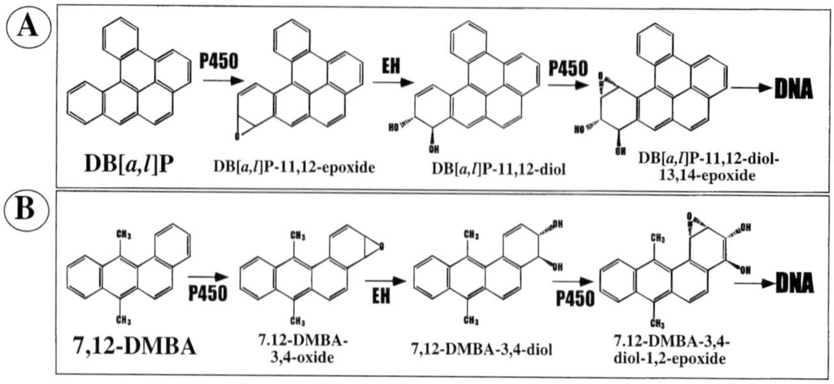

FIG. 2. Metabolic activation of DB[*a*, *l*]P (A) and 7, 12-DMBA (B) to bay region epoxides by P450 and epoxide hydrolase

methylchrysene (*26, 28*). Indeed, the reactive intermediates of these PAH dihydrodiols were activated by human CYPs to DNA-modifying products in *S. typhimurium* NM2009 tester strain with the highest reaction rate for 5-methylchrysene 1, 2-diol as substrate (Fig. 3) (*3, 29*).

In this review, we wish to focus attention to the diol-epoxide pathway of PAHs metabolic activation by CYPs. Readers who are interested in further pathways of PAH metabolism other than those described above may refer to additional review articles (*1, 11, 17*).

Roles of CYP1A1 and 1B1 in the Metabolic Activation of PAHs

Until early 1990, when CYP1B1 was first identified in mouse embryonic fibroblast cells and rat adrenal glands (*30, 31*), CYP1A1 had been thought to be uniquely responsible for the metabolic activation of most of the carcinogenic PAHs (*1, 5, 32*). In 1991, mouse CYP1B1 protein was purified from C3H/10T1/2 CL8 cells derived from an embryonic fibroblast. The purified enzyme, when reconstituted with NADPH-P450 reductase on phospholipid vesicles, had a high turnover rate for the metabolism of 7, 12-DMBA (*31*). Subsequently, the cDNA clone for mouse CYP1B1 was obtained and an expression plasmid of the cDNA was engineered for protein production in *Escherichia coli* (*34*). The bacterially derived recombinant mouse CYP1B1 enzyme was found to transform 7, 12-DMBA to several oxidized products at high rates. Additional spectroscopical studies suggested that purified mouse CYP1B1 was able to interact with several polycyclic aromatic hydrocarbons such as B[*a*]P, benz[*a*]anthracene, 7, 12-DMBA, 3-methylcholanthrene and 1-ethynylpyrene (*34*). In rat, CYP1B1 was first identified in adrenal microsomes as a novel ACTH-inducible P450RAP and was found to oxidize several polycyclic aromatic hydrocarbons including 7, 12-DMBA (*30, 35*). RNA blot analysis using the isolated cDNA as probe demonstrated that the mRNA for CYP1B1 was expressed ubiquitously in various tissues of rat, including adrenal, ovary, liver, lung, uterus, and kidney (*14, 36*).

Human CYP1B1 cDNA was isolated in 1994 and was introduced into a yeast expression vector (*3, 37*). Yeast microsomes containing the expressed CYP1B1 protein activated diverse procarcinogens including PAHs, aryl- and heterocyclic amines

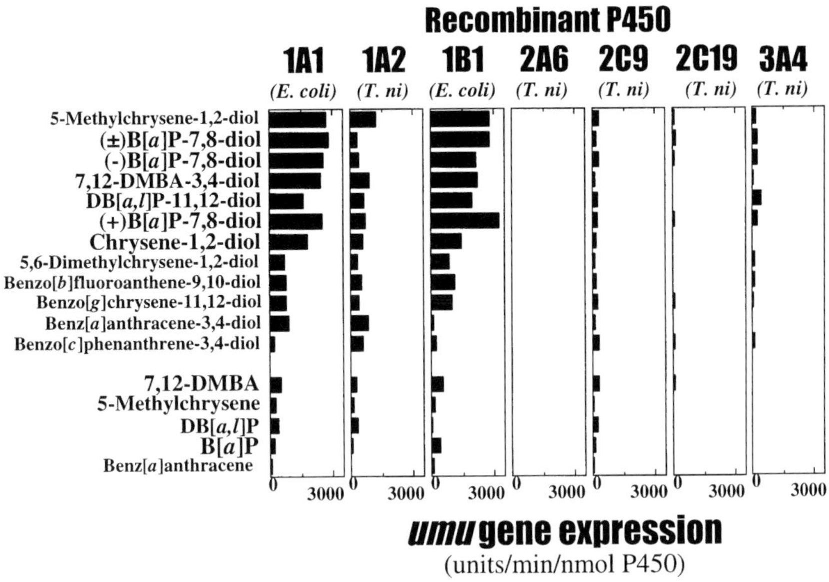

FIG. 3. Activation of PAHs and their dihydrodiol derivatives to DNA-damaging products by recombinant human P450 enzymes in *S. typhimurium* NM2009

Recombinant P450s from *Escherichia coli* (CYP1A1 and 1B1) and from *Trichoplusia ni* cells (CYP1A2, 2A6, 2C9, 2C19 and 3A4) were used. Data were obtained from Shimada *et al.* (*39*) with slight modifications.

and nitroarenes to mutagenic products as determined by the *umu* gene expression system using the *S. typhimurium* NM2009 tester strain (*3*, *29*, *38*). Interestingly, a close resemblance was found in the substrate specificities of CYP1A1 and 1B1 towards various procarcinogens and promutagens, particularly when dihydrodiol derivatives of PAHs were used as substrates (Fig. 3) (*3*, *39*). Human CYP1A2 displayed significant activity towards several PAH-diols, though to a lesser degree than CYP1A1 and 1B1. Other human CYPs such as CYP2A6, 2C9, 2C19 and 3A4 were all relatively weak at activating these PAH compounds (Fig. 3).

Is there any difference in the catalytic specificities of CYP1A1 and 1B1 toward the activation of PAHs? Buters *et al.* (*40*) reported that cultured embryonic fibroblast cells isolated from CYP1B1-null mice, which were incapable of metabolizing 7, 12-DMBA, were resistant to the cytotoxicity caused by 7, 12-DMBA. The inability of 7, 12-DMBA to produce malignant lymphomas and other tumors was also observed in CYP1B1-null mice (*40*). In a similar line of investigation, Doehmer and his associates reported that recombinant human CYP1A1 and 1B1 differ in their regio- and stereochemical selectivity for the activation of DB[*a*, *l*]P and further, that CYP1B1 played more important roles than CYP1A1 in the formation of bay (fjord) region DB[*a*, *l*]P-11, 12-diol-13, 14-epoxides (*27*, *41*, *42*). In support of these findings, Buters *et al.* reported that DB[*a*, *l*]P did not produce any type of malignant or benign tumor in ovaries or lymphoid tissues of CYP1B1-null mice (*43*). These results suggest that CYP1B1 may play important roles in the metabolic activation of two prototype carcinogens DB[*a*, *l*]P and 7, 12-DMBA to toxic and carcinogenic metabolites.

Carcinogenesis Induced by B[a]P in Wild-type and AhR Knockout Mice

AhR is responsible for the inducible expression of several xenobiotic-metabolizing enzymes including CYP1A1 and CYP1B1 by PAHs and 2, 3, 7, 8-tetrachlorodibenzo-*p*-dioxin (TCDD) (*1, 44–46*). Mechanisms of inducible expression of CYP1A1 by these compounds have been extensively studied using TCDD as a prototype inducer (*47, 48*). It has been reported that there is an enhancer region with five conserved, putative XREs (xenobiotic response elements) in the upstream 5′-flanking sequence of *CYP1B1* gene closely resembling those of the *CYP1A1* gene (*48–51*). Furthermore, CYP1B1 is induced by TCDD in human carcinoma cell lines such as mammary carcinoma (*52, 53*), renal adenocarcinoma (ACHN) (*54*) and squamous cell carcinoma (SCC12) (*55*). TCDD and other AhR agonists induce CYP1B1 by an AhR-dependent mechanism similar to CYP1A1 (*53, 56, 57*). However, some differences were reported in the mode of induction of CYP1A1 and 1B1 by TCDD (*52, 57*). For example, the dose response and the time course of CYP1B1 induction by TCDD was found to differ from that of CYP1A1 and CYP1A2 in rats (*58, 59*). Walker *et al.* (*36*) have also reported that there are sex-related differences in the induction of CYP1B1 and CYP1A1 by TCDD in several organs of rats (*36*). It remains unclear whether, in experimental animals and humans, different regulatory mechanisms govern the induction of CYP1A1 and CYP1B1 by TCDD and other chemicals (*16, 60*). Using a mouse Hepa-1 variant LA2 cell line defective in expression of Arnt, Eltom *et al.* (*56*) have shown that expression of CYP1A1 is extremely low and even unresponsive to TCDD, whereas basal CYP1B1 mRNA and protein levels were similar to those seen in wild type Hepa-1 cells treated with TCDD. It has been reported that in mouse fibroblast C3H/10T1/2CL8 cells, the expression of CYP1B1 relies upon both AhR-dependent transcription activation and protein stabilization (*60*). Different responses in the expressions of *CYP1A1* and *CYP1B1* genes to TCDD treatment have been reported in human breast cancer MCF-7 and MDA-MB 231 cell lines (*61*) and in human hepatoblastoma line HepG2 (*54*). AhR-dependent induction of CYP1A1, CYP1B1 and other genes has been reported to be influenced by interaction of AhR with negative and positive regulators, particularly in a tissue- and species-dependent manner (*46, 62*).

Shimizu *et al.* (*63*) have reported that topical application and subcutaneous injection of B[*a*]P induced skin tumors in AhR(+/+) mice but not in AhR(−/−) mice. They suggest a possible role for CYP1A1 in B[*a*]P-induced carcinogenesis in AhR(+/+) mice because they observed no expression of CYP1A1 in the skin of the AhR-null mice. It would be interesting to see whether or not CYP1B1 is expressed in the skin of the AhR-null mice. Our recent studies showed that B[*a*]P and other carcinogenic PAHs, such as 7, 12-DMBA, DB[*a*, *l*]P, 3-MC (3-methylcholanthrene), benzo[*b*]fluoranthene, 5-mrthylchrysene, and dibenz[*a*, *h*]anthracene, induce CYP1B1 as well as CYP1A1 in liver and lung of AhR(+/+) mice, but not in those of AhR(−/−) mice (Fig. 4) (*64*). Further studies on tissue-specific expression and induction of mRNAs of CYP1A1 and 1B1 by these PAHs suggested that CYP1A1 and CYP1B1 are differentially regulated in their expression in extrahepatic organs of mice (*65*). For example, CYP1B1 is expressed at significant levels in heart, kidney, intestine, testis and brain of AhR(−/−) mice as well as AhR(+/+) mice, contrasting with CYP1A1 whose expression is very low or below the detection limit of in these

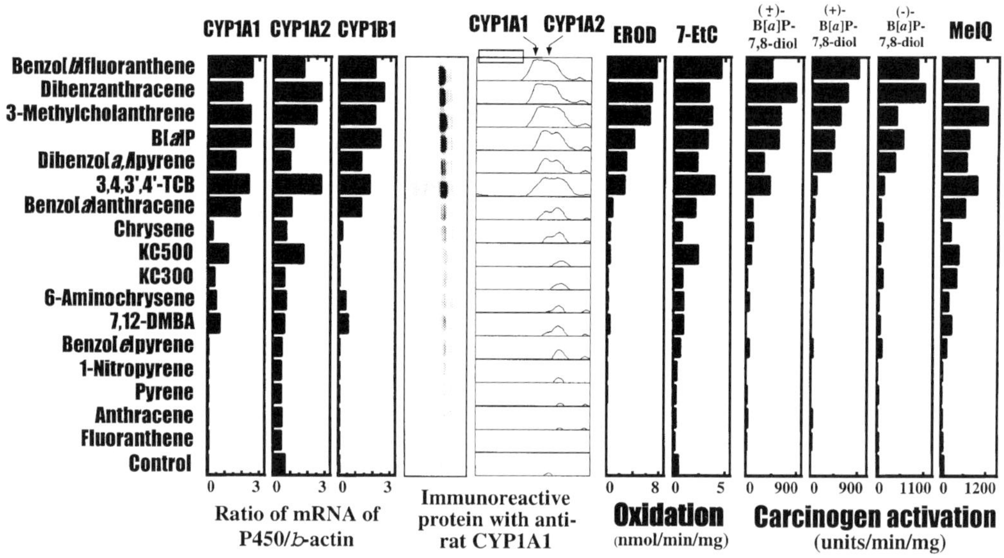

FIG. 4. Induction of mRNA, protein and catalytic activity of liver CYP1A1, 1A2 and 1B1 by PAHs and 3, 4, 3′, 4′-tetrachlorobiphenyl (3, 4, 3′, 4′-TCB) and PCB mixtures Kanechloro 300 and 500 (KC300 and KC500) in AhR(+/+) mice

Levels of liver P450 mRNAs were determined relative to β-actin mRNA. Immunoblotting analysis to detect P450 proteins in liver microsomes of PAH-treated mice was done with anti-rat CYP1A1 IgG. Liver microsomal xenobiotic oxidation activities were determined with the substrates 7-ethoxyresorufin, 7-ethoxycoumarin, (±)-B[*a*]P-7, 8-diol, (+)- B[*a*]P-7, 8-diol, (−)- B[*a*]P-7, 8-diol and MeIQ. Data were obtained from Shimada *et al.* (*64*) with slight modifications.

organs of AhR(−/−) mice (*65*). Further work will be required to determine whether CYP1A1 and 1B1 make different contributions to the occurrence of tumor formation in experimental animals and humans.

As described above, B[*a*]P is activated by CYPs to form bay region epoxides by two activation steps (*2*, *11*, *17*). The first step in the activation of B[*a*]P is the formation of B[*a*]P-7, 8-oxide by the action of CYP, followed by formation of B[*a*]P-7, 8-diol by microsomal epoxide hydrolase (*17*). It has been shown that recombinant human CYP1B1 is more active than CYP1A1 in catalyzing oxidation of B[*a*]P to B[*a*]P-7, 8-diol when human or rat liver epoxide hydrolase is present in the reaction mixture (*66*). The dihydrodiol metabolites thus produced are activated by CYP1A1 and CYP1B1 to DNA-damaging products at almost similar rates in the *S. typhimurium* NM2009 tester strain (*3*, *29*). Taken together, these results suggested that CYP1B1 may be more significant for the first step oxidation of B[*a*]P at the 7, 8-position and thus play a more important role than CYP1A1 in the tumorigenesis caused by B[*a*]P. In this regard, it is interesting to note the recent work by Uno *et al.* (*67*) who showed that CYP1A1-knockout mice produced increased levels of hepatic B[*a*]P-DNA adducts *in vivo*, as compared with those of wild-type mice.

Genetic Polymorphisms of CYP1A1 and 1B1 and Cancer Susceptibilities

Many types of genetic polymorphisms in *CYP1A1* and *1B1* have been identified in humans and some of them are reported to relate to susceptibilities in lung and breast cancer (*50*, *68–72*). On the contrary, results have also been reported that there is no relationship between genetic polymorphisms in *CYP1A1* and *1B1* and cancer sueceptibility in humans (*73–76*). Race-related differences in the occurrence of genetic polymorphisms in CYP species including CYP1A1 and 1B1 have been reported and these differences make it difficult to interpret the possible roles of CYP genetic polymorphisms in cancer susceptibility in humans (*76*, *77*). Biochemical studies have been carried out to investigate the catalytic activity variant forms of CYP1A1 and 1B1 exhibit towards a number of environmental carcinogens (*78–81*). Although much have been learned about the roles of variant forms of CYP1A1 and 1B1 in the metabolic activation of PAHs and other carcinogens, further work is required before any final conclusion can be drawn about the link between *CYP1A1* and *1B1* genetic polymorphisms and cancer susceptibility of individuals of the human population.

Chemoprevention

As described, most procarcinogenic PAHs require the metabolic activation by the oxidative action of CYPs to exhibit carcinogenicity and the chemicals which inhibit the CYP activity are expected to work as preventive agents against chemical carcinogonesis. Many chemicals including (*82*, *83*) α-naphthoflavone, synthetic chemopreventive organoselenium compounds such as 1, 2-, 1, 3 and 1, 4-phenylenebis(methylene) selenocyanate (*o*-, *m*- and *p*-XSC, respectively), vinylic and acetylenic polycyclic aromatic hydrocarbons such as 1-(1-propynyl) pyrene, 2-(1-propynyl) phenanthrene, 1-ethynylpyrene, 2-ethynylpyrene and 4-(1-propynyl) biphenyl have been identified as inhibitors of CYP1A1 and 1B1. Recently, Chun *et al.* have reported that the natural products, resveratrol and rhapontigenin, are potent inhibitors of human CYP1A1 (*84*, *85*). Resverotrol was shown to inhibit human CYP1B1 in a non-competitive manner, while it inhibits CYP1A1 competitively (*85*). Chun *et al.* have also revealed that 2, 4, 3′, 5′-tetramethoxystilbene is a potent and selective inhibitor of CYP1B1 (*86*).

It has been suggested that some of these inhibitors of CYP1A1 and 1B1 suppress tumorigenesis induced by a variety of chemical carcinogens (*87–91*). In a rat mammary tumor model system using 7, 12-DMBA as a prototype carcinogen, 1, 4-phenylenebis (methylene) selenocyanate (*p*-XSC) has been shown to have chemopreventive activity (*90*, *91*) and *o*- and *m*-XSC appear to be better inhibitors of 7, 12-DMBA-DNA adduct formation in rat mammary gland (*92*, *93*). These synthetic organoselenium compounds were found to be potent inhibitors of human CYP1A1 and CYP1B1 with more selectivity in inhibiting CYP1B1 activities (*82*). Likewise, 1-ethynylpyrene inhibits covalent binding of 7,12-DMBA and B[*a*]P to the epidermal DNA (*94*) and consequently prevents tumor formation caused by 7, 12-DMBA and B[*a*]P in mouse skin (*95*). 1- and 2-Ethynylpyrenes are relatively selective inhibitors for CYP1B1. As described above, resveratrol which is found in red grapes, shown to have cancer prevention activity, is a potent inhibitor of human CYP1A1 and 1B1 (*85*, *96*, *97*).

Conclusion

CYP1A1 and 1B1 are the two enzymes involved in the activation of a number of carcinogenic PAHs to reactive electrophiles that initiate cell transformation. These enzymes have similar, but not identical, substrate specificity towards various types of PAHs. CYP1A1 and 1B1 are expressed mainly in extrahepatic organs of animals and are highly induced by carcinogenic PAHs and TCDD through AhR. Genetic polymorphisms in CYP1A1 and 1B1 may determine the different susceptibilities of individual humans to carcinogenesis caused by the action of PAHs. Further study is needed to define the impact of variant forms of CYP1A1 on the incidence of cancers in humans.

Acknowledgment

We would like to thank Dr. V. Kelly (University of Tsukuba, TARA center) for critical reading of the manuscript and Mrs. Y. Nemoto (University of Tsukuba, TARA center) for typographical work.

REFERENCES

1. Conney AH. Induction of microsomal enzymes by foreign chemicals and carcinogenesis by polycyclic aromatic hydrocarbons: G.H.A. Clowes memorial lecture. *Cancer Res* 1982; **4**: 4875–917.
2. Guengerich FP, Shimada T. Oxidation of toxic and carcinogenic chemicals by human cytochrome P-450 enzymes. *Chem Res Toxicol* 1991; **4**: 391–407.
3. Shimada T, Hayes CL, Yamazaki H, Amin S, Hecht SS, Guengerich FP, Sutter TR. Activation of chemically diverse procarcinogens by human cytochrome P450 1B1. *Cancer Res* 1996; **56**: 2979–84.
4. Aeschbacher H-U Turesky RJ. Mammalian cell mutagenicity and metabolism of heterocyclic aromatic amines. *Mutat Res* 1991; **259**: 235–50.
5. Shimada T, Iwasaki M, Martin MV, Guengerich FP. Human liver microsomal cytochrome P-450 enzymes involved in the bioactivation of procarcinogens detected by *umu* gene response in *Salmonella typhimurium* TA1535/pSK1002. *Cancer Res* 1989; **49**: 3218–28.
6. Yamazaki H, Inui Y, Yun CH, Guengerich FP, Shimada T. Cytochrome P450 2E1 and 2A6 enzymes as major catalysts for metabolic activation of *N*-nitrosodialkylamines and tobacco-related nitrosamines in human liver microsomes. *Carcinogenesis* 1992; **13**: 1789–94.
7. Kushida H, Fujita K, Suzuki A, Yamada M, Endo T, Nohmi T, Kamataki T. Metabolic activation of *N*-alkylnitrosamines in genetically engineered *Salmonella typhimurium* expressing CYP2E1 or CYP2A6 together with human NADPH-cytochrome P450. *Carcinogenesis* 2000; **21**: 1227–32.
8. Guengerich FP, Kim DH, Iwasaki M. Role of human cytochrome P-450 IIE1 in the oxidation of many low molecular weight cancer suspects. *Chem Res Toxicol* 1991; **4**: 168–79.
9. Shimada T, Guengerich FP. Evidence for cytochrome P-450NF, the nifedipine oxidase, being the principal enzyme involved in the bioactivation of aflatoxins in human liver. *Proc Natl Acad Sci USA* 1989; **86**: 462–5.
10. Imaoka S, Hiroi T, Tamura Y, Yamazaki H, Shimada T, Komori M, Degawa M, Funae, Y. Mutagenic activation of 3-methoxy-4-aminoazobenzene by mouse renal cy-

tochrome P450 CYP4B1: cloning and characterization of mouse CYP4B1. *Arch Biochem Biophys* 1995; **321**: 255–62.

11. Pelkonen O, Nebert DW. Metabolism of polycyclic aromatic hydrocarbons: etiologic role in carcinogenesis. *Pharmacol Rev* 1982; **34**: 189–222.
12. Kapitulnik J, Wislocki PG, Levin W, Yagi H, Jerina DM, Conney AH. Tumorigenicity studies with diol-epoxides of benzo(*a*)pyrene which indicate that (±)-*trans*-7β, 8α-dihydroxy-9α, 10α-epoxy-7, 8, 9, 10-tetrahydrobenzo(*a*)pyrene is an ultimate carcinogen in newborn mice. *Cancer Res* 1978; **38**: 354–8.
13. Spink DC, Spink BC, Cao JQ, De Pasquale JA, Pentecost BT, Fasco MJ, Li Y, Sutter TR. Differential expression of CYP1A1 and CYP1B1 in human breast epithelial cells and breast tumor cells. *Carcinogenesis* 1998; **19**: 291–8.
14. Bhattacharyya KK, Brake PB, Eltom SE, Otto SA, Jefcoate CR. Identification of a rat adrenal cytochrome P450 active in polycyclic hydrocarbon metabolism as rat CYP1B1. *J Biol Chem* 1995; **270**: 11595–602.
15. Huang Z, Fasco MJ, Figge HL, Keyomars FK, Kaminsky LS. Expression of cytochromes P450 in human breast tissue and tumors. *Drug Metab Dispos* 1996; **24**: 899–905.
16. Hakkola J, Pasanen M, Pelkonen O, Hukkanen J, Evisalmi S, Anttila S, Rane A, Mantyla M, Purkunen R, Saarikoski S, Tooming M, Raunio H. Expression of CYP1B1 in human adult and fetal tissues and differential inducibility of CYP1B1 and CYP1A1 by Ah receptor ligands in human placenta and cultured cells. *Carcinogenesis* 1997; **18**: 391–7.
17. Gelboin HV. Benzo[*a*]pyrene metabolism, activation, and carcinogenesis: role and regulation of mixed-function oxidases and related enzymes. *Physiol Rev* 1980; **60**: 1107–66.
18. Miller JA. Carcinogenesis by chemicals: an overview. *Cancer Res* 1970; **30**: 559–76.
19. Jerina DM, Daly JW. Arene oxides: a new aspect of drug metabolism. *Science* 1974; **185**: 573–82.
20. Tang M-shong, Vulimiri SV, Viaje A, Chen JX, Bilolikar DS, Morris RJ, Harvey RG, Slaga TJ, DiGiovanni J. Both (±)*syn*- and (±)*anti*-7, 12-dimethylbenz[*a*]anthracene-3, 4-diol-1, 2-epoxides initiate tumors in mouse skin that possess -CAA- to CTA- mutations at codon 61 of c-H-*ras*. *Cancer Res* 2000; **60**: 5688–95.
21. Buening MK, Wislocki PG, Levin W, Yagi H, Thakker DR, Akagi H, Koreeda M, Jerina DM, Conney AH. Tumorigenicity of the optical enantiomers of the diastereomeric benzo[*a*]pyrene 7, 8-diol-9, 10-epoxides in newborn mice: exceptional activity of (+)-7β, 8α-dihydroxy-9α, 10α-epoxy-7, 8, 9, 10-tetrahy drobenzo[*a*]pyrene. *Proc Natl Acad Sci USA* 1978; **75**: 5358–61.
22. Wood AW, Chang RL, Levin W, Yagi H, Thakker DR, Jerina DM, Conney AH. Differences in mutagenicity of the optical enantiomers of the diastereomeric benzo[*a*]pyrene 7, 8-diol-9, 10-epoxides. *Biochem Biophys Res Commun* 1977; **77**: 1389–96.
23. Kapitulnik J, Levin W, Conney AH, Yagi H, Jerina DM. Benzo[*a*]pyrene 7, 8-dihydrodiol is more carcinogenic than benzo[*a*]pyrene in newborn mice. *Nature* 1977; **266**: 378–80.
24. Levin W, Wood AW, Yagi H, Jerina DM, Conney AH. (±)-*trnas*-7, 8-Dihydroxy-7,

8-dihydrobenzo[*a*]pyrene: a potent skin carcinogen when applied topically to mice. *Proc Natl Acad Sci USA* 1976; **73**: 3867–71.

25. Adams JD, Yagi H, Levin W, Jerina DM. Stereo-selectivity and regio-selectivity in the metabolism of 7, 8-dihydrobenzo[*a*]pyrene by cytochrome P450, epoxide hydrolase and hepatic microsomes from 3-methylcholanthrene-treated rats. *Chem Biol Interact* 1995; **95**: 57–77.
26. Marquardt H, Baker S, Tierney B, Crover PL, Sims P. Induction of malignant transformation and mutagenesis by dihydrodiols derived from 7, 12-dimethylbbenz[*a*]anthracene. *Biochem Biophys Res Commun* 1978; **85**: 357–62.
27. Luch A, Schober W, Soballa VJ, Raab G, Greim H, Jacob J, Doehmer J, Seidel A. Metabolic activation of dibenzo[*a, l*]pyrene by human cytochrome P450 1A1 and 1B1 expressed in V79 Chinese hamster cells. *Chem Res Toxicol* 1999; **12**: 353–64.
28. Yang SK. Stereoselectivity of cytochrome P-450 isozymes and epoxide hydrolase in the metabolism of polycyclic aromatic hydrocarbons. *Biochem Pharmacol* 1988; **37**: 61–70.
29. Shimada T, Watanabe J, Kawajiri K, Sutter TR. Guengerich FP, Gillam EMJ, Inoue K. Catalytic properties of polymorphic human cytochrome P450 1B1 variants. *Carcinogenesis* 1999; **20**: 1607–13.
30. Otto S, Bhattacharyya KK, Jefcoate CR. Polycyclic aromatic hydrocarbon metabolism in rat adrenal, ovary, and testis microsomes is catalyzed by the same novel cytochrome P450 (P450RAP). *Endocrinology* 1992; **131**: 3067–76.
31. Pottenger LH, Christou M, Jefcoate CR. Purification and immunological characterization of a novel cytochrome P450 from C3H/10T1/2 cells. *Arch Biochem Biophys* 1991; **286**: 488–97.
32. Guengerich FP. Roles of cytochrome P-450 enzymes in chemical carcinogenesis and cancer chemotherapy. *Cancer Res* 1988; **48**: 2946–54.
33. Savas U, Bhattacharyya KK, Christou M, Alexander DL, Jefcoate CR. Mouse cytochrome P-450EF, representative of a new *1B* subfamily of cytochrome P-450s. *J Biol Chem* 1994; **269**: 14905–11.
34. Savas U, Carstens C-P, Jefcoate CR. Recombinant mouse CYP1B1 expressed in *Eschericha coli* exhibits selective binding by polycyclic hydrocarbons and metabolism which parallels C3H10T1/2 cell microsomes, but differs from human recombinant CYP1B1. *Arch Biochem Biophys* 1997; **347**: 181–92.
35. Otto S, Marcus C, Pidgeon C, Jefcoate C. A novel adrenocorticotropin-inducible cytochrome P450 from rat adrenal microsomes catalyzes polycyclic aromatic hydrocarbon metabolism. *Endocrinology* 1991; **129**: 970–82.
36. Walker NJ, Gastel JA, Costa LT, Clark GC, Lucier GW, Sutter TR. Rat CYP1B1: an adrenal cytochrome P450 that exhibits sex dependent expression in livers and kidneys of TCDD-treated animals. *Carcinogenesis* 1995; **16**: 1319–27.
37. Sutter TR, Guzman K, Dold KM, Greenlee WF. Targets for dioxin: Genes for plasminogen activator inhibitor-2 and interleukin-1b. *Science* 1995; **254**: 415–8.
38. Shimada T, Wunsch RM, Hanna IH, Sutter TR, Guengerich FP, Gillam EMJ. Recombinant human cytochrome P450 1B1 expression in *Escherichia coli. Arch Biochem Biophys* 1998; **357**: 111–20.
39. Shimada T, Oda Y, Inoue K. Metabolic activation of polycyclic aromatic hydrocarbons and other procarcinogens by cytochromes P450 1A1 and P450 1B1 allelic variants and

other human cytochromes P450 in *Salmonella. Drug Metab Dispos* 2001; **29**: 1176–82.

40. Buters JTM, Sakai S, Richter T, Pineau T, Alexander DL, Savas U, Doehmer J, Ward JM, Jefcoate CR, Gonzalez FJ. Cytochrome P450 CYP1B1 determines susceptibility to 7, 12-dimethylbenz[*a*]anthracene-induced lymphomas. *Proc Natl Acad Sci USA* 1999; **96**: 1977–82.
41. Luch A, Coffing SL, Tang YM, Schneider A, Soballa V, Greim H, Jefcoate CR, Seidel A, Greenlee WF, Baird WM, Doehmer J. Stable expression of human cytochrome P450 1B1 in V79 Chinese hamster cells and metabolically catalyzed DNA adduct formation of dibenzo[*a*, *l*]pyrene. *Chem Res Toxicol* 1998; **11**: 686–95.
42. King LC, Adams L, Allison J, Kohan MJ, Nelson G, Desai D, Amin S, Ross JA. A quantitative comparison of dibenzo[*a*, *l*]pyrene-DNA adduct formation by recombinant human cytochrome P450 microsomes. *Mol Carcinogenesis* 1999; **26**: 74–82.
43. Buters JTM, Mahadevan B, Quintanilla-Martinez L, Gonzalez FJ, Greim H, Baird WM, Luch A. Cytochrome P450 1B1 determines susceptibility to dibenzo[*a*, *l*]pyrene-induced tumor formation. *Chem Res Toxicol* 2002; **15**: 1127–35.
44. Nebert DW, Eisen HJ, Negishi M, Lang MA, Hjelmeland LM. Genetic mechanisms controlling the induction of polysubstrate monooxygenase (P-450) activities. *Annu Rev Pharmacol Toxicol* 1981; **21**: 431–62.
45. Gonzalez FJ. Molecular genetics of the P-450 superfamily. *Pharmacol Ther* 1990; **45**: 1–38.
46. Hankinson O. The aryl hydrocarbon receptor complex. *Annu Rev Pharmacol Toxicol* 1995; **35**: 307–40.
47. Zhang L, Savas U, Alexander DL, Jefcoate CR. Characterization of the mouse *Cyp1B1* gene: identification of an enhancer region that directs aryl hydrocarbon receptor-mediated constitutive and induced expression. *J Biol Chem* 1998; **273**: 5174–83.
48. Whitlock JP. Induction of cytochrome P4501A1. *Annu Rev Pharmacol Toxicol* 1999; **39**: 103–25.
49. Sogawa K, Fujisawa-Sehara A, Yamane M, Fujii-Kuriyama Y. Location of regulatory elements responsible for drug induction in the rat cytochrome P-450c gene. *Proc Natl Acad Sci USA* 1986; **83**: 8044–8.
50. Kawajiri K, Fujii-Kuriyama Y. P450 and human cancer. *Jpn J Cancer Res* 1991; **82**: 1325–35.
51. Kubota M, Sogawa K, Kaizu Y, Sawaya T, Watanabe J, Kawajiri K, Gotoh O, Fujii-Kuriyama Y. Xenobiotic responsive element in the 5′-upstream region of the human P-450c gene. *J Biochem (Tokyo)* 1991; **110**: 232–6.
52. Eltom SE, Larsen MC, Jefcoate CR. Expression of CYP1B1 but not CYP1A1 by primary cultured human mammary stromal fibroblasts constitutively and in response to dioxin exposure: role of the Ah receptor. *Carcinogenesis* 1998; **19**: 1437–44.
53. Christou M, Savas U, Spink DC, Gierthy JF, Jefcoate CR. Co-expression of human CYP1A1 and a human analog of cytochrome P450-EF in response to 2, 3, 7, 8-tetrachlorodibenzo-*p*-dioxin in the human mammary carcinoma-derived MCF-7 cells. *Carcinogenesis* 1994; **15**: 725–32.
54. Kress S, Greenlee WF. Cell-specific regulation of human *CYP1A1* and *CYP1B1* genes. *Cancer Res* 1997; **57**: 1264–9.
55. Sutter TR, Tang YM, Hayes CL, Wo Y-YP, Jabs W, Li X, Yin H, Cody CW, Greenlee

WF. Complete cDNA sequence of a human dioxin-inducible mRNA identifies a new gene subfamily of cytochrome P450 that maps to chromosome 2. *J Biol Chem* 1994; **269**: 13092–9.

56. Eltom SE, Zhang L, Jefcoate CR. Regulation of cytochrome P-450 (CYP) 1B1 in mouse hepa-1 variant cell lines: a possible role for aryl hydrocarbon receptor nuclear translocator (ARNT) as a suppressor of *CYP1B1* gene expression. *Mol Pharmacol* 1999; **55**: 594–604.
57. Brake PB, Zhang L, Jefcoate CR. Aryl hydrocarbon receptor regulation of cytochrome P4501B1 in rat mammary fibroblasts: evidence for transcriptional repression by glucocorticoids. *Mol Pharmacol* 1998; **54**: 825–33.
58. Walker NJ, Crofts FG, Li Y, Lax SF, Hayes CL, Strickland PT, Lucier GW, Sutter TR. Induction and localization of cytochrome P450 1B1 (CYP1B1) protein in the livers of TCDD-treated rats: detection using polyclonal antibodies raised to histidine-tagged fusion proteins produced and purified from bacteria. *Carcinogenesis* 1998; **19**: 395–402.
59. Warker NJ, Portier CJ, Lax SF, Crofts FG, Li Y, Lucier GW, Sutter TR. Characterization of the dose-response of CYP1B1, CYP1A1, and CYP1A2 in the liver of female Sprague-Dawley rats following chronic eposure to 2, 3, 7, 8-tetrachlorodibenzo-*p*-dioxin. *Toxicol Appl Pharmacol* 1999; **154**: 279–86.
60. Savas U, Jefcoate CR. Dual regulation of cytochrome P450EF expression via the aryl hydrocarbon receptor and protein stabilization in C3H/10T1/2 cells. *Mol Pharmacol* 1994; **45**: 1153–9.
61. Dohr O, Vogel C, Abel J. Different response of 2, 3, 7, 8-tetrachlorodibenzo-*p*-dioxin (TCDD)-sensitive genes in human breast cancer MCF-7 and MDA-MB 231 cells. *Arch Biochem Biophys* 1995; **321**: 405–12.
62. Takahashi Y, Nakayama K, Itoh S, Fujii-Kuriyama Y, Kamataki T. Inhibition of the transcription of *CYP1A1* gene by the upstream stimulatory factor 1 in rabbits. *J Biol Chem* 1997; **272**: 30025–31.
63. Shimizu Y, Nakatsuru Y, Ichinose M, Takahashi Y, Kume H, Mimura J, Fujii-Kuriyama Y, Ishikawa T. Benzo[*a*]pyrene carcinogenicity is lost in mice lacking the aryl hydrocarbon receptor. *Proc Natl Acad Sci USA* 2000; **97**: 779–82.
64. Shimada T, Inoue K, Suzuki Y, Kawai T, Azuma E, Nakajima T, Shindo M, Kurose K, Sugie A, Yamagishi Y, Fujii-Kuriyama Y, Hashimoto M. Arylhydrocarbon receptor-dependent induction of liver and lung cytochromes P450 1A1, 1A2, and 1B1 by polycyclic aromatic hydrocarbons and polychlorinated biphenyls in genetically engineered C57BL/6J mice. *Carcinogenesis* 2002; **23**: 1199–207.
65. Shimada T, Sugie A, Shindo M, Nakajima T, Azuma E, Hashimoto M, Inoue K. Tissue-specific induction of cytochromes P450 1A1 and 1B1 by polycyclic aromatic hydrocarbons and polychlorinated biphenyls in engineered C57BL/6J mice of *Arylhydrocarbon Receptor* gene. *Toxicol Appl Pharmacol* 2003; **187**: 1–10.
66. Shimada T, Gillam EMJ, Oda Y, Tsumura F, Sutter TR, Guengerich FP, Inoue K. Metabolism of benzo[*a*]pyrene to *trans*-7, 8-dihydroxy-7, 8-dihydrobenzo[*a*]pyrene by recombinant human cytochrome P450 1B1 and purified liver epoxide hydrolase. *Chem Res Toxicol* 1999; **12**: 623–9.
67. Uno S, Dalton TP, Shertzer HG, Genter MB, Warshawsky D, Talaska G, Nebert DW.

Benzo[*a*]pyrene-induced toxicity: paradoxical protection in *Cyp1a1* (−/−) knockout mice having increased hepatic BaP-DNA adduct levels. *Biochem Biophys Res Commun* 2001; **289**: 1049–56.

68. Kawajiri K, Nakachi K, Imai K, Yoshii A, Shinoda N, Watanabe J. Identification of genetically high risk individuals to lung cancer by DNA polymorphisms of the cytochrome P4501A1 gene. *FEBS Lett* 1990; **263**: 131–3.
69. Nakachi K, Imai K, Hayashi S, Kawajiri K. Genetic susceptibility to squamous cell carcinoma of the lung in relation to cigarette smoking dose. *Cancer Res* 1991; **51**: 5177–80.
70. Hayashi S, Watanabe J, Kawajiri K. High susceptibility to lung cancer analyzed in terms of combined genotypes of P4501A1 and Mu-class glutathione *S*-transferase genes. *Jpn J Cancer Res* 1992; **83**: 866–70.
71. Nakachi K, Imai K, Hayashi S, Kawajiri K. Polymorphisms of the *CYP1A1* and glutathione S-transferase genes associated with susceptibility to lung cancer in relation to cigarette dose in a Japanese population. *Cancer Res* 1993; **53**: 2994–9.
72. Watanabe J, Shimada T, Gillam EMJ, Ikuta T, Suemasu K, Higashi Y, Gotoh O, Kawajiri K. Association of *CYP1B1* genetic polymorphism with incidence to breast and lung cancer. *Pharmacogenetics* 2000; **10**: 25–33.
73. Wedlund PJ, Kimura S, Gonzalez FJ, Nebert DW. 1462V mutation in the human *CYP1A1* gene: lack of correlation with either the Msp I 1.9kb (M2) allele or CYP1A1 inducibility in a three-generation family of east mediterranean descent. *Pharmacogenetics* 1994; **4**: 21–6.
74. Kelsey KT, Wiencke JK, Spitz, MR. A race-specific genetic polymorphism in the CYP1A1 gene is not associated with lung cancer in African Americans. *Carcinogenesis* 1994; **15**: 1121–4.
75. Tefre T, Ryberg D, Haugen A, Nebert DW, Skaug V, Brogger A, Borresen AL. Human *CYP1A1* (cytochrome P1450) gene: lack of association between the *Msp* I restriction fragment length polymorphism and incidence of lung cancer in a Norwegian population. *Pharmacogenetics* 1991; **1**: 20–5.
76. Nebert DW, Ingelman-Sundberg M, Daly AK. Genetic epidemiology of environmental toxicity and cancer susceptibility: human allelic polymorphisms in drug metabolizing enzyme genes, their functional importance, and nomenclature issues. *Drug Metab Rev* 1999; **31**: 467–87.
77. Inoue K, Asao T, Shimada T. Ethnic-related differences in the frequency distribution of genetic polymorphisms in the *CYP1A1* and *CYP1B1* genes in Japanese and Caucasian populations. *Xenobiotica* 2000; **30**: 285–95.
78. Battula N, Sagara J, Gelboin HV. Expression of P1-450 and P3-450 DNA coding sequences as enzymatically active cytochromes P-450 in mammalian cells. *Proc Natl Acad Sci USA* 1987; **84**: 4073–7.
79. Ching MS, Lennard MS, Tucker GT, Woods HF, Kelly DE, Kelly SL. The expression of human cytochrome P450IA1 in the yeast Saccharomyces cerevisiae. *Biochem Pharmacol* 1991; **42**: 753–8.
80. Komori M, Kikuti O, Kitada T, Kamataki T. Molecular cloning of monkey P450 1A1 cDNA and expression in yeast. *Biochim Biophys Acta* 1992; **1131**: 23–9.
81. Guo Z, Gillam E, Ohmori S, Tukey RH, Guengerich FP. Expression of modified hu-

man cytochrome P450 1A1 in *Escherichia coli*: effects of 5′ substitution, stabilization, purification, spectral characterization, and catalytic properties. *Arch Biochem Biophys* 1994; **312**: 436–46.

82. Shimada T, El-Bayoumy K, Upadhyaya P, Sutter TR, Guengerich FP, Yamazaki H. Inhibition of human cytochrome P450-catalyzed oxidations of xenobiotics and procarcinogens by synthetic organoselenium compounds. *Cancer Res* 1997; **57**: 4757–64.
83. Shimada T, Yamazaki H, Foroozesh M, Hopkins NE, Alworth WL, Guengerich FP. Selectivity of polycyclic inhibitors for human cytochromes P450 1A1, 1A2, and 1B1. *Chem Res Toxicol* 1998; **11**: 1048–56.
84. Chun YJ, Ryu SY, Jeong TC, Kim MY. Mechanism-based inhibition of human cytochrome P450 1A1 by rhapontigenin. *Drug Metab Dispos* 2001; **29**: 389–93.
85. Chun YJ, Kim MY, Guengerich FP. Resveratrol is a selective human cytochrome P450 1A1 inhibitor. *Biochem Biophys Res Commun* 1999; **262**: 20–4.
86. Chun Y-J, Kim S, Kim D, Lee S-K, Guengerich FP. A new selective and potent inhibitor of human cytochrome P450 1B1 and its application to antimutagenesis. *Cancer Res* 2001; **61**: 8164–70.
87. Kinoshita N, Gelboin HV. The role of aryl hydrocarbon hydroxylase in 7, 12-dimethylbenz(*a*)anthracene skin tumorigenesis: on the mechanism of 7, 8-benzoflavone inhibition of tumorigenesis. *Cancer Res* 1972; **32**: 1329–39.
88. Kinoshita N, Gelboin HV. Aryl hydrocarbon hydroxylase and polycyclic hydrocarbon tumorigenesis: effect of the enzyme inhibitor 7, 8-benzoflavone on tumorigenesis and macromolecule binding. *Proc Natl Acad Sci USA* 1972; **69**: 824–8.
89. Gelboin HV, Wiebel F. Dimethylbenzanthracene tumorigenesis and aryl hydrocarbon hydroxylase in mouse skin: inhibition by 7, 8-benzoflavone. *Science* 1970; **170**: 169–71.
90. El-Bayoumy K, Chae Y-H, Upadhyaya P, Meschter C, Cohen LA, Reddy BS. Inhibition of 7, 12-dimethylbenzo[*a*]anthracene-induced tumors and DNA adduct formation in the mammary glands of female Sprague-Dawley rats by the synthetic organoselenium compound, 1,4-phenylenebis(methylene)selenocyanate. *Cancer Res* 1992; **52**: 2402–7.
91. Ip C, El-Bayoumy K, Upadhyaya P, Ganther H, Vadhanavikit S, Thompson H. Comparative effect of inorganic and organic selenocyanate derivatives in mammary cancer chemoprevention. *Carcinogenesis* 1994; **15**: 187–92.
92. El-Bayoumy K, Upadhyaya P, Chae Y-H, Sohn O-S, Rao CV, Faila E, Reddy BS. Chemoprevention of cancer by organoselenium compounds. *J Cell Biochem* 1995; **22**: 92–100.
93. Upadhyaya P, Sohn O-S, Fiala ES, El-Bayoumy K. *In vitro* and *in vivo* metabolism of [U-^{14}C]1, 4-phenylenebis(methylene)selenocyanate, a chemopreventive organoselenium compound, in female CD rats. *Am Assoc Cancer Res* 1996; **37**: 1876.
94. Viaje A, Lu J-YL, Hopkins NE, Nettikumara AN, DiGiovanni J, Alworth WL, Slaga TJ. Inhibition of the binding of 7, 12-dimethylbenz[*a*]anthracene and benzo[*a*]pyrene to DNA in mouse skin epidermis by 1-ethynylpyrene. *Carcinogenesis* 1990; **11**: 1139–43.
95. Alworth WL, Viaje A, Sandoval A, Warren BS, Slaga TJ. Potent inhibitory effects of suicide inhibitors of P450 isozyme on 7, 12-dimethylbenz[*a*]anthracene and

benzo[*a*]pyrene initiated skin tumors. *Carcinogenesis* 1991; **12**: 1209–15.

96. Jang M, Cai L, Udeani GO, Slowing KV, Thomas CF, Beecher CWW, Fong HHS, Fransworth NR, Kinghorn AD, Mehta RG, Moon RC, Pezzuto JM. Cancer chemopreventive activity of resveratrol, a natural product derived from grapes. *Science* 1997; **275**: 218–20.
97. Potter GA, Patterson LH, Wanogho E, Perry PJ, Butler PC, Ijaz T, Ruparelia KC, Lamb JH, Farmer PB, Stanley LA, Burke MD. The cancer preventative agent resveratrol is converted to the anticancer agent piceatannol by the cytochrome P450 enzyme CYP1B1. *Brit J Cancer* 2002; **86**: 774–8.

CELL BIOLOGY

NK4 (HGF-ANTAGONIST/ANGIOGENESIS INHIBITOR) IN CANCER BIOLOGY AND THERAPEUTICS

Kunio MATSUMOTO and Toshikazu NAKAMURA

*Division of Molecular Regenerative Medicine, Course of Advanced Medicine, Osaka University Graduate School of Medicine**

Invasion and subsequent establishment of metastasis are devastating events for patients with cancer, but past therapeutic approaches have paid relatively little attention to these important issues. Hepatocyte growth factor (HGF) and its receptor, the c-Met tyrosine kinase, play roles in cancer invasion and metastasis in a wide variety of tumor cells. Activation of the c-Met receptor integrates multiple signal transduction pathways involved in cell-cell and cell-matrix interactions, cellular migration, and breakdown of the extracellular scaffold. Paracrine activation of the c-Met receptor by stromal-derived HGF mediates tumor-stromal interactions that facilitate invasion and metastasis. Likewise, aberrant expression of the c-Met receptor and autocrine or mutational activation of c-Met receptor tyrosine kinase are closely associated with the progression of malignant tumors. Based on this background, NK4, a competitive antagonist of HGF-c-Met association was prepared so as to block cancer invasion and metastasis. NK4, an internal fragment of HGF, binds to but does not activate the c-Met receptor, thereby competitively antagonizing the biological activities of HGF. Unexpectedly, NK4 was subsequently shown to be an angiogenesis inhibitor as well, and this angioinhibitory activity is independent of its action as an HGF-antagonist. Importantly, NK4 protein or *NK4* gene therapy have been shown to inhibit tumor invasion, metastasis and angiogenesis, effectively converting malignant tumors into benign tumors. Targeting tumor invasion-metastasis and angiogenesis with NK4 seems to have considerable therapeutic potential for cancer patients.

Though knowledge of the molecular mechanisms of tumorigenesis has greatly advanced in recent years, the cure rate of cancer has not been substantially improved. Cancers are still the first or second most common cause of death in developed countries. Tumor metastasis is the most important factor affecting the survival of cancer patients. Many cancer patients die as a consequence of a metastatic, not a primary tumor. If metastasis could be controlled, the rate of cancer cures should show a marked improvement.

The dissociation and migration of tumor cells, adhesive interaction of cancer

* Suita, Osaka 565-0871, Japan

This paper is dedicated to the memory of late Dr. Tomizo Yoshida on the occasion of the 100th anniversary of his birth. It was originally published in Cancer Science in April, 2003.

cells towards the extracellular matrix (ECM), and extracellular proteolysis of ECM proteins all play key roles in tumor invasion and metastasis. Although mutational alterations that occur in oncogenes and tumor suppressor genes are responsible for tumorigenic transformation of cells, the metastatic behavior of tumor cells is largely regulated by extracellularly acting growth factors. Among these factors, hepatocyte growth factor (HGF), a ligand for the c-met protooncogene product, affects metastatic behavior in a wide variety of cells (*1–3*).

HGF was first identified and cloned as a mitogenic polypeptide for hepatocytes (*4–6*). HGF is a heterodimeric molecule composed of a 69 kDa α-chain and a 34 kDa β-chain. The α-chain contains the N-terminal hairpin domain and four kringle domains, while the β-chain contains a serine protease-like domain (Fig. 1). Subsequent studies revealed that HGF has multiple biological effects on a wide variety of cells, including mitogenic, motogenic, morphogenic, and anti-apoptotic activities (Fig. 1). The receptor for HGF is a c-met protooncogene product (*7*). The c-Met receptor is composed of a 50 kDa α-chain and a 145 kDa β-chain. The α-chain is exposed extracellularly, while the β-chain is a transmembrane subunit containing an intracellular tyrosine kinase domain (Fig. 1). Binding of HGF to the c-Met receptor induces phosphorylation of C-terminally clustered tyrosine residues and these residues recruit intracellular signaling molecules containing the src homology (SH) domain (Fig. 1) (*1*).

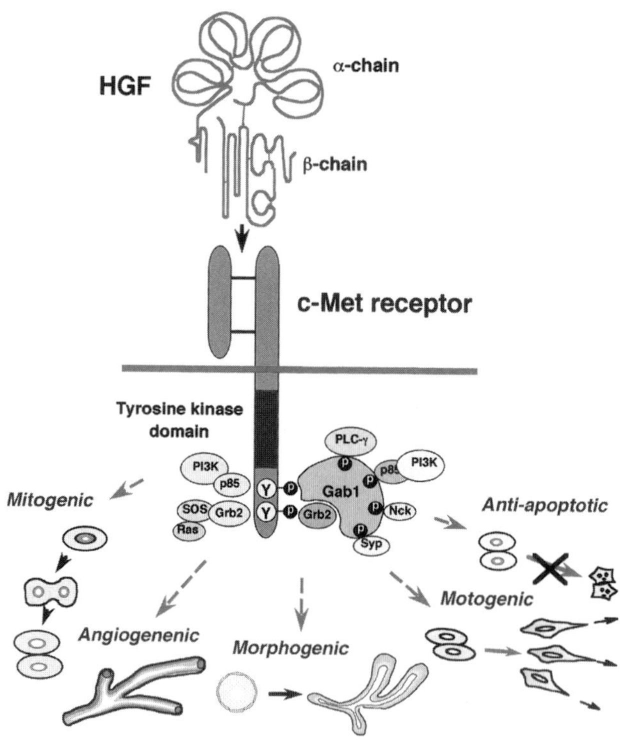

FIG. 1. Schematic structure of HGF and c-Met receptor, and typical biological activities of HGF (see the text for detail)

In normal tissues, HGF plays roles in dynamic construction and reconstruction of tissues during organogenesis and tissue regeneration (*8*, *9*). HGF is involved in development of embryonic tissues, including the liver, kidney, lung, mammary gland, teeth, placenta, and skeletal muscle (*8*). In mature tissues, HGF has an organotrophic role in regeneration and protection of various tissues, including the liver, lung, kidney, gastrointestinal tissues, nervous tissue, pancreas, and heart (*9*). HGF has angiogenic activity for vascular endothelial cells (*10*). In tumor tissues, however, tumor cells utilize the biological actions of HGF for their dissociative, invasive and metastatic behavior. The abrogation of HGF-c-Met receptor coupling or c-Met receptor-mediated signalling events seems to be a highly promising strategy for prevention of tumor metastasis.

NK4 was isolated as a competitive antagonist for HGF and the c-Met receptor (*11*), and subsequent studies showed that NK4 is bifunctional: it is an HGF-antagonist and an angiogenesis inhibitor (*12*). NK4 has potential value in cancer treatment by targeting the malignant behavior of tumor cells, rather than by direct killing of the tumor cells. This review focuses on tumor invasion and metastasis regulated by the HGF-c-Met system, and interference with these processes by NK4 as an approach to cancer treatment.

c-Met Receptor-Mediated Signals in Invasion and Metastasis

Invasion of tumor cells is regulated by distinct cellular functions, including cell-cell adhesion, cell-matrix association, proteolytic breakdown of the extracellular matrix, and cellular locomotion. HGF affects these processes and exhibits profound effects on the invasive behavior of a wide variety of tumor cells. Fig. 2A summarizes HGF-induced signaling events involved in the invasive behavior of tumor cells.

Among various cell adhesion molecules, epithelial cadherin (E-cadherin)-mediated cell-cell adhesion contributes to the invasive characteristics of variety of tumor cells of epithelial origin. E-Cadherin binds to β-catenin, plakoglobin/γ-catenin, and $p120^{ctn}$, and the complex associates with α-catenin, which links cadherin complexes to the actin cytoskeleton. HGF induces tyrosine phosphorylation of β-catenin, plakoglobin/γ-catenin and $p120^{ctn}$ (*13*), thereby facilitating dissociation of cells mediated by the E-cadherin complex. As c-Met receptor associates with E-cadherin (*14*), the rapid and direct tyrosine phosphorylation of the E-cadherin/catenin complex by the activated c-Met receptor seems to occur.

Cellular migration is regulated by multiple extracellular and intracellular processes organized by complex signaling cascades. Cells adhere to extracellular matrix (ECM) components via integrin family receptors and integrin-mediated attachment of cells transduces signals through focal adhesion complex for ECM-dependent cell shape arrangement and cell movement. Coupled with active turnover (association and dissociation) of focal adhesion complexes, rearrangement and retraction of cytoskeletal networks occur in migrating cells. HGF induces tyrosine phosphorylation of focal adhesion kinase (FAK) and paxillin (*15*, *16*). Because expression of kinase-negative FAK in cells and antibody against α2 integrin inhibited HGF-induced migration of cells (*16*), integrin-dependent cell-ECM binding and intracellular tyrosine phosphorylation of FAK is required for cell migration. Together with cell-substratum interactions, HGF activates Rho family small GTP-binding proteins (Rho, Rac, Cdc42)

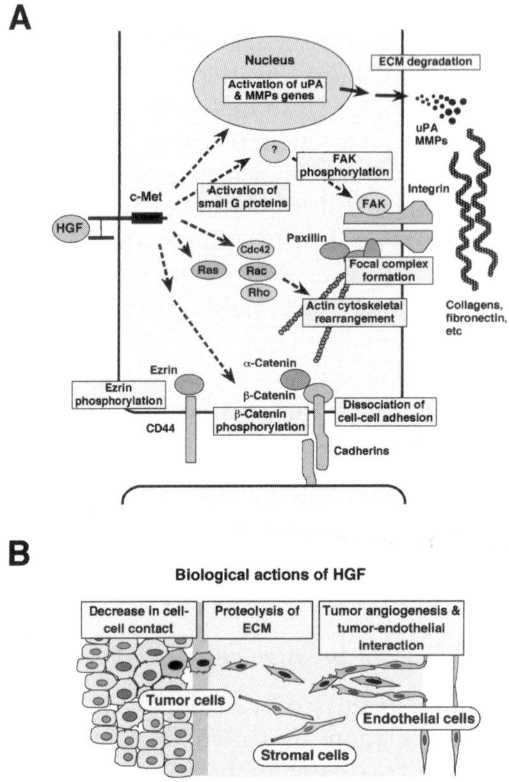

FIG. 2. Intracellular and extracellular mechanisms for tumor invasion and metastasis mediated by HGF-c-Met pathway

A: Signal transduction pathways involved in tumor invasion by activation of the c-Met receptor. B: Involvement of the HGF-c-Met system in tumor invasion and metastasis. For details, see the text. HGF enhances dissociation of tumor cells in primary sites, invasion through basement membrane and stroma, angiogenesis, and interactions between tumor and endothelial cells.

involved in the regulation of cell shape and movement through remodeling of cytoskeletal networks. Utilizing dominant-negative approaches, activation of Rho, Rac, and Cdc42 was found to be essential for HGF-induced dissociation and spreading of cells (*17–19*). HGF induces tyrosine phosphorylation of ezrin, thereby facilitating actin cytoskeletal rearrangement in cadherin- and integrin-based adhesion complexes (*20*).

Among various types of proteases, the urokinase-type plasminogen activator (uPA)-dependent proteolytic network and matrix metalloproteinases (MMPs) affect invasiveness of tumor cells. HGF induces *uPA* gene expression and strongly stimulates uPA production in many types of both normal and tumor cells (*21–23*). Establishment of an autocrine activation loop of HGF-c-Met in human cells resulted in marked activation of uPA and concomitant acquisition of invasiveness and metastatic potential of the cells (*21*). In addition, HGF stimulates the production of MMPs, including membrane-type MMP-1, collagenase-1, MMP-2, MMP-3, and MMP-9 (*22–24*).

Angiogenesis is critical for tumor growth, and increased angiogenesis coincides with increased tumor cell entry into the blood circulation, and thus facilitates metastasis (*25*). When the *HGF* gene was stably expressed in human breast cancer cells and in glioma cells, these tumor cells exhibited more extensive tumor angiogenesis and enhanced growth in nude mice (*26*). Therefore, HGF is one of the growth factors affecting tumor angiogenesis. In addition to angiogenesis, HGF stimulates attachment of tumor cells to endothelial cells by increasing 1) endothelial expression of CD44, a molecule which may play a critical role in tumor-endothelial interactions and the establishment of metastasis (*27*), or 2) $\alpha2\beta1$ integrin expression in cancer cells (*28*).

Fig. 2B schematically describes the participation of HGF in early steps leading to cancer metastasis. HGF stimulates 1) dissociation of cancer cells at the primary site, 2) invasion through the basement membrane and host stroma by enhancing cell-matrix interactions, protease networks for breakdown of ECM proteins, and motogenic responses, 3) angiogenesis in tumor tissues, and 4) interaction of cancer cells with blood vessels.

c-Met Receptor Activation Pathways in Cancer Cells

1. Paracrine activation through tumor-stromal interaction

Host stromal influence on epithelial neoplasia, tumor angiogenesis and malignant behavior in carcinomas is evident in various types of cancers, including prostate, stomach, skin, oral cavity, mammary gland, and colon cancers (*2, 3*). *In vitro* and *in vivo* growth and invasiveness of carcinoma cells were enhanced by the co-existence of stromal fibroblasts. Thus, the host stromal-derived factor(s) is a key molecule that enhances invasive and metastatic potential of cancer cells.

Fig. 3A shows *in vitro* invasion of human carcinoma cells through Matrigel basement membrane, in the absence or presence of stromal fibroblasts (*22*). Without

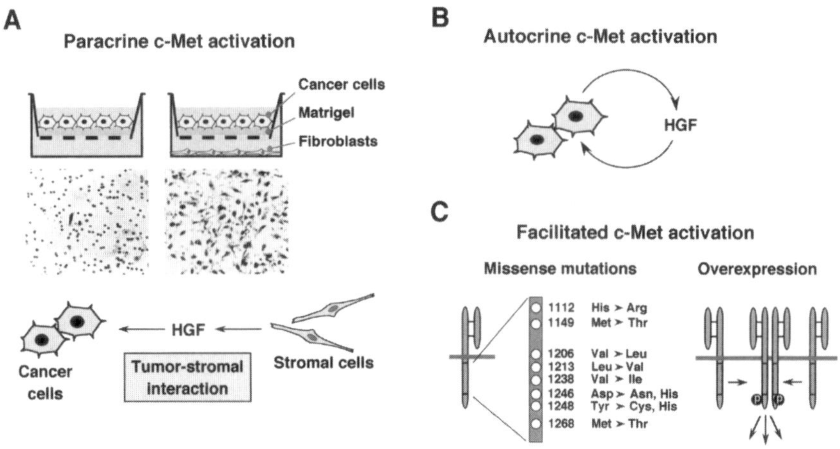

FIG. 3. Distinct mechanisms for c-Met receptor activation in tumor cells

A: Invasion of human carcinoma cells in co-culture with stromal fibroblasts (upper figures) and paracrine activation of the c-Met receptor through tumor-stromal interaction (lower figure). Human gallbladder cancer cells were cultured on Matrigel basement membrane components in the absence or presence of stromal fibroblasts (*22*). Photographs show the appearance of cancer cells beneath the filter membrane. B: Autocrine activation of the c-Met receptor. C: Facilitated activation of the c-Met receptor, through mutational alteration (left) or over-expression (right). The left figure indicates localization of missense mutations in *c-met* gene in patients with hereditary and sporadic papillary renal carcinoma (*34*).

stromal fibroblasts, only a few cancer cells invaded, whereas invasion of cancer cells was potently enhanced by co-cultivation with stromal fibroblasts. Importantly, an antibody against HGF and a competitive antagonist of HGF almost completely abrogated invasion of the cancer cells in the co-culture system (see below). Similar results were noted with various types of cancer cells, including oral squamous cell carcinoma cells, mammary carcinoma, gallbladder carcinoma, esophageal, and prostate cancers (*3, 15, 22, 29*). These results indicate that invasion of tumor cells depends on a fibroblast-derived factor and that HGF is a major stromal-derived paracrine factor that confers invasive potential in a wide variety of cancers.

Consistent with a lack of autonomous potential of many carcinoma cells to aggressively invade the scaffold of ECM, most carcinoma cells do not secrete HGF. However, many types of tumor cells secrete a variety of HGF-inducers, through which HGF production in stromal fibroblasts is up-regulated (*3, 29*). These tumor-derived HGF-inducers were identified as interleukin-1, basic fibroblast growth factor (bFGF), platelet-derived growth factor, transforming growth factor-α, and prostaglandin E2. These observations suggest a mutual interaction between tumor cells and stromal fibroblasts: tumor cells secrete HGF-inducers for stromal cells, while stromal cells secrete HGF that may stimulate tumor invasion, angiogenesis, and metastasis.

2. *Autocrine activation*

Since the c-Met receptor is predominantly expressed in epithelial cells but not in stromal cells, while HGF is predominantly expressed in stromal cells but not in epithelial cells, autocrine activation of the c-Met receptor is the result of expression of HGF in the c-Met-positive (but HGF-negative) epithelial cells, or expression of the c-Met receptor in HGF-positive (but c-Met-negative) stromal cells. Stable expression of the c-Met receptor gene in fibroblasts conferred invasive and metastatic characteristics in mice (*30*). Transfection of the *HGF* gene into epithelial cells induced tumorigenic transformation or conferred invasive and metastatic behavior (*31, 32*).

Tumorigenesis and invasive and metastatic progression in cells through experimental establishment of the HGF-c-Met autocrine loop suggest the presence of an HGF-c-Met autocrine loop in naturally developed cancer cells. Indeed, co-expression of HGF and the c-Met receptor has been detected in a variety of human tumors, including breast, pancreatic and thyroid cancers, glioma, meningioma, myeloma, lymphoma, and sarcoma/fibroma (*1–3*). Thus, autocrine activation of the c-Met receptor is closely associated with malignant progression of tumor cells (Fig. 3B).

3. *Over-expression and mutational activation*

Over-expression of the c-Met receptor was noted in a wide variety of tumor cells and tissues, including various carcinomas, lymphomas, and soft tissue tumors (*2, 3*). In colorectal cancers, over-expression of the c-Met receptor was related to transcriptional activation in 90% of the primary tumors, whereas 8 of 9 cases of metastases of colorectal cancers showed amplification of the *c-met* gene (*33*). Amplification of the *c-met* gene may occur more frequently in late-stage metastatic tumors than in primary tumors, presumably due to chromosomal instability of the advanced cancers. The level of c-Met receptor expression tends to correlate with progression of many types of tumors; a higher expression of the c-Met receptor is seen in the late stage or in metastatic tumors (*2*). Thus, over-expression of c-Met receptor is likely to increase susceptibility to ligand-independent or -dependent activation of the receptor (Fig. 3C).

Genetic analysis of papillary renal carcinoma in patients indicated that missense mutations in the *c-met* gene are causative in inherited and some sporadic papillary renal carcinomas (*34*). All mutations that occur in eight distinct positions in the *c-met* gene are missense and are located in the tyrosine kinase domain of the c-Met receptor (Fig. 3C). Because the c-Met receptor with these mutations has enhanced tyrosine kinase activity (*35*), c-Met receptor mutations identified in patients with papillary renal carcinoma are likely to be gain-of-function mutations, and thus may play a determinant role in papillary renal carcinoma.

Identification of NK4 as an HGF-Antagonist

Close involvement of c-Met receptor activation in acquisition of malignant characteristics in a wide variety of tumors suggests possible therapeutic strategies for prevention of tumor invasion, and metastasis, through blockage of c-Met receptor-mediated signaling. For this purpose, NK4, a specific antagonist of the HGF-c-Met pathway was prepared (*11*).

NK4 is composed of the N-terminal 447 amino acids of the α-chain of HGF and contains the N-terminal hairpin domain and four kringle domains (thus having been designated NK4) (Fig. 4A). Because NK4 has receptor binding domains (i.e., NK1), NK4 can bind to the c-Met receptor, but it does not activate the c-Met receptor and is devoid of c-Met-mediated agonistic activities (Fig. 4A). It is noteworthy that NK1, NK2, and NK3, all variants of the α-chain containing binding domains to the c-Met receptor, retain agonistic activity, not fully, but in part (*36–38*). NK4 itself is a complete competitive antagonist for HGF and for the c-Met receptor. Fig. 4B illustrates the effect of NK4 on HGF-induced invasion of cancer cells. When human pancreatic cancer cells were co-cultured with stromal fibroblasts, invasion of the cells was strongly enhanced compared to that seen in the culture of cancer cells alone. In contrast, NK4 almost completely inhibited invasion of cancer cells in the co-culture system.

NK4 as an Angiogenesis Inhibitor

Since vascular endothelial cells express the c-Met receptor and HGF has angiogenic activity, it was considered that NK4 might inhibit the angiogenic responses induced by HGF. However, NK4 inhibits the angiogenic responses induced by bFGF, vascular endothelial cell growth factor (VEGF), and HGF (*12*). NK4 inhibits endothelial proliferation and migration stimulated by bFGF and VEGF, as well as by HGF. Fig. 4C shows the inhibitory effects of NK4 on bFGF-induced angiogenesis. When a pellet containing bFGF was implanted under the rabbit cornea, bFGF induced extensive angiogenesis, whereas the co-existence of NK4 with bFGF in the pellet potently inhibited the bFGF-induced angiogenesis.

Subsequent studies showed that deletion of the N-terminal hairpin domain (an essential domain for c-Met receptor binding in NK4 and HGF) in NK4 led to a selective loss of HGF-antagonist activity, while the remaining four-kringle variant of HGF (K1-4) retained the angioinhibitory effects (*39*). Thus, NK4 is considered to be

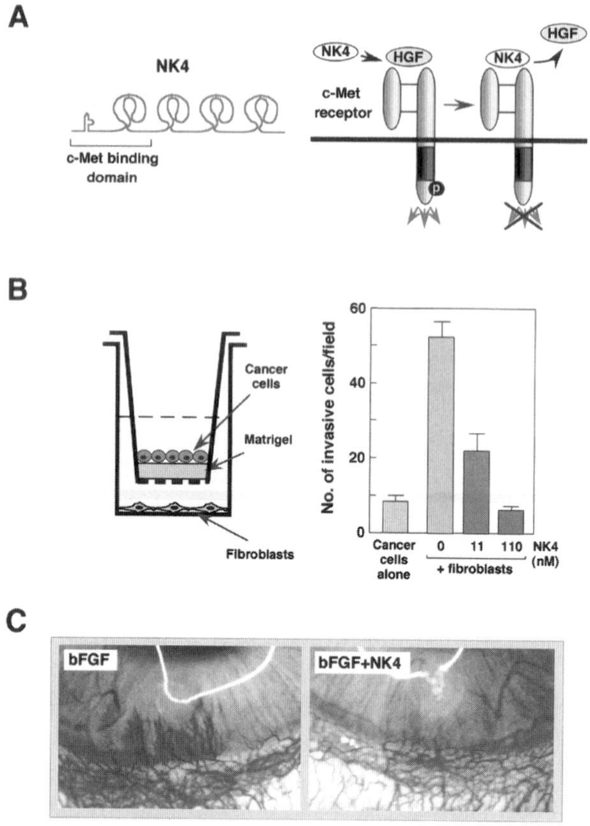

FIG. 4. Structure and functions of NK4

A: Schematic structure of NK4 (left) and the biological action of NK4, as a competitive HGF-antagonist (right). B: Inhibitory effect of NK4 on invasion of pancreatic cancer cells. Cancer cells were cultured on Matrigel basement membrane components in the absence or presence of stromal fibroblasts and the number of invading cells was determined. C: Inhibition of bFGF-induced angiogenesis by NK4 in rabbit cornea.

bifunctional, as it is an HGF-antagonist and an angiogenesis inhibitor, and the domains responsible for angiogenesis inhibition reside in the four kringles. In this context, it is noteworthy that kringle domains in some other kringle-containing proteins have angioinhibitory activity, including those of angiostatin (*40*), the fifth kringle domain of plasminogen (*41*), and the kringle-2 of prothrombin (*42*). It is noteworthy that angiostatin is composed of three or four kringle domains (1st to 3rd or 4th) of plasminogen (*40*) and NK4 has 47% amino acid homology with angiostatin. Angiostatin inhibits endothelial proliferation by disrupting the G2/M transition and induces endothelial apoptosis (*43*). It binds to the endothelial cell surface ATP synthase (*44*) and $\alpha v\beta 3$ integrin (*45*). Inhibition of cell surface ATP synthesis and/or interaction between $\alpha v\beta 3$ integrin and plasmin via angiostatin were suggested to be mechanisms responsible for angiogenesis inhibition by angiostatin. On the other hand, NK4 inhibits the G1/S transition in endothelial cells, and angiostatin has no antagonistic activity to HGF (our unpublished data), suggesting that NK4 inhibits angiogenesis through a distinct mechanism(s) from that of angiostatin. Although the mechanisms by which some kringle domains in distinct kringle-containing proteins inhibit angiogenic responses remain an open question, they may exert angiostatic signals through putative binding molecules expressed on endothelial cells.

Experimental Cancer Treatment with NK4

The bifunctional character of NK4 as an HGF-antagonist and angiogenesis inhibitor means that NK4 treatment of patients might effectively suppress the malignant behavior of cancer. Studies on cancer treatment with NK4 in experimental models have supported the unique therapeutic potential of NK4 (*12*, *22*, *46–50*).

Among malignant tumors, pancreatic cancer is one of the major causes of cancer-related deaths in industrialized countries. Only 3–4% of all patients with pancreatic cancer survive 5 years after the diagnosis, and this morbidity is because of the highly invasive and metastatic characteristics of pancreatic cancer cells. Even if patients are correctly diagnosed at an early stage, pancreatic cancer frequently exhibits highly malignant phenotypes characterized by extensive invasion into surrounding tissues and metastasis to distant organs. It is our view that treatment of such patients with NK4 would be an appropriate approach to evaluate the therapeutic value of the bifunctionality of NK4, targeting both tumor angiogenesis and HGF-mediated invasion-metastasis (*46*).

When human pancreatic cancer cells (SUIT-2 cell line) were orthotopically inoculated into the pancreas of nude mice, the cells were engrafted in the pancreas 3 days after the tumor inoculation (*46*). Four weeks later, the pancreatic cancer was large, and had spontaneously disseminated into the peritoneal cavity. Accumulation of cancerous ascites was apparent, thereby indicating that the pancreatic cancer had reached an advanced stage. Human recombinant NK4 was daily administered intraperitoneally to mice with pancreatic cancer from day 3 to day 28 after tumor inoculation (Fig. 5A).

Four weeks after tumor inoculation, NK4 treatment suppressed the growth of pancreatic tumor by 61% (Fig. 5B). Further, the treatment decreased microvessel density to 35% of that seen in control mice (Fig. 5B). Moreover, blood vessels in tumor tissues of NK4-treated mice were much smaller than those in control mice, suggesting that the ability of the blood vessels to supply oxygen and nutrients to tumor tissues might be inhibited by NK4 treatment. Because the number of apoptotic cancer cells was increased by NK4 treatment to 2.4-fold over the control, the treatment may possibly have inhibited tumor growth through the inhibitory actions of NK4 on tumor angiogenesis. In addition to inhibition of the primary tumor growth, NK4 treatment inhibited metastasis into the peritoneal cavity and the accumulation of cancerous ascites (*46*).

On the other hand, early detection of pancreatic cancer is generally difficult. At the time of diagnosis, >80% of patients with pancreatic cancer have locally advanced or metastatic disease. In the clinical situation, NK4 treatment for patients with pancreatic cancer probably should be started from the advanced rather than from an early stage. In the second model, NK4 treatment was initiated from day 24 after tumor inoculation, a time when peritoneal dissemination and accumulation of cancerous ascites became apparent, yet all the mice survived (Fig. 5C) (*46*). Control mice started to die due to pancreatic cancer from 26 days post-inoculation, and all of the

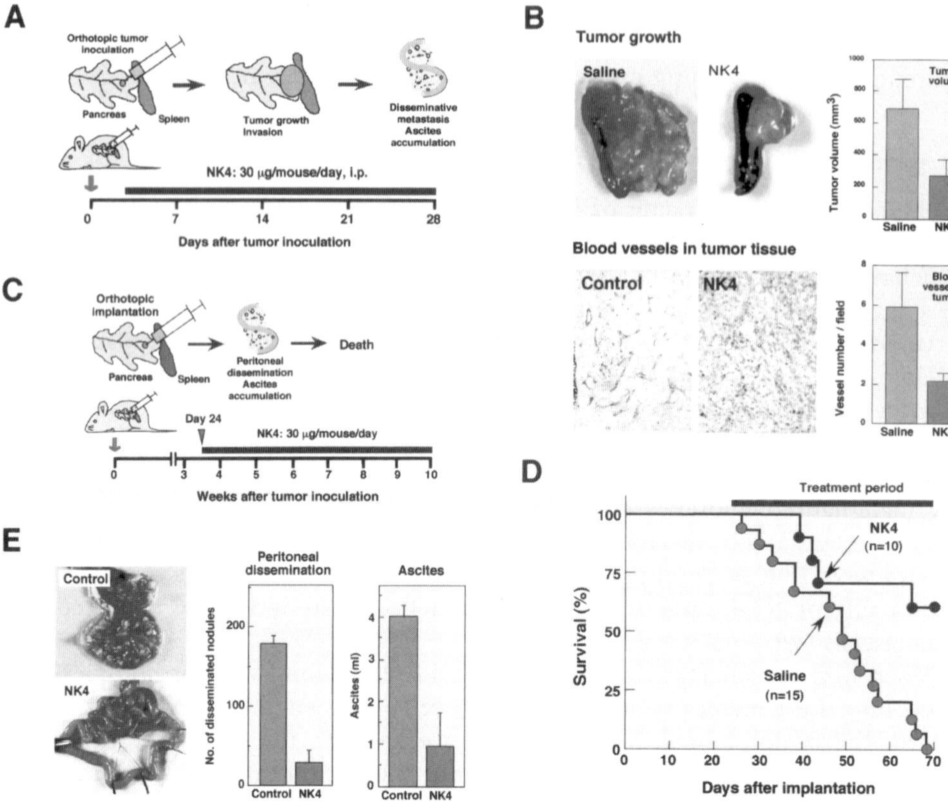

FIG. 5. Therapeutic effects of NK4 on human pancreatic cancer in mice (*46*)
A: Experimental model to examine the effects of NK4 on tumor growth and angiogenesis. B: Suppression of tumor growth and angiogenesis by NK4 treatment. Blood vessels in tumor tissues were immunohistochemically stained using antibody to platelet-endothelial cell adhesion molecule. C: Experimental model to examine effects of NK4 on survival. D: Prolonged survival of mice treated with NK4. E: Inhibitions of disseminated metastasis into peritoneal cavity and ascites accumulation by NK4 treatment. Left panels show appearance of mesentery.

mice died within 69 days after the inoculation (Fig. 5D). In mice treated with NK4, 60% of mice survived for more than 70 days. When moribund control mice were examined, the peritoneum, diaphragm, and mesentery were occupied with numerous metastatic nodules, and the mean number of disseminated metastatic nodules reached 180 (Fig. 5E). In contrast, the number of disseminated metastatic nodules was only 29 in NK4-treated mice. Furthermore, NK4 treatment inhibited ascites accumulation to 24.5% of the control levels (Fig. 5E). Thus, NK4 treatment has unique and potent anti-metastasis and anti-growth effects, the result being prolonged survival of the mice, even in the case of treatment from an advanced stage.

Cancer treatment with NK4 protein or *NK4* gene therapy has been given in a laboratory setting for distinct types of cancers, including pancreatic, lung, breast, colon, gallbladder, gastric, and ovarian cancers (*12*, *22*, *46–50*). NK4 treatment, including *NK4* gene therapy had anti-metastatic, anti-angiogenic and anti-growth effects in these cancers. In the case of *NK4* gene therapy using recombinant adenovirus for *NK4* gene expression, systemic treatment with intraperitoneal administration of recombinant adenoviruses, as well as intratumoral administration, resulted in inhibition of tumor angiogenesis and tumor growth (*48*). Likewise, intraperitoneal administration of recombinant adenoviruses inhibited disseminated metastasis of pancreatic cancer (*50*). These results suggest that systemic treatment with *NK4* gene therapy may possibly inhibit metastasis and growth of invisible tumors, through the action of circulating NK4 protein in the bloodstream. This strategy could be considered as a kind of "gene drug" for cancer treatment.

Perspective

Undoubtedly, the final objective of cancer research is to cure patients with cancer. The many past approaches used to treat cancer patients have been less than satisfactory. Since both chemo- and radiotherapies are based on the concept of directly killing cancer cells, these therapies have severe side effects, which result in a reduction in the quality of life and/or impaired immune responses. The surgical removal of cancer after early detection can be associated with disease-free survival of patients with some malignant cancers, yet surgical treatment often results in incomplete removal of cancer cells, leading to regrowth and metastasis. NK4, as an HGF-antagonist/angiogenesis inhibitor, can inhibit tumor invasion, growth, angiogenesis, and metastasis of tumors in laboratory animals. It may therefore offer a new therapeutic approach for cancer patients.

HGF has biological activities that are involved in dynamic tissue remodeling during embryogenesis and tissue regeneration. Breakdown of the ECM scaffold and concomitant cellular migration, mitogenesis, and morphogenesis driven by the HGF-c-Met system make way for construction and reconstruction of tissues through epithelial-mesenchymal (or -stromal) interactions for organogenesis and organ regeneration. The functioning of the HGF-c-Met system in embryonic, wounded and cancer tissues may imply some similarity in gene expression profiles among these tissues. The simile that "cancer is a never-healing wound" seems pertinent here.

Acknowledgments

We are grateful to M. Ohara for helpful comments.

REFERENCES

1. Vande Woude GF, Jeffers M, Cortner J, Alvord G, Tsarfaty I, Resau J. Met-HGF/SF: tumorigenesis, invasion and metastasis. In: Gherardi E, editor. Plasminogen-related growth factors. Chichester (UK): John Wiley & Sons; 1997. p. 119–32.
2. Jiang WG, Hiscox S, Matsumoto K, Nakamura T. Hepatocyte growth factor/scatter factor, its molecular, cellular and clinical implications in cancer. *Crit Rev Oncol Hematol* 1999; **29**: 209–48.
3. Matsumoto K, Nakamura T. HGF-c-Met receptor pathway in tumor invasion-metastasis and potential cancer treatment with NK4. In: Jiang WG, Matsumoto K, Nakamura T, editors. Growth factors and their receptors in cancer metastasis. Dordrecht (The Netherland): Kluwer Academic Publisher; 2001. p. 241–76.
4. Nakamura T, Nawa K, Ichihara A. Partial purification and characterization of hepato-

cyte growth factor from serum of hepatectomized rats. *Biochem Biophys Res Commun* 1984; **122**: 1450–9.

5. Nakamura T, Nishizawa T, Hagiya M, Seki T, Shimonishi M, Sugimura A, Tashiro K, Shimizu S. Molecular cloning and expression of human hepatocyte growth factor. *Nature* 1989; **342**: 440–3.
6. Miyazawa K, Tsubouchi H, Naka D, Takahashi K, Okigaki M, Arakaki N, Nakayama H, Hirono S, Sakiyama O, Takahashi K, Gohda E, Daikuhara Y, Kitamura N. Molecular cloning and sequence analysis of cDNA for human hepatocyte growth factor. *Biochem Biophys Res Commun* 1989; **163**: 967–73.
7. Bottaro DP, Rubin JS, Faletto DL, Chan AMI, Kmiecik TE, Vande Woude GF, Aaronson SA. Identification of hepatocyte growth factor receptor as the c-met protooncogene product. *Science* 1991; **251**: 802–4.
8. Birchmeier C, Gherardi E. Developmental roles of HGF/SF and its receptor, the c-Met tyrosine kinase. *Trends Cell Biol* 1998; **8**: 404–11.
9. Matsumoto K, Nakamura T. Hepatocyte growth factor (HGF) as a tissue organizer for organogenesis and regeneration. *Biochem Biophys Res Commun* 1997; **239**: 639–44.
10. Bussolino F, Di Renzo MF, Ziche M, Bochietto E, Olivero M, Naldini L, Gaudino G, Tamagnone L, Coffer A, Comoglio PM. Hepatocyte growth factor is a potent angiogenic factor which stimulates endothelial cell motility and growth. *J Cell Biol* 1992; **119**: 629–41.
11. Date K, Matsumoto K, Shimura H, Tanaka M, Nakamura T. HGF/NK4 is a specific antagonist for pleiotrophic actions of hepatocyte growth factor. *FEBS Lett* 1997; **420**: 1–6.
12. Kuba K, Matsumoto K, Date K, Shimura H, Tanaka M, Nakamura T. HGF/NK4, a four-kringle antagonist of hepatocyte growth factor, is an angiogenesis inhibitor that suppresses tumor growth and metastasis in mice. *Cancer Res* 2000a; **60**: 6737–43.
13. Shibamoto S, Hayakawa M, Takeuchi K, Hori T, Oku N, Miyazawa K, Kitamura N, Tekeichi M, Ito F. Tyrosine phosphorylation of β-catenin and plakoglobin enhanced by hepatocyte growth factor and epidermal growth factor in human carcinoma cells. *Cell Adhes Commun* 1994; **1**: 295–305.
14. Hiscox S, Jiang WG. Association of the HGF/SF receptor, c-met, with the cell-surface adhesion molecule, E-cadherin, and catenins in human tumor cells. *Biochem Biophys Res Commun* 1999; **261**: 406–11.
15. Matsumoto K, Matsumoto K, Nakamura T, Kramer RH. Hepatocyte growth factor/scatter factor induces tyrosine phosphorylation of focal adhesion kinase (p125FAK) and promotes migration and invasion by oral squamous cell carcinoma cells. *J Biol Chem* 1994; **269**: 31807–13.
16. Lai JF, Kao SC, Jiang ST, Tang MJ, Chan PC, Chen HC. Involvement of focal adhesion kinase in hepatocyte growth factor-induced scatter of Madin-Darby canine kidney cells. *J Biol Chem* 2000; **275**: 7474–80.
17. Takaishi K, Sasaki T, Kato M, Yamochi W, Kuroda S, Nakamura T, Takeichi M, Takai Y. Involvement of Rho p21 small GTP-binding protein and its regulator in the HGF-induced cell motility. *Oncogene* 1994; **9**: 273–9.
18. Ridley AJ, Comoglio PM, Hall A. Regulation of scatter factor/hepatocyte growth factor responses by Ras, Rac, and Rho in MDCK cells. *Mol Cell Biol* 1995; **15**: 1110–22.

19. Royal I, Lamarche-Vane N, Lamorte L, Kaibuchi K, Park M. Activation of cdc42, rac, PAK, and rho-kinase in response to hepatocyte growth factor differentially regulates epithelial cell colony spreading and dissociation. *Mol Biol Cell* 2000; **11**: 1709–25.
20. Jiang WG, Hiscox S, Singharo SK, Puntis MC, Nakamura T, Mansel RE, Hallett MB. Induction of tyrosine phosphorylation and translocation of ezrin by hepatocyte growth factor (HGF/SF). *Biochem Biophys Res Commun* 1995; **217**: 1062–9.
21. Jeffers M, Rong S, Vande Woude GF. Enhanced tumorigenicity and invasion-metastasis by hepatocyte growth factor/scatter factor-met signaling in human cells concomitant with induction of the urokinase proteolysis network. *Mol Cell Biol* 1996; **16**: 1115–25.
22. Date K, Matsumoto K, Kuba K, Shimura H, Tanaka M, Nakamura T. Inhibition of tumor growth and invasion by a four-kringle antagonist (HGF/NK4) for hepatocyte growth factor. *Oncogene* 1998; **17**: 3045–54.
23. Rosenthal EL, Johnson TM, Allen ED, Apel IJ, Punturieri A, Weiss SJ. Role of the plasminogen activator and matrix metalloproteinase system in epidermal growth factor- and scatter factor-stimulated invasion of carcinoma cells. *Cancer Res* 1998; **58**: 5221–30.
24. Nabeshima K, Inoue T, Shimao Y, Okada Y, Itoh Y, Seiki M, Koono M. Front-cell-specific expression of membrane-type 1 matrix metalloproteinase and gelatinase A during cohort migration of colon carcinoma cells induced by hepatocyte growth factor/ scatter factor. *Cancer Res* 2000; **60**: 3364–9.
25. Hanahan D, Folkman J. Patterns and emerging mechanisms of the angiogenesis switch during tumorigenesis. *Cell* 1996; **86**: 353–64.
26. Laterra J, Nam M, Rosen EM, Rao JS, Lamszus K, Goldberg ID, Johnston P. Scatter factor/hepatocyte growth factor gene transfer enhances glioma growth and angiogenesis *in vivo*. *Lab Invest* 1997; **76**: 565–77.
27. Hiscox SE, Jiang WG. Regulation of endothelial CD44 expression and endothelium-tumour cell interactions by hepatocyte growth factor-scatter factor. *Biochem Biophys Res Commun* 1997; **233**: 1–5.
28. Kawakami-Kimura N, Narita T, Ohmori K, Yoneda T, Matsumoto K, Nakamura T, Kannagi R. Involvement of hepatocyte growth factor in increased integrin expression on HepG2 cells triggered by adhesion to endothelial cells. *Br J Cancer* 1997; **75**: 47–53.
29. Nakamura T, Matsumoto K, Kiritoshi A, Tano Y, Nakamura T. Induction of hepatocyte growth factor in fibroblasts by tumor-derived factors affects invasive growth of tumor cells: *in vitro* analysis of tumor-stromal interactions. *Cancer Res* 1997; **57**: 3305–13.
30. Rong S, Segal S, Anver M, Resau JH, Vande Woude GF. Invasiveness and metastasis of NIH 3T3 cells induced by Met-hepatocyte growth factor/scatter factor autocrine stimulation. *Proc Natl Acad Sci USA* 1994; **91**: 4731–5.
31. Kanda H, Tajima H, Lee G, Nomura K, Ohtake K, Matsumoto K, Nakamura T, Kitagawa T. Hepatocyte growth factor transforms immortalized mouse liver epithelial cells. *Oncogene* 1993; **8**: 3047–53.
32. Johnson M, Koukoulis G, Kochhar K, Kubo C, Nakamura T, Iyer A. Selective tumorigenesis in non-parenchymal liver epithelial cell lines by hepatocyte growth factor transfection. *Cancer Lett* 1995; **96**: 37–48.

33. Di Renzo MF, Olivero M, Giacomini A, Porte H, Chastre E, Mirossay L, Nordlinger B, Bretti S, Bottardi S, Giordano S, Plebani M, Gespach C, Comoglio PM. Overexpression and amplification of the met/HGF receptor gene during the progression of colorectal cancer. *Clin Cancer Res* 1995; **1**: 147–54.
34. Schmidt L, Duh F, Chan F, Kishida T, Glenn G, Choyke P, Scherer SW, Zhuang Z, Lubensky I, Dean M, Allikmets R, Chidambaram A, Bergerheim UR, Feltis JT, Casadevall C, Zamarron A, Bernues M, Richard S, Lips CJM, Walther MM, Tsui L, Geil L, Orcutt ML, Stackhouse T, Lipan J, Slife L, Brauch H, Decker J, Niehans G, Hughson MD, Moch H, Storkel S, Lerman MI, Linehan WM, Zbar B. Germline and somatic mutations in the tyrosine kinase domain of the MET proto-oncogene in papillary renal carcinomas. *Nat Genet* 1997; **16**: 68–73.
35. Jeffers M, Schmidt L, Nakagawa N, Webb CP, Weirich G, Kishida T, Zbar B, Vande Woude GF. Activating mutations for the Met tyrosine kinase receptor in human cancer. *Proc Natl Acad Sci USA* 1997; **94**: 11445–50.
36. Schwall RH, Chang LY, Godowski PJ, Kahn DW, Hillan KJ, Bauer KD, Zioncheck TH. Heparin induces dimerization and confers proliferative activity onto the hepatocyte growth factor antagonists NK1 and NK2. *J Cell Biol* 1996; **133**: 709–18.
37. Silvagno F, Follenzi A, Arese M, Prat M, Giraudo E, Gaudino G, Camussi G, Comoglio PM, Bussolino F. *In vivo* activation of met tyrosine kinase by heterodimeric hepatocyte growth factor molecule promotes angiogenesis. *Arterioscler Thromb Vasc Biol* 1995; **15**: 1857–65.
38. Cioce V, Csaky KG, Chan AML, Bottaro DP, Taylor WG, Jensen R, Aaronson SA, Rubin JS. Hepatocyte growth factor (HGF)/NK1 is a naturally occurring HGF/scatter factor variant with partial agonist/antagonist activity. *J Biol Chem* 1996; **271**: 13110–5.
39. Kuba K, Matsumoto K, Ohnishi K, Shiratsuchi T, Tanaka M, Nakamura T. Kringle 1-4 of hepatocyte growth factor inhibits proliferation and migration of human microvascular endothelial cells. *Biochem Biophys Res Commun* 2000; **279**: 846–52.
40. O'Reilly MS, Holmgren L, Shing Y, Chen C, Rosenthal RA, Moses M, Lane WS, Cao Y, Sage EH, Folkman J. Angiostatin: a novel angiogenesis inhibitor that mediates the suppression of metastases by a Lewis lung carcinoma. *Cell* 1994; **79**: 315–28.
41. Cao Y, Chen A, An SSA, Ji RW, Davidson D, Llinas M. Kringle 5 of plasminogen is a novel inhibitor of endothelial cell growth. *J Biol Chem* 1997; **272**: 22924–8.
42. Lee TH, Rhim T, Kim SS. Prothrombin kringle-2 domain has a growth inhibitory activity against basic fibroblast growth factor-stimulated capillary endothelial cells. *J Biol Chem* 1998; **273**: 28805–12.
43. Claesson-Welsh L, Welsh M, Ito N, Anand-Apte B, Soker S, Zetter B, O'Reilly M, Folkman J. Angiostatin induces endothelial cell apoptosis and activation of focal adhesion kinase independently of the integrin-binding motif RGD. *Proc Natl Acad Sci USA* 1998; **95**: 5579–83.
44. Moser TL, Stack MS, Asplin I, Enghild JJ, Hojrup P, Everitt L, Hubchak S, Schnaper HW, Pizzo SV. Angiostatin binds ATP synthase on the surface of human endothelial cells. *Proc Natl Acad Sci USA* 1999; **96**: 2811–6.
45. Tarui T, Majumdar M, Miles LA, Ruf W, Takada Y. Plasmin-induced migration of endothelial cells. A potential target for the anti-angiogenic action of angiostatin. *J Biol Chem* 2002; **277**: 33564–70.

46. Tomioka D, Maehara N, Kuba K, Mizumoto K, Tanaka M, Matsumoto K, Nakamura T. Inhibition of growth, invasion, and metastasis of human pancreatic carcinoma cells by NK4 in an orthotopic mouse model. *Cancer Res* 2001; **61**: 7518–24.
47. Saga Y, Mizukami H, Suzuki M, Urabe M, Kume A, Nakamura T, Sato I, Ozawa K. Expression of HGF/NK4 in ovarian cancer cells suppresses intraperitoneal dissemination and extends host survival. *Gene Ther* 2001; **8**: 1450–5.
48. Maemondo M, Narumi K, Saijo Y, Usui K, Tahara M, Tazawa R, Hagiwara K, Matsumoto K, Nakamura T, Nukiwa, T. Targeting angiogenesis and HGF function using an adenoviral vector expressing the HGF-antagonist NK4 for cancer therapy. *Mol Ther* 2002; **5**: 177–85.
49. Hirao S, Yamada Y, Koyama F, Fujimoto H, Takahama Y, Ueno M, Kamada K, Mizuno T, Maemondo M, Nukiwa T, Matsumoto K, Nakamura T, Nakajima Y. Tumor suppression effect using NK4, a molecule acting as an antagonist of HGF, on human gastric carcinomas. *Cancer Gene Ther* 2002; **9**: 700–7.
50. Saimura M, Nagai E, Mizumoto K, Maehara N, Okino H, Katano M, Matsumoto K, Nakamura T, Narumi K, Nukiwa T, Tanaka M. Intraperitoneal injection of adenovirus-mediated NK4 gene suppresses peritoneal dissemination of pancreatic cancer cell line AsPC-1 in nude mice. *Cancer Gene Ther* 2002; **9**: 799–806.

NEW ASPECTS OF IFN-α/β SIGNALLING IN IMMUNITY, ONCOGENESIS AND BONE METABOLISM

Akinori TAKAOKA and Tadatsugu TANIGUCHI

*Department of Immunology, Graduate School of Medicine and Faculty of Medicine, University of Tokyo**

Although interferons (IFNs) were originally identified as humoral factors that confer an antiviral state upon cells, they have been demonstrated to be multifunctional in a variety of biological systems. The IFN-α/β system modulates not only the cellular immune response to viral and bacterial infections, but also the oncogenic process and bone metabolism. Further studies have revealed additional unique facets of the IFN-α/β system. A weak signal by constitutively produced IFN-α/β is critical not only for the regulation of cellular amplification of IFN-α/β production upon viral infection or the enhancement of signalling by other cytokines, but also for the regulation of adaptive immune responses, such as the enhancement of $CD8^+$ T cell activation. Furthermore, IFN-β signalling is critical for the regulation of the bone-resorbing osteoclasts. In this review, we focus on the newly discovered roles of the IFN-α/β system in host defense and bone remodeling, particularly on the functions of the weak IFN-α/β signalling in the context of what we refer to as the "revving-up" model.

Biological systems have acquired adaptability to, and robustness against rapid environmental changes, and one typical example is the immune system, which eradicates invading pathogens such as viruses. Type I interferons, i.e., IFN-α and IFN-β, the production of which is induced upon viral infection, are essential components of this system (*1*, *2*). Production is induced *en masse* in many types of cells upon infection by a variety of viruses, and this induction is primarily controlled at the transcriptional level. As well as eliciting strong antiviral activities in target cells, IFN-α/β also activates effector cells of the innate immune system, such as natural killer (NK) cells and macrophages (*1–4*). Given the essential function of IFN-α/β as mediators of innate immune responses against viruses, it is interesting that there are many reports on IFN-α/β production occurring in the absence of viral infection, albeit at very low levels, both *in vitro* and *in vivo* (*1*, *5*, *6*). However, in this article, we focus on other unique facets of the IFN-α/β system. A weak IFN-α/β signal, transmitted independently of viral infection, is critical for priming cells to enhance their response to other stimuli. In fact, the weak signal renders cells "ready-to-go," by stimulating amplified IFN-α/β production in response to viral infection, and enhances responses to other cytokines (*7*, *8*). Spontaneous IFN-α/β signalling is also critical for enhancing the

* 7-3-1 Hongo, Bunkyo-ku, Tokyo 113-0033, Japan

This paper is dedicated to the memory of late Dr. Tomizo Yoshida on the occasion of the 100th anniversary of his birth. It was originally published in Cancer Science in May, 2003.

activation of CD8⁺ T cells, but it needs to be properly attenuated to maintain homeostatic CD8⁺ T-cell responses (*9*). These observations offer interesting examples of how weak signals elicited by a given stimulus contribute to eliciting strong cellular responses to other stimuli. The role of continuous, weak IFN-α/β signalling, described here in the context of our newly proposed "revving-up model," may point to a broad operation of similar mechanisms in other biological systems. On the other hand, even a weak dysregulation of such a signalling system can also be the basis for disease development.

IFN-β has also recently been shown to be an essential regulator of osteoclastogenesis, wherein the IFN-β signalling makes a balance with RANKL (receptor activator of nuclear factor κB ligand) signalling through a unique signalling crosstalk mechanism to properly regulate the differentiation of osteoclasts (*10*).

IFN-α/β System in Viral Immunity

1. *IFN-α/β gene induction by viral infection: operation of a positive feedback regulation for robust IFN production*

Type I IFNs are produced by a variety of cells in response to viral infections. The type I IFNs comprise a number of species of IFN-α and one IFN-β. All IFN-α/β species interact with the same receptor complex, termed the IFN-α/β receptor (IFNAR), which consists of at least two subunits, IFNAR-1 and IFNAR-2 (Fig. 1). The intracellular domains of these two subunits. IFNAR-1 and IFNAR-2, are associated with Jak PTKs (Janus protein tyrosine kinases), Tyk2 and Jak1, respectively. Binding of IFN-α/β to IFNAR results in cross-activation of these Jak PTKs, which then phosphorylate their downstream substrates, two members of the family of signal transducers and activators of transcription (Stats), namely, Stat1 and Stat2 (*11–14*). The tyrosine phosphorylation of these Stats leads to formation of two transcriptional activator complexes, IFN-α-activated factor (AAF) and IFN-stimulated gene factor 3 (ISGF3) (Fig. 1). AAF is a homodimer of tyrosine-phosphorylated Stat1, whereas ISGF3 is a heterotrimeric complex of tyrosine-phosphorylated Stat1, Stat2 and another transcription factor member, IFN-regulatory factor (IRF)-9/p48/ISGF3γ (Fig. 1). These complexes translocate into the nucleus; subsequently, AAF and ISGF3 bind to their specific DNA sequences containing each common motif, namely, the IFN-γ-activated sequence (GAS) and the IFN-stimulated response element (ISRE), respectively. IFN stimulation of promoters containing ISRE and GAS results in the transcriptional induction of a large number of target genes (ISGs; IFN-stimulated genes) to evoke antiviral activity.

The mechanism for the induction of *IFN-α/β* gene transcription in virus-infected cells has been extensively studied (reviewed in Refs. 15, 16). The promoter region of the *IFN-β* gene contains at least four regulatory *cis*-elements; the positive regulatory domains (PRDs) I, II, III and IV (Fig. 2). Analysis of the promoter region revealed that the transcriptional activators NF-κB and ATF-2/c-Jun bind to PRD II and PRD IV elements, respectively, and activate, in cooperation with PRD I and PRD III, the *IFN-β* gene in virus-infected cells (*17*). On the other hand, PRD I and PRD III elements, which members of the IRF family can recognize, are essential as virus-inducible enhancers of IFN-β induction (*18–21*). As for the *IFN-α* genes, it was reported that PRD-like elements (PRD-LEs), which are similar to the PRD I

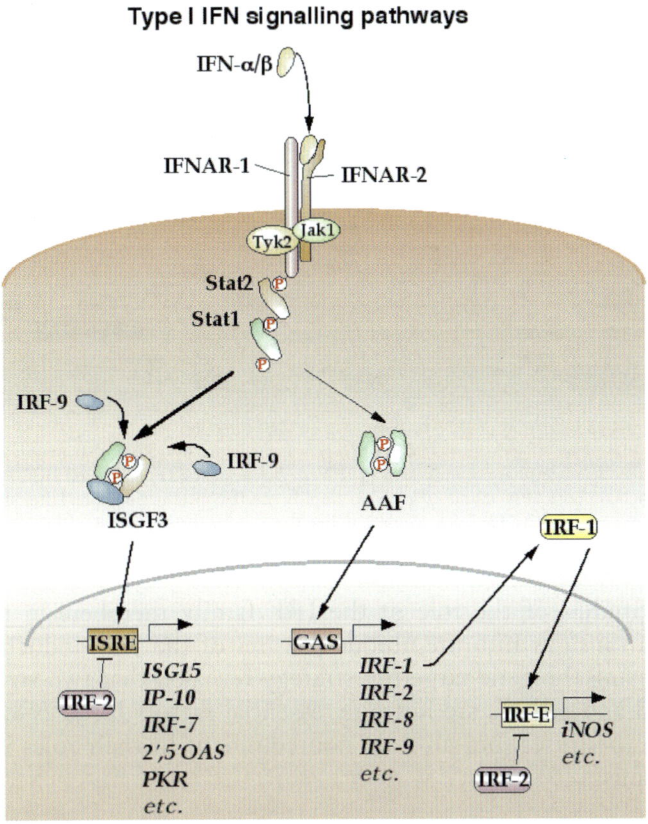

FIG. 1. Cardinal features of the IFN-α/β signalling pathway

IFN-α/β transmits signals via its homologous receptor complex, IFNAR (*13*, *14*). IFNAR is composed of at least two subcomponents, IFNAR-1 and IFNAR-2, of which IFNAR-2 is the major ligand-binding subunit. Ligand binding results in the formation of a signalling complex with IFNAR-1 and IFNAR-2, leading to activation of the receptor-associated Tyk2 and Jak1, respectively (*11–14*). This is followed by the tyrosine phosphorylations of Stat1 and Stat2, leading to the formation of the heterotrimeric ISGF3 transcription factor together with an IRF-family member of transcription factors, IRF-9 (also referred to as p48). In addition, a Stat1 homodimer, termed AAF, is formed. Subsequently, these transcriptional activator complexes translocate into the nucleus and activate the interferon-stimulated response element (ISRE) or the IFN-γ-activated site (GAS). The human IFNAR-1 subunit contains within the cytoplasmic region four tyrosine residues, of which the tyrosine residue 466 (Y466) provides the main docking site for Stat2/Stat1. Of note in this review is the *IRF-7* gene, the expression of which is totally dependent on ISGF3. On the other hand, another IRF-family member, IRF-2, is a nuclear factor that also binds to ISRE, and this factor interferes with the ISGF3 action, thereby functioning as a transcriptional attenuator (*9*). Although not depicted in this figure, it has been suggested that Stat1 and Stat2 are associated with IFNAR-2 before stimulation (*14*).

and PRD III elements in the IFN-β promoter, are found within IFN-α promoters (*22*).

Since IRF-1 was first discovered as a transcriptional activator that binds to virus-inducible enhancer-like elements of the human *IFN-β* gene (*19*), other IRFs have been found to constitute a family of transcriptional factors, which now consists of nine members (IRF-1 to -9; reviewed in Refs. *16*, *23*, *24*). In a series of studies on *IFN-α/β* gene regulation, IRF-1, IRF-3, IRF-7 and IRF-9 among the above IRFs, were shown to be implicated in *IFN-α/β* gene induction by viral infection

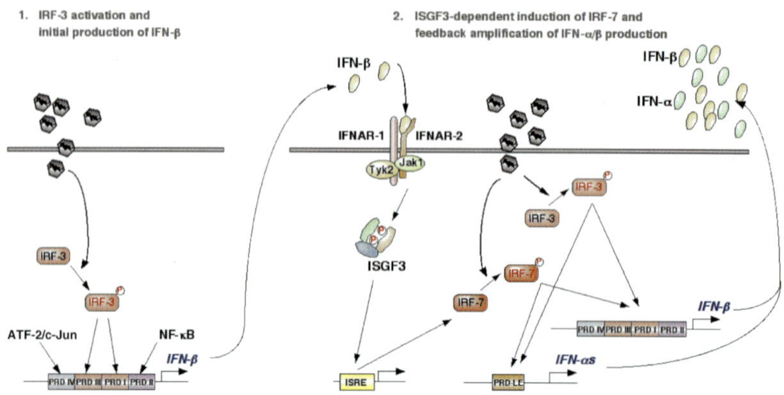

FIG. 2. Two-step induction of *IFN-α/β* genes upon viral infection
1. The initial phase of induction *of IFN-α/β* genes, mediated by IRF-3 that mainly acts on the *IFN-β* gene. 2. The late phase of induction of *IFN-α/β* genes. The IFN-induced IRF-7 is activated and IRF-7 acts on both *IFN-α* and *-β* genes to amplify the IFN production. The latter step is therefore considered as a positive feedback regulation. See the text for further explanation.

(*7, 20, 21, 25*). Studies of the role of the IRF family members in the IFN system should provide an insight into the unique features of the IFN induction mechanism. A recent study using the gene targeting strategy revealed that two structurally related members, IRF-3 and IRF-7, are not only essential factors for *IFN-α/β* gene induction in response to viruses, but also are nonredundant in their roles in the IFN-α/β induction mechanism (*7*).

2. *Roles of IRF-3 and IRF-7 in two-step induction of IFN-α/β genes*

In the initial phase (Fig. 2 (1)), IRF-3, which is constitutively expressed in normally growing cells, plays a dominant part in the initial induction of *IFN-α/β* genes (*7, 26–28*). In fact, virus infection results in the serine/threonine phosphorylation of IRF-3 at its carboxyl-terminal region by an unknown kinase(s) to become an active form (See "Added-in-proof"). The activated IRF-3 undergoes nuclear translocation, and binds to IRF-Es in the IFN-β promoter. Since, unlike IRF-3, IRF-7 expression is inducible by IFN-α/β stimulation (*29, 30*), IRF-7, which is induced by IFN-α/β secreted in the initial phase, mainly participates in the late phase of *IFN-α/β* gene induction (Fig. 2 (2)), particularly in mouse embryonic fibroblasts expressing IRF-7 at a low level in the absence of infection. This indicates the two-step induction of *IFN-α/β* genes by virus infection, wherein each of IRF-3 and IRF-7 plays a distinctive role in regulation of virus-induced IFN production (*7*). In addition, there is a unique positive feedback mechanism in the late phase, where signalling by *de novo* synthesized IFN-α/β amplifies IFN-α/β production through its enhancement of the intracellular expression level of IRF-7 (*7, 29, 30*). Interestingly, a further study showed that the expression level of IRF-7 before infection was critical for triggering the positive feedback system for efficient induction of *IFN-α/β* genes by viruses (*31*), which we will discuss in detail below.

3. *Spontaneous IFN-α/β production*

IFN-α/β is known to be massively produced upon viral infection, and functions in innate immune responses, but evidence has also been presented that the expression of IFN-α/β is constitutive, albeit at a very low level, in the absence of infection (*1*, *5*, *6*). Although there is evidence that these IFNs contribute to antiviral, anti-tumor activities and cell growth control (*1*, *5*, *32*) in a manner similar to the virus-induced IFNs, recent studies have revealed a unique molecular machinery of this system (*8*, *31*, *33*, *34*). In fact, the weak signal renders cells "ready-to-go" for the amplification or enhancement of cellular responses to rapid environmental changes, such as viral infection. This machinery is similar to a car engine revving up before the car starts moving and accelerating. The "revving up" of cells by a weak signal is implicated in eliciting robust and efficient cellular responses against infections (Fig. 3; Ref. *34*). This "revving-up" system is a unique signal-dependent regulatory mechanism for the responsiveness, particularly in host defense. Recent evidence has been shown that a weak IFN-α/β signal by the constitutively produced IFN-α/β is critical for eliciting strong responses of cells to IFN-γ and interleukin (IL)-6, which are major cytokines involved in adaptive immune responses (*8*, *33*). In addition, evidence has also been presented for a role of weak IFN-α/β signalling in the absence of viral infection in the regulation of innate immune responses against viruses; this signalling was found to play an important role in efficient production of IFN-α/β upon viral infection (*31*).

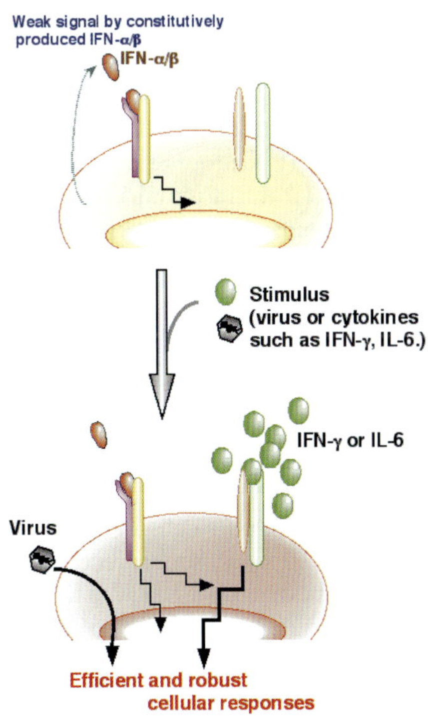

FIG. 3. "Revving up the cellular engine" by spontaneously produced IFN-α/β

A weak IFN-α/β signal by constitutively produced IFN-α/β plays an important role in the efficient and robust responses to IFN-γ, IL-6 or viral infection (*8*, *31*, *33*). The IFN-α/β continuously transmit weak signals to elicit from cells strong responses to these other cytokines. Therefore, somewhat analogous to revving up the engine in car racing, this signalling may provide the foundation for efficient cellular responses in the immune system.

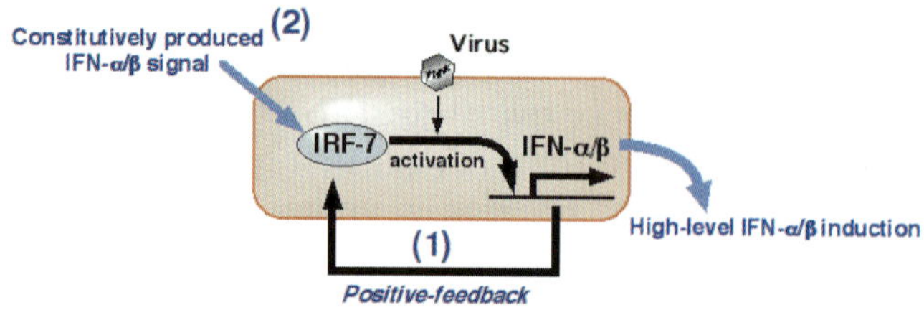

FIG. 4. Two amplification mechanisms for efficient *IFN-α/β* gene induction upon viral infection
There are two regulatory mechanisms for the amplification of virus-induced IFN-α/β production, both of which are dependent upon the expression of IRF-7. One is a postinfection positive feedback mechanism (1). The other is a preinfection regulatory mechanism that is controlled by a weak signal of constitutively produced IFN-α/β (2).

4. Two amplification mechanisms for efficient IFN-α/β gene induction by virus

Analysis of the roles of IRF-7 in the regulation of virus-induced IFN-α/β production revealed that there are two regulatory mechanisms for the efficient amplification of the IFN-α/β production system (Fig. 4). One is an IRF-7-mediated positive feedback mechanism that is triggered by IFN-α/β initially produced after infection (Fig.4 (1)). The other is a regulatory mechanism that is controlled by a weak signal by constitutively produced IFN-α/β before infection (Fig.4 (2)). The latter mechanism is also mediated by IRF-7. As mentioned above, both IRF-3 and IRF-7 are essential factors for virus-induced IFN-α/β production. On the other hand, the nonredundant roles of these two factors in IFN-α/β induction were clarified by a recent gene disruption/introduction study (*7*). Unlike constitutively expressed IRF-3, IRF-7 is short-lived and its gene expression is dependent on IFN-α/β signalling (*7, 29, 30*); hence, the IFN-α/β-dependency of IRF-7 provides an underlying mechanism for the autoamplification of IFN production, whereby induction of the *IRF-7* gene by *de novo* produced IFN-α/β during viral infection results in a positive feedback enhancement of *IFN-α/β* gene induction (Fig.4 (1)). In addition, there is another unique signal-amplification mechanism that is mediated by the weak IFN-α/β signalling in the absence of infection (Fig.4 (2)). This weak IFN-α/β signalling contributes to setting the IRF-7 expression level beyond an appropriate threshold for the activation of the positive-feedback loop upon infection (*31*). In fact, in splenocytes, which express a relatively high level of IRF-7 even before infection, this induction mechanism is more effective than in fibroblasts with a much lower level of IRF-7 expression (*31*). These expression levels of IRF-7 were found to be correlated with the expression level of the constitutive IFN-α/β. Thus, in advance of viral invasion, the constitutive, weak IFN-α/β signalling puts cells in a "revving up" state for the robust and efficient production of IFN-α/β upon viral infection (*34*).

Furthermore, recent reports have shown that the activation of Toll-like receptors (TLRs) by several pathogen-associated molecular patterns (PAMPs) resulted in the induction of the *IFN-α/β* genes. Among these TLRs, TLR3 is known to bind to double-stranded RNA (dsRNA), leading to the induction of *IFN-α/β* genes (*35*). Our recent data show that TLR3 itself is induced by type I IFNs in an ISGF3-dependent manner (*71*). In this regard, it may be suggested that TLR3 signalling is positively regulated through *Tlr3* gene induction by *de novo*-produced IFN-α/β, and that IFN-α/β-induced TLR3, as well as IRF-7, is one of the targets in the "IFN priming." (*36*) More interestingly, this may provide a possible explanation for a mechanism by which uninfected cells neighboring infected cells can get ready for the recognition of invading pathogens and for efficient cellular responses.

These observations offer an interesting example of how weak signals by a given stimulus contribute to eliciting strong cellular responses to other stimuli. Thus, the role of constitutive, weak IFN-α/β signalling, described here in the context of the "revving-up model," may point to a broad operation of similar mechanisms in other biological systems.

5. *Role of the weak IFN-α/β-mediated signals for efficient CD8$^+$ T cell activation upon T-cell receptor (TCR) stimulation*

Recently, interesting data have shown that spontaneous IFN-α/β expression was only marginally augmented upon stimulation of CD8$^+$ T cells by a mixed lymphocyte reaction (*37*). In fact, different from the case of viral infections, induction of IFN-α/β mRNAs upon TCR stimulation is not efficient less than 1/200 the level of gene induction by viral infection (*31*). In the context of the revving-up system based on the constitutively produced IFN-α/β, one can postulate that the low levels of IFN-α/β expression, which are only slightly induced upon T cell activation, play a similar role to the more efficient TCR signalling in CD8$^+$ T cells. In addition, the augmentation of the local IFN-α/β concentration at the site of T-cell activation may contribute to a more efficient operation of this mechanism for the activation of TCR signalling in CD8$^+$ T cells. During viral infections, it is known that CD8$^+$ T cells can be activated in a CD4$^+$ T-cell-independent manner, concomitant with the massive production of IFN-α/β (Refs. *38–40*). Our recent results obtained with ovalbumin (OVA)-specific activation assays show that exogenous treatment with recombinant IFN-β enhances the proliferation of CD8$^+$ T cells in a dose-dependent manner (*37*). On the other hand, CD8$^+$ T cells lacking the IFN-α/β signalling are hyporesponsive to antigen stimulation. Further evidence showed that IFN-α/β-mediated signals are required for the induction of chemokines, IFN-γ-inducible protein (IP)-10/CXC chemokine ligand (CXCL) 10 and IFN-inducible T-cell α chemoattractant (I-TAC)/CXCL11, as well as their common receptor, CXC chemokines receptor (CXCR) 3; this in turn provides evidence that CXCR3-mediated signals subsequently contribute to the efficient induction of activation markers such as CD25 and CD69, thereby leading to the efficient proliferation of CD8$^+$ T cells (*37*). These observations offer another indication of possible involvement of the constitutive, weak IFN-α/β signalling in the efficient activation of CD8$^+$ T cell upon the engagement of TCR with major histocompatibility complex (MHC)/peptide complexes on antigen-presenting cells.

6. *Dysregulation of weak IFN-α/β signalling*

As described above, it was found that the weak IFN-α/β signalling is critical for efficiently eliciting robust cellular responses in the immune system, and may point to a broad operation of similar mechanisms in other biological systems. One can infer that dysregulation of this weak signalling may give rise to potentially serious disruption of these biological systems. Recent studies on IRF-2$^{-/-}$ mice provided an interesting model for clarifying this issue (*9*). IRF-2, a stable nuclear protein expressed in a variety of cells, is found to be a transcriptional attenuator of IFN-α/β signalling, which is known to function negatively on ISRE sites of IFN-inducible genes by competition with ISGF3 for these sites (*21*). Accordingly, in the absence of IRF-2, the action of ISGF3 becomes dominant, leading to the continual, elevated expression of ISGF3-dependent IFN-inducible genes, such as *IRF-7*. Our recent report showed that IRF-$2^{-/-}$ mice spontaneously develop an inflammatory skin lesion, which is similar to lesions observed in patients with psoriasis (*9*). It was also found that the development of this skin disease results from selective $CD8^{+}$ T-cell hyperactivation, with a remarkable upregulation of ISGF3-dependent IFN-α/β-stimulated genes. Other pathological conditions observed in IRF-2-null mice, such as impaired hematopoiesis and autoimmune-like pancreatitis, may be caused by dysregulated weak IFN-α/β-signalling. These abnormal findings in IRF-$2^{-/-}$ mice suggest that the constitutive, weak IFN-α/β signalling should be controlled by a proper regulatory mechanism for maintaining homeostasis in the host. In this context, IRF-2 is one of the essential regulators that properly set the level of constitutive, weak IFN-α/β signalling to balance the beneficial and harmful effects of this signalling. Thus, dysregulation of such a signalling system can also be the basis for disease development.

The IFN-α/β System in Oncogenesis

Much evidence regarding anti-tumor activities of IFNs has been reported (reviewed in Refs. *41*, *42*). Most of their antitumor functions are explained in terms of modulatory actions on the immune system. At least hundreds of cellular genes are transcriptionally activated after IFN stimulation (*43*). Several of these ISGs were shown to encode proteins that mediate tumor suppressor activities directly or indirectly: for example, IRF-1, dsRNA-dependent protein kinase (PKR), and 2′-5′oligoadenylate synthetase (OAS) (*44–51*). They modulate the functional activities of the immune system against tumors in various ways and affect cell proliferation and differentiation. Recent studies on the immunomodulatory activity of type I IFNs have shown that IFNs act on T-lymphocytes or dendritic cells to modulate their functions, which may explain IFN-induced tumor immunity (reviewed in Ref. *52*).

On the other hand, in the context of the antiviral actions of IFNs themselves, evidence points also to the potential benefits of IFNs against tumors of viral origin, such as hairy cell leukemia, Kaposi's sarcoma, hepatitis B or C virus-related hepatomas, HPV-related condylomata acuminatum and juvenile laryngeal papillomatosis, and others (*53*, *54*).

Different from the aspects mentioned above, we have recently found a novel aspect of the anti-tumor activities induced by IFN-α/β. As discussed above, low levels of IFN-α/β production in the absence of viral infection were previously observed in mouse embryonic fibroblasts (MEFs) and other cells, and IFN-α/β mRNAs can be detected in MEFs and other cells/tissues of the mouse by reverse transcriptase-polymerase chain reaction (RT-PCR) analysis. Evidence has also been provided that, very similar to virus-induced IFN-α/β, these low-level IFN-α/β expressions indeed contribute to anti-tumor activities and to the control of cell growth. Recently, we have made an interesting observation regarding the involvement of a weak signal by the constitutively produced IFN-α/β in the regulation of oncogenesis. Long-term cultures of IFNAR-1-deficient MEFs as well as IFN-β-deficient MEFs, both of which show little or no signalling by constitutively produced IFN-α/β, resulted in the formation of transformed colonies, albeit at a low incidence, which could form tumors in nude mice (Takaoka and Taniguchi, unpublished data). Moreover, IFNAR-1-deficient mice showed papilloma formation on the skin after chemical induction (Takaoka and Taniguchi, unpublished data). These findings suggest a novel biological significance of the weak signal by constitutively produced IFN-α/β, which may be implicated in homeostatic host defense mechanisms for preventing cells from developing tumors. Furthermore, it can be speculated that this weak IFN-α/β signalling might be involved in maintaining the constitutive expression level of some molecule(s) which might be a regulator(s) in the surveillance system against oncogenesis. Therefore, IFNs seem to be essential mediators not only for the host defense in the innate immune responses against microbial infections, but also for a host defense system against oncogenesis.

The IFN-α/β System in Bone Metabolism

Several recent studies have revealed a novel facet of the IFN system in bone metabolism (*10*, *55*), which led to the development of a new field, termed osteoimmunology, that is, the overlapping of bone metabolism and the immune system (*56*, *57*). Maintenance of bone homeostasis is widely known to be regulated by a mechanism that balances bone formation and bone resorption, wherein osteoblasts and osteoclasts, respectively, are the essential effector cells (*58*). In osteoclastogenesis, RANKL, a member of the TNF (tumor necrosis factor) family, is a critical cytokine for the differentiation of monocyte/macrophage precursors to osteoclasts (*59–61*). It was demonstrated that osteoclastogenesis is strictly regulated by activated T-cell-derived IFN-γ via its counterbalancing action on RANKL signalling (*55*) (Fig. 5). In this regulatory system, IFN-γ negatively regulates RANKL signalling through the degradation of TRAF6 (TNF-receptor-associated factor 6), one of the major downstream molecules in RANKL signalling. Further extensive analyses revealed that IFN-β is also a critical mediator during osteoclast differentiation (*10*). Both IFNAR-

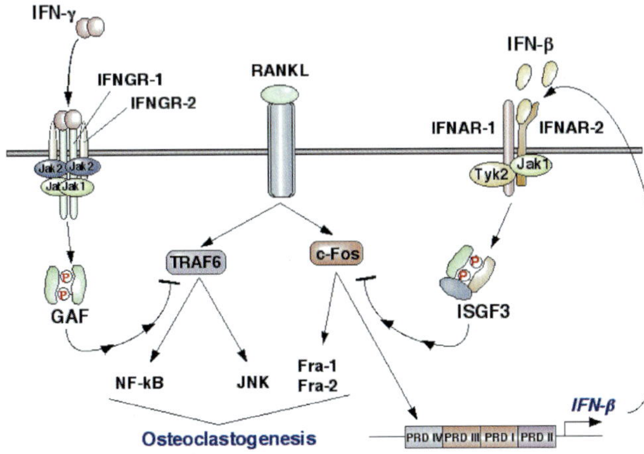

FIG. 5. Role of the IFN-β system in the negative regulation of osteoclastogenesis through crosstalk with RANKL signalling

During osteoclastogenesis, the IFN-β system is utilized in negative feedback regulation for shaping the RANKL signalling. IFN-β is induced by RANKL stimulation in a c-Fos-dependent manner. See the text for details.

1-deficient mice and IFN-β-deficient mice showed a significant reduction in trabecular bone mass, with an increase in the number of osteoclasts. This observation indicates that type I IFN signalling is required for the negative regulation of osteoclastogenic bone resorption. Further analysis of the mechanism underlying the inhibitory action of type I IFN revealed that as yet unidentified protein(s) encoded by an IFN-stimulated gene(s) may posttranslationally suppress the expression of c-*fos*, one of the critical target genes for RANKL-induced osteoclast differentiation (Fig. 5). In bone marrow-derived macrophages (BMMs), which are known to be osteoclast precursor cells, RANKL stimulates the induction of the *IFN-β* gene, but not that of *IFN-α* genes, which suggests a unique signalling crosstalk wherein RANKL signalling finely regulates osteoclastogenesis by controlling the balance via the utilization of the IFN system with the RANKL-induced IFN-β. It is of interest that the mechanism of IFN-β induction by RANKL is totally different from that of the type I IFN induction by viral infection. The induction of the *IFN-β* gene by RANKL in BMMs is still detected even in the absence of two IRF transcriptional factors, IRF-3 and IRF-7, which are essential factors for the virus-mediated induction of IFN-α/β, as discussed above. However, the RANKL-induced IFN-β mRNA expression was no longer observed in cells lacking c-Fos. Actually, the (weak) induction of *IFN-β* gene by RANKL requires c-Fos, perhaps in the context of the AP-1 transcription factor complex that binds to the promoter. These results indicate a hitherto unrecognized new role of IFN-β, beyond its function in anti-viral immunity, whereby the IFN-β system is utilized for the negative regulation of RANKL signalling for osteoclastogenesis.

Conclusions and Future Prospects

In this article, we reviewed new aspects of the IFN-α/β system, highlighting the functional implication of the weak signalling by constitutively produced IFN-α/β in the regulation of cellular responses to other extracellular stimuli.

As described in this article, it was found that the weak IFN-α/β signal provides unique signal regulatory mechanisms for its own IFN-α/β signalling system and signalling systems of other cytokines such as IFN-γ and IL-6, as well as the TCR signalling system. In this regulatory system, the weak IFN-α/β signalling by the constitutively produced IFN-α/β allows the cell to rev up for efficient and robust responses to various stimuli (the "revving-up" model (*34*)). In this regard, the weak IFN-α/β signalling in the absence of infection contributes to the control of the IRF-7 expression level beyond a certain threshold that is crucial for triggering the autoamplification mechanism for IFN-α/β production upon viral infection (*31*). This IFN-α/β signal-mediated "revving-up" mechanism through IRF-7 expression enables cells to efficiently produce IFN-α/β to achieve a robust immune response to viral infections.

In the IFN-α/β signalling system described here, signalling molecules remain constantly activated, albeit weakly, and the expression of target genes is maintained, thereby providing a foundation for more efficient signalling, either in that pathway or in different pathways. Thus, consumption of cellular resources is a regulated "trade-off" to provide the cell with a greater dynamic range (signal-to-noise) in its response to stimuli. The IFN-α/β system may also provide an interesting illustration of the feedback loops required when such a function is operational. The advantages of highly efficient IFN-γ/IL-6 responses and the disadvantages of the failure of the IRF-2-mediated attenuation (autoimmune, psoriasis-like syndrome) indicate that the selective advantages of "revving up" the response can also be the basis of disease states when it is dysregulated. The possibility that this may be a key theme in the overall setting of host defense and autoimmunity opens exciting avenues for future research.

The host defense mechanism comprises two major defense systems: innate and adaptive immunities. Innate immunity initiates protection of the host organism against invasion and subsequent multiplication of microbes by recognition of the PAMPs (*62, 63*). In this regard, several microbial pattern recognition receptors have been recently identified as TLRs, the mammalian homologues of the *Drosophila* Toll receptor (reviewed in Refs. *64, 65*). Recently, much attention has been focused on the roles of the IFN and IRF systems in relation to TLRs. In fact, it was reported that several microbial products, such as dsRNA, lipopolysaccharide (LPS), and oligodeoxyribonucleotides containing unmethylated CpG motifs (CpG-DNA), activate the induction of *IFN-α/β* genes through their respective TLRs (*66–70*). Recent studies led us to envisage the sequence of IFN-α/β-mediated events that operate during the maturation of dendritic cells (DCs) (*71*). The newly discovered role of IFN-α/β in DC maturation may provide practical approaches to an adjuvant for vaccines that enhance anti-tumor and anti-viral immunity.

Acknowledgments

This work was supported in part by a grant for Advanced Research on Cancer from the Ministry of Education, Culture, Sports, Science, and Technology of Japan, Grants-in-Aid from the Ministry of Education, Science, and Culture (Scientific Research on Priority Areas), Research Grant of the Princess Takamatsu Cancer Research Fund, The Nakajima Foundation, The Sumitomo Foundation, and Research Fund of Mitsukoshi Health and Welfare Foundation.

REFERENCES

1. De Maeyer E, De Maeyer-Guignard J. In: Interferons and other regulatory cytokines. New York: John Wiley and Sons; 1988.
2. Vilcek J, Sen GS. Interferons and other cytokines. In: Fields DM, Knipe PM, Howley PM, editors. Fields virology. 3rd ed. Philadelphia: Lippincott-Raven; 1996. p. 375–99.
3. Pestka S, Langer JA, Zoon KC, Samuel CE. Interferons and their actions. *Annu Rev Biochem* 1987; **56**: 727–77.
4. Biron CA, Nguyen KB, Pien GC, Cousens LP, Salazar-Mather TP. Natural killer cells in antiviral defense: function and regulation by innate cytokines. *Annu Rev Immunol* 1999; **17**: 189–220.
5. Bocci V. The physiological interferon response. *Immunol Today* 1985; **6**: 7–9.
6. Tovey MG, Streuli M, Gresser I, Gugenheim J, Blanchard B, Guymarho J, Vignaux F, Gigou M. Interferon messenger RNA is produced constitutively in the organs of normal individuals. *Proc Natl Acad Sci USA* 1987; **84**: 5038–42.
7. Sato M, Suemori H, Hata N, Asagiri M, Ogasawara K, Nakao K, Nakaya T, Katsuki M, Noguchi S, Tanaka N, Taniguchi T. Distinct and essential roles of transcription fac-

tors IRF-3 and IRF-7 in response to viruses for *IFN-α/β* gene induction. *Immunity* 2000; **13**: 539–48.

8. Takaoka A, Mitani Y, Suemori H, Sato M, Yokochi T, Noguchi S, Tanaka N, Taniguchi T. Cross talk between interferon-γ and -α/β signaling components in caveolar membrane domains. *Science* 2000; **288**: 2357–60.
9. Hida S, Ogasawara K, Sato K, Abe M, Takayanagi H, Yokochi T, Sato T, Hirose S, Shirai T, Taki S, Taniguchi T. CD8(+) T cell-mediated skin disease in mice lacking IRF-2, the transcriptional attenuator of interferon-α/β signaling. *Immunity* 2000; **13**: 643–55.
10. Takayanagi H, Kim S, Matsuo K, Suzuki H, Suzuki T, Sato K, Yokochi T, Oda H, Nakamura K, Ida N, Wagner EF, Taniguchi T. RANKL maintains bone homeostasis through c-Fos-dependent induction of interferon-β. *Nature* 2002; **416**: 744–9.
11. Darnell JE Jr, Kerr IM, Stark GR. Jak-STAT pathways and transcriptional activation in response to IFNs and other extracellular signaling proteins. *Science* 1994; **264**: 1415–21.
12. Ihle JN, Kerr IM. Jaks and Stats in signaling by the cytokine receptor superfamily. *Trends Genet* 1995; **11**: 69–74.
13. Schindler C, Darnell JE Jr. Transcriptional responses to polypeptide ligands: the JAK-STAT pathway. *Annu Rev Biochem* 1995; **64**: 621–51.
14. Stark GR, Kerr IM, Williams BR, Silverman RH, Schreiber RD. How cells respond to interferons. *Annu Rev Biochem* 1998; **67**: 227–64.
15. Maniatis T, Whittermore LA, Du W, Fan CM, Keller A, Palmobella V, Thanos D. In: McKnight SL, Yamamoto KR, editors. Transcriptional regulation. Part 2. Positive and negative control of human *interferon-β* gene expression, New York, Cold Spring Harbor: Cold Spring Harbor Laboratory Press; 1992, p. 1193–220.
16. Taniguchi T, Ogasawara K, Takaoka A, Tanaka N. IRF family of transcription factors as regulators of host defense. *Annu Rev Immunol* 2001; **19**: 623–55.
17. Du W, Thanos D, Maniatis T. Mechanisms of transcriptional synergism between distinct virus-inducible enhancer elements. *Cell* 1993; **74**: 887–98.
18. Fujita T, Sakakibara J, Sudo Y, Miyamoto M, Kimura Y, Taniguchi T. Evidence for a nuclear factor(s), IRF-1, mediating induction and silencing properties to human *IFN-β* gene regulatory elements. *EMBO J* 1988; **7**: 3397–405.
19. Miyamoto M, Fujita T, Kimura Y, Maruyama M, Harada H, Sudo Y, Miyata T, Taniguchi T. Regulated expression of a gene encoding a nuclear factor, IRF-1, that specifically binds to *IFN-β* gene regulatory elements. *Cell* 1988; **54**: 903–13.
20. Fujita T, Kimura Y, Miyamoto M, Barsoumian EL, Taniguchi T. Induction of endogenous *IFN-α* and *IFN-β* genes by a regulatory transcription factor, IRF-1. *Nature* 1989; **337**: 270–2.
21. Harada H, Fujita T, Miyamoto M, Kimura Y, Maruyama M, Furia A, Miyata T, Taniguchi T. Structurally similar but functionally distinct factors, IRF-1 and IRF-2, bind to the same regulatory elements of IFN and IFN-inducible genes. *Cell* 1989; **58**: 729–39.
22. Ryals J, Dierks P, Ragg H, Weissmann C. A 46-nucleotide promoter segment from an *IFN-α* gene renders an unrelated promoter inducible by virus. *Cell* 1985; **41**: 497–507.
23. Nguyen H, Hiscott J, Pitha PM. The growing family of interferon regulatory factors.

Cytokine Growth Factor Rev 1997; **8**: 293–312.
24. Mamane Y, Heylbroeck C, Genin P, Algarte M, Servant MJ, LePage C, DeLuca C, Kwon H, Lin R, Hiscott J. Interferon regulatory factors: the next generation. *Gene* 1999; **237**: 1–14.
25. Harada H, Matsumoto M, Sato M, Kashiwazaki Y, Kimura T, Kitagawa M, Yokochi T, Tan RS, Takasugi T, Kadokawa Y, Schindler C, Schreiber RD, Noguchi S, Taniguchi T. Regulation of *IFN-α/β* genes: evidence for a dual function of the transcription factor complex ISGF3 in the production and action of IFN-α/β. *Genes Cells* 1996; **1**: 995–1005.
26. Juang Y, Lowther W, Kellum M, Au WC, Lin R, Hiscott J, Pitha PM. Primary activation of *interferon α and interferon β* gene transcription by interferon regulatory factor 3. *Proc Natl Acad Sci USA* 1998; **95**: 9837–42.
27. Yoneyama M, Suhara W, Fukuhara Y, Fukuda M, Nishida E, Fujita T. Direct triggering of the type I interferon system by virus infection: activation of a transcription factor complex containing IRF-3 and CBP/p300. *EMBO J* 1998; **17**: 1087–95.
28. Lin R, Heylbroeck C, Pitha PM, Hiscott J. Virus-dependent phosphorylation of the IRF-3 transcription factor regulates nuclear translocation, transactivation potential, and proteasome-mediated degradation. *Mol Cell Biol* 1998; **18**: 2986–96.
29. Marie I, Durbin JE, Levy DE. Differential viral induction of distinct *interferon-α* genes by positive feedback through interferon regulatory factor-7. *EMBO J* 1998; **17**: 6660–9.
30. Sato M, Hata N, Asagiri M, Nakaya T, Taniguchi T, Tanaka N. Positive feedback regulation of type I *IFN* genes by the IFN-inducible transcription factor IRF-7. *FEBS Lett* 1998; **441**: 106–10.
31. Hata N, Sato M, Takaoka A, Asagiri M, Tanaka N, Taniguchi T. Constitutive IFN-α/β signal for efficient *IFN-α/β* gene induction by virus. *Biochem Biophys Res Commun* 2001; **285**: 518–25.
32. Gresser I, Maury C, Kaido T, Bandu MT, Tovey MG, Maunoury MT, Fantuzzi L, Gessani S, Greco G, Belardelli F. The essential role of endogenous IFN α/β in the anti-metastatic action of sensitized T lymphocytes in mice injected with Friend erythroleukemia cells. *Int J Cancer* 1995; **63**: 726–31.
33. Mitani Y, Takaoka A, Kim SH, Kato Y, Yokochi T, Tanaka N, Taniguchi T. Cross talk of the interferon-α/β signalling complex with gp130 for effective interleukin-6 signalling. *Genes Cells* 2001; **6**: 631–40.
34. Taniguchi T, Takaoka A. A weak signal for strong responses: interferon-α/β revisited. *Nat Rev Mol Cell Biol* 2001; **2**: 378–86.
35. Alexopoulou L, Holt AC, Medzhitov R, Flavell RA. Recognition of double-stranded RNA and activation of NF-kappaB by Toll-like receptor 3. *Nature* 2001; **413**: 732–8.
36. Stewart WE 2nd, Gosser LB, Lockart RZ Jr. Priming: a nonantiviral function of interferon. *J Virol* 1971; **7**: 792–801.
37. Ogasawara K, Hida S, Weng Y, Saiura A, Sato K, Takayanagi H, Sakaguchi S, Yokochi T, Kodama T, Naitoh M, De Martino JA, Taniguchi T. Requirement of the IFN-α/β-induced CXCR3 chemokine signalling for $CD8^+$ T cell activation. *Genes Cells* 2002; **7**: 309–20.
38. Buller RM, Holmes KL, Hugin A, Frederickson TN, Morse HC 3rd. Induction of cy-

totoxic T-cell responses *in vivo* in the absence of CD4 helper cells. *Nature* 1987; **328**: 77–9.

39. Hou S, Mo XY, Hyland L, Doherty PC. Host response to Sendai virus in mice lacking class II major histocompatibility complex glycoproteins. *J Virol* 1995; **69**: 1429–34.
40. Ridge JP, Di Rosa F, Matzinger P. A conditioned dendritic cell can be a temporal bridge between a CD4$^+$ T-helper and a T-killer cell. *Nature* 1998; **393**: 474–8.
41. Strander H, Einhorn S. Interferons and the tumor cell. *Biotherapy* 1996; **8**: 213–8.
42. Belardelli F, Ferrantini M, Proietti E, Kirkwood JM. Interferon-α in tumor immunity and immunotherapy. *Cytokine Growth Factor Rev* 2002; **13**: 119–34.
43. Der SD, Zhou A, Williams BR, Silverman RH. Identification of genes differentially regulated by interferon α, β, or γ using oligonucleotide arrays. *Proc Natl Acad Sci USA* 1998; **95**: 15623–8.
44. Kimchi A, Shure H, Lapidot Y, Rapoport S, Panet A, Revel M. Antimitogenic effects of interferon and (2′-5′)-oligoadenylate in synchronized 3T3 fibroblasts. *FEBS Lett* 1981; **134**: 212–6.
45. Koromilas AE, Roy S, Barber GN, Katze MG, Sonenberg N. Malignant transformation by a mutant of the IFN-inducible dsRNA-dependent protein kinase. *Science* 1992; **257**: 1685–9.
46. Harada H, Kitagawa M, Tanaka N, Yamamoto H, Harada K, Ishihara M, Taniguchi T. Anti-oncogenic and oncogenic potentials of interferon regulatory factors-1 and -2. *Science* 1993; **259**: 971–4.
47. Meurs EF, Galabru J, Barber GN, Katze MG, Hovanessian AG. Tumor suppressor function of the interferon-induced double-stranded RNA-activated protein kinase. *Proc Natl Acad Sci USA* 1993; **90**: 232–6.
48. Harada H, Kondo T, Ogawa S, Tamura T, Kitagawa M, Tanaka N, Lamphier MS, Hirai H, Taniguchi T. Accelerated exon skipping of IRF-1 mRNA in human myelodysplasia/leukemia; a possible mechanism of tumor suppressor inactivation. *Oncogene* 1994; **9**: 3313–20.
49. Tanaka N, Ishihara M, Lamphier MS, Nozawa H, Matsuyama T, Mak TW, Aizawa S, Tokino T, Oren M, Taniguchi T. Cooperation of the tumor suppressors IRF-1 and p53 in response to DNA damage. *Nature* 1996; **382**: 816–8.
50. Nozawa H, Oda E, Ueda S, Tamura G, Maesawa C, Muto T, Taniguchi T, Tanaka N. Functionally inactivating point mutation in the tumor-suppressor *IRF-1* gene identified in human gastric cancer. *Int J Cancer* 1998; **77**: 522–7.
51. Nozawa H, Oda E, Nakao K, Ishihara M, Ueda S, Yokochi T, Ogasawara K, Nakatsuru Y, Shimizu S, Ohira Y, Hioki K, Aizawa S, Ishikawa T, Katsuki M, Muto T, Taniguchi T, Tanaka N. Loss of transcription factor IRF-1 affects tumor susceptibility in mice carrying the Ha-*ras* transgene or nullizygosity for *p53*. *Genes Dev* 1999; **13**: 1240–5.
52. Belardelli F, Ferrantini M. Cytokines as a link between innate and adaptive antitumor immunity. *Trends Immunol* 2002; **23**: 201–8.
53. Gutterman JU. Cytokine therapeutics: lessons from interferon α. *Proc Natl Acad Sci USA* 1994; **91**: 1198–205.
54. Pfeffer LM, Dinarello CA, Herberman RB, Williams BR, Borden EC, Bordens R, Walter MR, Nagabhushan TL, Trotta PP, Pestka S. Biological properties of recombi-

nant α-interferons: 40th anniversary of the discovery of interferons. *Cancer Res* 1998; **58**: 2489–99.
55. Takayanagi H, Ogasawara K, Hida S, Chiba T, Murata S, Sato K, Takaoka A, Yokochi T, Oda H, Tanaka K, Nakamura K, Taniguchi T. T-cell-mediated regulation of osteoclastogenesis by signalling cross-talk between RANKL and IFN-γ. *Nature* 2000; **408**: 600–5.
56. Arron JR, Choi Y. Bone versus immune system. *Nature* 2000; **408**: 535–6.
57. Takayanagi H, Kim S, Taniguchi T. Signaling crosstalk between RANKL and interferons in osteoclast differentiation. *Arthritis Res* 2002; **4** Suppl 3: S227–32.
58. Manolagas SC. Birth and death of bone cells: basic regulatory mechanisms and implications for the pathogenesis and treatment of osteoporosis. *Endocr Rev* 2000; **21**: 115–37.
59. Lacey DL, Timms E, Tan HL, Kelley MJ, Dunstan CR, Burgess T, Elliott R, Colombero A, Elliott G, Scully S, Hsu H, Sullivan J, Hawkins N, Davy E, Capparelli C, Eli A, Qian YX, Kaufman S, Sarosi I, Shalhoub V, Senaldi G, Guo J, Delaney J, Boyle WJ. Osteoprotegerin ligand is a cytokine that regulates osteoclast differentiation and activation. *Cell* 1998; **93**: 165–76.
60. Yasuda H, Shima N, Nakagawa N, Yamaguchi K, Kinosaki M, Mochizuki S, Tomoyasu A, Yano K, Goto M, Murakami A, Tsuda E, Morinaga T, Higashio K, Udagawa N, Takahashi N, Suda T. Osteoclast differentiation factor is a ligand for osteoprotegerin/osteoclastogenesis-inhibitory factor and is identical to TRANCE/RANKL. *Proc Natl Acad Sci USA* 1998; **95**: 3597–602.
61. Kong YY, Yoshida H, Sarosi I, Tan HL, Timms E, Capparelli C, Morony S, Oliveira-dos-Santos AJ, Van G, Itie A, Khoo W, Wakeham A, Dunstan CR, Lacey DL, Mak TW, Boyle WJ, Penninger JM. OPGL is a key regulator of osteoclastogenesis, lymphocyte development and lymph-node organogenesis. *Nature* 1999; **397**: 315–23.
62. Medzhitov R, Janeway CA Jr. Innate immunity: the virtues of a nonclonal system of recognition. *Cell* 1997; **91**: 295–8.
63. Medzhitov R, Janeway C Jr. Innate immune recognition: mechanisms and pathways. *Immunol Rev* 2000; **173**: 89–97.
64. Aderem A, Ulevitch RJ. Toll-like receptors in the induction of the innate immune response. *Nature* 2000; **406**: 782–7.
65. Akira S, Takeda K, Kaisho T. Toll-like receptors: critical proteins linking innate and acquired immunity. *Nat Immunol* 2001; **2**: 675–80.
66. Doyle S, Vaidya S, O'Connell R, Dadgostar H, Dempsey P, Wu T, Rao G, Sun R, Haberland M, Modlin R, Cheng G. IRF3 mediates a TLR3/TLR4-specific antiviral gene program. *Immunity* 2002; **17**: 251–63.
67. Ito T, Amakawa R, Kaisho T, Hemmi H, Tajima K, Uehira K, Ozaki Y, Tomizawa H, Akira S, Fukuhara S. Interferon-α and interleukin-12 are induced differentially by Toll-like receptor 7 ligands in human blood dendritic cell subsets. *J Exp Med* 2002; **195**: 1507–12.
68. Krieg AM. CpG motifs in bacterial DNA and their immune effects. *Annu Rev Immunol* 2002; **20**: 709–60.
69. Shinobu N, Iwamura T, Yoneyama M, Yamaguchi K, Suhara W, Fukuhara Y, Amano F, Fujita T. Involvement of TIRAP/MAL in signaling for the activation of interferon

regulatory factor 3 by lipopolysaccharide. *FEBS Lett* 2002; **517**: 251–6.
70. Yamamoto M, Sato S, Mori K, Hoshino K, Takeuchi O, Takeda K, Akira S. Cutting edge: a novel Toll/IL-1 receptor domain-containing adapter that preferentially activates the IFN-β promoter in the Toll-like receptor signaling. *J Immunol* 2002; **169**: 6668–72.
71. Honda K, Sakaguchi S, Nakajima C, Watanabe A, Yanai H, Matsumoto M, Ohteki T, Kaisho T, Takaoka A, Akira S, Seya T, Taniguchi T. Selective contribution of IFN-α/β signaling to the maturation of dendritic cells induced by double-stranded RNA or viral infection. *Proc Nalt Acad Sci USA* 2003; **100**: 10872–7.

Added in proof: It has recently been reported that IκB kinase (IKK)-related kinases, IKKε and TANK-binding kinase 1, are components of the virus-activated kinase responsible for IRF-3/7 phosphorylation (Fitzgerald, K. A. *et al. Nat Immunol* 2003; **4**: 491–6, and Sharma, S. *et al. Science* 2003; **300**: 1148–51.

TUMOR FORMATION BY GENETIC MUTATIONS OF β-CATENIN, APC, AND AXIN IN THE WNT SIGNALING PATHWAY

Akira KIKUCHI, Shosei KISHIDA, Hideki YAMAMOTO and Shin-ichiro HINO

*Department of Biochemistry, Graduate School of Biomedical Sciences, Hiroshima University**

The genetics of development and cancer have converged in the identification of intra- and extra-cellular signaling pathways that are aberrantly regulated in cancer and are also central to embryonic patterning. The Wnt signaling pathway has provided an outstanding example of this. The genes for β-catenin, APC, and Axin in the Wnt signaling pathway are often mutated in human cancers. In all such cases, the common denominator is the activation of gene transcription by β-catenin. The resulting gene expression profile should provide a significant clue as to those cancers carrying defects in the Wnt signaling pathway. The post-translational modification of β-catenin and other components in the Wnt signaling pathway is important for the regulation of this signaling pathway. In this review, the functions of β-catenin, APC, and Axin and their genetic alterations in human cancers are described. Furthermore, the physiological significance of the post-translational modification in the components of the Wnt signaling pathway is also discussed.

Outline of the Wnt Signaling Pathway

Wnt proteins constitute a large family of cysteine-rich secreted ligands that control development in organisms ranging from nematode worms to mammals (*1*). The intracellular signaling pathway of Wnt is also conserved evolutionally and regulates cellular proliferation, morphology, motility, fate, axis formation, and organ development (*1, 2*). Wnt regulates at least three distinct pathways; the canonical β-catenin pathway, planar cell polarity pathway, and Ca^{2+} pathway. It has been shown that abnormalities of the canonical β-catenin pathway lead to tumor formation. According to the most widely accepted current model of the β-catenin pathway, casein kinase Iα (CKIα) and glycogen synthase kinase-3β (GSK-3β) phosphorylate β-catenin in the Axin complex (Fig. 1) (*3–5*). Phosphorylated β-catenin is ubiquitinated, resulting in the degradation of β-catenin by the proteasome (Fig. 2) (*6*). As a result, the cytoplasmic β-catenin level is low.

When Wnt acts on its cell-surface receptor consisting of Frizzled and lipoprotein receptor-related protein 5/6 (LRP5/6) (*7*), CKIε phosphorylates Dvl, and the

* 1-2-3 Kasumi, Minami-ku, Hiroshima 734-8551, Japan

This paper is dedicated to the memory of late Dr. Tomizo Yoshida on the occasion of the 100th anniversary of his birth. The essential part of this article was originally published in Cancer Science in March, 2003.

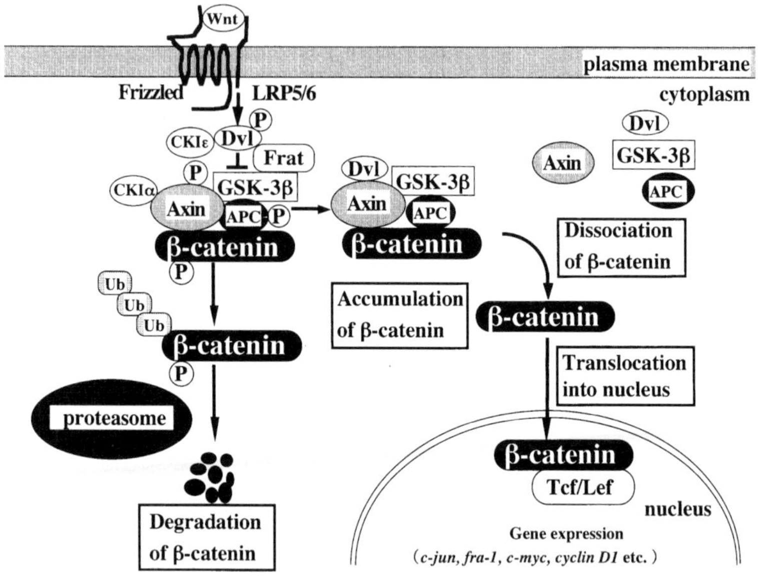

FIG. 1. Wnt signaling pathway
Ub, ubiquitin; P, phosphorylation.

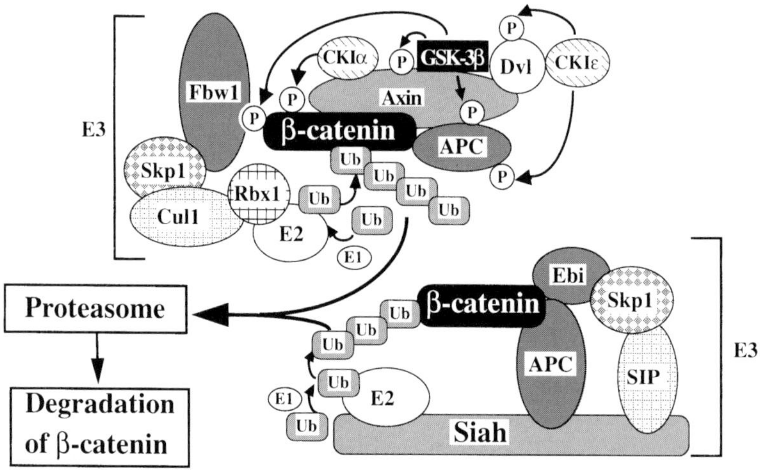

FIG. 2. Regulation of the stability of β-catenin
There are two distinct mechanisms to degrade β-catenin. Ub, ubiquitin; P, phosphorylation.

phosphorylation antagonizes the action of GSK-3β in the Axin complex (*8*). Once the phosphorylation of β-catenin is reduced, β-catenin dissociates from the Axin complex and is no longer degraded, resulting in its accumulation in the cytoplasm (Fig. 2). Accumulated β-catenin is translocated to the nucleus, where it binds to the transcription factor T cell factor (Tcf)/lymphoid enhancer factor (Lef) and thereby stimulates the expression of various genes (*2*, *9*).

Thus, Wnt increases the stability of β-catenin, thereby stimulating Tcf/Lef-me-

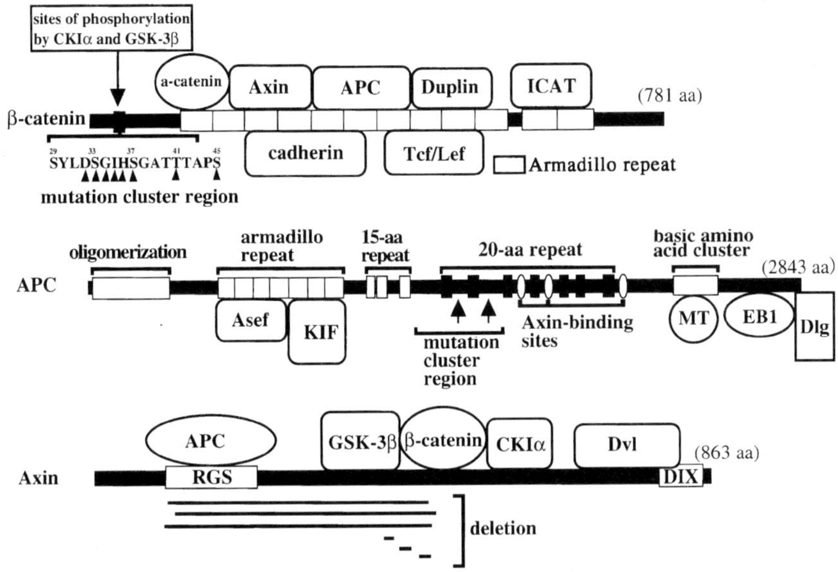

FIG. 3. Mutations of β-catenin, APC, and Axin in human cancers
The proteins binding to and the positions of mutations of β-catenin, APC, and Axin are described. MT, microtubules.

diated gene expression in the canonical β-catenin pathway. Among various molecules involved in this pathway, alterations in the *β-catenin*, *adenomatous polyposis coli* (*APC*), and *Axin* genes have been frequently found in several human cancers. β-Catenin is abnormally accumulated in the cytoplasm and nucleus of these cancer cells and Tcf-mediated gene expression is increased. Since APC and Axin induce the degradation of β-catenin, it is conceivable that β-catenin functions as an oncogene product, while APC and Axin act as tumor suppressor gene products.

β-Catenin

1. *Identification and structure of β-catenin*

β-Catenin was originally identified as a protein which interacts with the cytoplasmic domain of cadherin and links cadherin to α-catenin, which in turn mediates the anchorage of the cadherin complex to the cortical actin cytoskeleton (*10*). Many binding partners of β-catenin have been found, suggesting that β-catenin has other functions in addition to its role in cell-cell adhesion (Fig. 3). Genetic and embryological studies have revealed that β-catenin is a component of the Wnt signaling pathway and that it exhibits signaling functions (*1, 2, 4*). The primary structure of β-catenin is characterized by a central region that contains 12 repeats of 42 amino acids known as armadillo repeats. β-Catenin interacts with cadherin and α-catenin through the armadillo repeats on the plasma membranes. In addition to these proteins, β-catenin also associates with Axin and APC in the cytoplasm and Tcf/Lef in the nucleus. Thus, β-catenin has different binding partners in distinct subcellular fractions.

2. Degradation of β-catenin in a phosphorylation-dependent manner

Cytoplasmic β-catenin is a target for the ubiquitin-proteasome pathway and the phosphorylation by GSK-3β and CKIα is required for its ubiquitination. In general, degradation of proteins by the ubiquitin-proteasome pathway involves an ubiquitin-activation enzyme (E1), an ubiquitin-conjugating enzyme (E2), and an ubiquitin ligase (E3) (*11*). The ubiquitin ligase is generally thought to be directly involved in substrate recognition and consists of a multiprotein complex. An F-box protein Fbw1, which is a component of the ubiquitin ligase for β-catenin, associates with β-catenin phosphorylated by GSK-3β and CKIα and stimulates ubiquitination and degradation of β-catenin (*5*, *6*) (Fig. 2). The amino acid sequence for the phosphorylation of β-catenin is D^{32}SGXXSXXXTXXXS^{45} (D, asparatate; S, serine; G, glycine; T, threonine; X, any amino acid). CKIα-dependent phosphorylation of S^{45} proceeds and the phosphorylation enhances subsequent GSK-3β-dependent phosphorylation of T^{41}, S^{37}, and S^{33}. D^{32} and G^{34} are necessary for the interaction of phosphorylated β-catenin with Fbw1. Therefore, Fbw1 directly links the phosphorylation machinery to the ubiquitination apparatus.

3. Degradation of β-catenin in a phosphorylation-independent manner

Although CKIα- and GSK-3β-dependent phosphorylation is essential for the degradation of β-catenin, a phosphorylation-independent pathway has been recently found (*12*, *13*). Siah binds to the ubiquitin-conjugating enzyme with its N-terminal RING domain and forms a complex with Ebi through SIP and Skp1 (Fig. 2). Ebi is an F-box protein and binds to β-catenin. The complex of SIP, Skp1, and Ebi functions as an ubiquitin ligase. Since Siah downregulates the β-catenin mutant, in which serine and threonine residues between codons 33 and 45 are mutated, and a dominant negative form of Fbw1 does not block Siah-mediated downregulation of β-catenin, Siah is likely to promote degradation of β-catenin through a mechanism independent of GSK-3β-mediated phosphorylation and the Fbw1-mediated proteasome pathway. Interestingly, Siah binds to the C-terminal region of APC, and downregulation of β-catenin is dependent on APC. Another interesting aspect of this pathway is that Siah is a p53-inducible regulator of cell cycle arrest and apoptosis. Indeed, Siah mediates p53-inducible degradation of β-catenin. Although it is clear that there is a novel pathway by which Siah and APC mediate β-catenin degradation linked to the p53 response, the physiological role of this pathway in the regulation of β-catenin stability is not fully understood.

4. Activation of Tcf/Lef by β-catenin

Tcf and Lef bind directly to DNA through their high mobility group (HMG) domains, but they can not activate gene expression, rather, they suppressed it (*9*). Repression of gene expression by Tcf may be due to its direct interaction with co-repressors such as Groucho/TLE, CtBP, and CBP (*9*). Since β-catenin activates Tcf/Lef and stimulates gene expression, it is thought that β-catenin supplies additional cofactors required for transcriptional activation and that this might involve additional proteins that bridge the Tcf/β-catenin complex to the basal transcriptional machinery. Candidates may be Pontin52 (*14*) and *Drosophila* tearshirt (*15*). Furthermore, two novel molecules that interfere with the complex formation of β-catenin with Tcf have been isolated (*16–18*). They are ICAT and Duplin, both of which bind to β-catenin directly and inhibit β-catenin-dependent gene expression. ICAT and Duplin may function to establish a threshold to prevent premature and inappropriate signaling events and accumulation of β-catenin would compete with them for binding to Tcf/Lef.

The DNA-binding HMG domains of the Tcf/Lef family proteins have a high affinity for the DNA sequence (A/T)(A/T)CAA(A/T)GG. Tcf/Lef activated by β-catenin stimulates the expression of various genes, including *c-myc*, *cyclin D1*, *fra1*, *c-jun*, *peroxisome proliferator-activated receptor* δ, *matrilysin*, *CD44*, and *urokinase-type plasminogen activator receptor* (*2*, *9*), which contain the Tcf/Lef binding sites in their promoters.

5. *Genetic mutations of β-catenin in cancers*

Mutations in the β-catenin gene that affect specific serine and threonine residues and amino acids adjacent to them, which are essential for the targeted degradation of β-catenin, are found in a wide variety of human cancers including colon cancers, desmoid, gastric cancer, hepatocarcinoma, medulloblastoma, melanoma, ovarian cancer, pancreatic cancer, and prostate cancer (*2*) (Fig. 3). The β-catenin mutants occur at D^{32}, S^{33}, G^{34}, S^{37}, T^{41}, and S^{45}. As described above, S^{45} is a phosphorylation site of CKIα, and S^{33}, S^{37}, and T^{41} are phosphorylation sites of GSK-3β. D^{32} and G^{34} are necessary for the interaction of β-catenin with Fbw1. Since these mutations abrogate the phosphorylation-dependent interaction of β-catenin with Fbw1, thereby stabilizing β-catenin, the mutated β-catenin is accumulated in the nucleus and activates Tcf/Lef. Myc and cyclin D1 are clearly relevant in tumor formation, because of their roles in proliferation, apoptosis, and cell-cycle regulation. Changes in the normal expression of Myc and cyclin D1 are likely to increase the overall proliferating rate. The proteins of other target genes, matrilysin, CD44, and urokinase-type plasminogen activator receptor, seem more likely to be involved in tumor proliferation, rather than initiation.

APC

1. *Identification and structure of APC*

APC is a tumor suppressor linked to familial adenomatous polyposis coli (FAP) and to the initiation of sporadic human colorectal cancer (*2*, *19*). APC encodes a 300-kDa multifunctional protein with several structural domains (Fig. 3). The N-terminus contains an oligomerization domain followed by seven repeats of an armadillo motif. The armadillo motif binds to two proteins that provide new functions of APC. One is Asef, which is a GDP/GTP exchange protein for the small G protein Rac (*20*). The other is KIF3, which is known to bind to kinesin and regulate vesicle transport on microtubules (*21*). Although the binding site is not identified, the catalytic subunit of protein phosphatase 2A binds to the N-terminal third of APC. The middle portion of APC contains three successive 15-amino acid (aa) repeats followed by seven related but distinct 20-aa repeats, and both of these repeat regions are able to bind independently to β-catenin (*2*, *19*). The Axin-binding sites reside between the 20-aa repeat numbers 3 and 4, 4 and 5, and downstream of repeat 7 (*22*, *23*). Following the 20-aa repeats is a basic amino acid cluster region, which directly binds to microtubules (*24*), and a binding site for EB1 (*25*), another microtubule-binding protein. The C-terminus has an S/TXV (V, valine)motif that interacts with the PDZ domain-containing the human Dlg homolog (*26*).

2. Role of APC in downregulation of β-catenin

APC appears to be a critical component for β-catenin destruction (Fig. 2) (*2, 19*). In colon cancers, mutations of APC correlate with high levels of β-catenin and transcriptionally active Tcf/β-catenin complexes. Expression of wild-type APC in colorectal cancer cells reduces β-catenin levels, and the fragment of APC containing the 20-aa repeats is sufficient for the activity (*2, 19*). However, an APC fragment with either mutated β-catenin-binding sites or Axin-binding sites fails to induce degradation of β-catenin (*27*). Therefore, the interaction of APC with both Axin and β-catenin is required for the ability of APC to degrade β-catenin. In the complex, GSK-3β bound to Axin efficiently phosphorylates APC, which enhances the binding of β-catenin to APC (*28, 29*), and GSK-3β also phosphorylates β-catenin bound to APC in addition to β-catenin bound to Axin (*30*). The molecular mechanism by which APC downregulates β-catenin has not yet been fully elucidated, however, it is likely that APC activates Axin in a manner that facilitates the phosphorylation of β-catenin by GSK-3β.

3. Role of APC in the regulation of cytoskeleton

Several studies using APC knockout mice have suggested that APC mutations affect the directionality of cell migration in epithelial layers (*19, 31*). The migration of epithelial layers is intricately linked to the cytoskeletal organization. Functional interactions of APC with actin filaments and microtubules have been recently studied extensively.

A basic amino acid cluster region of APC binds to microtubules and induces microtubule bundling *in vitro*. APC localizes to clusters at the ends of microtubules (*32, 33*). The clusters result from movement of APC along microtubules towards the growing ends, where APC accumulates near the plasma membrane. APC also interacts with the kinesin superfamily (KIF) proteins, microtubule plus-end-directed motor proteins, through an association with the kinesin superfamily-associated protein (KAP3) (*21*). The interaction of APC with KAP3 through its armadillo repeats is required for the accumulation of APC in clusters, and the C-terminal truncated form of APC does not accumulate in clusters. Therefore, APC is transported along microtubules by KAP3-KIF3, and accumulates in the tips of membrane protrusions.

Furthermore, APC localizes to the external face of kinetochores where microtubules attach to chromosomes (*19*). Interestingly, cells expressing a mutant APC that lacks the C-terminal region are prone to errors in chromosome segregation and develop aneuploidy. Therefore, APC has a role in microtubule attachment and stabilization at kinetochores, and truncated mutation in APC, an early event in colorectal cancer, may be linked to the genetic instability that also occurs early in colorectal cancer.

In addition to associating with microtubules, APC is likely to connect to the actin filaments. The armadillo domain of APC interacts with Asef (*20*), which is a GDP/GTP exchange protein for the small G protein Rac. APC activates the ability of Asef to stimulate the GDP/GTP exchange of Rac, and induces lamellipodia formation and ruffling of the plasma membrane as the activated Rac does, thereby stimulating cell migration. Although APC localizes mainly to microtubules, when this interaction is disrupted, APC associates with the actin filaments. Which cytoskeletal element is favored by a particular APC protein is not known, however, it is possible that APC can link and coordinate actin and tubulin dynamics locally.

4. *Genetic mutations of APC in cancers*

Mutations of APC are frequently identified in FAP and colorectal cancers, but quite rare in other cancers (*2, 19*). Most APC mutations result in truncated proteins that lack all Axin-binding motifs and a variable number of the 20-aa repeats (Fig. 3). In FAP, germ-line mutations are scattered throughout the 5' half of the APC gene. By contrast, most somatic mutations are clustered between codons 1286 and 1513. In any case, mutations of APC relate strongly to the regulation of the stability of β-catenin. Selective pressure is directed against the presence of Axin-binding sites, because the presence of Axin-binding sites is critical to APC in the regulation of β-catenin levels. Furthermore, the remaining N-terminal truncated form of APC may affect cell migration by activating Asef, thereby leading to metastasis.

Importantly, the overall frequency of β-catenin mutations is quite low in colorectal cancers with APC mutations, and those with an intact APC gene contain mutations of β-catenin that alter phosphorylation sites (*2*). The exclusivity of β-catenin and APC mutations in colorectal cancers is also evident from the analysis of replication error-positive tumors identified by microsatellite instability. Both the hereditary and sporadic forms of replication error-positive colorectal cancers have a relatively high frequency of β-catenin mutations, where APC mutations are relatively rare (*34*).

Axin

1. *Identification and structure of Axin*

Axin was originally identified as the product of the mouse gene called *Fused* (*35*). An intriguing feature of many homozygous Axin mutant embryos is a duplication of the embryonic axis, suggesting that Axin normally plays a negative regulatory role in the response to an axis-inducing signal in the developmental process (*36*).

The N-terminal region of Axin, called the RGS domain, shares 31% amino acid identity with RGS4, which has been identified as a GTPase-activating protein for heterotrimeric GTP-binding protein (Fig. 3). The C-terminal region of Axin called the DIX domain shares 37% amino acid identity with the N-terminal region of Dvl. The site phosphorylated by GSK-3β is adjacent to the N-terminal region of the GSK-3β-binding site (*3*).

2. *Roles of Axin as a scaffold protein in the Wnt signaling pathway*

Axin binds to various components of the Wnt signaling pathway (Figs. 2 and 3) (*4*). APC binds to the RGS domain (*22, 23*). GSK-3β, β-catenin, and CKIα interact with the different sites of the central region of Axin (*3, 5*). Dvl binds to the following C-terminal region of Axin including the DIX domain (*37, 38*).

In the Axin complex, CKIα and GSK-3β phosphorylate β-catenin efficiently and phosphorylated β-catenin is ubiquitinated and degraded by the proteasome (*3, 5*). Indeed, expression of Axin induces the downregulation of β-catenin in various cell lines (*23, 39*). Thus, Axin plays important roles in the Wnt signaling pathway as a negative regulator. Dvl binds to CKIε and Axin (*38, 40*). CKIε mediates Wnt-3a-dependent phosphorylation of Dvl and phosphorylated Dvl has a high affinity for Frat, which binds to and inhibits GSK-3 (Fig. 1) (*8, 40, 41*). Disruption of CKIε by RNA interference reduces the Wnt-3a-induced binding of Dvl to Frat and accumulation of β-catenin (*8*). Therefore, when Wnt acts on the cells, Frat bound to Dvl phosphorylated by CKIε may prevent GSK-3β that has interacted with Axin from phosphorylating β-catenin, thereby stabilizing β-catenin. Taken together, Axin binds to positive and negative regulators of the Wnt signaling pathway and regulates the stability of β-catenin.

3. Receptor-mediated endocytosis and Axin

The mechanism by which Frizzled and LRP5/6 transduce the signals remains elusive. *Drosophila* genetics have shown that the fly dynamin dominant negative form abolishes cuticle deposition, indicating that receptor-mediated endocytosis triggers the Wnt signaling (*42*). Wnt causes the translocation of Axin to the membrane and enhances the interaction between Axin and LRP5 (*43*). Furthermore, the LRP5 sequences involved in the interaction with Axin are required for Lef activation. Therefore, the binding of Axin to LRP5 may be important for the Wnt signaling pathway. Dvl and Axin have the DIX domain that is necessary for the binding of Dvl and Axin to intracellular vesicles and actin filaments (*44*). Although whether the intracellular vesicles are derived from endocytotic vesicles is not known, Axin and Dvl may collaborate to regulate receptor-mediated endocytosis of the Wnt signaling pathway.

4. Genetic mutations of Axin in cancers

Axin was expected to be a tumor suppressor based on its ability to downregulate β-catenin, and this has been indeed verified by documentation of its biallelic inactivation in human hepatocarcinoma (*45*). Importantly, these mutations of Axin are found in hepatocarcinomas with intact genes for β-catenin and APC. All of the mutations generate a truncated form of Axin eliminated the β-catenin binding site (Fig. 3). Therefore, Axin is now regarded as a tumor suppressor, and constitutes the third genetic defect in the Wnt signaling pathway.

There exists an Axin homolog, termed rat Axil (*46*), mouse conductin (*22*), or human Axin2 (*47*). The biochemical characteristics of Axil are similar to those of Axin, and Axil is able to downregulate β-catenin under conditions of overexpression. However, this redundant protein does not suppress Axin mutations in hepatocarcinoma. Therefore, Axil/conductin/Axin2 is either not functionally equivalent to Axin or not expressed at levels sufficient to compensate for its loss in hepatocarcinoma. Although mutations in the C-terminal region of Axin2 are found in colorectal cancers with defective DNA mismatch repair (*47*), the mechanism by which these Axin2 mutations are involved in tumorgenesis is unclear.

Regulation of the Wnt Signaling Pathway by the Post-translational Modifications

1. Phosphorylation

As described already, the phosphorylation of β-catenin by CKIα and GSK-3β is important for the degradation of β-catenin. It has been recently shown that the phos-

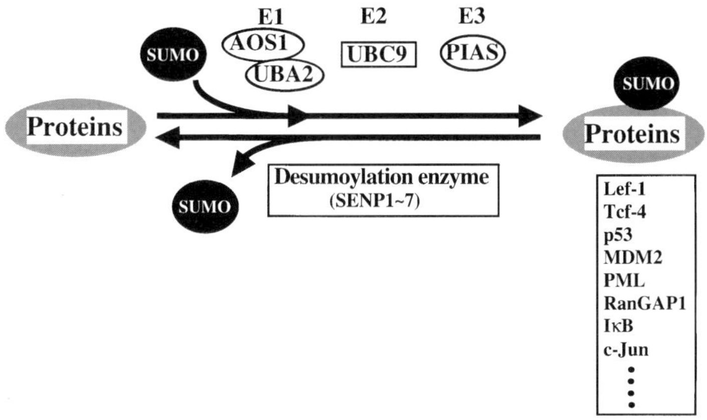

FIG. 4. Modification of proteins with SUMO

phorylation of β-catenin by cyclic AMP-dependent protein kinase (PKA) is also involved in the β-catenin degradation.

The Alzheimer's disease-linked gene *presenilin1* forms a complex with GSK-3β, β-catenin, and the catalytic domain of PKA (*48*, *49*). In the presenilin1 complex, PKA phosphorylates S^{45} and enhances the GSK-3β-dependent phosphorylation of β-catenin (*48*), suggesting that PKA and presenilin1 induce the downregulation of β-catenin independently of the Wnt-controlled Axin complex. Indeed, nuclear accumulation of β-catenin is observed in epidermis of *presenilin1*-deficient mice (*48*). Several evidences support the concept that presenilin1 is an important negative regulator of β-catenin. In a genetic screen, the *Drosophila presenilin* was identified a negative regulator of the wingless/Wnt signaling pathway (*50*), and *Drosophila presenilin* deficiency resulted in cytoplasmic accumulation of Armadillo, a *Drosophila* β-catenin homolog (51). In contrast to the findings that PKA might function as a negative regulator of the β-catenin stability, it has been shown that stimulation with prostaglandin E2, which activates PKA, increases the transcriptional activity of Tcf in HEK-293 cells probably through direct phosphorylation and inhibition of GSK-3β by PKA (*52*). However, the molecular mechanism of the cross-talk between the Wnt and PKA signaling pathways is largely unknown.

In addition to β-catenin and Dvl, Tcf and Lef are also phosphorylated. NEMO-like kinase (NLK), which acts downstream of TAK1 kinase activated by TGF-β, associates with and phosphorylates Tcf-4 (*53*). The phosphorylation of Tcf-4 by NLK inhibits the binding of β-catenin-Tcf-4 complex to DNA, thereby suppressing the Wnt signaling pathway (*53*).

2. *Sumoylation*

The small ubiquitin-related modifier (SUMO) modification (sumoylation) pathway resembles the ubiquitin conjugation pathway, but the enzymes involved in these two processes are distinct (Fig. 4) (*54–56*). SUMO is activated for conjugation by the E1 enzyme Aos/Uba2, subsequently transferred to the E2 conjugation enzyme Ubc9, and finally conjugated to target proteins by either of the E3 ligases: protein inhibitor of activated STAT (PIAS) or RanBP2 (*57*). Known target proteins of sumoylation include p53, MDM2, PML, RanGAP1, IκBα, and c-Jun. Modification of these proteins by sumoylation changes their subcellular localization, transcriptional activation, and protein stability. Sumoylation is reversible, and there are at least seven mammalian SUMO-specific proteases, which are designated the SENP family proteins (*54–56*).

It has been suggested that PIASy (an E3 ligase) and Axam (a desumoylation enzyme, SENP2) are involved in the Wnt signaling pathway. PIASy interacts with Lef-1, resulting in the sumoylation of Lef-1, and inhibits the transcriptional activity of Lef-1 (*58*). Tcf-4 is also sumoylated and PIASy enhances the sumoylation of Tcf-4 (*59*). In contrast to Lef-1, sumoylation of Tcf-4 enhances its transcriptional activity (*59*). Axam has been identified as an Axin-binding protein and regulates the Wnt signaling pathway negatively by inducing the degradation of β-catenin (*60*). This action of Axam requires its desumoylation activity (*61*). Axam inhibits sumoylation of Tcf-4 and its activity (*59*). Although the precise molecular mechanism by which sumoylation and desumoylation regulate the Wnt signaling pathway is not known, it is likely that sumoylation is involved in the Wnt signaling pathway as well as phosphorylation and ubiquitination.

3. *Acetylation*

Nuclear histone acetyltransferases play important roles in gene regulation (*62*). They catalyze the reversible acetylation of histones to alleviate chromatin-mediated restrictions imposed on promoter activation. Adenovirus E1A-associated p300 and the closely related CREB-binding protein (CBP) are well-characterized acetyltransferases. CBP and p300 can form larger protein complexes that include other acetylases and serve as coactivators of numerous transcriptional factors. They can accomplish their task not only by utilizing their intrinsic histone acetyltransferase activity but also as adaptor proteins that link activators to the basal transcriptional machinery.

Drosophila CBP (dCBP) has been shown to regulate Wingless signaling negatively by acetylating Tcf (*63*). The acetylation inhibits the binding of Tcf to Armadillo in *Drosophila*. In contrast, p300 and CBP serve as coactivators for β-catenin in vertebrates (*64*). Furthermore, the intrinsic acetylase activity of p300 is not required for its function as a coactivator of β-catenin. dCBP and mammalian orthologs may be functionally different from each other.

Conclusion

The growth of animal cells is directed by mechanisms that have evolved to establish and maintain the optimal size and function of interdependent organs. Cancer cells subvert these evolutionary adaptations to multicellularity and revert to a largely nutrient-limited style of growth. From this perspective, an understanding of the mechanisms of normal growth control should help to explain the deranged cell growth associated with cancer.

It is apparent that genetic mutations in the Wnt signaling pathway cause cancers and that tumor promotion by this pathway can proceed through a number of different genetic defects. The manifestation of cancer by aberrant Wnt signaling results

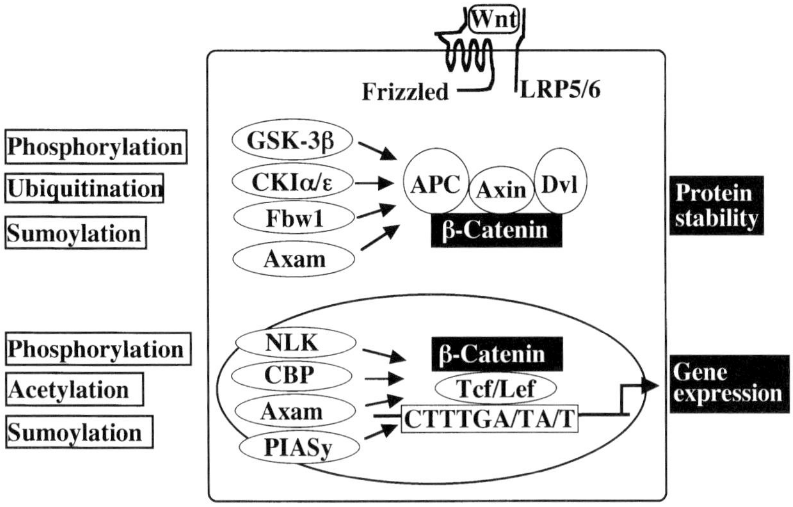

FIG. 5. Regulation of Wnt signaling pathway by post-translational modification

from inappropriate gene activation mediated by stabilized β-catenin. Several target genes of β-catenin signaling have been identified and some of their functions are consistent with control of cellular growth, differentiation, and apoptosis. However, the identification of target genes that do not contain Tcf/Lef binding sites in their promoters would provide a new model of gene activation by Wnt signaling.

The post-translational modification of β-catenin, Dvl, and Tcf/Lef regulates the β-catenin stability and β-catenin-dependent Tcf transcriptional activity (Fig. 5). Since phosphorylation occurs at serine or threonine residue and ubiquitination, sumoylation, and acetylation occur at lysine residue, it is important to identify target amino acids modified post-translationally and to find the abnormalities of these amino acids in human cancers.

Acknowledgments

Work in the authors' laboratory was supported by Grants-in-Aid for Scientific Research and for Scientific Research on priority areas from the Ministry of Education, Science, and Culture, Japan.

REFERENCES

1. Wodarz A, Nusse R. Mechanisms of Wnt signaling in development. *Annu Rev Cell Dev Biol* 1998; **14**: 59–88.
2. Polakis P. Wnt signaling and cancer. *Genes Dev* 2000; **14**: 1837–51.
3. Ikeda S, Kishida S, Yamamoto H, Murai H, Koyama S, Kikuchi A. Axin, a negative regulator of the Wnt signaling pathway, forms a complex with GSK-3β and β-catenin and promotes GSK-3β-dependent phosphorylation of β-catenin. *EMBO J* 1998; **17**: 1371–84.
4. Kikuchi A. Roles of Axin in the Wnt signalling pathway. *Cell Signal* 1999; **11**: 777–88.
5. Liu C, Li Y, Semenov M, Han C, Baeg G-H, Tan Y, Zhang Z, Lin X, He X. Control

of β-catenin phosphorylation/degradation by a dual-kinase mechanism. *Cell* 2002; **108**: 837–47.

6. Kitagawa M, Hatakeyama S, Shirane M, Matsumoto M, Ishida N, Hattori K, Nakamichi I, Kikuchi A, Nakayama K-I, Nakayama K. An F-box protein, FWD1, mediates ubiquitin-dependent proteolysis of β-catenin. *EMBO J* 1999; **18**: 2401–10.
7. Howell BW, Herz J. The LDL receptor gene family: signaling functions during development. *Curr Opin Neurobiol* 2001; **11**: 74–81.
8. Hino S-I, Michiue T, Asashima M, Kikuchi A. Casein kinase Iε enhances the binding of Dvl-1 to Frat-1 and is essential for Wnt-3a-induced accumulation of β-catenin. *J Biol Chem* 2003; **278**: 14066–73.
9. Hurlstone A, Clevers H. T-cell factors: turn-ons and turn-offs. *EMBO J* 2002; **21**: 2303–11.
10. Takeichi M. Cadherin cell adhesion receptors as a morphogenetic regulator. *Science* 1991; **251**: 1451–5.
11. Ciechanover A. The ubiquitin-proteasome pathway: on protein death and cell life. *EMBO J* 1998; **17**: 7151–60.
12. Liu J, Stevens J, Rote CA, Yost HJ, Hu YL, White RL, Matsunami N. Siah-1 mediates a novel β-catenin degradation pathway linking p53 to the adenomatous polyposis coli protein. *Mol Cell* 2001; **7**: 927–36.
13. Matsuzawa S-I, Reed JC. Siah-1, SIP, and Ebi collaborate in a novel pathway for β-catenin degradation linked to p53 responses. *Mol Cell* 2001; **7**: 915–26.
14. Bauer A, Chauvet S, Huber O, Usseglio F, Rothbacher U, Aragnol D, Kemler R, Pradel J. Pontin52 and Reptin52 function as antagonistic regulators of β-catenin signalling activity. *EMBO J* 2000; **19**: 6121–30.
15. Gallet A, Angelats C, Erkner A, Charroux B, Fasano L, Kerridge S. The C-terminal domain of armadillo binds to hypophosphorylated teashirt to modulate wingless signalling in *Drosophila*. *EMBO J* 1999; **18**: 2208–17.
16. Kobayashi M, Kishida S, Fukui A, Michiue T, Miyamoto Y, Okamoto T, Yoneda Y, Asashima M, Kikuchi A. Nuclear localization of duplin, a beta-catenin-binding protein, is essential for its inhibitory activity on the Wnt signaling pathway. *J Biol Chem* 2001; **277**: 5816–22.
17. Sakamoto I, Kishida S, Fukui A, Kishida M, Yamamoto H, Hino S-I, Michiue T, Takada S, Asashima M, Kikuchi A. A novel β-catenin-binding protein inhibits β-catenin-dependent Tcf activation and axis formation. *J Biol Chem* 2000; **275**: 32871–8.
18. Tago K-I, Nakamura T, Nishita M, Hyodo J, Nagai S-I, Murata Y, Adachi S, Ohwada S, Morishita Y, Shibuya H, Akiyama T. Inhibition of Wnt signaling by ICAT, a novel β-catenin-interacting protein. *Genes Dev* 2000; **14**: 1741–9.
19. Fodde R, Smits R, Clevers H. APC, signal transduction and genetic instability in colorectal cancer. *Nat Rev Cancer* 2001; **1**: 55–67.
20. Kawasaki Y, Senda T, Ishidate T, Koyama R, Morishita T, Iwayama Y, Higuchi O, Akiyama T. Asef, a link between the tumor suppressor APC and G-protein signaling. *Science* 2000; **289**: 1194–7.
21. Jimbo T, Kawasaki Y, Koyama R, Sato R, Takada S, Haraguchi K, Akiyama T. Identification of a link between the tumour suppressor APC and the kinesin superfamily. *Nat Cell Biol* 2002; **4**: 323–7.

22. Behrens J, Jerchow B-A, Würtele M, Grimm J, Asbrand C, Wirtz R, Kühl M, Wedlich D, Birchmeier W. Functional interaction of an Axin homolog, conductin, with β-catenin, APC, and GSK3β. *Science* 1998; **280**: 596–9.
23. Kishida S, Yamamoto H, Ikeda S, Kishida M, Sakamoto I, Koyama S, Kikuchi A. Axin, a negative regulator of the Wnt signaling pathway, directly interacts with Adenomatous Polyposis Coli and regulates the stabilization of β-catenin. *J Biol Chem* 1998; **273**: 10823–6.
24. Smith KJ, Levy DB, Maupin P, Pollard TD, Vogelstein B, Kinzler KW. Wild-type but not mutant APC associates with the microtubule cytoskeleton. *Cancer Res* 1994; **54**: 3672–5.
25. Su LK, Burrell M, Hill DE, Gyuris J, Brent R, Wiltshire R, Trent J, Vogelstein B, Kinzler KW. APC binds to the novel protein EB1. *Cancer Res* 1995; **55**: 2972–7.
26. Matsumine A, Ogai A, Senda T, Okumura N, Satoh K, Baeg GH, Kawahara T, Kobayashi S, Okada M, Toyoshima K, Akiyama T. Binding of APC to the human homolog of the *Drosophila* discs large tumor suppressor protein. *Science* 1996; **272**: 1020–3.
27. Kawahara K, Morishita T, Nakamura T, Hamada F, Toyoshima K, Akiyama T. Down-regulation of β-catenin by the colorectal tumor suppressor APC requires association with axin and β-catenin. *J Biol Chem* 2000; **275**: 8369–74.
28. Ikeda S, Kishida M, Matsuura Y, Usui H, Kikuchi A. GSK-3β-dependent phosphorylation of adenomatous polyposis coli gene product can be modulated by β-catenin and protein phosphatase 2A complexed with Axin. *Oncogene* 2000; **19**: 537–45.
29. Rubinfeld B, Albert I, Porfiri E, Fiol C, Munemitsu S, Polakis P. Binding of GSK3β to the APC-β-catenin complex and regulation of complex assembly. *Science* 1996; **272**: 1023–6.
30. Hinoi T, Yamamoto H, Kishida M, Takada S, Kishida S, Kikuchi A. Complex formation of adenomatous polyposis coli gene product and Axin facilitates glycogen synthase kinase-3β-dependent phosphorylation of β-catenin and downregulates β-catenin. *J Biol Chem* 2000; **275**: 34399–406.
31. Oshima H, Oshima M, Kobayashi M, Tsutsumi M, Taketo MM. Morphological and molecular processes of polyp formation in Apc(Δ716) knockout mice. *Cancer Res* 1997; **57**: 1644–9.
32. Mimori-Kiyosue Y, Shiina N, Tsukita S. Adenomatous polyposis coli (APC) protein moves along microtubules and concentrates at their growing ends in epithelial cells. *J Cell Biol* 2000; **148**: 505–18.
33. Nathke IS, Adams CL, Polakis P, Sellin JH, Nelson WJ. The adenomatous polyposis coli tumor suppressor protein localizes to plasma membrane sites involved in active cell migration. *J Cell Biol* 1996; **134**: 165–79.
34. Miyaki M, Iijima T, Kimura J, Yasuno M, Mori T, Hayashi Y, Koike M, Shitara N, Iwama T, Kuroki T. Frequent mutation of β-catenin and APC genes in primary colorectal tumors from patients with hereditary nonpolyposis colorectal cancer. *Cancer Res* 1999; **59**: 4506–9.
35. Zeng L, Fagotto F, Zhang T, Hsu W, Vasicek TJ, Perry III WL, Lee JJ, Tilghman SM, Gumbiner BM, Costantini F. The mouse *Fused* locus encodes Axin, an inhibitor of the Wnt signaling pathway that regulates embryonic axis formation. *Cell* 1997; **90**: 181–92.

36. Jacobs-Cohen RJ, Spiegelman M, Cookingham JC, Bennett D. Knobbly, a new dominant mutation in the mouse that affects embryonic ectoderm organization. *Genet Res* 1984; **43**: 43–50.
37. Hino S-I, Kishida S, Michiue T, Fukui A, Sakamoto I, Takada S, Asashima M, Kikuchi A. Inhibition of the Wnt signaling pathway by Idax, a novel Dvl-binding protein. *Mol Cell Biol* 2001; **21**: 330–42.
38. Kishida S, Yamamoto H, Hino S-I, Ikeda S, Kishida M, Kikuchi A. DIX domains of Dvl and Axin are necessary for protein interactions and their ability to regulate β-catenin stability. *Mol Cell Biol* 1999; **19**: 4414–22.
39. Kishida M, Koyama S, Kishida S, Matsubara K, Nakashima S, Higano K, Takada R, Takada S, Kikuchi A. Axin prevents Wnt-3a-induced accumulation of β-catenin. *Oncogene* 1999; **18**: 979–85.
40. Kishida M, Hino S-I, Michiue T, Yamamoto H, Kishida S, Fukui A, Asashima M, Kikuchi A. Synergistic activation of the Wnt signaling pathway by Dvl and casein kinase Iε. *J Biol Chem* 2001; **276**: 33147–55.
41. Lee E, Salic A, Kirschner MW. Physiological regulation of β-catenin stability by Tcf3 and CK1ε. *J Cell Biol* 2001; **154**: 983–93.
42. Moline MM, Southern C, Bejsovec A. Directionality of wingless protein transport influences epidermal patterning in the *Drosophila* embryo. *Development* 1999; **126**: 4375–84.
43. Mao J, Wang J, Liu B, Pan W, Farr GHI, Flynn C, Yuan H, Takada S, Kimelman D, Li L, Wu D. Low-density lipoprotein receptor-related protein-5 binds to Axin and regulates the canonical Wnt signaling pathway. *Mol Cell* 2001; **7**: 801–9.
44. Capelluto DG, Kutateladze TG, Habas R, Finkielstein CV, He X, Overduin M. The DIX domain targets dishevelled to actin stress fibres and vesicular membranes. *Nature* 2002; **419**: 726–9.
45. Satoh S, Daigo Y, Furukawa Y, Kato T, Miwa N, Nishiwaki T, Kawasoe T, Ishiguro H, Fujita M, Tokino T, Sasaki Y, Imaoka S, Murata M, Shimano T, Yamaoka Y, Nakamura Y. *AXIN1* mutations in hepatocellular carcinomas, and growth suppression in cancer cells by virus-mediated transfer of *AXIN1*. *Nat Genet* 2000; **24**: 245–50.
46. Yamamoto H, Kishida S, Uochi T, Ikeda S, Koyama S, Asashima M, Kikuchi A. Axil, a member of the Axin family, interacts with both glycogen synthase kinase-3β and β-catenin and inhibits axis formation of *Xenopus* embryos. *Mol Cell Biol* 1998; **18**: 2867–75.
47. Liu W, Dong X, Mai M, Seelan RS, Taniguchi K, Krishnadath KK, Halling KC, Cunningham JM, Qian C, Christensen E, Roche PC, Smith DI, Thibodeau SN. Mutations in *AXIN2* cause colorectal cancer with defective mismatch repair by activating β-catenin/TCF signalling. *Nat Genet* 2000; **26**: 146–7.
48. Kang DE, Soriano S, Xia X, Eberhart CG, De Strooper B, Zheng H, Koo EH. Presenilin couples the paired phosphorylation of β-catenin independent of axin: implications for β-catenin activation in tumorigenesis. *Cell* 2002; **110**: 751–62.
49. Soriano S, Kang DE, Fu M, Pestell R, Chevallier N, Zheng H, Koo EH. Presenilin 1 negatively regulates β-catenin/T cell factor/lymphoid enhancer factor-1 signaling independently of β-amyloid precursor protein and notch processing. *J Cell Biol* 2001; **152**: 785–94.

50. Cox RT, McEwen DG, Myster DL, Duronio RJ, Loureiro J, Peifer M. A screen for mutations that suppress the phenotype of *Drosophila* armadillo, the β-catenin homolog. *Genetics* 2000; **155**: 1725–40.
51. Noll E, Medina M, Hartley D, Zhou J, Perrimon N, Kosik KS. Presenilin affects arm/β-catenin localization and function in *Drosophila*. *Dev Biol* 2000; **227**: 450–64.
52. Fujino H, West KA, Regan JW. Phosphorylation of glycogen synthase kinase-3 and stimulation of T-cell factor signaling following activation of EP2 and EP4 prostanoid receptors by prostaglandin E2. *J Biol Chem* 2002; **277**: 2614–9.
53. Ishitani T, Ninomiya-Tsuji J, Nagai S-I, Nishita M, Meneghini M, Barker N, Waterman M, Bowerman B, Clevers H, Shibuya H, Matsumoto K. The TAK1-NLK-MAPK-related pathway antagonizes signalling between β-catenin and transcription factor TCF. *Nature* 1999; **399**: 798–802.
54. Hochstrasser M. Evolution and function of ubiquitin-like protein-conjugation systems. *Nat Cell Biol* 2000; **2**: E153–7.
55. Müller S, Hoege C, Pyrowolakis G, Jentsch S. SUMO, ubiquitin's mysterious cousin. *Nat Rev Mol Cell Biol* 2001; **2**: 202–10.
56. Yeh ET, Gong L, Kamitani T. Ubiquitin-like proteins: new wines in new bottles. *Gene* 2000; **248**: 1–14.
57. Jackson PK. A new RING for SUMO: wrestling transcriptional responses into nuclear bodies with PIAS family E3 SUMO ligases. *Genes Dev* 2001; **15**: 3053–8.
58. Sachdev S, Bruhn L, Sieber H, Pichler A, Melchior F, Grosschedl R. PIASy, a nuclear matrix-associated SUMO E3 ligase, represses LEF1 activity by sequestration into nuclear bodies. *Genes Dev* 2001; **15**: 3088–103.
59. Yamamoto H, Ihara M, Matsuura Y, Kikuchi A. Sumoylation is involved in β-catenin-dependent activation of Tcf-4. *EMBO J* 2003; **22**: 2047–59.
60. Kadoya T, Kishida S, Fukui A, Hinoi T, Michiue T, Asashima M, Kikuchi A. Inhibition of Wnt signaling pathway by a novel Axin-binding protein. *J Biol Chem* 2000; **275**: 37030–7.
61. Kadoya T, Yamamoto H, Suzuki T, Yukita A, Fukui A, Michiue T, Asahara T, Tanaka K, Asashima M, Kikuchi A. Desumoylation activity of Axam, a novel Axin-binding protein, is involved in downregulation of β-catenin. *Mol Cell Biol* 2002; **22**: 3803–19.
62. Workman JL, Kingston RE. Alteration of nucleosome structure as a mechanism of transcriptional regulation. *Annu Rev Biochem* 1998; **67**: 545–79.
63. Waltzer L, Bienz M. *Drosophila* CBP represses the transcription factor TCF to antagonize Wingless signalling. *Nature* 1998; **395**: 521–5.
64. Hecht A, Vleminckx K, Stemmler MP, van Roy F, Kemler R. The p300/CBP acetyltarnsferases function as transcriptional coactivators of β-catenin in vertebrates. *EMBO J* 2000; **19**: 1839–50.

REGULATION OF TGF-β SIGNALING AND ITS ROLES IN PROGRESSION OF TUMORS

Kohei MIYAZONO[*1, *2], Hiroyuki SUZUKI[*1] and Takeshi IMAMURA[*2]

*Department of Molecular Pathology, Graduate School of Medicine, University of Tokyo[*1] and Department of Biochemistry, The Cancer Institute of the Japanese Foundation for Cancer Research (JFCR)[*2]*

Transforming growth factor-β (TGF-β) is a potent growth inhibitor of most types of cells; therefore, perturbations of TGF-β signaling are believed to result in progression of various tumors. On the other hand, TGF-β has been shown to act as an oncogenic cytokine through induction of extracellular matrices, angiogenesis, and immune suppression. A wide variety of effects of TGF-β are mediated by physical interaction of signal transducer Smad proteins with various transcription factors. Among these, Runx3 plays a pivotal role in prevention of gastric cancer. TGF-β signaling is regulated by various mechanisms in the cytoplasm and nucleus. Inhibitory Smads (I-Smads) repress TGF-β signaling mainly by interacting with activated TGF-β receptors. Smad ubiquitin regulatory factors (Smurfs) play important roles in facilitating the inhibitory signals induced by I-Smads. In addition, the transcriptional co-repressors c-Ski and SnoN interact with Smads, and repress transcription induced by TGF-β. Abnormalities of these regulators of TGF-β signaling may thus participate in the progression of various tumors.

Transforming growth factor-β (TGF-β) is a member of a large family of disulfide-bonded cytokines. Three isoforms of TGF-β, termed TGF-β1, -β2, and -β3, are present in mammals. Since TGF-β is a potent growth inhibitor of most types of cells, perturbations of TGF-β signaling result in progression of various tumors (*1*). Mutations of one of the TGF-β receptors, TGF-β type II receptor (TβR-II), have been identified in patients with hereditary nonpolyposis colon cancer (HNPCC) (*2*). Moreover, mutations of a signaling component of TGF-β, Smad4 (originally termed "deleted in pancreatic carcinoma, locus 4" or DPC4), have been found in patients with pancreatic carcinoma and those with advanced colon carcinoma (*3*, *4*). On the other hand, TGF-β induces extracellular matrix accumulation, angiogenesis, and immunosuppression, indicating that TGF-β facilitates progression of tumors under certain conditions (*5*, *6*). In order to elucidate the roles of TGF-β in tumor progression, it is thus important to understand the mechanisms of the TGF-β signaling system. In this review, we discuss the signaling pathways activated by TGF-β, focusing in

[*1] 7-3-1 Hongo, Bunkyo-ku, Tokyo 113-0033, Japan

[*2] 1-37-1 Kami-ikebukuro, Toshima-ku, Tokyo 170-8455, Japan

This paper is dedicated to the memory of late Dr. Tomizo Yoshida on the occasion of the 100th anniversary of his birth. It was originally published in Cancer Science in March, 2003.

particular on the roles of molecules that modulate TGF-β signaling, i.e. Runx proteins, inhibitory Smads (I-Smads) and Smad ubiquitin regulatory factors (Smurfs), and c-Ski and SnoN.

TGF-β Signaling Through Serine/Threonine Kinase Receptors

TGF-βs are synthesized as latent high-molecular-weight complexes from producer cells, and are activated by various mechanisms, including effects of plasmin and thrombospondin. Active TGF-β then binds to two different serine/threonine kinase receptors, termed type II and type I, both of which are required for signaling (*7*). Upon binding of TGF-β to type II and type I receptors, the former transphosphorylates the GS domain of the latter, resulting in the activation of type I receptor kinase (Fig. 1). The type II and type I receptors form hetero-tetramers composed of two type II and two type I receptors (*8*). Many growth factor receptors contain tyrosine kinase domains in their intracellular domains; thus, TGF-β receptors are unique compared to growth factor receptors. TGF-β belongs to the TGF-β superfamily, which includes activins, nodal, bone morphogenetic proteins (BMPs) and anti-Müllerian hormone. Members of the TGF-β superfamily bind to their cognate type II and type I receptors, and transduce signals in a manner essentially similar to TGF-β. Only one type II receptor for TGF-β (TβR-II) is present in mammals, whereas two receptors, termed activin receptor-like kinase (ALK)-5 and ALK-1, serve as type I receptors for TGF-β (*9*). ALK-5 (also termed TβR-I) is ubiquitously expressed in TGF-β-responsive cells, and transduces signals for growth inhibition and extracellular matrix formation. In contrast, ALK-1 is preferentially expressed in endothelial cells, and does not transmit the typical TGF-β signals. Instead, ALK-1 activates signals similar to BMP type I receptors and induces migration of endothelial cells (*10*).

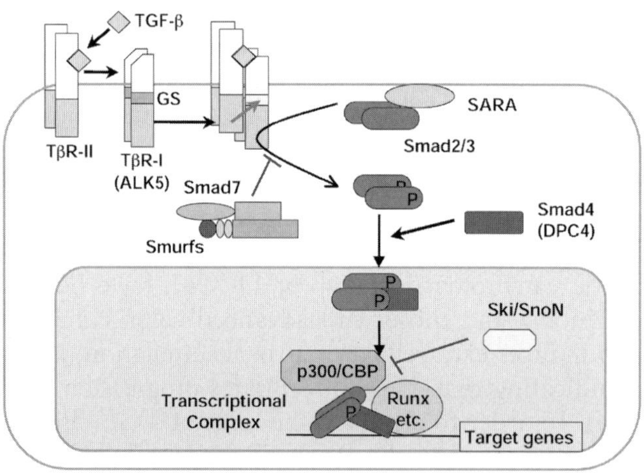

FIG. 1. TGF-β signaling by type II and type I serine/threonine kinase receptors and Smad proteins TGF-β induces hetero-tetrameric complex of TβR-II and TβR-I. R-Smads (Smad2 and Smad3) are anchored to the plasma membrane by SARA, and activated by the TβR-I kinase. R-Smads then form complexes with Co-Smad, and translocate into the nucleus, where they regulate transcription of target genes by interacting with other transcription factors, e.g. Runx proteins, and transcriptional co-activators p300/CBP. TGF-β signaling is suppressed by the action of I-Smad-Smurf complexes and transcriptional co-repressors c-Ski and SnoN.

Since ALK-1 is activated only in certain types of cells, we will focus on the signals induced by ALK-5/TβR-I in this review article.

Signaling by Smad Proteins

Once the type I receptor kinase is activated, TGF-β triggers various intracellular signaling pathways, including the Erk and p38 mitogen-activated protein (MAP) kinase pathways (*11*). Among those signaling molecules, Smad proteins are activated in all TGF-β-responsive cells, and play central roles in manifestation of the biological activities of TGF-β. Smad proteins can be classified into three subtypes, e.g. receptor-regulated Smads (R-Smads), common-partner Smads (Co-Smads), and inhibitory Smads (I-Smads). Of the eight different Smad proteins in mammals, Smad2 and Smad3 serve as R-Smads for TGF-β signaling pathways, Smad4 acts as a Co-Smad, and Smad7 functions as an I-Smad for TGF-β signaling. Smads 1, 5, and 8 are R-Smads activated by BMP receptors, and Smad6 is an I-Smad preferentially inhibiting BMP signaling (*12*). Smad4 is the only Co-Smad in mammals, and is shared by the TGF-β and BMP pathways.

Smad proteins have conserved N- and C-terminal regions, termed the MH1 and MH2 domains, respectively. The MH1 and MH2 domains are bridged by linker regions. In all three subtypes of Smads, MH2 domains are highly conserved. In contrast, MH1 domains are conserved in R-Smads and Co-Smads, whereas the N-terminal regions of I-Smads are highly divergent from those of R- and Co-Smads.

R-Smads are anchored to the plasma membrane through various molecules, among which Smad anchor for receptor activation (SARA) has been most extensively studied (*13*). SARA has a FYVE domain, which is responsible for binding to phosphatidyl inositol-3-phosphate in the plasma membrane. SARA preferentially binds to the MH2 domains of Smad2 and Smad3, but not to those of other Smads. SARA forms a dimer in cells, and anchors two molecules of Smad2/3 to the plasma membrane (*14*), which may be important for efficient activation of R-Smads by the hetero-tetrameric TβR-II and TβR-I complexes.

The activated TβR-I kinase phosphorylates the last two serine residues at the C-terminal Ser-Ser-X-Ser motif of R-Smads. R-Smads then form heteromeric complexes with Co-Smad through their MH2 domains, and translocate into the nucleus (Fig. 1). Although the exact structures of the R-Smad/Co-Smad heteromers have not been fully determined (*15*), a hetero-trimer composed of two molecules of R-Smads and one molecule of Co-Smad (*16*), or a hetero-dimer composed of one molecule each of R-Smad and Co-Smad (*17*), has been proposed. R-Smads and Co-Smads shuttle between the nucleus and cytoplasm. Nuclear localization signals (NLSs) in the MH1 domains of R-Smads play pivotal roles in translocation of Smads into the nucleus, whereas nuclear export signals (NESs) in the MH2 domains of R-Smads and those in the linker region of Co-Smads are responsible for nuclear export of the complex (*18–20*).

In the nucleus, the R-Smad-Co-Smad heteromers interact with various transcription factors and transcriptional co-activators or co-repressors, resulting in transduction of a wide variety of intracellular signals in target cells (*21*). R-Smads and Co-Smads also directly bind to specific DNA sequences, although with relatively low affinities. Thus, Smads and other transcription factors cooperatively regulate transcription of target genes through binding to their promoters. Transcriptional co-activators, including p300, CBP, and P/CAF, contain histone acetyl transferase (HAT) domains. Through acetylation of histones and probably other proteins, these transcriptional co-activators help Smads activate the transcription of target genes.

Cooperation of TGF-β Signaling with Runx3 in Gastric Mucosa

A wide variety of biological activities of TGF-β may result from the ability of Smads to interact with various transcription factors (*21, 22*). More than 30 transcription factors, including FAST1, TFE3, Mixer, c-Jun, Sp1, and vitamin D3 receptor, have been reported to interact with Smads. By selecting these transcription factors as partners, Smads may exhibit specific biological effects on target cells. Of these transcription factors, Runx proteins appear to play unique roles in TGF-β/BMP signaling (*23*).

Runx proteins have a Runt domain, which is responsible for DNA binding. Runx was originally given three different names, i.e. polyomavirus enhancer binding protein (PEBP) 2α, core binding factor a (Cbfa), and acute myeloid leukemia (AML). Three Runx proteins, termed Runx1 (PEBP2αB/Cbfa2/AML1), Runx2 (PEBP2αA/Cbfa1/AML3) and Runx3 (PEBP2αC/Cbfa3/AML2), are present in mammals. The β subunit of PEBP2, PEBP2β, interacts with Runx proteins (the α subunits of PEBP2) through the Runt domains, and stabilizes the Runx proteins by preventing ubiquitination of the Runt domain. Mutations in Runx1 have been found in ~30% of human acute leukemias, while haploinsufficiency of Runx2 results in the autosomal dominant bone disease cleidocranial dysplasia. Importantly, recent studies have revealed that alterations of expression of the *Runx3* gene product result in progression of gastric cancer (*24*).

R-Smads have been shown to interact with all three Runx proteins (*25, 26*). Smad1 activated by BMPs physically interacts with Runx2, and facilitates the differentiation of mesenchymal cells into osteoblasts (*27*). Smads 2 and 3 activated by TGF-β interact with Runx1–3, and induce transcriptional activation of target genes, e.g. *IgA*. On the TGF-β-responsive element (TβRE) of the immunoglobulin Cα region, Runx binding sites and Smad binding sites are located in close vicinity; thus, the Runx-Smad complexes bind to TβRE, and upregulate the transcription of IgA (*25, 26*).

Runx3-null mice exhibit hyperplasia of gastric mucosa (*24*). The gastric epithelial cells of the Runx3$^{-/-}$ mice are resistant to the growth-inhibitory and apoptosis-inducing activities of TGF-β, suggesting that Runx3 plays important roles in these processes. Approximately half of human gastric cancer cells lack expression of Runx3 due to hemizygous deletion and DNA methylation of the promoter of Runx3 (*24*). Runx3 inhibited the tumor growth of human gastric cancer inoculated into nude mice, and a mutant Runx3 found in a gastric cancer patient abolished the tumor-suppressive effect of Runx3. Thus, Runx3 plays a pivotal role in tumorigenesis of gastric cancer, and alterations of its function may affect the signaling activities of TGF-β.

Roles of I-Smads and Smurfs in TGF-β Signaling

I-Smads are structurally related to R-Smads and Co-Smads, especially in the

MH2 domains. However, their N-terminal regions (N-domains) are highly distinct from those of other Smads, and I-Smads inhibit the signaling activities induced by TGF-β superfamily proteins. Smad7 inhibits both TGF-β and BMP signaling, whereas Smad6 preferentially inhibits BMP signaling (*12*). I-Smads physically interact with type I receptors activated by type II receptor kinases (*28–30*). Thus, I-Smads compete with R-Smads for activation by type I receptors, and inhibit signaling by the TGF-β superfamily proteins. The MH2 domain of Smad7 directly binds to the type I receptor kinases, while its N-domain physically interacts with the MH2 domain, and facilitates the interaction of the MH2 domain with the receptors (*31*). In addition to inhibiting TGF-β superfamily signaling by preventing activation of R-Smads by the receptors, I-Smads also interact with R-Smads activated by the receptors, and interfere with the complex formation of R-Smads with Co-Smads (*32*). Moreover, Smad6 has been reported to repress transcription of certain genes in the nucleus (*33*). Thus, I-Smads inhibit TGF-β superfamily signaling through multiple mechanisms.

Inhibitory activities of I-Smads are facilitated by HECT type E3 ubiquitin ligases Smurf1 and Smurf2. Smurfs were originally identified as E3 ligases that interact with R-Smads and induce their degradation (*34*), but recent findings have revealed that Smurfs interact with I-Smads with higher affinities than R-Smads (*35*). Importantly, I-Smads are mainly located in the nucleus in most cells. Smurfs induce the export of Smad7 from the nucleus to the cytoplasm, and allow it to associate with the activated type I receptors at the plasma membrane (*35, 36*) (Fig. 2). Although I-Smads do not have NES, Smurfs appear to have functional NESs. Smurfs induce polyubiquitination and degradation not only of Smad7, but also of type I receptors. Thus, the Smad7-Smurf complexes inhibit TGF-β signaling through down-regulation of the amounts of receptors on cells surface. In addition to degradation of the

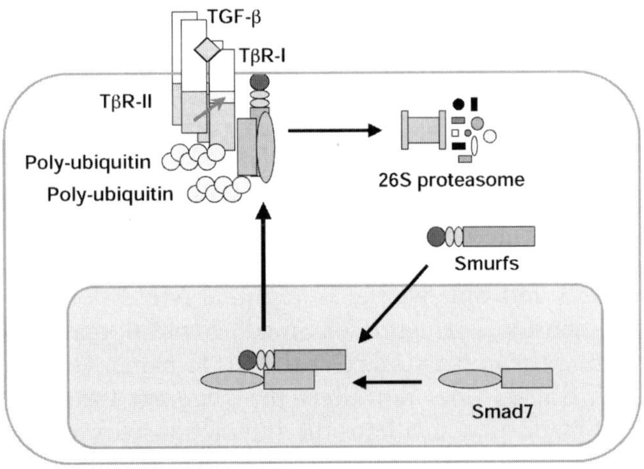

FIG. 2. Inhibition of TGF-β signaling by Smad7 and Smurfs (Smurf1 and Smurf2)
Smad7 inhibits TGF-β signaling through multiple mechanisms. Of those, interaction of Smad7 with activated TβR-I may be one of the most important ones. However, Smad7 is mainly located in the nucleus. Smurf1 and Smurf2 interact with Smad7 and induce the nuclear export of Smad7. Smurfs then induce association of Smad7 with TβR-I, and enhance the Smad7-induced repression of TGF-β signaling. Smurfs also induce polyubiquitination and degradation of TβR-I, as well as that of Smad7, in the 26S proteasome, resulting in further repression of TGF-β signaling.

cell surface receptors, Smurfs directly degrade R-Smads as originally reported (*34*). Moreover, Smurfs induce degradation of R-Smads indirectly through binding to R-Smads via I-Smads (*37*).

Expression of I-Smads is induced by various stimuli (*21*). Expression of Smad7 has been reported to be induced by TGF-β, BMP, interferon-γ, growth factors, nuclear factor kappa B (NF-κB) signals, laminar shear stress, and ultraviolet irradiation. Since Smad6 and Smad7 are induced by TGF-β and BMP, their expression levels are regulated by negative feed-back loops. Overexpression of Smad7 has been found in pancreatic carcinoma. Moreover, Smurf2 has been reported to be expressed in patients with esophageal squamous carcinoma (*38*), and its high expression is correlated with poor prognosis of esophageal cancer.

Transcriptional Co-Repressors, c-Ski and SnoN

Ski was originally identified as the oncogene of the avian Sloan-Kettering retrovirus. When v-Ski is expressed at high levels in fibroblasts, it induces their transformation. v-Ski is truncated in both the N- and C-termini of c-Ski. SnoN was identified as a molecule structurally related to c-Ski. Both c-Ski and SnoN interact with N-CoR/SMRT and mSin3A, and form complexes with histone deacetylases (HDACs). c-Ski and SnoN thus induce deacetylation of histones, and repress transcription of target genes (*39*). It has been shown that c-Ski interacts with nuclear hormone receptors and tumor suppressor gene products, e.g. *retinoblastoma* (*Rb*) gene product and Mad, and that it regulates transcription of their target genes.

c-Ski and SnoN interact with Smad2, Smad3, and Smad4. c-Ski and SnoN thus repress transcription induced by TGF-β. They also interact with BMP-activated R-Smads (*40*), but only very weakly (*41*). However, interaction of c-Ski and Smad4 may be strong enough, and therefore signaling of BMPs is potently inhibited by c-Ski.

Domains responsible for interaction between c-Ski and Smad3 or Smad4 have been determined in detail (Fig. 3). The N-terminal region of c-Ski (amino acids 16–40) is most important for the interaction with Smad3 (*14*), but another region located in the middle portion of c-Ski may also participate in the interaction with Smad3 (*41*). In contrast, the I-loop of c-Ski is responsible for the interaction with Smad4 (*42*). Thus, c-Ski binds to Smad3 and Smad4 through multiple regions, and the regions responsible for interaction with Smad3 are distinct from that for interaction with Smad4.

In both Smad2/3 and Smad4, the C-terminal MH2 domains interact with c-Ski. In the three-dimensional structure of Smad3 MH2 domain, the c-Ski-interacting surface is located at the upper surface of the MH2 trimer (Fig. 3) (*43*). The interaction of c-Ski with Smad3 does not affect the oligomer formation of Smad3, and oligomerization of Smad3 may facilitate the interaction with c-Ski (*14, 43*). The c-Ski-binding site in Smad3 overlaps with that of transcriptional co-activators p300 and CBP. In contrast to Smad3, the surface of interaction of Smad4 with c-Ski is located in the L3 loop of Smad4 (*42*). The L3 loop in Smad4 is responsible for oligomer formation with Smad3. Thus, interaction of c-Ski with Smad4 may disrupt the formation of hetero-oligomers between Smad3 and Smad4. TGF-β represses the expression of c-myc, and c-Ski counteracts the effect of TGF-β. This may not occur by recruitment of HDACs, and may instead be induced by disruption of the hetero-oligomerization of Smad2/3 and Smad4.

Expression of SnoN is regulated in a biphasic fashion upon TGF-β treatment. It is down-regulated immediately following the addition of TGF-β, and up-regulated thereafter (*44*). The early down-regulation of SnoN is induced by a ternary complex of SnoN, Smad2 and Smurf2 (*45*). Although Smurf2 does not directly bind to SnoN, it can indirectly bind to SnoN via activated Smad2. Smurf2 in the complex induces polyubiquitination and degradation of SnoN; thus, after stimulation by TGF-β, the expression level of SnoN protein decreases, allowing TGF-β to act efficiently in target cells. Thereafter, expression of SnoN is induced at the mRNA level. c-Ski is also up-regulated by TGF-β later, although less remarkably than SnoN (*46*). Thus, like I-Smads, c-Ski and SnoN regulate the effects of TGF-β through negative feedback loops.

Since SnoN inhibits TGF-β signaling, regulation of the expression of SnoN is important for efficient signaling of TGF-β. Degradation of SnoN through Smurf2 may be one such mechanism. In addition, Smad3 has been shown to interact with the anaphase-promoting complex (APC), a cell-cycle regulated ubiquitin ligase (*47*). Smad3 recruits APC during cell cycle progression and induces ubiquitination and degradation of SnoN.

When treated with a chemical carcinogen, both c-Ski$^{+/-}$ and SnoN$^{+/-}$ mice exhibit higher levels of tumor formation than wild-type mice (*48*, *49*). The SnoN$^{+/-}$ mice develop lymphomas at low frequency. Thus, c-Ski and SnoN act as tumor suppressors in certain cells. TGF-β has been reported to play bidirectional roles in tumor-

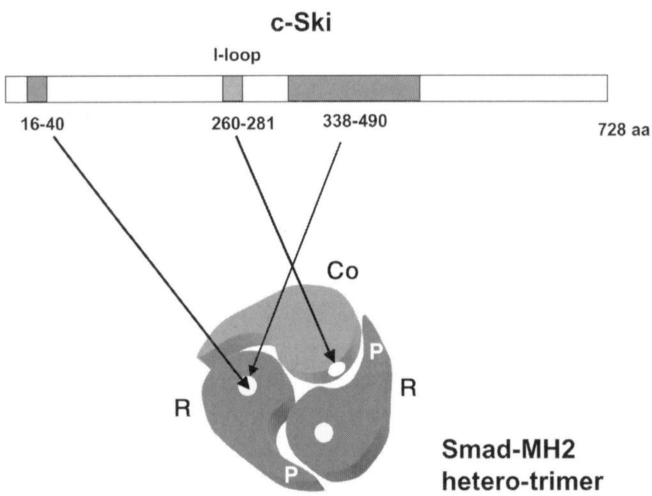

FIG. 3. c-Ski interacts with Smads and inhibit TGF-β signaling
Structures of c-Ski and hetero-trimer formed by the MH2 domains of R-Smads and Co-Smad are shown. Hetero-trimer and hetero-dimer models have been proposed for the R-Smad and Co-Smad complexes; only hetero-trimeric Smad oligomer is shown in this figure. c-Ski has two Smad2/3 interacting domains. The region containing amino acids 16–40 is important for interaction with c-Ski, while that containing amino acids 338–490 may support the interaction of the c-Ski (16–40) region with Smad3. The I-loop is responsible for interaction with Smad4. c-Ski interacts with the upper surface of the R-Smad MH2 trimer, whereas it binds to the L3 loop of Smad4. Thus, when c-Ski binds to Smad4, it may disrupt formation of the R-Smad and Co-Smad complexes. It is currently unknown whether a single c-Ski molecule can bind to R-Smads and Co-Smad at the same time.

igenesis. Although perturbations of TGF-β signaling result in the development of cancers in certain tissues, TGF-β induces tumor formation under other conditions. Similarly, c-Ski and SnoN have both oncogenic and anti-oncogenic properties depending on the target cells. It will be interesting to determine how these bidirectional oncogenic signals are switched in various tissues.

Perspectivies

Recent progress in research on TGF-β signaling mechanisms has revealed that TGF-β signaling is regulated by various mechanisms, and that many oncogenic and anti-oncogenic proteins play roles in development of tumors by modulating TGF-β signaling activities. Since TGF-β is a potent growth inhibitor, loss of TGF-β signaling is involved in the progression of certain tumors. However, in certain tissues, TGF-β produced in tumor tissues induces progression of tumors. In fact, inhibition of TGF-β signaling has been shown to prevent progression of tumors in some animal models (*5*, *6*). Since chemical TGF-β inhibitors have recently been generated (*50*), it will be very interesting to determine whether these TGF-β inhibitors can be used for treatment of certain human cancers.

Acknowledgments

There are many important papers in this field, and for reasons of space, we have not been able to mention all of them. We apologize to those investigators whose papers could not be cited. This study was supported by Grants-in-Aid for Scientific Research from the Ministry of Education, Culture, Sports, Science and Technology of Japan.

REFERENCES

1. Blobe GC, Schiemann WP, Lodish HF. Role of transforming growth factor-β in human disease. *N Engl J Med* 2000; **342**: 1350–8.
2. Markowitz S, Wang J, Myeroff L, Parsons R, Sun L, Lutterbaugh J, Fan RS, Zborowska E, Kinzler KW, Vogelstein B, Brattain M, Willson JKV. Inactivation of the type II TGF-β receptor in colon cancer cells with microsatellite instability. *Science* 1995; **268**: 1336–8.
3. Hahn SA, Schutte M, Hoque ATMS, Moskaluk CA, da Costa LT, Rozenblum E, Weinstein CL, Fischer A, Yeo CJ, Hruban RH, Kern SE. *DPC4*, a candidate tumor suppressor gene at human chromosome 18q21.1. *Science* 1996; **271**: 350–3.
4. Miyaki M, Iijima T, Konishi M, Sakai K, Ishii A, Yasuno M, Hishima T, Koike M, Shitara N, Iwama T, Utsunomiya J, Kuroki T, Mori T. Higher frequency of Smad4 gene mutation in human colorectal cancer with distant metastasis. *Oncogene* 1999; **18**: 3098–103.
5. Derynck R, Akhurst RJ, Balmain A. TGF-β signaling in tumor suppression and cancer progression. *Nat Genet* 2001; **29**: 117–29.
6. Wakefield LM, Roberts AB. TGF-β signaling: positive and negative effects on tumorigenesis. *Curr Opin Genet Dev* 2002; **12**: 22–9.
7. Heldin C-H, Miyazono K, ten Dijke P. TGF-β signalling from cell membrane to nucleus through SMAD proteins. *Nature* 1997; **390**: 465–71.

8. Hart PJ, Deep S, Taylor AB, Shu Z, Hinck CS, Hinck AP. Crystal structure of the human TβR2 ectodomain-TGF-β3 complex. *Nat Struct Biol* 2002; **9**: 203–8.
9. Oh SP, Seki T, Goss KA, Imamura T, Yi Y, Donahoe PK, Li L, Miyazono K, ten Dijke P, Kim S, Li E. Activin receptor-like kinase 1 modulates transforming growth factor-β1 signaling in the regulation of angiogenesis. *Proc Natl Acad Sci USA* 2000; **97**: 2626–31.
10. Goumans M-J, Valdimarsdottir G, Itoh S, Rosendahl A, Sideras P, ten Dijke P. Balancing the activation state of the endothelium via two distinct TGF-β type I receptors. *EMBO J* 2002; **21**: 1743–53.
11. Takekawa M, Tatebayashi K, Itoh F, Adachi M, Imai K, Saito H. Smad-dependent GADD45β expression mediates delayed activation of p38 MAP kinase by TGF-β. *EMBO J* 2002; **21**: 6473–82.
12. Itoh S, Landstrom M, Hermansson A, Itoh F, Heldin C-H, Heldin N-E, ten Dijke P. Transforming growth factor β1 induces nuclear export of inhibitory Smad7. *J Biol Chem* 1998; **273**: 29195–201.
13. Tsukazaki T, Chiang TA, Davison AF, Attisano L, Wrana JL. SARA, a FYVE domain protein that recruits Smad2 to the TGFβ receptor. *Cell* 1998; **11**: 779–91.
14. Qin BY, Lam SS, Correia JJ, Lin K. Smad3 allostery links TGF-β receptor kinase activation to transcriptional control. *Genes Dev* 2002; **16**: 1950–63.
15. Kawabata M, Inoue H, Hanyu A, Imamura T, Miyazono K. Smad proteins exist as monomers *in vivo* and undergo homo- and hetero-oligomerization upon activation by serine/threonine kinase receptors. *EMBO J* 1998; **17**: 4056–65.
16. Qin BY, Chacko BM, Lam SS, de Caestecker MP, Correia JJ, Lin K. Structural basis of Smad1 activation by receptor kinase phosphorylation. *Mol Cell* 2001; **6**: 1303–12.
17. Wu JW, Hu M, Chai J, Seoane J, Huse M, Li C, Rigotti DJ, Kyin S, Muir TW, Fairman R, Massagué J, Shi Y. Crystal structure of a phosphorylated Smad2. Recognition of phosphoserine by the MH2 domain and insights on Smad function in TGF-β signaling. *Mol Cell* 2001; **8**: 1277–89.
18. Kurisaki A, Kose S, Yoneda Y, Heldin C-H, Moustakas A. Transforming growth factor-β induces nuclear import of Smad3 in an importin-β1 and Ran-dependent manner. *Mol Biol Cell* 2001; **12**: 1079–91.
19. Xiao Z, Watson N, Rodriguez C, Lodish HF. Nucleocytoplasmic shuttling of Smad1 conferred by its nuclear localization and nuclear export signals. *J Biol Chem* 2001; **276**: 39404–10.
20. Watanabe M, Masuyama N, Fukuda M, Nishida E. Regulation of intracellular dynamics of Smad4 by its leucine-rich nuclear export signal. *EMBO Rep* 2000; **1**: 176–82.
21. Miyazono K, ten Dijke P, Heldin C-H. TGF-β signaling by Smad proteins. *Adv Immunol* 2000; **75**: 115–57.
22. Miyazawa K, Shinozaki M, Hara T, Furuya T, Miyazono K. Two major Smad pathways in TGF-β superfamily signalling. *Genes Cells* 2002; **7**: 1191–204.
23. Ito Y, Miyazono K. RUNX transcription factors as key targets of TGF-β superfamily signaling. *Curr Opin Genet Dev* 2003; **13**: 43–7.
24. Li QL, Ito K, Sakakura C, Fukamachi H, Inoue K, Chi XZ, Lee KY, Nomura S, Lee CW, Han SB, Kim HM, Kim WJ, Yamamoto H, Yamashita N, Yano T, Ikeda T, Itohara S, Inazawa J, Abe T, Hagiwara A, Yamagishi H, Ooe A, Kaneda A, Sugimura

T, Ushijima T, Bae SC, Ito Y. Causal relationship between the loss of RUNX3 expression and gastric cancer. *Cell* 2002; **109**: 113–24.

25. Hanai J-i, Chen LF, Kanno T, Fujita N, Kim WY, Imamura T, Ishidou Y, Fukuchi M, Shi M-J, Stavnezer J, Kawabata M, Miyazono K, Ito Y. Interaction and functional cooperation of PEBP2/CBF with Smads: synergistic induction of the immunoglobulin germline Cα promoter. *J Biol Chem* 1999; **274**: 31577–82.
26. Pardali E, Xie XQ, Tsapogas P, Itoh S, Arvanitidis K, Heldin C-H, ten Dijke P, Grundstrom T, Sideras P. Smad and AML proteins synergistically confer transforming growth factor β1 responsiveness to human germ-line IgA genes. *J Biol Chem* 2000; **275**: 3552–60.
27. Zhang Y-W, Yasui N, Huang G, Fujii M, Hanai J-i, Nogami H, Ochi T, Miyazono K, Ito Y. A RUNX2/PEBP2αA/CBFA1 mutation displaying impaired transactivation and Smad interaction in cleidocranial dysplasia. *Proc Natl Acad Sci USA* 2000; **97**:10549–54.
28. Imamura T, Takase M, Nishihara A, Oeda E, Hanai J, Kawabata M, Miyazono K. Smad6 inhibits signalling by the TGF-β superfamily. *Nature* 1997; **389**: 622–6.
29. Nakao A, Afrakhte M, Moren A, Nakayama T, Christian JL, Heuchel R, Itoh S, Kawabata M, Heldin NE, Heldin CH, ten Dijke P. Identification of Smad7, a TGFβ-inducible antagonist of TGF-β signalling. *Nature* 1997; **389**: 631–5.
30. Hayashi H, Abdollah S, Qiu Y, Cai J, Xu YY, Grinnell BW, Richardson MA, Topper JN, Gimbrone MA Jr, Wrana JL, Falb D. The MAD-related protein Smad7 associates with the TGFβ receptor and functions as an antagonist of TGFβ signaling. *Cell* 1997; **89**: 1165–73.
31. Hanyu A, Ishidou Y, Ebisawa T, Shimanuki T, Imamura T, Miyazono K. The N-domain of Smad7 is essential for specific inhibition of transforming growth factor-β signaling. *J Cell Biol* 2001; **155**: 1017–28.
32. Hata A, Lagna G, Massague J, Hemmati-Brivanlou A. Smad6 inhibits BMP/Smad1 signaling by specifically competing with the Smad4 tumor suppressor. *Genes Dev* 1998; **12**: 186–97.
33. Bai S, Shi X, Yang X, Cao X. Smad6 as a transcriptional corepressor. *J Biol Chem* 2000; **275**: 8267–70.
34. Zhu H, Kavsak P, Abdollah S, Wrana JL, Thomsen GH. A SMAD ubiquitin ligase targets the BMP pathway and affects embryonic pattern formation. *Nature* 1999; **400**: 687–93.
35. Ebisawa T, Fukuchi M, Murakami G, Chiba T, Tanaka K, Imamura T, Miyazono K. Smurf1 interacts with transforming growth factor-β type I receptor through Smad7 and induces receptor degradation. *J Biol Chem* 2001; **276**: 12477–80.
36. Kavsak P, Rasmussen RK, Causing CG, Bonni S, Zhu H, Thomsen GH, Wrana JL. Smad7 binds to Smurf2 to form an E3 ubiquitin ligase that targets the TGFβ receptor for degradation. *Mol Cell* 2000; **6**: 1365–75.
37. Murakami G, Watabe T, Takaoka K, Miyazono K, Imamura T. Cooperative inhibition of BMP signaling by Smurf1 and inhibitory Smads. *Mol Biol Cell* 2003; **14**: 2809–17.
38. Fukuchi M, Fukai Y, Masuda N, Miyazaki T, Nakajima M, Sohda M, Manda R, Tsukada K, Kato H, Kuwano H. High-level expression of the Smad ubiquitin ligase Smurf2 correlates with poor prognosis in patients with esophageal squamous cell carci-

noma. *Cancer Res* 2002; **62**: 7162–5.
39. Liu X, Sun Y, Weinberg RA, Lodish HF. Ski/Sno and TGF-β signaling. *Cytokine Growth Factor Rev* 2001; **12**: 1–8.
40. Wang W, Mariani FV, Harland RM, Luo K. Ski represses bone morphogenetic protein signaling in *Xenopus* and mammalian cells. *Proc Natl Acad Sci USA* 2000; **97**: 14393–9.
41. Akiyoshi S, Inoue H, Hanai J-i, Kusanagi K, Nemoto N, Miyazono K, Kawabata M. c-Ski acts as a transcriptional co-repressor in transforming growth factor-β signaling through interaction with Smads. *J Biol Chem* 1999; **274**: 35269–77.
42. Wu JW, Krawitz AR, Chai J, Li W, Zhang F, Luo K, Shi Y. Structural mechanism of Smad4 recognition by the nuclear oncoprotein Ski: insights on Ski-mediated repression of TGF-β signaling. *Cell* 2002; **111**: 357–67.
43. Mizuide M, Hara T, Furuya T, Takeda M, Kusanagi K, Inada Y, Mori M, Imamura T, Miyazawa K, Miyazono K. Two short segments of Smad3 are important for specific interaction of Smad3 with c-Ski and SnoN. *J Biol Chem* 2003; **278**: 531–6.
44. Stroschein SL, Wang W, Zhou S, Zhou Q, Luo K. Negative feedback regulation of TGF-β signaling by the SnoN oncoprotein. *Science* 1999; **286**: 771–4.
45. Bonni S, Wang HR, Causing CG, Kavsak P, Stroschein SL, Luo K, Wrana JL. TGF-β induces assembly of a Smad2-Smurf2 ubiquitin ligase complex that targets SnoN for degradation. *Nat Cell Biol* 2001; **3**: 587–95.
46. Sun Y, Liu X, Ng-Eaton E, Lodish HF, Weinberg RA. SnoN and Ski protooncoproteins are rapidly degraded in response to transforming growth factor β signaling. *Proc Natl Acad Sci USA* 1999; **96**: 12442–7.
47. Stroschein SL, Bonni S, Wrana JL, Luo K. Smad3 recruits the anaphase-promoting complex for ubiquitination and degradation of SnoN. *Genes Dev* 2001; **15**: 2822–36.
48. Shinagawa T, Dong HD, Xu M, Maekawa T, Ishii S. The *sno* gene, which encodes a component of the histone deacetylase complex, acts as a tumor suppressor in mice. *EMBO J* 2000; **19**: 2280–91.
49. Shinagawa T, Nomura T, Colmenares C, Ohira M, Nakagawara A, Ishii S. Increased susceptibility to tumorigenesis of *ski*-deficient heterozygous mice. *Oncogene* 2001; **20**: 8100–8.
50. Inman GJ, Nicolas FJ, Callahan JF, Harling JD, Gaster LM, Reith AD, Laping NJ, Hill CS. SB-431542 is a potent and specific inhibitor of transforming growth factor-β superfamily type I activin receptor-like kinase (ALK) receptors ALK4, ALK5, and ALK7. *Mol Pharmacol* 2002; **62**: 65–74.

VASCULAR ENDOTHELIAL GROWTH FACTOR RECEPTOR-2: ITS UNIQUE SIGNALING AND SPECIFIC LIGAND, VEGF-E

Masabumi SHIBUYA

*Division of Genetics, Institute of Medical Science, University of Tokyo**

Vascular endothelial growth factor receptor-2 (VEGFR-2/KDR/Flk-1) is a high-affinity receptor for vascular endothelial growth factor-A (VEGF-A), and mediates most of the endothelial growth and survival signals from VEGF-A. VEGFR-2 has a typical tyrosine kinase receptor structure with seven immunoglobulin (Ig)-like domains in the extracellular region, as well as a long kinase insert in the tyrosine kinase domain. It utilizes a unique signaling system for DNA synthesis in vascular endothelial cells, i.e. a phospholipase Cγ-protein kinaseC-Raf-MAP kinase pathway. Although VEGF-A binds two receptors, VEGFR-1 and -2, a newly isolated ligand VEGF-E (Orf-virus-derived VEGF) binds and activates only VEGFR-2. Transgenic mice expressing VEGF-E_{NZ-7} showed a dramatic increase in angiogenesis with very few side effects (such as edema and hemorrhagic spots), suggesting strong angiogenic signaling and a potential clinical utility of VEGF-E. VEGF family members bear three loops produced via three intramolecular disulfide bonds, and cooperation between loop-1 and loop-3 is necessary for the specific binding and activation of VEGFR-2 for angiogenesis. As it directly upregulates tumor angiogenesis, VEGFR-2 is an appropriate target for suppression of solid tumor growth using exogenous antibodies, small inhibitory molecules and *in vivo* stimulation of the immune system.

Background

Angiogenesis is an important biological process not only under physiological conditions but also in a variety of diseases including cancer, diabetic retinopathy and rheumatoid arthritis (*1*, *2*). Among angiogenic factors reported so far, vascular endothelial growth factor-A (VEGF-A) appears to mediate the basic signaling of angiogenesis, particularly signals for endothelial cell growth and survival *in vivo* (*3*). VEGF-A belongs to the platelet-derived growth factor (PDGF) supergene family, and as a homodimer, binds to, and activates two tyrosine kinase receptors, vascular endothelial growth factor receptor (VEGFR)-1 (Flt-1) and VEGFR-2 (KDR/Flk-1 in mice) (*4*) (Fig. 1). In addition to these tyrosine kinase receptors, a subtype of VEGF-A, VEGF-A_{165}, binds another membrane protein, neuropilin-1 (*5*). Knockout studies indicate that VEGFR-2 is the major signal transducer for the differentiation

* 4-6-1 Shirokane-dai, Minato-ku, Tokyo 108-8639, Japan

This paper is dedicated to the memory of late Dr. Tomizo Yoshida on the occasion of the 100th anniversary of his birth. It was originally published in Cancer Science in September, 2003.

of endothelial cells from precursor mesodermal cells and the growth of endothelial cells in early embryogenesis, whereas VEGFR-1 plays different roles, negative and regulatory, in angiogenesis at this stage (*6, 7*). Questions to answer are (1) what signaling pathways does VEGFR-2 utilize for a variety of VEGF-A-mediated biological activities? and (2) what biological effects are generated after the activation of VEGFR-2 alone without activation of VEGFR-1? Furthermore, (3) which receptor, VEGFR-1 or VEGFR-2, is responsible for stimulating pathological angiogenesis? Accumulating evidence suggests that more than half of pathological angiogenesis involves the activation of VEGFR-2. While VEGFR-1 mediates signaling for less than half, it plays a major role in the inflammatory cell/macrophage-dependent process in a variety of diseases such as rheumatoid arthritis and atherosclerosis (*8, 9*). This mini-review focuses on the structure, specific ligand and functions of VEGFR-2.

Structure and Gene Expression of VEGFR-2

1. Domain structure of VEGFR-2

VEGFR-2 was first isolated by Terman *et al.* in 1991 (*10*) and was named Kinase-insert domain containing receptor (KDR), its overall structure being highly homologous to that of Flt-1/VEGFR-1 (*11*). The murine *VEGFR-2* gene was independently isolated by two research groups (*12, 13*) and named *flk-1*. Like VEGFR-1, VEGFR-2 bears an extracellular region with seven immunoglobulin (Ig)-like domains, a transmembrane domain and a tyrosine kinase domain with an about 70-amino-acid insert. The approximately 40-amino-acid stretch at the carboxyl terminus of murine Flk-1 originally reported highly diverged from those of human

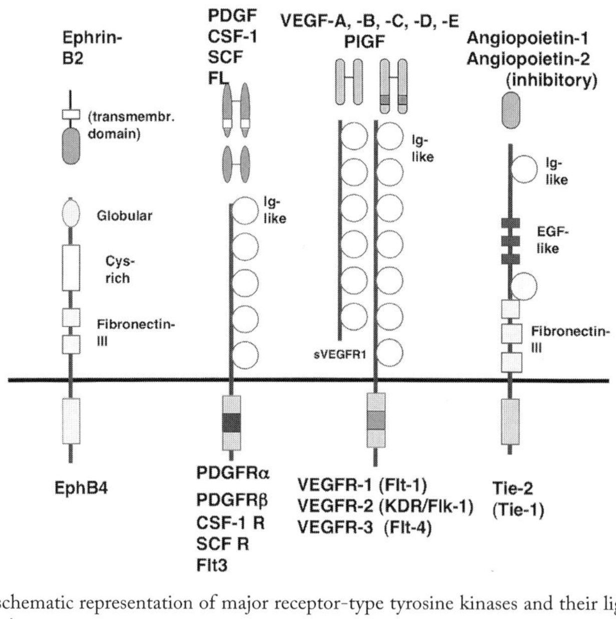

FIG. 1. A schematic representation of major receptor-type tyrosine kinases and their ligands related to angiogenesis

VEGF-A binds VEGFR-1 and -2, VEGF-C and -D bind VEGFR-3 (and weakly bind VEGFR-2), whereas VEGF-E specifically binds VEGFR-2. PlGF and VEGF-B are ligands specific to VEGFR-1.

VEGFR-2 and VEGFR-1. However, this apparent heterogeneity was due to extreme difficulty in nucleotide sequencing of this region, and revision of the amino acid sequence resulted in higher homology to both human VEGFR-2 and -1.

Non-vertebrate animals such as *Drosophila* carry a single 7-Ig type tyrosine kinase receptor (*D-VEGFR*) gene without the 5-Ig type receptor genes (*14*). Therefore, it is likely that all of the 7-Ig/5-Ig tyrosine kinase receptors in mammals, including the three VEGFRs and five PDGFR-related receptors (two PDGFRs and three Fms family members, c-Fms/c-Kit/Flt-3), were phylogenetically generated from a single ancestral 7-Ig tyrosine kinase receptor gene (*15*).

Unlike the *VEGFR-1* gene, which encodes a short message for a soluble form in addition to the full-length message (*11, 16*), the *VEGFR-2* gene encodes only one message for the full-length receptor of 1357 amino acids. Within the cell, VEGFR-2 protein is produced as a 150-kDa protein without significant glycosylation, then rapidly processed to a protein of about 200 kDa with glycosylation. This 200-kDa molecule is further glycosylated to a mature 230-kDa form, and expressed on the cell surface (*17*). The 200-kDa VEGFR-2 is mostly expressed within the cell, possibly in the Golgi apparatus, since exogenously added VEGF-A usually induces autophosphorylation of only the 230-kDa form of VEGFR-2 (*17*).

2. Ligand binding region

Previous studies on the PDGFR family revealed that the first three Ig-like domains constitute the region for direct binding with the ligand, while the fourth Ig-domain is responsible for dimerization of the receptor and an increase in affinity to the ligand. As in the case of PDGFR, deletion analysis of the VEGFR-2 ligand binding domain has shown that the second and third Ig-like domains compose the high-affinity ligand binding region (*18, 19*). The first Ig-like domain appears to have a negative regulatory role. Interestingly, the K_d of VEGFR-2 for VEGF-A expressed on the cell surface is about one order of magnitude weaker than that of VEGFR-1. Furthermore, the K_d of artificially created soluble forms of VEGFR-2 such as 7-Ig-s-VEGFR-2 without an immunoglobulin Fc region at the carboxyl terminus was much (about 100-fold) lower than that of the soluble form of VEGFR-1. The biological significance of this large difference in the affinity to VEGF-A between VEGFR-2 and -1 is not clear, but one possible explanation is that a third molecule such as neuropilin could upregulate the affinity between VEGFR-2 and VEGF-A ligand, creating flexibility in the intracellular signaling from VEGFR-2.

3. Tyrosine kinase domain and carboxyl terminal region

The structure of the VEGFR-2 tyrosine kinase domain is typical, with about 35% identity at the amino acid level to v-Src and 56% to PDGFR. An important characteristic of VEGFR-2 is the presence of a long kinase insert (KI) in the middle of the tyrosine kinase domain, and the length and position of the KI are very similar to those in PDGFR. However, as Kondo *et al.* (*20*) first showed for *VEGFR-1*, the exon-intron organization of the KI region in the VEGFR family is different from that in PDGFR family genes. This suggests that significant genomic rearrangement occurred during the formation of 5-Ig tyrosine kinase receptor genes such as *PDGFR* from 7-Ig receptor (*VEGFR*) genes in the phylogenetic development of animals.

In agreement with this hypothesis, the amino acid sequence of the KI in

VEGFR-2 is highly divergent from that of the KI in PDGFR. For example, two tyrosine residues with the motif Y-x-x-M or Y-M-x-M in the KI of PDGFR, which are crucial for the binding of the PI3K-p85 subunit and activation of PI3K, do not exist in the KI of VEGFR-2.

In the carboxyl-terminal region, 6 tyrosine residues are present in VEGFR-2, and most of them are conserved among the vertebrates (Fig. 2). As discussed below, at least one of the tyrosines is essential for the critical signaling for DNA synthesis.

4. *Gene expression of VEGFR-2*

The gene expression of VEGFR-2 in mice starts around E7.0 in the posterior mesodermal area of the embryo, appearing as a broad band, then a part of the VEGFR-2-expressing cells migrate into the yolk sac to form blood islands (*6*, *21*). The primitive endothelial cells surrounding hematopoietic cells in each blood island express a high level of VEGFR-2, and start to form a primitive blood vessel network with a tubular structure. VEGFR-2 is specifically expressed on the endothelial cells, endothelial cell progenitor cells at embryonal stages and a variety of vascular endothelial cells at adult stages (*22*, *23*). Furthermore, the endothelial cells with filopodia guiding the neovascularization in murine neonatal retina also appear to express VEGFR-2, even though these cells have yet to form a typical tubular structure (*24*). In hematopoietic cells, Eichmann *et al.* demonstrated that hematopoietic stem cell-like cells budding from endothelial cells in chicken embryo express VEGFR-2 (*25*). Similar phenomena were reported in mouse embryo.

At adult stages, endothelial cell progenitor cells were reported to exist among bone marrow cells which express VEGFR-2. However, it is not yet clear what percentage of bone marrow cells is endothelial cell progenitor cells, or how strongly

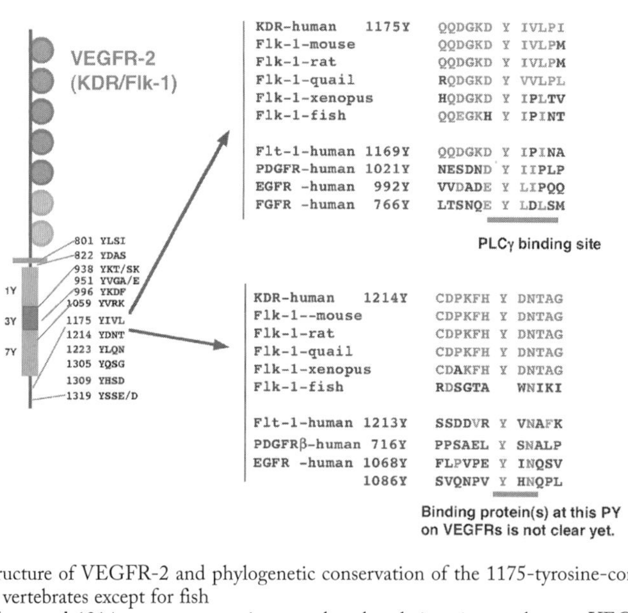

FIG. 2. Structure of VEGFR-2 and phylogenetic conservation of the 1175-tyrosine-containing region among vertebrates except for fish

The 1175-tyr and 1214-tyr are two major autophosphorylation sites on human VEGFR-2. The 1175-PY region is the PLCγ binding site, but the protein(s) that binds to the 1214-PY region is unknown.

these cells express VEGFR-2 (*26*).

Signal Transduction via VEGFR-2

The tyrosine kinase receptor family has about 50 members, including Insulin R/IGF-1R, the EGFR family, 7-Ig/5-Ig receptors (VEGFRs and the PDGFR family), FGFRs, HGF-Rs, NGFRs, and Eph receptors. Most of these tyrosine kinase receptors, except for VEGFRs and Eph receptors, have the potential to transform non-transformed cells, such as NIH3T3 cells. Also, basically all the transforming tyrosine kinases utilize the Ras activation pathway for cell transformation.

Since overexpression of VEGFR-1 or VEGFR-2 in NIH3T3 cells failed to transform these cells even in the presence of a high concentration of VEGF-A (*27–29*), we hypothesized that VEGFRs, particularly the major positive signal transducer VEGFR-2, utilize a unique signaling pathway for endothelial cell proliferation. Xia *et al.* suggested the possible involvement of a protein kinase C pathway downstream from VEGF-A based on experiments using a PKC inhibitor (*30*). We have directly shown that the binding with VEGF-A and activation of VEGFR-2 induce the binding of phospholipase Cγ (PLCγ) to VEGFR-2 via its carboxyl-terminal SH2 domain, as well as strong phosphorylation at tyrosine (*31*). Then, the activated PLCγ efficiently activates protein kinase C (particularly PKCβ), and stimulates the Raf-MEK-MAP kinase pathway (*31*) (Fig. 3).

To our surprise, given the general pathway of cell growth signaling via tyrosine

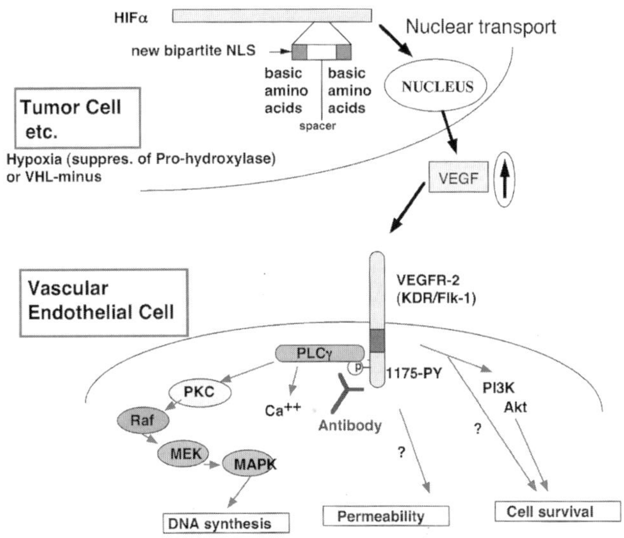

FIG. 3. Signal transduction of VEGFR-2 for endothelial cell proliferation via the PLCγ-PKC-MAP kinase pathway

Inhibitors specific to VEGFR-2 tyrosine kinase or antibodies which block the PLCγ binding to 1175-PY region efficiently suppress this signaling pathway. In a normoxic condition, HIFα proteins (HIF1α, 2α, 3α) are structurally modified by prolyl hydroxylase, and degraded via the ubiquitin ligase pathway in a VHL-dependent manner. In a hypoxic condition, which suppresses prolyl hydroxylase activity, or in VHL-minus genetic background (von Hippel-Lindau disease), HIFα proteins are stabilized, resulting in nuclear localization and induction of hypoxia-responsive genes such as VEGF-A.

kinases (but consistent with the lack of transforming activity of VEGFR-2), after stimulation with VEGF-A, Ras was activated only very weakly, if at all, in both primary endothelial cells and VEGFR-2-overexpressing NIH3T3 cells (*32*). In general when tyrosine kinases activate Ras, the tyrosine kinase itself or a tyrosine kinase-adaptor complex recruits Grb2 or Shc-Grb2 complex, which further recruits Sos, a nucleotide exchange factor for Ras, to stimulate Ras to GTP-bound form. However, after binding with VEGF-A, the activated VEGFR-2 did not efficiently recruit Grb2 or Shc-Grb2 to the receptor. This is consistent with the very weak activation of Ras downstream of VEGF-A signaling (*32*).

A PI3K inhibitor, wortmannin, did not significantly suppress VEGF-dependent DNA synthesis of endothelial cells in a 20-h culture system. However, treatment of cells with PI3K inhibitor for longer than 48 h suppressed endothelial cell proliferation, most likely due to its strong inhibition of the survival signal from focal adhesion.

In a series of analyses on the effects of tyrosine to phenylalanine mutation in VEGFR-2 and tryptic phosphotyrosine-containing peptides, we have determined that a single autophosphorylation site, the 1175-tyrosine residue in human VEGFR-2, is the major site for the activation of the PLCγ-PKC-MAP kinase pathway (*31*) (Fig. 3). As expected, 1175-tyr or the corresponding tyrosine (for example, 1173-tyr in mice) is well conserved in VEGFR-2 in vertebrates (except for fish Flk-1). On the other hand, one report suggested that Ras is activated downstream from VEGFR (*33*). The reason for this discrepancy is not clear.

One should point out, however, that primary endothelial cells do contain Ras protein. It is well known that Ras is deeply involved in the focal adhesion-FAK/c-Src/actin pathway in many cell types. Thus, it is reasonable that Ras in endothelial cells functions in the cell-to-matrix and cell-to-cell attachment and signaling of cell migration. Survival signaling for endothelial cells from the VEGF receptor is reported to involve the PI3K-Akt pathway (*34*). Since the signal to activate PI3K by VEGFR-2 is usually not very strong, it is possible that another pathway is also used for this signal.

Biological Functions of VEGFR-2

VEGF-A which activates both VEGFR-1 and -2 stimulates (1) endothelial cell proliferation, (2) tubular formation, (3) endothelial cell survival, (4) endothelial cell migration, (5) vascular permeability *in vivo*, (6) gene expression of Ets-1, tissue factor, PAI-1, matrix metalloproteinases, etc., and (7) monocyte/macrophage migration. Based on the results obtained using VEGF-E (see below), receptor-specific VEGF-A mutants and VEGFR-1-specific ligand PlGF and VEGF-B, part of the signaling for (1) to (6) and most of that for (7) appear to be mediated by VEGFR-1, while most of the signaling for (1) to (6) is mediated through VEGFR-2 (*35*).

VEGFR-2-specific Ligand, VEGF-E

To clarify the biological functions influenced by each VEGFR, we searched for a novel type of VEGF, and found that the Orf virus genome-encoded VEGF-like gene (*36*) encodes a protein (designated VEGF-E_{NZ-7}) that specifically binds at high affinity and activates VEGFR-2 (*37*). Consistent with the lack of ability of radio-labeled VEGF-E_{NZ-7} to bind VEGFR-1 overexpressed in NIH3T3 cells, soluble VEGFR-1 (sFlt-1), a potent inhibitor of VEGF-A, failed to suppress the biological activity of VEGF-E_{NZ-7}. Interestingly, VEGF-E_{NZ-7} does not bear a typical heparin-binding domain with a basic amino acid stretch, or bind neuropilin, but it still exhibits high-affinity binding to VEGFR-2. VEGF-E_{NZ-7} showed activity to promote endothelial cell growth and survival at similar levels to VEGF-A_{165}, and had a slightly less potent effect on vascular permeability than VEGF-A_{165}.

Two other VEGF-E family members, VEGF-E_{NZ-2} and VEGF-E_{D1701} were subsequently isolated (*38*, *39*), both with essentially the same activity as VEGF-E_{NZ-7}. However, VEGF-E_{NZ-2} was reported to have heparin-binding activity, although it is not yet clear which amino acid stretch is responsible for this activity. It should be noted that VEGF-E family members show only 20 to 25% amino acid identity with VEGF-A, though the K_d for VEGFR-2 is almost the same as that of VEGF-A_{165} for

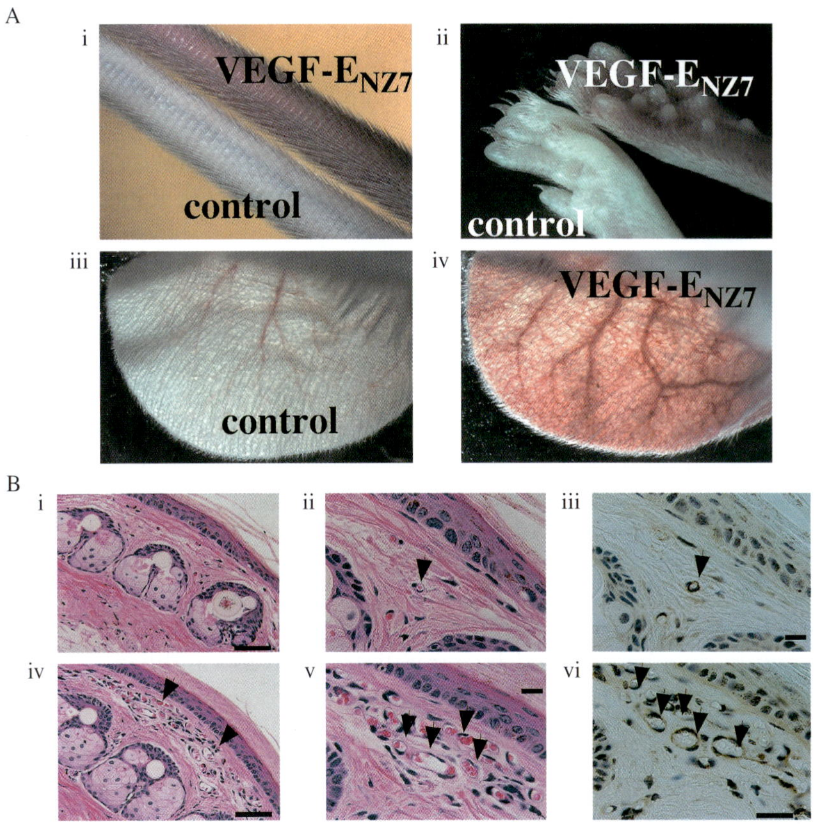

FIG. 4. VEGF-E_{NZ-7} transgenic mice show significant neovascularization in the skin without clear side effects

A. Tail (i), toes (ii), and ear (iv) of VEGF-E_{NZ-7} transgenic mice exhibit significant neovascularization without clear edema or hemorrhagic spots. B. Microscopic analysis of the tail in VEGF-E_{NZ-7} transgenic mice. About a 10-fold increase in angiogenesis was observed in the transgenic mice (iv–vi) compared with control mice (i–iii). i, ii, iv and v, H-E staining; iii and vi, immunostaining for vWF (*40*).

VEGFR-2.

To further compare the biological activities of VEGF-E and VEGF-A, we generated K14-promoter driven VEGF-E_{NZ-7} transgenic (Tg) mice (*40*). Gene expression of VEGF-E_{NZ-7} in the basal cell layer of the skin of these mice induced a strong angiogenic response, about a 10-fold increase compared to the control mice. To our surprise, edematous lesions and hemorrhagic spots on the ear and other dermal tissues which were reported as side effects in VEGF-A Tg mice (*41*) were not detectable in VEGF-E Tg mice (Fig. 4). The endothelial cell-cell junction as well as the recruitment of pericytes to endothelial cells was well organized. The mechanisms behind the strong angiogenic activity with fewer side effects of VEGF-E_{NZ-7} *in vivo* are worthy of further study. At least two explanations are possible: (1) without the support of neuropilin, VEGF-E_{NZ-7} binds at high affinity with and continuously activates VEGFR-2, resulting in a tight endothelial cell-to-cell junction with less leakage, and (2) the functions of lymphatic vessels such as the absorption of fluid in tissues are well maintained in VEGF-E Tg mice, leading to an appropriate balance between leaks from newly formed blood vessels and absorption by lymph vessels.

One significant characteristic of VEGF-E_{NZ-7} is its very strong affinity to VEGFR-2 despite a low amino acid homology to VEGF-A. Thus, we attempted to clarify which domain in VEGF-E is essential for the construction and organization of a high-affinity tertiary structure for the ligand-binding region of VEGFR-2. All of the VEGF/PDGF supergene family products have eight cysteines in a monomer polypeptide. Six cysteines are used for intramolecular S-S bonds, and the other two for inter-molecular S-S bonds to form a dimer structure (*42*). Thus, three loops are formed within a monomer, loop-1, loop-2 and loop-3.

Keyt *et al.* showed that a few basic amino acids in loop-3 of VEGF-A are essential for binding to VEGFR-2 since mutation of these amino acids removed the binding activity (*43*). However, none of these basic amino acids is conserved at the same position in the VEGF-E family, suggesting that they are not an absolute requirement for ligand-VEGFR-2 binding. Using a series of chimeric constructs of VEGF-E, VEGF-A and PlGF, we found that cooperation between loop-1 and loop-3 in VEGF-E or VEGF-A is crucial for the appropriate tertiary structure needed for high-affinity binding to VEGFR-2 (*44*). A combination of loop-1 from VEGF-E and loop-3 from VEGF-A or *vice versa* did not work, suggesting that combining loop-1 and loop-3 from the same molecule, VEGF-E or VEGF-A, is important (Fig. 5).

Since VEGF-E_{NZ-7} induces significant angiogenesis *in vivo* with few side effects, VEGF-E family members should be carefully studied as candidates for a potential angiogenic factor for clinical use in pro-angiogenic therapy.

VEGFR-2 as a Target for Suppression of Solid Tumor Growth

A large body of evidence indicates that the VEGF-VEGFR system is involved in the pathological angiogenesis which promotes the malignancy of solid tumors, diabetic retinopathy and rheumatoid arthritis. VEGFR-1 (Flt-1) is involved in inflammatory diseases and tissue-specific metastasis of cancer (*45*, *46*), while the VEGF-A and VEGFR-2 system is a direct target in the suppression of pathological angiogenesis. Anti-VEGF-A monoclonal antibody is now under phase III clinical trial, and

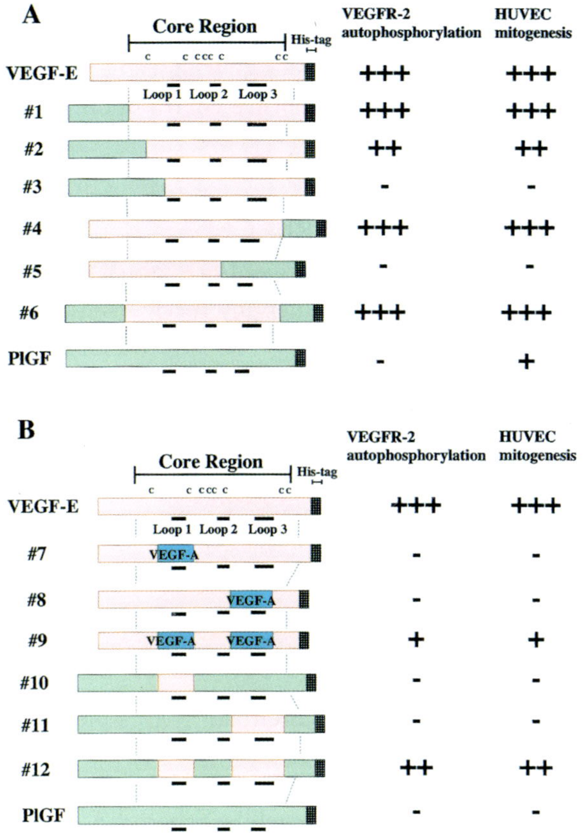

FIG. 5. The set of loop-1 and -3 structures in VEGF-E_{NZ-7} is essential for the activation of VEGFR-2 signaling

A. The amino-terminal and carboxyl-terminal regions can be replaced with the corresponding sequences of PlGF without suppression of VEGFR-2-stimulatory activity. B. Cooperation between loop-1 and -3 in VEGF-E (chimera #12) or VEGF-A (chimera #9) is crucial for the binding and activation of VEGFR-2 (*44*). Sequences derived from VEGF-E, PlGF and VEGF-A are indicated by light-brown, green and blue color, respectively.

monoclonal antibody against VEGFR-2 also has a suppressive effect on solid tumor growth in mice (*47*). Many pharmaceutical companies are developing small molecules which specifically block the tyrosine kinase activity of VEGFR-2 (*48*, *49*), although most compounds block in parallel the tyrosine kinase activity of VEGFR-1 due to the high structural homology between the two receptors.

Another target for regulating VEGFR-2 signaling could be the critical autophosphorylation site on the receptor. Downstream signaling is an important target for the suppression of endothelial cell proliferation via the VEGF-A-VEGFR-2 pathway (*31*). Furthermore, a recent report suggests that oral administration of a bacterial-type vector (non-toxic *Salmonella typhimurium*) containing VEGFR-2-expressing vector DNA induces an immune response to VEGFR-2, leading to an efficient inhibition of solid tumor growth in the immunized animals (*50*). In the near future we may have an appropriate tool or strategy for regulating the activity of VEGFR-2 and thereby blocking severe pathological angiogenesis.

Acknowledgments

I thank all the members in my laboratory in the Institute of Medical Science, University of Tokyo, particularly Drs. Tomoko Takahashi, Sachiyo Ogawa, Atsushi Kiba, Sachiko Yamaguchi and Asako Sawano, for their extensive contributions to the studies on VEGF and VEGFR-2 signaling.

REFERENCES

1. Risau W. Mechanism of angiogenesis. *Nature* 1997; **386**: 671–4.
2. Hanahan D, Folkman J. Patterns and emerging mechanisms of the angiogenic switch during tumorigenesis. *Cell* 1996; **86**: 353–64.
3. Ferrara N, Davis-Smyth T. The biology of vascular endothelial growth factor. *Endocr Rev* 1997; **18**: 4–25.
4. Shibuya M. Role of VEGF-Flt receptor system in normal and tumor angiogenesis. *Adv Cancer Res* 1995; **67**: 281–316.
5. Soker S, Takashima S, Miao HQ, Neufeld G, Klagsbrun M. Neuropilin-1 is expressed by endothelial and tumor cells as an isoform-specific receptor for vascular endothelial growth factor. *Cell* 1998; **92**: 735–45.
6. Shalaby F, Rossant J, Yamaguchi TP, Gertsenstein M, Wu X-F, Breitman ML, Schuh AC. Failure of blood-island formation and vasculogenesis in Flk-1-deficient mice. *Nature* 1995; **376**: 62–6.
7. Fong G-H, Rossant J, Gertsentein M, Breitman ML. Role of the Flt-1 receptor tyrosine kinase in regulating the assembly of vascular endothelium. *Nature* 1995; **376**: 66–70.
8. Luttun A, Tjwa M, Moons L, Wu Y, Angelillo-Scherrer A, Liao F, Nagy JA, Hooper A, Priller J, De Klerck B, Compernolle V, Daci E, Bohlen P, Dewerchin M, Herbert JM, Fava R, Matthys P, Carmeliet G, Collen D, Dvorak HF, Hicklin DJ, Carmeliet P. Revascularization of ischemic tissues by PlGF treatment, and inhibition of tumor angiogenesis, arthritis and atherosclerosis by anti-Flt1. *Nat Med* 2002; **8**: 831–40.
9. Sawano A, Iwai S, Sakurai Y, Ito M, Shitara K, Nakahata T, Shibuya M. Vascular endothelial growth factor receptor-1 (Flt-1) is a novel cell surface marker for the lineage of monocyte-macrophages in humans. *Blood* 2001; **97**: 785–91.
10. Terman BI, Carrion ME, Kovacs E, Rasmussen BA, Eddy R, Shows TB. Identification of a new endothelial cell growth factor receptor tyrosine kinase. *Oncogene* 1991; **6**: 1677–83.
11. Shibuya M, Yamaguchi S, Yamane A, Ikeda T, Tojo A, Matsushime H, Sato M. Nucleotide sequence and expression of a novel human receptor-type tyrosine kinase gene (flt) closely related to the fms family. *Oncogene* 1990; **5**: 519–24.
12. Matthews W, Jordan CT, Gavin M, Jenkins NA, Copeland NG, Lemischka IR. A receptor tyrosine kinase cDNA isolated from a population of enriched primitive hematopoietic cells and exhibiting close genetic linkage to c-kit. *Proc Natl Acad Sci USA* 1991; **88**: 9026–30.
13. Millauer B, Wizigmann-Voos S, Schnurch H, Martinez R, Moller NPH, Risau W, Ullrich A. High affinity VEGF binding and developmental expression suggest flk-1 as a major regulator of vasculogenesis and angiogenesis. *Cell* 1993; **72**: 835–46.
14. Duchek P, Somogyi K, Jekely G, Beccari S, Rorth P. Guidance of cell migration by the

Drosophila PDGF/VEGF receptor. *Cell* 2001; **107**: 17–26.

15. Shibuya M. Vascular endothelial growth factor receptor family genes: when did the three genes phylogenetically segregate? *Biol Chem* 2002; **383**: 1573–9.
16. Kendall RL, Thomas KA. Inhibition of vascular endothelial cell growth factor activity by an endogenously encoded soluble receptor. *Proc Natl Acad Sci USA* 1993; **90**: 10705–9.
17. Takahashi T, Shibuya M. The 230 kDa mature form of KDR/Flk-1 (VEGF receptor-2) activates the PLCγ pathway and partially induces mitotic signals in NIH3T3 fibroblasts. *Oncogene* 1997; **14**: 2079–89.
18. Fuh G, Li B, Crowley C, Cunningham B, Wells JA. Requirements for binding and signaling of the kinase domain receptor for vascular endothelial growth factor. *J Biol Chem* 1998; **273**: 11197–204.
19. Shinkai A, Ito M, Anazawa H, Yamaguchi S, Shitara K, Shibuya M. Mapping of the sites involved in ligand-association and dissociation at the extracellular domain of vascular endothelial growth factor receptor KDR. *J Biol Chem* 1998; **273**: 31283–8.
20. Kondo K, Hiratsuka S, Subbalakshmi E, Matsushime H, Shibuya M. Genomic organization of the *flt-1* gene encoding for vascular endothelial growth factor (VEGF) receptor-1 suggests an intimate evolutionary relationship between the 7-Ig and the 5-Ig tyrosine kinase receptors. *Gene* 1998; **208**: 297–305.
21. Yamashita J, Itoh H, Hirashima M, Ogawa M, Nishikawa S, Yurugi T, Naito M, Nakao K, Nishikawa S. Flk1-positive cells derived from embryonic stem cells serve as vascular progenitors. *Nature* 2000; **408**: 92–6.
22. Kaipainen A, Korhonen J, Pajusola K, Aprelikova O, Persico MG, Terman BI, Alitalo K. The related FLT4, FLT1, and KDR receptor tyrosine kinases show distinct expression patterns in human fetal endothelial cells. *J Exp Med* 1993; **178**: 2077–88.
23. Yamane A, Seetharam L, Yamaguchi S, Gotoh N, Takahashi T, Neufeld G, Shibuya M. A new communication system between hepatocytes and sinusoidal endothelial cells in liver through vascular endothelial growth factor and Flt tyrosine kinase receptor family (Flt-1 and KDR/Flk-1). *Oncogene* 1994; **9**: 2683–90.
24. Ruhrberg C, Gerhardt H, Golding M, Watson R, Ioannidou S, Fujisawa H, Betsholtz C, Shima DT. Spatially restricted patterning cues provided by heparin-binding VEGF-A control blood vessel branching morphogenesis. *Genes Dev* 2002; **16**: 2684–98.
25. Eichmann A, Corbel C, Nataf V, Vaigot P, Breant C, Le Douarin NM. Ligand-dependent development of the endothelial and hemopoietic lineages from embryonic mesodermal cells expressing vascular endothelial growth factor receptor 2. *Proc Natl Acad Sci USA* 1997; **94**: 5141–6.
26. Asahara T, Masuda H, Takahashi T, Kalka C, Pastore C, Silver M, Kearne M, Magner M, Isner JM. Bone marrow origin of endothelial progenitor cells responsible for postnatal vasculogenesis in physiological and pathological neovascularization. *Circ Res* 1999; **85**: 221–8.
27. Waltenberger J, Claesson-Welsh L, Siegbahn A, Shibuya M, Heldin C-H. Different signal transduction properties of KDR and Flt1, two receptors for vascular endothelial growth factor. *J Biol Chem* 1994; **269**: 26988–95.
28. Seetharam L, Gotoh N, Maru Y, Neufeld G, Yamaguchi S, Shibuya M. A unique signal transduction from FLT tyrosine kinase, a receptor for vascular endothelial growth

factor VEGF. *Oncogene* 1995; **10**: 135–47.

29. Sawano A, Takahashi T, Yamaguchi S, Aonuma T, Shibuya M. Flt-1 but not KDR/Flk-1 tyrosine kinase is a receptor for placenta growth factor (PlGF), which is related to vascular endothelial growth factor (VEGF). *Cell Growth Diff* 1996; **7**: 213–21.
30. Xia P, Aiello LP, Ishii H, Jiang ZY, Park DJ, Robinson GS, Takagi H, Newsome WP, Jirousek MR, King GL. Characterization of vascular endothelial growth factor's effect on the activation of protein kinase C, its isoforms, and endothelial cell growth. *J Clin Invest* 1996; **98**: 2018–26.
31. Takahashi T, Yamaguchi S, Chida K, Shibuya M. A single autophosphorylation site on KDR/Flk-1 is essential for VEGF-A-dependent activation of PLCγ and DNA synthesis in vascular endothelial cells. *EMBO J* 2001; **20**: 2768–78.
32. Takahashi T, Ueno H, Shibuya M. VEGF activates protein kinase C-dependent, but Ras-independent Raf-MEK-MAP kinase pathway for DNA synthesis in primary endothelial cells. *Oncogene* 1999; **18**: 2221–30.
33. Meadows KN, Bryant P, Pumiglia K. Vascular endothelial growth factor induction of the angiogenic phenotype requires Ras activation. *J Biol Chem* 2001; **276**: 49289–98.
34. Gerber HP, McMurtrey A, Kowalski J, Yan M, Keyt BA, Dixit V, Ferrara N. Vascular endothelial growth factor regulates endothelial cell survival through the phosphatidylinositol 3-kinase/Akt signal transduction pathway. Requirement for Flk-1/KDR activation. *J Biol Chem* 1998; **273**: 30336–43.
35. Shibuya M, Ito N, Claesson-Welsh L. Structure and function of VEGF receptor-1 and -2. *Curr Topics Microbiol Immunol* 1999; **237**: 59–83.
36. Lyttle DJ, Fraser KM, Fleming SB, Mercer AA, Robinson AJ. Homologs of vascular endothelial growth factor are encoded by the poxvirus orf virus. *J Virol* 1994; **68**: 84–92.
37. Ogawa S, Oku A, Sawano A, Yamaguchi S, Yazaki Y, Shibuya M. A novel type of vascular endothelial growth factor: VEGF-E (NZ-7 VEGF) preferentially utilizes KDR/Flk-1 receptor and carries a potent mitotic activity without heparin-binding domain. *J Biol Chem* 1998; **273**: 31273–82.
38. Meyer M, Clauss M, Lepple-Wienhues A, Waltenberger J, Augustin HG, Ziche M, Lanz C, Buttner M, Rziha HJ, Dehio C. A novel vascular endothelial growth factor encoded by Orf virus, VEGF-E, mediates angiogenesis via signalling through VEGFR-2 (KDR) but not VEGFR-1 (Flt-1) receptor tyrosine kinases. *EMBO J* 1999; **18**: 363–74.
39. Wise LM, Veikkola T, Mercer AA, Savory LJ, Fleming SB, Caesar C, Vitali A, Makinen T, Alitalo K, Stacker SA. Vascular endothelial growth factor (VEGF)-like protein from orf virus NZ2 binds to VEGFR2 and neuropilin-1. *Proc Natl Acad Sci USA* 1999; **96**: 3071–6.
40. Kiba A, Sagara H, Hara T, Shibuya M. VEGFR-2-specific ligand VEGF-E induces non-edematous hyper-vascularization in mice. *Biochem Biophys Res Commun* 2003; **301**: 371–7.
41. Larcher F, Murillas R, Bolontrade M, Conti CJ, Jorcano JL. VEGF/VPF overexpression in skin of transgenic mice induces angiogenesis, vascular hyperpermeability and accelerated tumor development. *Oncogene* 1998; **17**: 303–11.
42. Wiesmann C, Fuh G, Christinger HW, Eigenbrot C, Wells JA, de Vos AM. Crystal

structure at 1.7 A resolution of VEGF in complex with domain 2 of the Flt-1 receptor. *Cell* 1997; **91**: 695–704.
43. Keyt BA, Nguyen HV, Berleau LT, Duarte CM, Park J, Chen H, Ferrara N. Identification of vascular endothelial growth factor determinants for binding KDR and FLT-1 receptors. *J Biol Chem* 1996; **271**: 5638–46.
44. Kiba A, Yabana N, Shibuya M. A set of loop-1 and -3 structures in the novel VEGF family member, VEGF-E_{NZ-7}, is essential for the activation of VEGFR-2 signaling. *J Biol Chem* 2003; **278**: 13453–61.
45. Carmeliet P, Moons L, Luttun A, Vincenti V, Compernolle V, De Mol M, Wu Y, Bono F, Devy L, Beck H, Scholz D, Acker T, DiPalma T, Dewerchin M, Noel A, Stalmans I, Barra A, Blacher S, Vandendriessche T, Ponten A, Eriksson U, Plate KH, Foidart JM, Schaper W, Charnock-Jones DS, Hicklin DJ, Herbert JM, Collen D, Persico MG. Synergism between vascular endothelial growth factor and placental growth factor contributes to angiogenesis and plasma extravasation in pathological conditions. *Nat Med* 2001; **7**: 575–83.
46. Hiratsuka S, Nakamura K, Iwai S, Murakami M, Itoh T, Kijima H, Shipley JM, Senior RM, Shibuya M. MMP9 induction by vascular endothelial growth factor receptor-1 is involved in lung specific metastasis. *Cancer Cell* 2002; **2**: 289–300.
47. Lyden D, Hattori K, Dias S, Costa C, Blaikie P, Butros L, Chadburn A, Heissig B, Marks W, Witte L, Wu Y, Hicklin D, Zhu Z, Hackett NR, Crystal RG, Moore MA, Hajjar KA, Manova K, Benezra R, Rafii S. Impaired recruitment of bone-marrow-derived endothelial and hematopoietic precursor cells blocks tumor angiogenesis and growth. *Nat Med* 2001; **7**: 1194–201.
48. Wedge SR, Ogilvie DJ, Dukes M, Kendrew J, Curwen JO, Hennequin LF, Thomas AP, Stokes ES, Curry B, Richmond GH, Wadsworth PF. ZD4190: an orally active inhibitor of vascular endothelial growth factor signaling with broad-spectrum antitumor efficacy. *Cancer Res* 2000; **60**: 970–5.
49. Wood JM, Bold G, Buchdunger E, Cozens R, Ferrari S, Frei J, Hofmann F, Mestan J, Mett H, O'Reilly T, Persohn E, Rosel J, Schnell C, Stover D, Theuer A, Towbin H, Wenger F, Woods-Cook K, Menrad A, Siemeister G, Schirner M, Thierauch KH, Schneider MR, Drevs J, Martiny-Baron G, Totzke F. PTK787/ZK 222584, a novel and potent inhibitor of vascular endothelial growth factor receptor tyrosine kinases, impairs vascular endothelial growth factor-induced responses and tumor growth after oral administration. *Cancer Res* 2000; **60**: 2178–89.
50. Niethammer AG, Xiang R, Becker JC, Wodrich H, Pertl U, Karsten G, Eliceiri BP, Reisfeld RA. A DNA vaccine against VEGF receptor 2 prevents effective angiogenesis and inhibits tumor growth. *Nat Med* 2002; **8**: 1369–75.

ROLES OF PERICELLULAR PROTEOLYSIS BY MEMBRANE TYPE-1 MATRIX METALLOPROTEINASE IN CANCER INVASION AND ANGIOGENESIS

Motoharu SEIKI and Ikuo YANA

*Division of Cancer Cell Research, Institute of Medical Science, University of Tokyo**

Behavior of cancer cells is profoundly affected by their microenvironment, which is often controlled by pericellular proteolysis or the processing of protein components, including extracellular matrices, growth factors, cytokines, receptors, cell adhesion molecules, and so on. Matrix metalloproteinases (MMPs) are a family of zinc-dependent proteases responsible for the proteolytic events in the extracellular milieu. Among the multiple MMPs expressed in a wide range of tumors, membrane type-1 MMP (MT1-MMP), which is expressed especially in tumor cells with significant invasive properties, is thought to be particularly important for pericellular proteolysis. Recent studies have elucidated in part how MT1-MMP is regulated biologically for the promotion of invasion by tumors or for angiogenesis by endothelial cells. Understanding of the proteolysis by, and the regulation of MT1-MMP, which probably promotes cell invasion, could provide a therapeutic hint as to how to block or delay the progression of cancer.

Tissue architecture is composed of cells and extracellular matrix (ECM), which not only acts as a scaffold, but also profoundly affects cellular functions associated with cell adhesion molecules, such as integrins. For cancers, the ECM is a barrier to their growth, invasion, and metastasis. Further, it markedly affects the behavior of cancer cells not only at early stages of carcinogenesis, but also throughout the progression of the disease. Therefore, it is important to understand how cancers, as well as normal cells, remodel the ECM.

The major proteases responsible for turnover of the ECM belong to either the serine protease or matrix metalloproteinase (MMP) family. MMPs are zinc-binding endopeptidases that collectively degrade most of the components of the ECM, including collagens, glycoproteins, and proteoglycans, in the normal range of pH. Aggressive cancer cells express multiple MMPs that have been implicated in growth, invasion, and metastasis of tumors by degrading the surrounding tissue. Angiogenesis around cancer nests also requires remodeling of the ECM by the proteases, including MMPs, expressed in endothelial cells. Thus, inhibition of the MMPs might be a possible approach to reduce tumor malignancy. Based on this idea, different types of

* 4-6-1 Shirokane-dai, Minato-ku, Tokyo 108-8639, Japan

This paper is dedicated to the memory of late Dr. Tomizo Yoshida on the occasion of the 100th anniversary of his birth. It was originally published in Cancer Science in July, 2003.

MMP inhibitors (MMPIs) have been developed and some have been demonstrated to work effectively in several cancer models using animals. Unfortunately, however, recent clinical trials using MMPIs to treat human malignant diseases have failed to provide greater benefit than conventional therapies such as surgery and chemotherapy (*1*). Why do MMPIs fail to work against human tumors? Based on the results of animal experiments, it seems unlikely that MMPs do not play a key role. One possible explanation is a difference in the sensitivity of tumors to MMPIs depending on tumor stage, as suggested by Hanahan's group (*2*). In animal models, administration of an MMPI sufficiently impaired angiogenesis to the tumor islets and subsequent tumor growth, but was not effective in late-stage tumors, indicating that MMP activity is required for tumor proliferation or invasion in the early stages, but not at the advanced stage. Actually, most clinical studies have been conducted with late stage tumors. In this regard, a trial of MMPIs should be conducted in patients with early stage cancers, even though most early cancers can be effectively treated using conventional therapies. Another important consideration is the possibility that MMPs play significant roles in host defense. In immune cells, MMPs may regulate cytokines and cell adhesion molecules in the post-translational period. In addition, the host defense system is stimulated during tumor progression, so that MMPIs might impair the immune system more severely in late than in early stages of tumor growth. From our experience in clinical trials, we have realized that knowledge about MMPs (or MMPIs) is still too fragmentary to allow us to take advantage of MMPIs in cancer therapy. Here, we will give a brief overview of MMPs, focusing especially on membrane type-1 MMP (MT1-MMP), a crucial enzyme on the cell surface. A better understanding of this enzyme could provide new ideas for suppressing cancer progression.

MT1-MMP as a Key Enzyme for Tumor Invasion

During cancer cell invasion, the ECM barrier has to be removed in the direction of the invasion. Among the MMPs expressed in tumors, MMP-2 and MMP-9, both of which have type IV collagenase activity, have been considered to play an important role in the cell invasion through the basement membrane (BM), because type IV collagen is a unique component of the BM. These MMPs are usually secreted from normal cells, while in invasive tumor cells, the breaching activity against type IV collagen is thought to be associated with the cell surface. In particular, proMMP-2, mainly secreted by stromal cells, becomes localized at the cell membrane of cancer cells (*3*). Like other MMPs, MMP-2 is produced as a zymogen (proMMP-2) and the activation is strictly controlled by a membrane-associated event. Whether the MMP-2 is provided by the host or not, the activation step in cancer is believed to be important, and to be correlated with invasion and metastasis.

MT1-MMP was the first membrane-anchored MMP expressed in tumors to be identified as possessing the ability to activate proMMP-2 (*4*). Expression of MT1-MMP enables cells to activate proMMP-2 *in vitro* and *in vivo*. In clinical specimens, expression of MT1-MMP has been detected both in tumor and in surrounding stroma. The expression levels of MT1-MMP in tissue correlate well with the rate of MMP-2 activation and with a poor prognosis of patients.

Structure of MT-MMPs

The MMP family in mammals includes 23 different enzymes that share a common domain structure composed of a propeptide, catalytic domain, hinge, and hemopexin-like (PEX) domain, except MMP-7, -23, and -26 which lack PEX (Fig. 1). Among the MMPs so far identified, MMP-14, -15, -16, -17, -24, and -25 form a subgroup; membrane-type MMPs, MT1–6 MMP, respectively. A hydrophobic sequence at the C-terminus in each of MT1-, MT2-, MT3-, and MT5-MMP acts as a type I transmembrane domain with a short cytoplasmic tail (*5*). A similar sequence in MT4- or MT6-MMP has been characterized as a signal anchoring to glycosyl phosphatidyl inositol (GPI). In terms of amino acid sequence and biochemical properties, MT4- and MT6-MMP are clearly different from the transmembrane-type molecules. MT-MMPs, being anchored to the cell membrane, are thought to play a role in pericellular proteolysis. In contrast, secreted MMPs may act on substrates remote from the producer cells. Thus, MT-MMPs presumably regulate various cell functions directly through their roles in pericellular proteolysis. The MT-MMPs also have other characteristic features. For example, a conserved motif, YGYL, in the propeptide has been demonstrated to act as an intramolecular chaperon (*6*). A four basic amino acid stretch (*4*), RXK/RR, has been suggested to be a site processed intracellularly by furin or other related proprotein convertases (PCs) for molecular activation. An insertion of 8 amino acids in the catalytic domain of MT1-MMP could

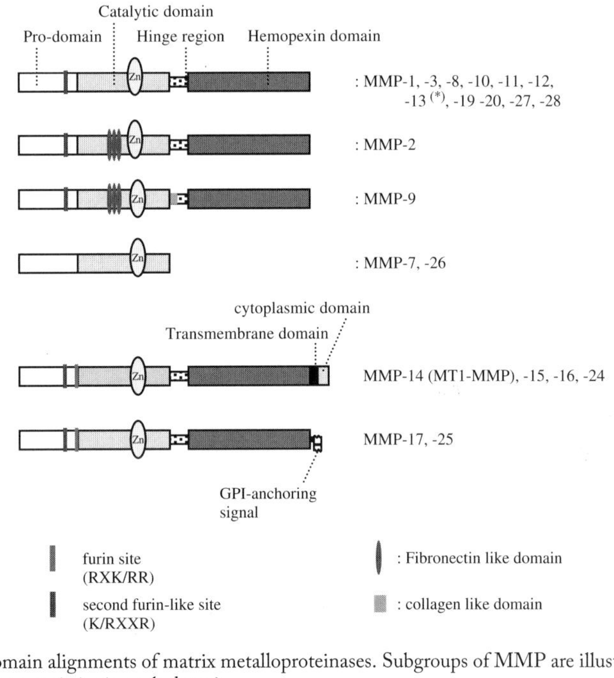

FIG. 1. Domain alignments of matrix metalloproteinases. Subgroups of MMP are illustrated according to the characteristics in each domain

Basic components of pro-, catalytic-, and hinge domains are common in almost all MMPs. MMP-7 and MMP-26 lack the hemopexin domain. MMP-14, -15, -16, -24, -17, and -25 belong to the membrane-anchored type. MMP-23 has been characterized as a type-II membrane type MMP (not classified in the figure). MMP-13(*) is considered to have a furin site and exceptionally, to be activated before secretion. Either RXXR or KXXR motifs, as a second furin-like site, are found in all MMPs except metalloelastase (MMP-12) and Matrilysin I/II (MMP-7/-26).

play a role in the activation of MMP-2 (*7*). The 2.75 Å crystal structure of the complex between the human MT1-MMP catalytic domain and bovine TIMP-2 has been solved (*8*).

Regulation of MT1-MMP

1. Gene expression

During murine development, MT1-MMP is mainly expressed in the cells from mesenchyme, including fibroblasts, muscular cells, and osteoblasts, and the expression decreases with maturation after birth (*9*). Expression can be re-induced, however, when the cells require remodeling of the ECM. For example, the expression of MT1-MMP is induced in the fibroblasts of injured tissue and continues throughout the wound healing process, together with the expression of MMP-2 (*10*). MT1-MMP is also expressed in endothelial cells, forming new vessels during angiogenesis (*11*). In tumors, both cancer and surrounding stromal cells express MT1-MMP. Since normal epithelial cells, even during the wound-healing process, rarely express MT1-MMP (*10*), the genetic events that render normal epithelial cells cancerous cause the abnormal induction of MT1-MMP in cancer.

Gene expression is regulated through specific transcription factors assembled in the promoter region. Each promoter in the *MMP-1*, *-3*, *-7*, and *-9* genes contains a typical TATA box and binding sites for transcription factors including AP-1, Ets, and NF-κB, which are thought to be the sites responsible for mediating the actions of growth factors or cytokines. The MT1-MMP promoter is characteristically different (*12*), rather resembling the *MMP-2* gene promoter, but lacking both the typical TATA box and the binding motifs for the transcription factors (*13*). Therefore, although the expression of MT1-MMP takes place under influence of growth factors or TPA in certain situations (*14*), it is unlikely that the gene expression occurs directly downstream of the signaling. Additionally, in the *MT1-MMP* gene, a GC-rich sequence lies immediately upstream of the cluster of multiple transcription start sites, which contains overlapping binding sites for Egr-1 and Sp1. Expression of MT1-MMP can be induced in endothelial cells cultured within collagen gel, in which the Egr-1 is thought to play a critical role (*12*). On the other hand, stress on endothelial cells down-regulates MT1-MMP expression. In the latter case, Sp1 is thought to play a negative role via its phosphorylation, thereby enhancing the affinity for the same targets as those of Egr-1, which intrinsically stimulates them in a "*cis*-acting" manner, finally resulting in a "*trans*-acting" overall effect.

It has been demonstrated that several genetic changes in cancer alter gene expression in a way that affects the cancer cell phenotype. One example could be the alteration of the *APC* (*adenomatus polyposis coli*) gene, which is associated with colorectal adenomas and cancers. Aberrant APC causes the accumulation of β-catenin in the nucleus, inducing expression of a variety of genes regulated downstream of the Wnt (wingless-type MMTV integration) signal (*15*). The targets include genes for c-Myc, cyclin D1, and AF17 that affect cell growth. Expression of genes related to the malignant phenotype of cancer cells could also be induced by β-catenin. These include genes for CD44, laminin-5 γ2-chain, MMP-7, and uPAR (urokinase, urokinase-type plasminogen activator receptor). It has recently been demonstrated that MT1-MMP expression is also regulated by β-catenin, as the depletion of β-catenin in colorectal carcinoma SW480 cells expressing the wild-type *APC* gene down-regulated the expression of MT1-MMP (*16*). A binding site of the β-catenin/Tcf4 (transcription factor) complex was identified in the promoter region of the *MT1-MMP* gene. Another oncogene, *v-Src*, could also induce MT1-MMP expression at the transcriptional level (*17*).

2. Activation and inhibition

Like other MMPs, MT1-MMP is expressed in a latent form (proMT1-MMP composed of 582 aa) and the propeptide sequence has to be removed to generate the active enzyme. The major cleavage for activation probably takes place downstream of the basic amino acid motif (RRKR↓Y), mediated by furin or other proprotein convertases, though an additional processing has also been suggested to occur before a cysteine residue within the propeptide (Fig. 1). It is generally accepted that the processing for activation of MT1-MMP occurs intracellularly, followed by transfer of the active enzyme to the cell surface, though it was also suggested that a PC-independent activation of MT1-MMP could occur. It is still not clear how the latency or the enzymatic activity of MT1-MMP is physiologically regulated.

Tissue inhibitors of metalloproteinases (TIMP-1, -2, -3, and -4) inhibit the enzymatic activity of MMPs by binding to the catalytic site. TIMP-1 and TIMP-2 are the major inhibitors in the body fluids. TIMP-1 enables to inhibit almost all of secreted MMPs but the transmembrane-type, whereas TIMP-2 acts as a major inhibitor of MT1-MMP in tissue (*18*). It is of note that TIMP-2 plays a role in the activation of proMMP-2 while inhibiting MT1-MMP, as described below (Fig. 2). TIMP-1 cannot inhibit the transmembrane-type, but unexpectedly inhibits GPI-type MT-MMPs.

RECK is another interesting inhibitor of MT1-MMP on the cell surface. RECK was originally isolated due to its activity to cause reversion of the transformed phenotype of K-ras-transfected cells. It was considered to be a GPI-anchored MMP inhibitor, as mice lacking the *RECK* gene, which was lethal within E10.5, showed a severe impairment of ECM turnover and vascular development (*19*).

Expression cloning has identified Testican 3 including its variant N-Tes (*20*) and claudin (*21*); Testican 3 inhibits MT1-MMP, while claudin enhances the activity, though the mechanisms involved are not well understood. Thus, not only TIMP-2, but also these molecules could modulate the activity of MT1-MMP on the cell surface.

3. Regulation of localization

MT1-MMP is localized at the leading edge of migrating cells, which is appropriate for the degradation of the ECM barrier to facilitate tumor invasion. A relatively stable association of MT1-MMP with the actin cytoskeleton is observed when the cells are treated with cytochalasin D, which disrupts polymerization of actin and generates actin aggregates (*22*). The domain responsible for the association was mapped to the PEX domain, but not to the cytoplasmic tail. Therefore, the link between MT1-MMP and actin must involve some other cell surface molecule anchoring to actin. CD44, a major hyaluronan receptor that associates with actin within the cells, is also localized at the leading edge. CD44 was identified as a linker that mediates the association of MT1-MMP with actin (*22*) (Fig. 3). The PEX domain of

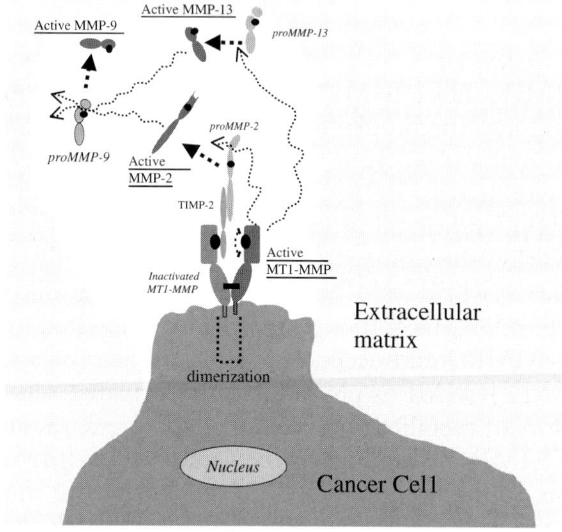

FIG. 2. Activation cascade of proteases at the cell invasion front
MT1-MMP degrades ECM directly or indirectly through the activation of MMP-2, which is thought to play a role in breaching a basement membrane component, type IV collagen. An assembly of at least two molecules of MT1-MMP located in close proximity to each other provides a system to trap and activate MMP-2 at the front. First, one of the MT1-MMP molecules binding directly to TIMP-2 acts as a trapper of MMP-2, the prodomain of which may then be clipped by another matured MT1-MMP located near the the trimolecular complex. Further, MT1-MMP could activate MMP-13, though the mechanism is poorly understood. Finally, MMP-9 could be activated subsequently by the activated MMP-2 or MMP-13.

MT1-MMP directly binds to CD44 and a mutant MT1-MMP lacking PEX cannot form such a complex and does not localize at the leading edge. The cytoplasmic deletion of CD44 abrogated both the association with the actin cytoskeleton and localization at the leading edge. Overexpression of the mutant CD44 prevented MT1-MMP from localizing to the leading edge as well. Thus, CD44 plays a critical role in the regulation of the polarized distribution of MT1-MMP during cell migration and association with the actin cytoskeleton (*22*).

4. Down-regulation

Once MT1-MMP is displayed on the cell surface as a free active molecule, it is inactivated either by binding of natural inhibitors, TIMPs, RECK, and Testican, as mentioned above, or by proteolytic self-degradation. Cells expressing MT1-MMP at high levels generate degraded fragments in the range of 43–45 kDa in SDS-PAGE (*23*). The degradation is mainly caused by an autocatalytic mechanism, so that the appearance of the fragments indirectly demonstrates the existence of active MT1-MMP on the cell surface and the ability to activate proMMP-2. How are these molecules cleared from the surface and replaced with newly synthesized molecules? MT1-MMP has a short cytoplasmic tail composed of 20 amino acids which plays a role in the internalization (*24*). The cytoplasmic tail contains a binding site for the 2 subunits of adaptor protein 2 (AP2) that mediates incorporation of the target protein into a clathrin-coated pit (*24*). Although it is still not clear whether the degraded fragments are selectively removed from the cell surface, this mechanism thought to be important for the molecular turnover (Fig. 3).

Substrates in the Extracellular Milieu

1. ECM proteins

To promote cancer invasion, MT1-MMP has to degrade the ECM barrier. A set of major components, including fibronectin, vitronectin, laminin-1, fibrin, and collagens type-I, -II and -III, has been demonstrated to be degraded by MT1-MMP (*25*). Consistently, mice deficient in *MT1-MMP* gene show inadequate collagen turnover, resulting in dwarfism, osteopenia, arthritis, and connective tissue disease, probably owing to lack of the enzymatic activity (*26*). MT1-MMP also processes laminin-5 to produce a γ2 fragment, which behaves as a cytokine like EGF, thereby modulating cell-associated receptors, and finally promoting cell migration (*27*).

2. Non-ECM proteins

In addition to the ECM components, MT1-MMP digests cell adhesion molecules as well. CD44, a major hyaluronan receptor, is cleaved by MT1-MMP and its ectodomain is released from the cell surface accompanying the stimulation of cell migration (*28*). However, CD44 is not the only enzyme involved in shedding, although no other enzyme has yet been identified. The pro-α v integrin subunit is also processed by MT1-MMP into a functional mature form (*29*). Tissue transglutaminase

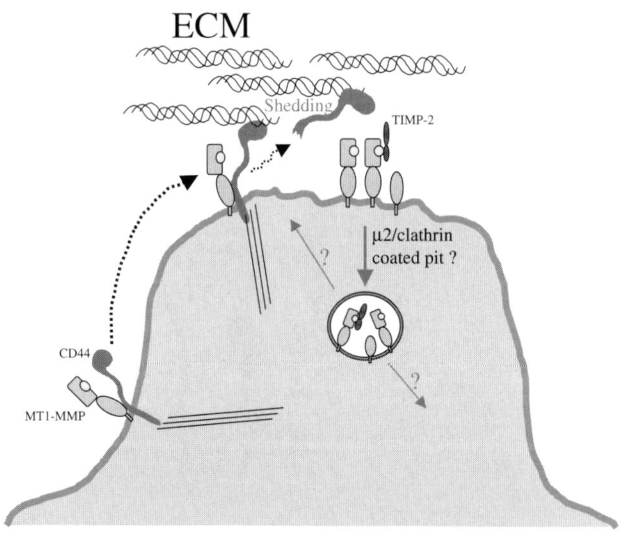

FIG. 3. Possible mechanisms for localization and turnover of MT1-MMP on the cell surface
MT1-MMP could be carried to the migration front with the shift of CD44 directly linked to the actin-cytoskeleton. MT1-MMP could also shed CD44 in migrating cells. In order to maintain the activity of MT1-MMP at the migration front, molecular turnover might be mediated by internalization through the cytoplasmic tail into clathrin coated pits.

(tTG) that acts as an integrin-binding adhesion co-receptor for fibronectin can be degraded by MT1-MMP as well (*30*) (Fig. 4). Since cell adhesion molecules bind the ECM ligands and mediate extracellular signaling to the cells, the processing of such molecules presumably regulates the ECM-cell communication.

Like other MMPs, some cytokines are also possible substrates of MT1-MMP as MCP-3 is converted to an antagonistic fragment to the receptor (*31*), stromal cell-derived factor (SDF) 1α is inactivated (*31*), and proTNF-α can be released and degraded further (*25*).

3. *Activation of proMMPs*

MT1-MMP triggers the activation cascade of proMMPs and this ability is likely to be important for invasion, which requires the cooperation of other MMPs to degrade a complex array of ECM proteins. For example, it binds to and activates proMMP-2 on the cell surface. The activation of proMMP-2 is uniquely and strictly regulated compared to that of other proMMPs, most of which are activated by serine proteases or active MMPs. MT1-MMP can cleave the propeptide sequence of proMMP-2, subsequently inducing an autocatalytic self-activation. Although this reaction occurs with only the two components in a test tube, the cell-mediated activation on the cell surface requires TIMP-2 as a co-factor. As a major inhibitor of MT1-MMP, it binds to the catalytic site of MT1-MMP with its N-terminal inhibitor domain. Concomitantly, the C-terminal domain of the TIMP-2 provides a specific site for the binding of the PEX domain in proMMP-2. Thus, MT1-MMP inhibited by TIMP-2 acts as a receptor for proMMP-2 on the cell surface (Fig. 2). The proMMP-2 in the complex is occasionally close enough to adjacent TIMP-2-free MT1-MMP, a matured form, for activation (*32*). An excess of TIMP-2 reduces

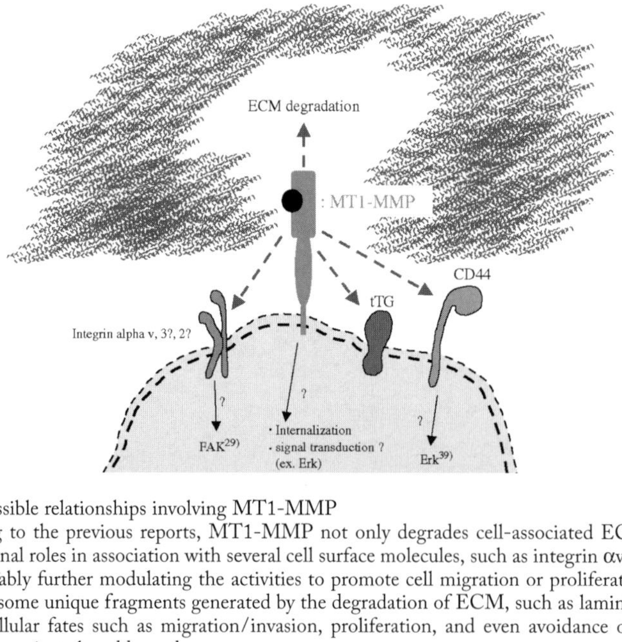

FIG. 4. Possible relationships involving MT1-MMP

According to the previous reports, MT1-MMP not only degrades cell-associated ECM but also plays additional roles in association with several cell surface molecules, such as integrin αv3, tTG, and CD44, probably further modulating the activities to promote cell migration or proliferation. On the other hand, some unique fragments generated by the degradation of ECM, such as laminin γ3, could modulate cellular fates such as migration/invasion, proliferation, and even avoidance of apoptosis. The details remain to be addressed.

the amount of "activator" MT1-MMP and inhibits the proMMP-2 activation as a result. Thus, the level of TIMP-2 on the cell surface plays a critical role in the activation of proMMP-2. Indeed, the tissue activation of MMP-2 in TIMP-2-deficient mice is significantly disturbed (*33*) compared to that of wild-type mice.

It has been generally assumed that in the cell-associated activation of MMP-2, at least two MT1-MMP molecules are required; an MT1-MMP combined with TIMP-2-MMP-2 close to another one free from TIMP2 (Fig. 2). It is possible that MT1-MMP forms homophilic oligomers through the PEX domain (*34*). The cytoplasmic portion of MT1-MMP may have an additional role in the oligomer formation (*35*) (Fig. 2). An interaction of MT1-MMP with ECM molecules such as type I collagen also causes clustering of MT1-MMP, enhancing the activation of proMMP-2 (*36*). It has also been demonstrated that both formation of the oligomers and activation of the proMMP-2 predominantly occur at the ruffled edge in the migration front of the cell. Thus, in epithelium, the activation of MMP-2 by cancer cells would contribute to the invasion of the basement membrane through the type IV collagenase activity. In stroma, MT1-MMP and MMP-2 could play a role in degrading type I collagen through the collagenase activity of MT1-MMP in combination with the gelatinase activity of MMP-2.

ProMMP-13 can also be activated by MT1-MMP in a cell-mediated manner. Subsequently, activation of proMMP-9 could be induced by the active MMP-2 or -13 (*37*).

Regulation of Cellular Functions

1. *Cell migration*

Several ECMs could modulate cancer cell motility, a driving force for the invasion. Laminin-5 is a major component of the basement membrane and regulates functions of epithelial cells. Through enzymatic modulation by MMP-2, laminin-5 promotes migration of breast epithelial cells (*38*). Recently, it has been demonstrated that several lines of cancer cells constitutively motile-dominantly express MT1-MMP rather than MMP-2, and this generates a unique fragment derived from the cryptic site of the γ2-chain of laminin-5, directly affecting the cellular signal, and finally promoting cell migration (*27*). Cancers which expresses both MT1-MMP and the γ2-chain *in vivo* could utilize the same system as above to stimulate and maintain cellular locomotion.

Processing of CD44 by MT1-MMP also accompanies stimulation of cell migration (*28*). Expression of a mutant without the processing site impairs the cell migration. Although the precise mechanism is not clear, the processing could make cell adhesion via CD44 favorable for migration. It is also possible that the processing couples with some signals from CD44, such as activation of extracellular signal-regulated kinase (ERK), to promote cell migration (*39*). The cytoplasmic portion of the processed CD44 is successively cleaved off, followed by a shift of the fragment into the nucleus to act as a transcription factor (*40*). Gene expression regulated by the fragment may also play a role in cell migration.

Integrins are well-known adhesion systems for cell migration. The integrin αvβ3, which binds vitronectin, is expressed in endothelial cells and invasive tumor cells. The αv chain, which is translated as a single polypeptide and converted into a two-chain form by PCs, is alternatively processed by MT1-MMP into a functional form (*41*). The expression of αvβ3 and MT1-MMP in a human breast carcinoma cell, MCF-7, did not alter the adhesion to vitronectin, but stimulated migration on the matrix accompanied by phosphorylation of FAK (*29*). The cell-surface tTG binds fibronectin as a co-receptor of integrins by associating with the β1 or β3 subunit. MT1-MMP cleaves tTG at multiple sites, suppressing cell adhesion to fibronectin and migration (*30*) (Fig. 3).

2. *Invasion*

Expression of MT1-MMP enhances the invasive and metastatic potential of cells (*4*, *32*). To act as an invasion-promoting enzyme, MT1-MMP has to be regulated appropriately. The catalytic domain is indispensable for its ECM-degrading activity, but other parts of MT1-MMP also play critical roles in promoting invasion. For example, the PEX domain of MT1-MMP is indispensable for invasion though Matrigel. Interestingly, overexpression of the PEX fragment inhibited invasion (*34*). A hinge sequence between the calalytic and PEX domains is also important for the collagenolytic activity of MT1-MMP, which is thought to be important for invasion of the type I collagen matrix (*36*).

Membrane anchoring is also an important part of the invasion-promoting activity of MT1-MMP. It has been demonstrated that MDCK cells stably transfected with a soluble form of wild-type MT1-MMP, lacking the C-terminal region, invaded 3D-collagen gel (*42*).

The cytoplasmic tail of MT1-MMP plays an important role in the invasion-promoting activity in Matrigel (*24*), but its role seems to be negligible in the invasion of type I collagen gel (*42*). Interestingly, mutations in the cytoplasmic tail that abolished internalization also abrogated the invasion- and migration-promoting activities of MT1-MMP (*24*). Internalization might be a mechanism to keep fresh enzyme at the leading edge of invasion by replacing inactivated enzyme.

3. *Cell morphology*

MDCK cells are known to form a tubular structure in collagen gel in response to HGF (hepatocyte growth factor). Although MT1-MMP is not expressed in cells cultured on a collagen-coated plastic dish, it is induced when the cells are cultured in 3D-collagen gel. The activity of MT1-MMP is indispensable for the tubule formation because blocking expression of the enzyme with an antisense oligonucleotide inhibited tubule formation (*43*). However, overexpression of MT1-MMP in the cells also disturbed the tubule formation (*42*). Thus, an appropriate amount of MT1-MMP is required for morphogenesis.

Human uveal melanoma cells also form a tubular structure resembling the microcirculatory system *in vivo* (vascular mimicry). A study using an antisense oligonucleotide against the gene for the γ2-chain and a neutralizing antibody against MT1-MMP demonstrated that both MT1-MMP and the γ2-chain of laminin-5 in the tumor cells play critical roles in the mimicry (*44*).

4. *Angiogenesis*

Like tumor cells, endothelial cells transmigrate through the ECM in response to angiogenic stimuli and this process requires degradation and remodeling of the

ECM. In collagen gel, expression of MT1-MMP is induced in endothelial cells and the collagen-degrading activity of MT1-MMP is required for the construction of a tubular network (*45*). MT1-MMP plays an important role in the formation of new vessels in both physiological and pathological situations (*46*). Indeed, angiogenesis was severely impaired in an *ex vivo* assay with mice cornea from MT1-MMP-deficient mice, compared to wild type (*47*). Vasculogenesis in the embryo is normal in MT1-MMP-deficient mice, but the formation of secondary ossification centers during bone formation is severely impaired, presumably by inhibition of angiogenesis around them (*47*). MT1-MMP also has fibrinolytic activity and supports the tubule formation of endothelial cells in fibrin gel in the absence of an uPA/plasminogen system (*11*). MMP-2 in association with αvβ3 integrin on endothelial cells is also evaluated as important in angiogenesis (*48*). Disruption of the interaction by a PEX fragment derived from MMP-2 inhibits angiogenesis *in vitro* and *in vivo* (*49*). The PEX domain is also expected to compete with proMMP-2 for binding to the C-terminal domain of TIMP-2 and eventually to inhibit the activation of the proMMP-2 by MT1-MMP. For the MMP-2/αvβ3 integrin system to work, MT1-MMP has to activate proMMP-2 in advance. In addition to its direct roles in endothelial cells, MT1-MMP may modulate the ability of cancer cells to induce angiogenesis. Tumor cells expressing MT1-MMP grow rapidly and form highly vascularized tumors. The angiogenic phenotype of MT1-MMP-producing cancer cells was found to be associated with the up-regulation of VEGF expression (*50*).

Conclusions

MT1-MMP is a potent ECM-degrading enzyme that forms a part of the invasion machinery of cancer cells. To promote invasion, MT1-MMP is delivered to the leading edge of the migratory cells and assembles other MMPs having different substrate specificities to degrade complex ECM components in the basement membrane and stroma. To promote cell migration, MT1-MMP also modulates several target molecules such as CD44, the integrin αv chain, tTg, and the laminin-5 γ2-chain (Fig. 3). Cell locomotion for tumor invasion probably requires the dynamic and appropriate actions of multiple molecules in time and space. Finally all the molecular events reviewed above should be more profoundly studied before we can assess whether they could form the basis of new cancer therapies.

Acknowledgments

Work on MMPs is progressing rapidly, and we regret that not all significant publications could be mentioned in this review because of limited space. Work in the author's laboratory has been supported by Grants-in-Aid for Scientific Research from the Ministry of Education, Culture, Sports, Science and Technology of Japan.

REFERENCES

1. Egeblad M, Werb Z. New functions for the matrix metalloproteinases in cancer progression. *Nat Rev Cancer* 2001; **2**: 163–76.
2. Bergers G, Javaherian K, Lo KM, Folkman J, Hanahan D. Effects of angiogenesis in-

hibitors on multistage carcinogenesis in mice. *Science* 1999; **284**: 808–12.

3. Tryggvason K, Hoyhtya M, Pyke C. Type IV collagenases in invasive tumors. *Breast Cancer Res Treat* 1993; **24** : 209–18.
4. Sato H, Takino T, Okada Y, Cao J, Shinagawa A, Yamamoto E, Seiki M. A matrix metalloproteinase expressed on the surface of invasive tumour cells. *Nature* 1994; **370**: 61–5.
5. Cao J, Sato H, Takino T, Seiki M. The C-terminal region of membrane type matrix metalloproteinase is a functional transmembrane domain required for pro-gelatinase A activation. *J Biol Chem* 1995; **270**: 801–5.
6. Pavlaki M, Cao J, Hymowitz M, Chen WT, Bahou W, Zucker S. A conserved sequence within the propeptide domain of membrane type 1 matrix metalloproteinase is critical for function as an intramolecular chaperone. *J Biol Chem* 2002; **277**: 2740–9.
7. English WR, Holtz B, Vogt G, Knauper V, Murphy G. Characterization of the role of the "MT-loop": an eight-amino acid insertion specific to progelatinase A (MMP2) activating membrane-type matrix metalloproteinases. *J Biol Chem* 2001; **276**: 42018–26.
8. Fernandez-Catalan C, Bode W, Huber R, Turk D, Calvete JJ, Lichte A, Tschesche H, Maskos K. Crystal structure of the complex formed by the membrane type 1-matrix metalloproteinase with the tissue inhibitor of metalloproteinases-2, the soluble progelatinase A receptor. *EMBO J* 1998; **17**: 5238–48.
9. Kinoh H, Sato H, Tsunezuka Y, Takino T, Kawashima A, Okada Y, Seiki M. MT-MMP, the cell surface activator of proMMP-2 (pro-gelatinase A), is expressed with its substrate in mouse tissue during embryogenesis. *J Cell Sci* 1996; **109**: 953–9.
10. Okada A, Tomasetto C, Lutz Y, Bellocq JP, Rio MC, Basset P. Expression of matrix metalloproteinases during rat skin wound healing: evidence that membrane type-1 matrix metalloproteinase is a stromal activator of pro-gelatinase A. *J Cell Biol* 1997; **137**: 67–77.
11. Hiraoka N, Allen E, Apel IJ, Gyetko MR, Weiss SJ. Matrix metalloproteinases regulate neovascularization by acting as pericellular fibrinolysins. *Cell* 1998; **95**: 365–77.
12. Haas TL, Stitelman D, Davis SJ, Apte SS, Madri JA. Egr-1 mediates extracellular matrix-driven transcription of membrane type 1 matrix metalloproteinase in endothelium. *J Biol Chem* 1999; **274**: 22679–85.
13. Huhtala P, Chow LT, Tryggvason K. Structure of the human type IV collagenase gene. *J Biol Chem* 1990; **265**: 11077–82.
14. Lohi J, Lehti K, Westermarck J, Kahari VM, Keski-Oja J. Regulation of membrane-type matrix metalloproteinase-1 expression by growth factors and phorbol 12-myristate 13-acetate. *Eur J Biochem* 1996; **239**: 239–47.
15. Fodde R, Smits R, Clevers H. APC, signal transduction and genetic instability in colorectal cancer. *Nat Rev Cancer* 2001; **1**: 55–67.
16. Takahashi M, Tsunoda T, Seiki M, Nakamura Y, Furukawa Y. Identification of membrane-type matrix metalloproteinase-1 as a target of the β-catenin/Tcf4 complex in human colorectal cancers. *Oncogene* 2002; **21**: 5861–7.
17. Cha HJ, Okada A, Kim KW, Sato H, Seiki M. Identification of cis-acting promoter elements that support expression of membrane-type 1 matrix metalloproteinase (MT1-MMP) in v-src transformed Madin-Darby canine kidney cells. *Clin Exp Metastasis* 2000; **18**: 675–81.

18. Strongin AY, Collier I, Bannikov G, Marmer BL, Grant GA, Goldberg GI. Mechanism of cell surface activation of 72-kDa type IV collagenase. Isolation of the activated form of the membrane metalloprotease. *J Biol Chem* 1995; **270**: 5331–8.
19. Oh J, Takahashi R, Kondo S, Mizoguchi A, Adachi E, Sasahara RM, Nishimura S, Imamura Y, Kitayama H, Alexander DB, Ide C, Horan TP, Arakawa T, Yoshida H, Nishikawa S, Itoh Y, Seiki M, Itohara S, Takahashi C, Noda M. The membrane-anchored MMP inhibitor RECK is a key regulator of extracellular matrix integrity and angiogenesis. *Cell* 2001; **107**: 789–800.
20. Nakada M, Yamada A, Takino T, Miyamori H, Takahashi T, Yamashita J, Sato H. Suppression of membrane-type 1 matrix metalloproteinase (MMP)-mediated MMP-2 activation and tumor invasion by testican 3 and its splicing variant gene product, N-Tes. *Cancer Res* 2001; **61**: 8896–902.
21. Miyamori H, Takino T, Kobayashi Y, Tokai H, Itoh Y, Seiki M, Sato H. Claudin promotes activation of pro-matrix metalloproteinase-2 mediated by membrane-type matrix metalloproteinases. *J Biol Chem* 2001; **276**: 28204–11.
22. Mori H, Tomari T, Koshikawa N, Kajita M, Itoh Y, Sato H, Tojo H, Yana I, Seiki M. CD44 directs membrane-type 1 matrix metalloproteinase to lamellipodia by associating with its hemopexin-like domain. *EMBO J* 2002; **21**: 3949–59.
23. Stanton H, Gavrilovic J, Atkinson SJ, d'Ortho MP, Yamada KM, Zardi L, Murphy G. The activation of ProMMP-2 (gelatinase A) by HT1080 fibrosarcoma cells is promoted by culture on a fibronectin substrate and is concomitant with an increase in processing of MT1-MMP (MMP-14) to a 45 kDa form. *J Cell Sci* 1998; **111**: 2789–98.
24. Uekita T, Itoh Y, Yana I, Ohno H, Seiki M. Cytoplasmic tail-dependent internalization of membrane-type 1 matrix metalloproteinase is important for its invasion-promoting activity. *J Cell Biol* 2001; **155**: 1345–56.
25. d'Ortho MP, Will H, Atkinson S, Butler G, Messent A, Gavrilovic J, Smith B, Timpl R, Zardi L, Murphy G. Membrane-type matrix metalloproteinases 1 and 2 exhibit broad-spectrum proteolytic capacities comparable to many matrix metalloproteinases. *Eur J Biochem* 1997; **250**: 751–7.
26. Holmbeck K, Bianco P, Caterina J, Yamada S, Kromer M, Kuznetsov SA, Mankani M, Robey PG, Poole AR, Pidoux I, Ward JM, Birkedal-Hansen H. MT1-MMP-deficient mice develop dwarfism, osteopenia, arthritis, and connective tissue disease due to inadequate collagen turnover. *Cell* 1999; **99**: 81–92.
27. Koshikawa N, Giannelli G, Cirulli V, Miyazaki K, Quaranta V. Role of cell surface metalloprotease MT1-MMP in epithelial cell migration over laminin-5. *J Cell Biol* 2000; **148**: 615–24.
28. Kajita M, Itoh Y, Chiba T, Mori H, Okada A, Kinoh H, Seiki M. Membrane-type 1 matrix metalloproteinase cleaves CD44 and promotes cell migration. *J Cell Biol* 2001; **153**: 893–904.
29. Deryugina EI, Ratnikov BI, Postnova TI, Rozanov DV, Strongin AY. Processing of integrin alpha v subunit by membrane type 1 matrix metalloproteinase stimulates migration of breast carcinoma cells on vitronectin and enhances tyrosine phosphorylation of focal adhesion kinase. *J Biol Chem* 2002; **277**: 9749–56.
30. Belkin AM, Akimov SS, Zaritskaya LS, Ratnikov BI, Deryugina EI, Strongin AY. Matrix-dependent proteolysis of surface transglutaminase by membrane-type metallo-

proteinase regulates cancer cell adhesion and locomotion. *J Biol Chem* 2001; **276**: 18415–22.

31. McQuibban GA, Gong JH, Wong JP, Wallace JL, Clark-Lewis I, Overall CM. Matrix metalloproteinase processing of monocyte chemoattractant proteins generates CC chemokine receptor antagonists with anti-inflammatory properties *in vivo*. *Blood* 2002; **100**: 1160–7.
32. Seiki M. The cell surface: the stage for matrix metalloproteinase regulation of migration. *Curr Opin Cell Biol* 2002; **14**: 624–32.
33. Wang Z, Juttermann R, Soloway PD. TIMP-2 is required for efficient activation of proMMP-2 *in vivo*. *J Biol Chem* 2000; **275**: 26411–5.
34. Itoh Y, Takamura A, Ito N, Maru Y, Sato H, Suenaga N, Aoki T, Seiki M. Homophilic complex formation of MT1-MMP facilitates proMMP-2 activation on the cell surface and promotes tumor cell invasion. *EMBO J* 2001; **20**: 4782–93.
35. Lehti K, Lohi J, Juntunen MM, Pei D, Keski-Oja J. Oligomerization through hemopexin and cytoplasmic domains regulates the activity and turnover of membrane-type 1 matrix metalloproteinase. *J Biol Chem* 2002; **277**: 8440–8.
36. Tam EM, Wu YI, Butler GS, Stack MS, Overall CM. Collagen binding properties of the membrane type-1 matrix metalloproteinase (MT1-MMP) hemopexin C domain. The ectodomain of the 44-kDa autocatalytic product of MT1-MMP inhibits cell invasion by disrupting native type I collagen cleavage. *J Biol Chem* 2002; **277**: 39005–14.
37. Murphy G, Gavrilovic J. Proteolysis and cell migration: creating a path? *Curr Opin Cell Biol* 1999; **11**: 614–21.
38. Giannelli G, Falk-Marzillier J, Schiraldi O, Stetler-Stevenson WG, Quaranta V. Induction of cell migration by matrix metalloprotease-2 cleavage of laminin-5. *Science* 1997; **277**: 225–8.
39. Gingras D, Bousquet-Gagnon N, Langlois S, Lachambre MP, Annabi B, Beliveau R. Activation of the extracellular signal-regulated protein kinase (ERK) cascade by membrane-type-1 matrix metalloproteinase (MT1-MMP). *FEBS Lett* 2001; **507**: 231–6.
40. Okamoto I, Kawano Y, Murakami D, Sasayama T, Araki N, Miki T, Wong AJ, Saya H. Proteolytic release of CD44 intracellular domain and its role in the CD44 signaling pathway. *J Cell Biol* 2001; **155**: 755–62.
41. Ratnikov BI, Rozanov DV, Postnova TI, Baciu PG, Zhang H, DiScipio RG, Chestukhina GG, Smith JW, Deryugina EI, Strongin AY. An alternative processing of integrin alpha v subunit in tumor cells by membrane type-1 matrix metalloproteinase. *J Biol Chem* 2002; **277**: 7377–85.
42. Hotary K, Allen E, Punturieri A, Yana I, Weiss SJ. Regulation of cell invasion and morphogenesis in a three-dimensional type I collagen matrix by membrane-type matrix metalloproteinases 1, 2, and 3. *J Cell Biol* 2000; **149**: 1309–23.
43. Kadono Y, Shibahara K, Namiki M, Watanabe Y, Seiki M, Sato H. Membrane type 1-matrix metalloproteinase is involved in the formation of hepatocyte growth factor/scatter factor-induced branching tubules in Madin-Darby canine kidney epithelial cells. *Biochem Biophys Res Commun* 1998; **251**: 681–7.
44. Seftor RE, Seftor EA, Koshikawa N, Meltzer PS, Gardner LM, Bilban M, Stetler-Stevenson WG, Quaranta V, Hendrix MJ. Cooperative interactions of laminin 5 gamma2 chain, matrix metalloproteinase-2, and membrane type-1-matrix/

metalloproteinase are required for mimicry of embryonic vasculogenesis by aggressive melanoma. *Cancer Res* 2001; **61**: 6322–7.

45. Haas TL, Davis SJ, Madri JA. Three-dimensional type I collagen lattices induce coordinate expression of matrix metalloproteinases MT1-MMP and MMP-2 in microvascular endothelial cells. *J Biol Chem* 1998; **273**: 3604–10.
46. Pepper MS. Role of the matrix metalloproteinase and plasminogen activator-plasmin systems in angiogenesis. *Arterioscler Thromb Vasc Biol* 2001; **21**: 1104–17.
47. Zhou Z, Apte SS, Soininen R, Cao R, Baaklini GY, Rauser RW, Wang J, Cao Y, Tryggvason K. Impaired endochondral ossification and angiogenesis in mice deficient in membrane-type matrix metalloproteinase I. *Proc Natl Acad Sci USA* 2000; **97**: 4052–7.
48. Brooks PC, Stromblad S, Sanders LC, von Schalscha TL, Aimes RT, Stetler-Stevenson WG, Quigley JP, Cheresh DA. Localization of matrix metalloproteinase MMP-2 to the surface of invasive cells by interaction with integrin alpha v beta 3. *Cell* 1996; **85**: 683–93.
49. Brooks PC, Silletti S, von Schalscha TL, Friedlander M, Cheresh DA. Disruption of angiogenesis by PEX, a noncatalytic metalloproteinase fragment with integrin binding activity. *Cell* 1998; **92**: 391–400.
50. Sounni NE, Devy L, Hajitou A, Frankenne F, Munaut C, Gilles C, Deroanne C, Thompson EW, Foidart JM, Noel A. MT1-MMP expression promotes tumor growth and angiogenesis through an up-regulation of vascular endothelial growth factor expression. *FASEB J* 2002; **16**: 555–64.

CHEMOTHERAPY

ANTITUMOR ACTIVITY OF SUGAR-MODIFIED CYTOSINE NUCLEOSIDES

Akira MATSUDA[*1] and Takuma SASAKI[*2]

*Graduate School of Pharmaceutical Sciences, Hokkaido University[*1] and Department of Experimental Therapeutics, Cancer Research Institute, Kanazawa University[*2]*

Nucleoside analogues which show antimetabolic activity in cells have been successfully used in the treatment of various tumors. Nucleosides such as cytosine arabinoside, 6-mercaptopurine, fludarabine and cladribine play an important role in the treatment of leukemias whereas gemcitabine, 5-fluorouracil and its prodrugs are used extensively in the treatment of many types of solid tumors. All of these nucleosides are metabolized similarly to endogenous nucleosides and nucleotides. Active metabolites interfere with the *de novo* synthesis of nucleosides and nucleotides or inhibit the DNA chain elongation after being incorporated into the DNA strand as terminators. Furthermore, nucleoside antimetabolites incorporated into the DNA strand induce strand-break and finally cause apoptosis. Nucleoside antimetabolites target one or more specific enzyme(s). The mode of inhibitory action on the target enzyme is not always similar even in nucleoside antimetabolites, which have the same nucleoside base, such as cytosine arabinoside and gemcitabine. Although both nucleosides are phosphorylated by deoxycytidine kinase and are also good substrates of cytidine deaminase, only gemcitabine shows antitumor activity against solid tumors. This suggests that differences in the pharmacological activity of these nucleoside antimetabolites may show a significant influence on different modes of action on target molecules. The design, *in vitro* cytotoxicity, *in vivo* antitumor activity, metabolism, and mechanism of action of sugar-modified cytosine nucleosides, such as (2′*S*)-2′-deoxy-2′-*C*-methylcytidine (SMDC), 1-(2-deoxy-2-methylene-β-D-*erythro*-pentofuranosyl)cytosine (DMDC), 1-(2-*C*-cyano-2-deoxy-1-β-D-*arabino*-pentofuranosyl)cytosine (CNDAC) and 1-(3-*C*-ethynyl-β-D-*ribo*-pentofuranosyl)cytosine (ECyd), developed by our groups, have already been described.

Introduction

Nucleoside antimetabolites, such as 1-β-D-arabinofuranosylcytosine (araC), 2-chloro-2′-deoxyadenosine (CldA), 9-β-D-arabinofuranosyl-2-fluoroadenine monophosphate (fludarabine, FaraAMP) and 2′-deoxy-2′,2′-difluorocytidine (gemcitabine,

---

[*1] Kita-12, Nishi-6, Kita-ku, Sapporo 060-0812, Japan

[*2] 13-1 Takara-machi, Kanazawa 920-0934, Japan

This paper is dedicated to the memory of late Dr. Tomizo Yoshida on the occasion of the 100th anniversary of his birth. The essential part of this article was originally published in Cancer Science in February, 2004.

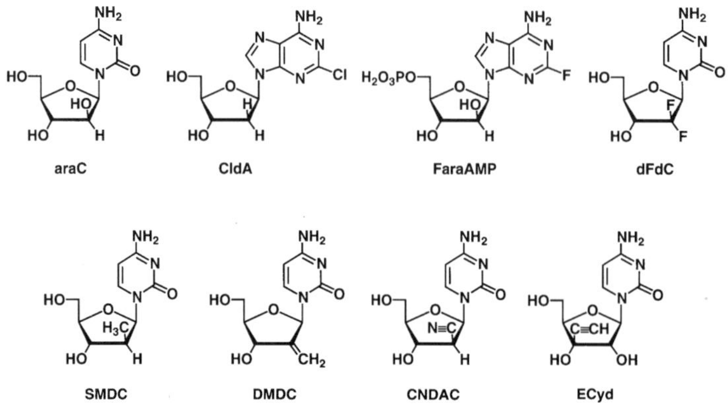

FIG. 1. Chemical structures of various sugar-modified nucleoside antimetabolites

dFdC) (Fig. 1), have been widely used not only as antileukemic agents but also as antitumor agents against solid tumors (*1*). Like other nucleoside antimetabolites, such as antiviral agents, these nucleosides are not active components themselves but have to be metabolically activated by phosphorylation. Therefore, two of the most important factors for effective clinical use are the substrate specificities of nucleoside kinases and their expression at tumor tissues in patients. The target enzymes of each metabolized nucleotide are slightly different. AraC 5′-triphosphate (araCTP) is incorporated into DNA, which becomes a trigger for apoptosis. 2-Chloro-2′-deoxyadenosine 5′-triphosphate (CldATP) is also incorporated into DNA by DNA polymerase and also potently inhibits ribonucleotide reductase (RDR) instead of dATP (*2*). Fludarabine 5′-triphosphate (FaraATP) is incorporated into both DNA and RNA, which causes inhibition of both enzyme activities of DNA and RNA polymerases. Moreover, FaraATP inhibits RDR as well as DNA ligase 1 and DNA primase (*2*). Gemcitabine 5′-diphosphate (dFdCDP) is a very potent inhibitor of RDR, and its corresponding 5′-triphosphate (dFdCTP) inhibits DNA polymerase (*3*). Such differences in target enzymes for nucleotide antimetabolites would reflect the target diseases. Therefore, further development of new types of nucleoside antimetabolites for use in fighting tumors is very important. In this review, we describe the design, *in vitro* cytotoxicity, *in vivo* antitumor activity, metabolism, and mechanism of action of new sugar-modified cytosine nucleosides, such as (2′*S*)-2′-deoxy-2′-*C*-methylcytidine (SMDC), 1-(2-deoxy-2-methylene-β-D-*erythro*-pentofuranosyl)cytosine (DMDC), 1-(2-*C*-cyano-2-deoxy-1-β-D-*arabino*-pentofuranosyl)cytosine (CNDAC) and 1-(3-*C*-ethynyl-β-D-*ribo*-pentofuranosyl)cytosine (ECyd), which we have been developing in our labs (*4*).

Deoxycytidine Kinase-dependent Chemotherapy

In mammalian cells and tissues, there are four nucleoside kinases, deoxycytidine kinase (dCK), thymidine kinase-1 (TK1), adenosine kinase (AK) and uridine/cytidine kinase (UCK) in cytosole and two nucleoside kinases, thymidine kinase-2 (TK2) and deoxyguanosine kinase (dGK) in mitochondria (*5–7*). Among the above mentioned nucleoside kinases, many of the antitumor nucleosides in clinical use, such as araC, CldA, gemcitabine and araG derivatives are phosphorylated by dCK to afford their corresponding 5′-monophosphates, which are further phosphorylated by nucleoside monophosphate kinases and then nucleoside diphosphate kinases (NDPK). Among the nucleoside kinases, dCK is believed to have a broader substrate specificity and has the following properties suitable for activation of the above described nucleosides to exhibit proper antitumor efficacy: 1) dCK is constitutively expressed both at the protein and mRNA levels, due to no cell cycle regulation. 2) dCK has the lowest substrate specificity among the nucleoside kinases. 3) Most solid tumor tissues express dCK activity with the exception of brain and liver tissue. 4) The average dCK content in most carcinomas is 3- to 5-fold higher than in normal tissues and about 5-fold lower than in normal or B-CLL lymphoid cells. These properties provided the basis for dCK dependent-chemotherapy.

dCK activity is regulated by a high concentration of dCTP, the end product of dCyd. Therefore, if a certain antitumor cytosine nucleoside is metabolized to its triphosphate, whether the triphosphate acts as a feedback inhibitor of dCK or not is very important for its antitumor activity. It is known that araCTP inhibits dCK like dCTP, which is therefore one of the drawbacks of araC. The cell lines resistant to dCyd nucleoside analogues such as araC, dFdC, DMDC and CNDAC underwent a mutation of the dCK gene (*8*).

Degradation of the Active Component

When a new cytosine nucleoside is selected as a candidate for antitumor nucleosides *in vitro*, the next step will be *in vivo* tests using tumor-bearing model animals such as mice and/or rats. However, these animals are largely different from humans in their enzyme activities of nucleotide biosynthesis, especially in their degradation of enzymes, such as cytidine deaminase (CDA), which degrades cytosine nucleosides to chemotherapeutically inactive uracil nucleosides. Since the activity is usually low in rodents and very high in humans, model pharmacokinetic studies using monkeys should be studied before clinical trials are carried out. AraC and gemcitabine are both very good substrates of CDA so that large amounts of the agents have to be administered to be effective. dCMP deaminase (dCMPDA) (*9*) is also responsible for the degradation of dCMP and its derivatives. However, its influence on antitumor activity has not been thoroughly studied.

The enzymatic stability of the nucleotide metabolites of a nucleoside in tumor cells is also important for its effectiveness, because a certain concentration of nucleotide metabolites is required to strongly inhibit a target enzyme for a certain period of time. AraCTP is known to be unstable in tumor cells, while ECTP (ECyd triphosphate) is stable, as will be discussed later. However, the enzymatic nature of such degradation activity has not been sufficiently elucidated.

AraC and Gemcitabine

When we started to design sugar-modified antitumor cytosine nucleosides, only araC (*10*) had been used in the clinic for the treatment of adult acute myeloblastic leukemia. AraC is a good substrate of dCK (K_m=8.8 μM, CHO cells) and further metabolized to araCTP, which inhibits DNA polymerization after incorporation into

DNA by DNA polymerase α. This inhibition could trigger apoptosis. However, araCTP at high concentrations acts as a feedback inhibitor of dCK and has a short half-life in tumor cells. These properties, together with the fact that araC and araCMP are good substrates of CDA and dCMPDA, respectively, cause araC to be ineffective against solid tumors. To overcome such drawbacks, a number of prodrugs of araC have been prepared (*11*). Although some of these are used against leukemias in the clinic in Japan, these araC-prodrugs are not yet effective against solid tumors.

Nevertheless, among sugar-modified cytosine nucleosides, gemcitabine (dFdCd) was originally designed as an antiviral agent mimicking FIAC (*12*). However, it proved too cytotoxic to be developed as an antiviral agent (*13*). dFdCyd is a good substrate of dCK (K_m=3.6 μM, CHO cells), which is further phosphorylated to its diphosphate (dFdCDP) and triphosphate (dFdCTP). dFdCDP is a potent inhibitor of RDR. On the other hand, dFdCTP inhibits DNA synthesis, the potency of which is lower than that of araCTP. dFdCTP also inhibits dCMPDA and CTP synthase, and is incorporated into RNA (*14*).

Although dFdCyd was initially approved by the FDA as an antitumor agent for pancreatic cancer to improve quality of life (QOL) but not to prolong life-span, in combination with other antitumor agents, such as cisplatin *etc.*, it does help prolong life-span in non-small lung carcinoma.

(2′S)-2′-Deoxy-2′-C-methylcytidine (SMDC)

We have synthesized (2′*S*)-2′-deoxy-2′-*C*-methylcytidine (SMDC), (2′*R*)-2′-deoxy-2′-*C*-methylcytidine (RMDC), and (2′*S*)-2′-deoxy-2′-*C*-ethylcytidine (SEDC) from uridine to elucidate the steric requirement of the substituent at the 2′β-position of 2′-deoxycytidine (*15*). Against mouse L1210 cells *in vitro*, SMDC was as potent

TABLE I. Cytotoxicity of araC, SMDC, DMDC, CNDAC and 5-FU against Various Tumor Cells

Cell line	IC_{50} (μg/mL)[a]			
	araC	SMDC	DMDC	5-FU
L1210	0.097	0.26	0.37	0.32
CCRF CEM	0.065	0.15	0.067	40
MOLT4	0.056	0.032	0.041	3.8
HL60	>0.1	0.65	0.040	ND
K562	3.2	2.2	ND	38
U937	0.31	0.38	0.44	3.5
PC10	>100	81.8	>100	>100
PC14	>100	>100	>100	>100
KATO III	>100	>100	8.3	10
SW480	>100	>100	3.8	3.7
TE2	>100	>100	2.9	3.3
T24	>100	1.1	1.1	6.1

[a] Tumor cells (2×10^3 cells/well) were incubated in the presence or absence of compounds for 72 h. MTT-reagent was added to each well and the plate was incubated for an additional 4 h. The resulting MTT-formazan was dissolved in DMSO and the OD (540 nm) was measured. Percent inhibition was calculated as follows: % inhibition = [1-OD (540 nm) of sample well/OD (540 nm) of control well] × 100. IC_{50} (μg/mL) is the concentration that inhibits cell growth by 50%.

as araC (Table I) but RMDC was 150-fold less effective than SMDC, and SECD was ineffective up to 100 μg/mL. Additionally, 2′-deoxy-2′-(methylthio)-β-D-arabinofuranosylcytosine did not show any cytotoxicity toward L5178Y cells *in vitro* up to 100 μg/mL. Therefore, it appears that increasing the bulkiness of the 2′-substituent in 2′-deoxycytidine greatly reduces cytotoxicity.

SMDC is a relatively good substrate of dCK (Table II) (*16*) and a very poor substrate of CDA. Chemically synthesized 5′-triphosphate (SMDCTP) is a potent competitive inhibitor of dCTP against DNA polymerase α, β, and γ with K_i values of 0.05, 0.10, and 0.07 μM, respectively (Table III). These values indicate that SM-

TABLE II. Relative Substrate Specificity of dCyd, araC, SMDC, DMDC and CNDAC toward Deoxycytidine Kinase (dCK) and Cytidine Deaminase (CDA)

	dCK			CDA	
Compd	Activity[a] (nmol/ min·mL)	Relative activity	Apparent K_m (μM)	Activity[b] (nmol/ min·mL)	Relative activity
dCyd	3.58	100	10	24.8	100
araC	6.13	170	17	6.12	25
SMDC	2.77	77	52	0.209	1
DMDC	2.27	63	33	0	0
CNDAC	1.79	50	49	1.03	4.2

[a] The reaction mixture containing 100 mM Tris-HCl buffer (pH 7.5), 50 μM each analog, 0.5 mM UTP, 2.4 mM $MgCl_2$, 1 mg/mL BSA, 0.5 mM DTT, 1 mM NaF, 1 mM tetrahydrouridine, and the enzyme in a total volume of 40 μL was incubated at 37 °C for 15 min, followed by HPLC analysis at 280 nm. Each phosphorylation was confirmed by conversion of the product to the substrate by alkaline phophatase, after incubation overnight.

[b] The reaction mixture containing 100 mM Tris-HCl buffer (pH 7.5), 0.05–1.0 mM of the substrate, 2.4 mM $MgCl_2$, 1 mg/mL BSA, 0.5 mM DTT, and the enzyme in a total volume of 40 μL was incubated at 37 °C for 5 min, followed by HPLC analysis at 260 nm.

TABLE III. Kinetic Data of DNA Polymerase Inhibition by 5′-triphosphates of Deoxycytidine Analogues[a]

Inhibitor	DNA pol α		DNA pol β		DNA pol γ	
	K_i (K_m)	K_i/K_m	K_i (K_m)	K_i/K_m	K_i (K_m)	K_i/K_m
(Substrate)	μM		μM		μM	
dCTP	(1.25)		(3.90)		(0.77)	
araCTP	1.10	0.88	No inhibition		No inhibition	
SMDCTP	0.05	0.04	0.10	0.02	0.07	0.08
DMDCTP	0.42	0.34	2.52	0.65	1.00	1.30
CNDACTP	0.16	0.14	ND[b]		ND[b]	

[a] DNA polymerases α and β were purified from calf thymus, and DNA polymerase γ was purified from bovine liver according to the methods described previously. DNA polymerase α activity was measured in a mixture (25 μL) containing 40 mM potassium phosphate (pH 7.5), 100 μg/mL of activated calf thymus DNA, 40 mM each of dCTP, dATP and dGTP, 5 mM of [methyl-^{3}H]TTP (4 Ci/mmol), 1 mM dithiothreitol, 8 mM $MgCl_2$, and an aliquot of the reaction mixture. In the case of DNA polymerase β, potassium phosphate was replaced by 40 mM Tris-HCl (pH 8.5). In the case of DNA polymerase γ, 200 mM KCl was added to the mixture for the assay. For kinetic analysis, the concentration of the inhibitor and dCTP were varied. After incubation, the reaction mixture was chilled in an ice bath and 20 μL was transferred to DEAE-cellulose paper disc. The discs were washed with 5% Na_2HPO_4 (×6), H_2O (×1), EtOH (×2) and ether, and dried. The remaining radioactivity was measured in a scintillation liquid.

[b] Not determined.

DCTP binds to DNA polymerase α, β, and γ about 25-, 39-, and 11-fold better than the natural substrate dCTP (*4*). Although these data were promising, indicating that SMDC should be effective *in vivo*, SMDC showed only marginal activity against a mouse leukemic P388 model with T/C values of 111% at 30 mg/kg/day and 126% at 100 mg/kg/day, while araC showed good activity with values of 184% at 10 mg/kg/day and 189% at 30 mg/kg/day.

On the basis of these data, we realized that SMDCMP (5′-monophosphate) and/or SMDCDP (5′-diphosphate) would not be good substrates for CMP/UMP kinase and/or NDP kinase to produce the active nucleotide, SMDCTP, which is a potent inhibitor of several DNA polymerases. Although the structural basis of this drawback is not clear, the preceding example of this type is 3′-azido-3′-deoxythymidine (AZT) 5′-monophosphate (AZTMP), which is not a good substrate of TMP kinase, although AZT is a good substrate of TK1 (*17*). We initially thought that nucleoside kinases had the most strict substrate specificity among various nucleoside and nucleotide kinases. However, now, we know that a nucleoside 5′-monophosphate kinase might also have rather strict substrate specificity.

1-(2-Deoxy-2-methylene-β-D-erythro-pentofuranosyl)cytosine (DMDC)

DMDC has an allylic alcohol system together with the 3′-secondary alcohol in the sugar moiety. This allylic alcohol in DMDC could be stable at the nucleoside level, but if it is phosphorylated to the 5′-polyphosphates by cellular kinases, the following chemical reactivities are expected. (i) At the 5′-diphosphate level (DMDCDP), it could be a mechanism-based inhibitor of ribonucleotide reductase if a 3′-radical were formed by enzyme action. (ii) The 5′-triphosphate (DMDCTP), which could be an inhibitor of DNA polymerases when incorporated into DNA molecules, becomes a more reactive allyl phosphate ester which could be cleaved by nucleophiles.

In vitro cytotoxicity of DMDC against various human tumor cell lines including mouse leukemic L1210 cells is shown in Table I (*18*, *19*). The cytotoxicity spectrum of DMDC is similar to that of 5-FU, but not to those of SMDC and araC. Unlike araC, DMDC was not a substrate of CDA from mouse kidney. In agreement with these characteristics, chemically synthesized DMDCTP was a potent inhibitor of DNA polymerase α, β, and γ with K_i values of 0.42, 2.52, and 1.00 μM, respectively, in a manner competitive with dCTP, while araCTP inhibited only DNA polymerase α with a K_i of 1.10 μM (*4*). It was also found that DMDCTP was incorporated into DNA molecules at the site complementary to guanine by the action of DNA polymerase α using a synthetic template-primer system. In this experiment, DMDCTP apparently acted as a chain-terminator, but whether it was a real chain-terminator or a result of strand-break after a further elongation of the chain, which we postulated, has not yet been proven. Moreover, while it did not inhibit RDR in L1210 murine leukemia and LX-1 human lung carcinoma cells (*20*), DMDCDP was reported to be a time-dependent inhibitor of *Escherichia coli* RDR (*21*).

In vivo antileukemic activity of DMDC was also examined using female $CD2F_1$ mice bearing i.p. inoculated L1210 cells. DMDC administered i.p. once a day for 5 days at 250 mg/kg had a T/C (%) of 235 (*22*). The activity of DMDC was schedule-dependent with much more therapeutic effect obtained by daily treatment than by a single treatment. DMDC was also effective against colon 26 murine carcinoma,

M5076 murine reticulum cell sarcoma, LX-1 human lung cancer xenograft, and SK-Mel-28 human melanoma xenograft, which are less sensitive or refractory to araC. The efficacy of DMDC correlates well with the tumor levels of CDA activity in human tumor xenograft models (*23, 24*). DMDC was highly effective in tumors with higher levels of CDA activity, whereas lower levels yielded only slight antitumor activity. In contrast, gemcitabine is only slightly effective in tumors with higher levels of the enzyme. The activation of DMDC to DMDCMP by dCK would be competitively inhibited by endogenous dCyd in cells. Therefore, the dCyd concentration in tumor cells, regulated by CDA, would be critical for phosphorylation of DMDC. On the other hand, since gemcitabine is a good substrate of CDA, in tumors with higher levels of CDA, both dCyd and gemcitabine are deaminated to uracil derivatives before phosphorylation.

Phase I clinical studies using DMDC with i.v. administration against solid tumors has already been carried out in Japan (*25*). The major dose-limiting toxicity was hematological depression, particularly leukopenia and neutropenia. The maximum tolerated dose for the 5-consecutive-day administration was 40 mg/m^2. Furthermore, a phase I clinical trial with p.o. administration has also been carried out (*26*). The dose-limiting toxicities were anorexia, leukopenia, thrombocytopenia and anemia. General fatigue was the common nonhematological toxicity. The maximum-tolerated dose was 18 $mg/m^2/day$. At the 18-$mg/m^2/day$ dose level, the mean terminal half-life, maximum plasma concentration (C_{max}), and the area under the plasma drug concentration-time curve on day 1 were 1.7496 h, 112.9 ng/mL, and 399.8 ng × h/mL, respectively. Forty to 50% of the administered dose was recovered in the urine, indicating its good bioavailability resulting in significant systemic exposure to the drug, which may enable chronic oral treatment. Details of the clinical pharmacokinetics were also reported (*27–29*).

All-*trans* retinoic acid (ATRA) differentiation therapy against acute promyelocytic leukemia (APL) greatly improved its prognosis. However, although complete remission can be achieved with ATRA alone, disease-free survival is still too short due to relapse. DMDC was found both to inhibit the growth and to induce differentiation of APL cell lines. ATRA combined treatment with DMDC induced differentiation of leukemia cells that had been freshly isolated from APL patients (*30*).

1-(2-C-Cyano-2-deoxy-1-β-D-arabino-pentofuranosyl)cytosine (CNDAC)

Introduction of an electron-withdrawing group (EWG) into the 2′β position would increase the acidity of the 2′α proton. If such a nucleoside is incorporated into DNA, after its enzymatic phosphorylation, the EWG becomes β to the phosphate diester in the DNA. In this case, β-elimination should produce (i) DNA strand-breaks or (ii) abasic site formation as illustrated in Fig. 2. Since strand-breaks in DNA by radiation therapy have been hypothesized to produce tumor cell death, it is worth examining whether the nucleoside having such chemical reactivities inhibits tumor cell growth or not. As an example of a nucleoside that has an EWG at the 2′β position of 2′-deoxycytidine, we synthesized 1-(2-*C*-cyano-2-deoxy-1-β-D-*arabino*-pentofuranosyl)cytosine (CNDAC) from cytidine (*31–35*).

In vitro cytotoxicity of CNDAC against various human tumor cell lines was compared with that of araC and DMDC and is summarized in Table IV. Although

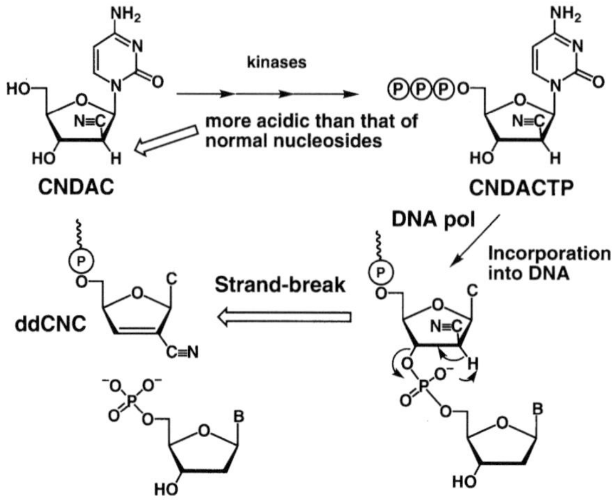

FIG. 2. A possible DNA strand-break mechanisms of DNA containing CNDAC

TABLE IV. Inhibitory Effects of araC, DMDC, CNDAC and ECyd on the Growth of Human Tumor Cell Lines *in vitro*

Cell line	IC_{50} (μg/mL)[a]			
	araC	DMDC	CNDAC	ECyd
PC8	0.28	1.0	4.6	0.024
PC9	1.6	<0.3	40	0.029
QG56	>100	3.4	40	0.012
QG95	50	>100	24	0.055
Lu65	ND	1.3	>100	0.0086
KKLS	>100	0.9	>100	0.0056
NUGC4	>100	0.85	5.2	0.0064
KATO III	>100	1.6	15	0.0082
NAKAJIMA	>100	51	2.8	0.046
ST-KM	>100	1.8	2.8	0.013
MKN45	14	0.46	4.6	0.0024
STSA1	0.34	1.0	1.1	0.039
SW48	>100	5.0	>100	>0.5
SW480	>100	3.8	>100	0.070
MG63	>100	0.45	28	0.040
HT1080	0.13	0.56	0.15	0.020
T24	0.50	1.1	9.4	0.0076

[a] See Table I.

the cytotoxicity spectrum of CNDAC is quite different from that of araC, the potency of CNDAC seemed to be no better than that of DMDC. *In vivo* antileukemic activity of CNDAC was compared with that of araC against i.p.-implanted P388 in CDF_1 mice. CNDAC administered i.p. 10 consecutive days at a dose of 20 mg/kg had a T/C of more than 600%, and 5 out of 6 mice survived more than 60 days, while araC on the same schedule showed a T/C of only 225%. CNDAC was phosphorylated to CNDACMP by dCK, but its relative activity was only half of the phosphorylation of 2′-deoxycytidine with about a 5-fold larger K_m value (Table II) (*16, 36*). Further phosphorylation of CNDACMP to its 5′-triphosphate (CN-

DACTP) was essential for its antitumor activity (*37*). Unlike araCTP, CNDACTP would not act as a feedback inhibitor of dCK, because its accumulation in cells was in a concentration-dependent manner over a 1000-fold range of CNDAC concentrations. On the other hand, CNDAC was a poor substrate of CDA from mouse kidney with 4.2% of the relative activity (Table II).

CNDACTP inhibited DNA polymerase α with a K_i value of 0.16 μM in a competitive manner with dCTP, the K_i value of which is about 7-fold more potent than that of araCTP (Table III). *In vitro* DNA primer extension experiments demonstrated that CNDACMP was incorporated into the *C* site of the elongating DNA strand, and seemed to cause termination of the primer DNA elongation at the site of the analog incorporation. CNDACTP was an effective substrate for DNA polymerase α, which exhibited a substrate efficiency that was similar to that for dCTP incorporation. After incorporation of CNDACMP in a DNA strand, further elongation was a rather slow process, because of its steric effect. However, once a nucleotide was elongated next to CNDACMP, β-elimination occurred to give 2′-*C*-cyano-2′,3′-didehydro-2′,3′-dideoxycytidine (ddCNC) at the 3′-terminus as we hypothesized (*34*, *37*, *38*). This β-elimination reaction was confirmed not only at an enzyme level but also at a tumor cell level. Since DNA replication in intact cells is much more complex than the simple *in vitro* model we have used, it is interesting to examine whether such a chemical reaction actually occurs *in vivo*. Moreover, CNDACTP inhibited T7 RNA polymerase with a K_i value of 0.25 mM, while the K_m value of CTP was 0.45 mM. Using whole cells, it was observed that CNDAC also inhibited RNA synthesis (*39*). However, the mechanism of this action in detail and its contribution to its antitumor activity are the subject of future studies.

The ability of CNDAC to induce DNA strand breaks by a β-elimination-mediated mechanism after its incorporation into the DNA strand is a novel mechanism. This unique strand-breaking action seems to be the basis of its ability to induce cell cycle arrest at the G_2 phase, as distinct from the S phase block seen in the cells treated with araC and gemcitabine. Since certain DNA-damaging agents, such as ionizing radiation and cisplatin, are known to block the cell cycle at the G_2 phase, it is logical to speculate that the β-elimination-mediated DNA strand breaks caused by CNDAC might activate similar signaling pathways (*38*, *39*).

Since CNDAC is a weak substrate of CDA, which is a major inactivating enzyme and is abundant in humans, further derivatives of CNDAC have been prepared. Oral administrations of N^4-palmitoyl CNDAC (PCNDAC, CS-682), among a number of derivatives, showed the most potent antitumor activity against s.c. implanted M5076 mouse reticulum cell sarcoma. Oral administration of PCNDAC exhibited more potent activity against human tumor xenografts with lower toxicity than CNDAC, 5′-deoxy-5-fluorouridine, 5-FU and gemcitabine. Moreover, PCNDAC was effective against P388 leukemic cells resistant to mitomycin-C, vincristine, 5-FU or cisplatin in syngeneic mice (*37*). Its promising antitumor activity in experimental systems has encouraged investigation of its activity in clinical trials with p.o. administration (*40*).

1-(3-C-Ethynyl-β-D-ribo-pentofuranosyl)cytosine (ECyd)

Tumor cells are well known to be heterogeneous. In this respect, the cell cycle of certain tumor tissues is not synchronized. If a certain antitumor agent has a mechanism of action inhibiting only DNA synthesis, such an agent only acts in the S phase of the cell cycle. Although solid tumor cells grow more rapidly than normal cells, their growth rate is much slower than blood cells. Therefore, such an antitumor agent can kill only part of the tumor cells. Inhibition of DNA synthesis is the most prominent activity of CNDAC. However, CNDAC also inhibits RNA synthesis to some extent depending on the cells used and this effect on RNA synthesis may also contribute to its cytotoxicity, particularly in more indolent cell populations in which RNA synthesis would assume more importance. Therefore, we have been looking for a nucleoside antimetabolite, which inhibits both DNA and RNA syntheses. We designed 1-(3-*C*-ethynyl-β-D-*ribo*-pentofuranosyl)cytosine (ECyd), and expected that ECyd 5′-diphosphate (ECDP) would inhibit ribonucleotide reductase and ECyd 5′-triphosphate (ECTP) would inhibit RNA polymerase to cause both DNA and RNA synthesis inhibition (*41–46*).

ECyd showed potent cytotoxicity *in vitro* against various human tumor cell lines with nanomolar to subnanomolar levels of IC_{50} values. The cytotoxic spectrum of ECyd was somewhat different from those of three DNA synthesis inhibitors, araC, DMDC and CNDAC (Table IV). ECyd exhibited strong antitumor activity against various human xenografts implanted into nude mice and nude rats via i.v. administration. Its antitumor potency was somewhat schedule independent and did not produce severe toxicities, such as diarrhea, myelosuppression or loss in body weight (*47*, *48*).

UCK is a key enzyme for the first phosphorylation of ECyd to ECyd 5′-monophosphate (ECMP) to show cytotoxicity. Further phosphorylation to its 5′-diphosphate (ECDP) and 5′-triphosphate (ECTP) occurred concomitantly. ECTP, the dead-end metabolite of ECyd, was accumulated in cells and was rather stable in mouse mammary FM3A cells with a half-life of about 81 h, while that of araCTP was less than 10 min. Therefore, intracellular ECTP was some 500-fold more stable than araCTP (*48*). RNA polymerase was inhibited competitively by ECTP in isolated nuclei of FM3A cells. The K_i value of ECTP was 21 nM, while the apparent K_m value of RNA polymerase for CTP was 8 μM (*47*). Since the IC_{50} value of ECyd in the growth of FM3A cells *in vitro* was 30 μM, the target enzyme responsible for its cytotoxicity would be RNA polymerase (*49*). There are three RNA polymerases (I, II and III) in eukaryotes. ECTP was found to be a no-selective inhibitor of these polymerases (*46*). This RNA inhibition could induce apoptosis in tumor cells (*50*). ECyd was a very poor substrate of CDA from mouse kidney *in vitro*. However, its deaminated analog, 1-(3-*C*-ethynyl-β-D-*ribo*-pentofuranosyl)uracil (EUrd), also exhibited similar cytotoxicity to ECyd, which also metabolized to its 5′-triphosphate (EUTP) and inhibited RNA polymerase with a K_i value of 84 nM (apparent K_m value of UTP was 13 μM) (*42*, *48*, *51*). Initially, ECDP was anticipated to inhibit ribonucleotide reductase, but it did not inhibit the enzyme from *E. coli* even at mM concentrations.

Since UCK activity in human tumor tissues is well known to be relatively high compared to its activity in normal tissues, tumor selective cytotoxicity of ECyd could therefore be expected clinically. Recently, a UCK family consisting of two members, UCK1 and UCK2, has been reported in human cells (*52*, *53*). Therefore, to determine which isozyme is responsible for the phosphorylation of ECyd is important for further development. We investigated the relationship between expression of UCK1 and UCK2 at both mRNA and protein levels, and ECyd phosphorylation activity in a panel of 10 human tumor cell lines (*54*). The UCK activity was found to be well correlated with the cells' sensitivity to ECyd. Furthermore, the mRNA or protein expression level of UCK2 was closely correlated with UCK activity in these cell lines, but neither the level of expression of UCK1 mRNA nor that of protein was correlated with the enzyme activity. Comparison of the protein expression level of UCK2 in several human tumor tissues and the corresponding normal tissues showed that the expression of UCK2 protein was barely detectable in 4 out of the 5 human tissues, but tended to be high in the pancreatic tumor tissue. In any of the normal tissues, the expression could not be detected at all. Therefore, expression of UCK2 seemed to be correlated with cellular sensitivity to ECyd, and it may contribute to the tumor-selective cytotoxicity of ECyd. ECyd is now under phase I clinical study against solid tumors in the U. S.

Conclusion

Since the great success of gemcitabine for the treatment of solid tumors in patients with a combination of other antitumor agents or radiation therapy has been achieved, the concept of a nucleoside antimetabolite, although it is an old idea, has been revived to further develop this class of compounds. The mechanism of action of gemcitabine is somewhat different from those of DMDC, CNDAC and ECyd. Therefore, these new nucleoside antimetabolites would act as different types of antimetabolites than gemcitabine against different tumors if suitable methods of administration or development of proper prodrugs for each of the nucleosides could be found. In particular, ECyd which is a novel antimetabolite targeting RNA polymerases and which is different in metabolic pathways from deoxycytidine analogues may be successful in combination chemotherapy.

REFERENCES

1. Montgomery JA, Ananthan S, Parker WB, Secrist III JA, Temple CG3. Antimetabolites. In: Foye WO, editor. Cancer Chemotherapy Agents. Series: ACS professional reference book. Washington, DC., American Chemical Society; 1995, p. 47–110.
2. Tsimberidou AM, Alvarado Y, Giles FJ. Evolving role of ribonucleoside reductase inhibitors in hematologic malignancies. *Expert Rev Anticancer Ther* 2002; **2**: 437–48 and references cited theirin.
3. Jacobs AD. Gemcitabine-based therapy in pancreas cancer. Gemcitabine-docetaxel and other novel combinations. *Cancer* 2002; **95**: 923–927 and references cited theirin.
4. Matsuda A, Azuma A, Nakajima Y, Takenuki K, Dan A, Iino T, Yoshimura Y, Minakawa N, Tanaka M, Sasaki T. In: Chu CK, Baker DC. editors. Nucleosides and Nucleotides as Antitumor and Antiviral Agents. Design of new types of antitumor nucleosides: The synthesis and antitumor activity of 2′-deoxy-(2′-*C*-substituted)cytidines, New York, Plenum Press; 1993, p. 1–22.
5. Arner ES, Eriksson S. Mammalian deoxyribonucleoside kinases. *Pharmacol Ther* 1995; **67**: 155–86.

6. Eriksson S, Munch-Petersen B, Johansson K, Eklund H. Structure and function of cellular deoxyribonucleoside kinases. *Cell Mol Life Sci* 2002; **59**: 1327–46.
7. Johansson NG, Eriksson S. Structure-activity relationships for phosphorylation of nucleoside analogs to monophosphates by nucleoside kinases. *Acta Biochim Pol* 1996; **43**: 143–60.
8. Obata T, Endo Y, Tanaka M, Uchida H, Matsuda A, Sasaki T. Deletion mutants of human deoxycytidine kinase mRNA in cells resistant to antitumor cytosine nucleoside. *Jpn J Cancer Res* 2001; **92**: 793–8.
9. Maley F, Maley GF. A tale of two enzymes, deoxycytidylate deaminase and thymidylate synthase. *Prog Nucleic Acid Res Mol Biol* 1990; **39**: 49–80.
10. Gmeiner WH. Antimetabolite incorporation into DNA: structural and thermodynamic basis for anticancer activity. *Biopolymers* 2002; **65**: 180–9.
11. Hadfield AF, Sartorelli AC. The pharmacology of prodrugs of 5-fluorouracil and 1-β-D-arabinofuranosylcytosine. *Adv Pharmacol Chemother* 1984; **20**: 21–67.
12. Lopez C, Watanabe KA, Fox JJ. 2′-Fluoro-5-iodo-aracytosine, a potent and selective anti-herpesvirus agent. *Antimicrob Agents Chemother* 1980; **17**: 803–6.
13. Hertel LW, Boder GB, Kroin JS, Rinzel SM, Poore GA, Todd GC, Grindey GB. Evaluation of the antitumor activity of gemcitabine (2′,2′-difluoro-2′-deoxycytidine). *Cancer Res* 1990; **50**: 4417–22.
14. Plunkett W, Huang P, Searcy CE, Gandhi V. Gemcitabine: preclinical pharmacology and mechanisms of action. *Semin Oncol* 1996; **23**: 3–15.
15. Matsuda A, Takenuki K, Sasaki T, Ueda T. Radical deoxygenation of *tert*-alcohols in 1-(2-*C*-alkylpentofuranosyl)pyrimidines: Synthesis of (2′*S*)-2′-deoxy-2′-*C*-methylcytidine, an antileukemic nucleoside. *J Med Chem* 1991; **34**: 234–9.
16. Uchida H, Morinaga H, Misaki T, Miyazaki T, Uwajima T, Obata T, Endo Y, Matsuda A, Sasaki T. A novel affinity chromatography method for the co-purification of deoxycytidine kinase and cytidine deaminase. *Nucleosides Nucleotides Nucleic Acids* 2001; **20**: 1647–54.
17. Agarwal RP, Mian AM. Thymidine and zidovudine metabolism in chronically zidovudine-exposed cells in vitro. *Biochem Pharmacol* 1991; **42**: 905–11.
18. Matsuda A, Takenuki K, Sasaki T, Ueda T. Synthesis of a new broad spectrum of antineoplastic nucleoside, 2′-deoxy-2′-methylidenecytidine (DMDC) and its derivatives. *J Med Chem* 1991; **34**: 812–9.
19. Ono T, Fujii A, Hosoya M, Okumoto T, Sakata S, Matsuda A, Sasaki T. Cell kill kinetics of an antineoplastic nucleoside, 1-(2-deoxy-2-methylene-β-D-*erythoro*-pentofuranosyl)cytosine. *Biochem Pharmacol* 1996; **52**: 1279–85.
20. Kanazawa J, Takahashi T, Akinaga S, Tamaoki T, Okabe M. The relationship between the antitumor activity and the ribonucleotide reductase inhibitory activity of (*E*)-2′-deoxy-2′-(fluoromethylene)cytidine, MDL 101,731. *Anticancer Drugs* 1998; **9**: 653–7.
21. Baker CH, Banzon J, Bollinger JM, Stubbe J, Samano V, Robins MJ, Lippert B, Jarvi E, Resvick R. 2′-Deoxy-2′-methylenecytidine and 2′-deoxy-2′,2′-difluorocytidine 5′-diphosphates: potent mechanism-based inhibitors of ribonucleotide reductase. *J Med Chem* 1991; **34**: 1879–84.
22. Yamagami K, Fujii A, Arita M, Okumoto T, Sakata S, Matsuda A, Ueda T, Sasaki T. Antitumor activity of 2′-deoxy-2′-methylidenecytidine, a new 2′-deoxycytidine deriva-

tive. *Cancer Res* 1991; **51**: 2319–23.

23. Eda H, Ura M, Ouchi KF, Tanaka Y, Miwa M, Ishitsuka H. The antiproliferative activity of DMDC is modulated by inhibition of cytidine deaminase. *Cancer Res* 1998; **58**: 1165–9.
24. Miwa M, Eda H, Ura M, Ouchi KF, Keith DD, Foley LH, Ishitsuka H. High susceptibility of human cancer xenografts with higher levels of cytidine deaminase to a 2′-deoxycytidine antimetabolite, 2′-deoxy-2′-methylidenecytidine. *Clin Cancer Res* 1998; **4**: 493–7.
25. Gemma A, Kudoh S, Fukuoka M, Kurita Y, Hasegawa K, Harada M, Mori K, Ariyoshi Y, Kurihara M, Furuse K, Horikoshi N, Kanamaru R, Fukuyama E, Yoneda S, Furue H, Taguchi T, Ota K, Wakui A, Tsukagoshi S, Niitani H. Phase I study on DMDC. *Gan To Kagaku Ryoho* 1996; **23**: 1799–811 (in Japanese).
26. Masuda N, Matsui K, Yamamoto N, Nogami T, Nakagawa K, Negoro S, Takeda K, Takifuji N, Yamada M, Kudoh S, Okuda T, Nemoto S, Ogawa K, Myobudani H, Nihira S, Fukuoka M. Phase I trial of oral 2′-deoxy-2′-methylidenecytidine: on a daily x 14-day schedule. *Clin Cancer Res* 2000; **6**: 2288–94.
27. Brindley CJ, Morrison R, Gordon RJ, Devlin AJ, van der Gaast A, Verweij L, Funaki T. Clinical pharmacokinetics of 2′-deoxy-2′-methylidenecytidine (DMDC), a deoxycytidine analogue antineoplastic agent. *Clin Pharmacokinet* 2000; **38**: 475–91.
28. Friberg LE, Brindley CJ, Karlsson MO, Devlin AJ. Models of schedule dependent haematological toxicity of 2′-deoxy-2′-methylidenecytidine (DMDC). *Eur J Clin Pharmacol* 2000; **56**: 567–74.
29. Friberg LE, Henningsson A, Maas H, Nguyen L, Karlsson MO. Model of chemotherapy-induced myelosuppression with parameter consistency across drugs. *J Clin Oncol* 2002; **20**: 4713–21.
30. Niitsu N, Ishii Y, Matsuda A, Honma Y. Induction of differentiation of acute promyelocytic leukemia cells by a cytidine deaminase-resistant analogue of 1-β-D-arabinofuranosylcytosine, 1-(2-deoxy-2-methylene-β-D-*erythro*-pentofuranosyl)cytidine. *Cancer Res* 2001; **61**: 178–85.
31. Azuma A, Nakajima Y, Nishizono N, Minakawa N, Suzuki M, Hanaoka K, Kobayashi T, Tanaka M, Sasaki T, Matsuda A. 2′-*C*-Cyano-2′-deoxy-1-β-D-arabinofuranosylcytosine and its derivatives: A new class of nucleoside with a broad antitumor spectrum. *J Med Chem* 1993; **36**: 4183–9.
32. Azuma A, Hanaoka K, Kurihara A, Kobayashi T, Miyauchi S, Kamo N, Tanaka M, Sasaki T, Matsuda A. Chemical stability of a new antitumor nucleoside, 2′-*C*-cyano-2′-deoxy-1-β-D-*arabino*-pentofuranosylcytosine (CNDAC) in alkaline medium: Formation of 2′-*C*-cyano-2′-deoxy-1-β-D-*ribo*-pentofuranosylcytosine (CNDC) and its antitumor activity. *J Med Chem* 1995; **38**: 3391–7.
33. Matsuda A, Nakajima Y, Azuma A, Tanaka M, Sasaki T. 2′-*C*-Cyano-2′-deoxy-1-β-D-arabinofuranosylcytosine (CNDAC): Design of a potential mechanism-based DNA-strand breaking antineoplastic nucleoside. *J Med Chem* 1991; **34**: 2917–9.
34. Matsuda A, Azuma A. 2′-*C*-Cyano-2′-deoxy-1-β-D-arabinofuranosylcytosine (CN-DAC): A mechanism-based DNA-strand-breaking antitumor nucleoside. *Nucleosides Nucleotides* 1995; **14**: 461–71.
35. Tanaka M, Matsuda A, Terao T, Sasaki T. Antitumor activity of a novel nucleoside, 2′-

C-cyano-2′-deoxy-1-β-D-arabinofuranosylcytosine (CNDAC) against murine and human tumors. *Cancer Lett* 1992; **64**: 67–74.

36. Uchida H, Chen YX, Morinaga H, Hayashi Y, Matsuda A, Obata T, Endo Y, Sasaki T. Isolation of deoxycytidine kinase from Ehrlich carcinoma cells by affinity chromatography based on a substrate analog, 2′-*C*-cyano-2′-deoxy-1-β-D-arabinofranosyl-N^4-palmitoylcytosine. *Bio Pharm Bull* 1999; **22**: 83–6.
37. Hanaoka K, Suzuki M, Kobayashi T, Tanzawa F, Tanaka K, Shibayama T, Miura S, Ikeda T, Iwabuchi H, Nakagawa A, Mitsuhashi Y, Hisaoka M, Kaneko M, Tomida A, Wataya Y, Nomura T, Sasaki T, Matsuda A, Tsuruo T, Kurakata S. Antitumor activity and novel DNA-self-strand-breaking mechanism of CNDAC (1-(2-*C*-cyano-2-deoxy-b-D-*arabino*-pentofuranosyl)cytosine) and its N^4-palmitoyl derivative (CS-682). *Int J Cancer* 1999; **82**: 226–36.
38. Azuma A, Huang P, Matsuda A, Plunkett W. 2′-*C*-Cyano-2′-deoxy-1-β-D-arabinopentofuranosylcytosine (CNDAC): a novel acting anticancer nucleoside analog that causes DNA strand-breaks and G2 arrest. *Mol Pharmacol* 2001; **59**: 725–31.
39. Azuma A, Huang P, Matsuda A, Plunkett W. Cellular pharmacokinetics and pharmacodynamics of the deoxycytidine analog 2′-*C*-cyano-2′-deoxy-1-β-D-*arabino*-pentofuranosylcytosine (CNDAC). *Biochem Pharmacol* 2001; **61**: 1497–507.
40. Donehower RC, Dees EC, Bakek SD, Summerson L, Carducci MA, Izumi T, Kobayashi T. A phase I study of CS-682, an oral antimetabolite, in patients with refractory solid tumors (Abstract). *Proc Am Soc Clin Oncol* 2000; **19**: 196a.
41. Azuma A, Matsuda A, Sasaki T, Fukushima T. 1-(3-*C*-Ethynyl-β-D-*ribo*-pentofuranosyl)cytosine (ECyd, TAS-106): Antitumor effect and mechanism of action. *Nucleosides Nucleotides Nucleic Acids* 2001; **20**: 609–19.
42. Hattori H, Tanaka M, Fukushima M, Sasaki T, Matsuda A. 1-(3-*C*-Ethynyl-β-D-*ribo*-pentofuranosyl)cytosine (ECyd), 1-(3-*C*-Ethynyl-β-D-*ribo*-pentofuranosyl)uracil (EUrd), and their Nucleobase Analogues as New Potential Multifunctional Antitumor Nucleosides with a Broad Spectrum of Activity. *J Med Chem* 1996; **39**: 5005–11.
43. Hattori H, Nozawa E, Iino T, Yoshimura Y, Shuto S, Shimamoto Y, Nomura M, Fukushima M, Tanaka M, Sasaki T, Matsuda A. The structural requirements of the sugar moiety for the antitumor activities of new nucleoside antimetabolites, 1-(3-*C*-ethynyl-β-D-*ribo*-pentofuranosyl)cytosine and -uracil. *J Med Chem* 1998; **41**: 2892–902.
44. Matsuda A, Fukushima M, Wataya Y, Sasaki T. A new antitumor nucleoside, 1-(3-*C*-ethynyl-β-D-*ribo*-pentofuranosyl)cytosine (ECyd), is a potent inhibitor of RNA polymerase. *Nucleosides Nucleotides* 1999; **18**: 811–4.
45. Tabata S, Tanaka M, Matsuda A, Fukushima M, Sasaki T. Antitumor effect of a novel multifunctional antitumor nucleoside, 3′-ethynylcytidine, on human cancers. *Oncology Rep* 1996; **3**: 1029–34.
46. Tabata S, Tanaka M, Endo Y, Obata T, Matsuda A, Sasaki T. Antitumor mechanisms of 3′-ethynyluridine and 3′-ethynylcytidine as RNA synthesis inhibitors: development and characterization of 3′-ethynyluridine-resistant cells. *Cancer Lett* 1997; **116**: 225–31.
47. Shimamoto Y, Fujioka A, Kazuno H, Murakami Y, Ohshimo H, Kato T, Matsuda A, Sasaki T, Fukushima M. Antitumor activity and pharmacokinetics of TAS-106, 1-(3-

C-ethynyl-β-D-*ribo*-pentofuranosyl)cytosine. *Jpn J Cancer Res* 2001; **92**: 343–51.

48. Takatori S, Kanda H, Takenaka K, Wataya Y, Matsuda A, Fukushima M, Shimamoto Y, Tanaka M, Sasaki T. Antitumor mechanisms and metabolism of novel antitumor nucleoside analogues, 1-(3-*C*-ethynyl-β-D-*ribo*-pentofuranosyl)cytosine and 1-(3-*C*-ethynyl-β-D-*ribo*-pentofuranosyl)uracil. *Cancer Chemother Pharmacol* 1999; **44**: 97–104.
49. Shimamoto Y, Kazuno H, Murakami Y, Azuma A, Koizumi K, Matsuda A, Sasaki T, Fukushima M. Cellular and biochemical mechanisms of the resistance of human cancer cells to a new anticancer *ribo*-nucleoside, TAS-106. *Jpn J Cancer Res* 2002; **93**: 445–52.
50. Takatori S, Tsutsumi S, Hidaka M, Kanda H, Matsuda A, Fukushima M, Wataya Y. The characterization of cell death induced by 1-(3-*C*-ethynyl-β-D-*ribo*-pentofuranosyl)cytosine (ECyd) in FM3A cells. *Nucleosides Nucleotides* 1998; **17**: 1309–17.
51. Matsuda A, Hattori H, Tanaka M, Sasaki T. 1-(3-*C*-Ethynyl-β-D-*ribo*-pentofuranosyl)uracil as a potential broad spectrum multifunctional antitumor nucleoside. *Bioorg Med Chem Lett* 1996; **6**: 1887–92.
52. Koizumi K, Shimamoto Y, Azuma A, Wataya Y, Matsuda A, Sasaki T, Fukushima M. Cloning and expression of uridine/cytidine kinase cDNA from human fibrosarcoma cells. *Int J Mol Med* 2001; **8**: 273–8.
53. Van Rompay AR, Norda A, Linden K, Johansson M, Krlsson A. Phosphorylation of uridine and cytidine nucleoside analogs by two human uridine-cytidine kinases. *Mol Pharmacol* 2001; **59**: 1181–6.
54. Shimamoto Y, Koizumi K, Okabe H, Kazuno H, Murakami Y, Nakagawa F, Matsuda A, Sasaki T, Fukushima M. Sensitivity of human cancer cells to the new anticancer *ribo*-nucleoside TAS-106 is correlated with expression of uridine-cytidine kinase 2. *Jpn J Cancer Res* 2002; **93**: 825–33.

MOLECULAR TARGETING THERAPY OF CANCER: DRUG RESISTANCE, APOPTOSIS AND SURVIVAL SIGNAL

Takashi TSURUO[*1,*2], Mikihiko NAITO[*1], Akihiro TOMIDA[*1], Naoya FUJITA[*1], Tetsuo MASHIMA[*2], Hiroshi SAKAMOTO[*1,*2] and Naomi HAGA[*1]

Institute of Molecular and Cellular Biosciences, The University of Tokyo[*1] *and Cancer Chemotherapy Center, Japanese Foundation for Cancer Research*[*2]

Recent progress in the development of molecular cancer therapeutics has revealed new types of antitumor drugs, such as Herceptin, Gleevec, and Iressa, as potent therapeutics for specific tumors. Our work has focused on molecular cancer therapeutics, mainly in the areas of drug resistance, apoptosis and apoptosis resistance, and survival-signaling, which is related to drug resistance. In this review, we describe our research on molecular cancer therapeutics, including molecular mechanisms and therapeutic approaches. Resistance to chemotherapeutic drugs is a principal problem in the treatment of cancer. P-Glycoprotein (P-gp), encoded by the *MDR1* gene, is a multidrug transporter and has a major role in multidrug resistance (MDR). Targeting of P-gp by small-molecular compounds and/or antibodies is an effective strategy to overcome MDR in cancer, especially hematologic malignancies. Several P-gp inhibitors have been developed and are currently under clinical phased studies. In addition to the multidrug transporter proteins, cancer cells have several drug resistance mechanisms. Solid tumors are often placed under stress conditions, such as glucose starvation and hypoxia. These conditions result in topo II poison resistance that is due to proteasome-mediated degradation of DNA topoisomerases. Proteasome inhibitors effectively prevent this stress-induced drug resistance. Glyoxalase I, which is often elevated in drug- and apoptosis-resistant cancers, offers another possibility for overcoming drug resistance. It plays a role in detoxification of methylglioxal, a side product of glycolysis, which is highly reactive with DNA and proteins. Inhibitors of glyoxalase I selectively kill drug-resistant tumors that express glyoxalase I. Finally, the susceptibility of tumor cells to apoptosis induced by antitumor drugs appears to depend on the balance between pro-apoptotic and survival (anti-apoptotic) signals. PI3K-Akt is an important survival signal pathway, that has been shown to be the target of various antitumor drugs, including UCN-01 and geldanamycin, new anticancer drugs under clinical evaluation. Our present studies provide novel targets for future effective molecular cancer therapeutics.

[*1] 1-1-1 Yayoi, Bunkyo-ku, Tokyo 113-0032, Japan

[*2] 1-37-1 Kami-Ikebukuro, Toshima-ku, Tokyo 170-8455, Japan

This paper is dedicated to the memory of late Dr. Tomizo Yoshida on the occasion of the 100th anniversary of his birth. It was originally published in Cancer Science in January, 2003.

Cancer chemotherapy has gradually improved with the development of novel antitumor drugs and has profound, positive results when applied to many hematologic malignancies, and some solid tumors, especially germ cell and some childhood malignancies. While treatment of certain malignancies with chemotherapy has been successful and encouraging, the effectiveness has often been limited by drug resistance of tumors and by side effects on normal tissues and cells. In fact, many tumors are intrinsically resistant to many of the more potent cytotoxic agents used in cancer therapy. Other tumors, initially sensitive, recur and are resistant not only to the initial therapeutic agents, but also to other drugs not used in the treatment. Because of the serious problem of clinical drug resistance, much effort has been expended to advance our understanding of the mechanisms of drug resistance in cancer cells. The molecular mechanisms of drug resistance, however, are not fully understood.

Apoptosis and anti-apoptosis pathways are also deeply related to drug sensitivity and resistance. A number of tumor cells have been reported to undergo apoptotic cell death when treated with such chemotherapeutic agents as etoposide, camptothecin, cisplatin, 1-β-D-arabinofuranosyl cytosine (Ara-C), mitomycin C, adriamycin, and vincristine. The findings indicate that apoptosis in tumor cells plays a critical role in chemotherapy-induced tumor cell killing and also suggest that blockade of the apoptosis-inducing pathway could be another mechanism for multidrug resistance (MDR). Based on the drug- and apoptosis-resistance mechanisms, we can design a rational strategy to target resistant cancers. In this review, we discuss several drug resistance mechanisms, including drug transporters, cellular stress responses, apoptosis regulation and cellular survival signals that have relevance to drug resistance. These pathways could provide new targets for effective cancer therapy.

MDR

1. *Mechanism of MDR by ATP-binding cassette (ABC) transporters*

Resistance to a broad spectrum of chemotherapeutic agents in cancer cell lines and human tumors has been called MDR (*1*). The MDR phenotype is associated with increased drug efflux from the cells that is mediated by an energy-dependent mechanism. Studies on the MDR phenotype have led to discovery of ABC transporters, such as P-glycoprotein (P-gp), and MDR-associated protein (MRP).

Overexpression of P-gp, encoded by the *MDR1* gene, confers resistance to a variety of structurally and functionally unrelated antitumor drugs, such as vinblastine, vincristine, doxorubicin, daunorubicin, etoposide, teniposide, paclitaxel, and many others (*2*). P-gp, localized on the plasma membrane of resistant cancer cells, can bind and transport the antitumor drugs in a ATP-dependent manner (Fig. 1) (*3–5*). The expression of P-gp is elevated in intrinsically drug-resistant cancers of the colon, kidney and adrenal, as well as in some tumors that acquire drug resistance after chemotherapy. The expression of MDR1 mRNA in tumors correlates well with certain kinds of clinical drug resistance. MDR1 promoter activity is up-regulated by various stimuli, such as anticancer drugs, DNA-damaging agents, heat shock, serum starvation, and ultraviolet irradiation. MDR1 expression can also be up-regulated as a consequence of tumor progression, such as mutation of tumor suppressor gene *p53* and activation of *ras* oncogene.

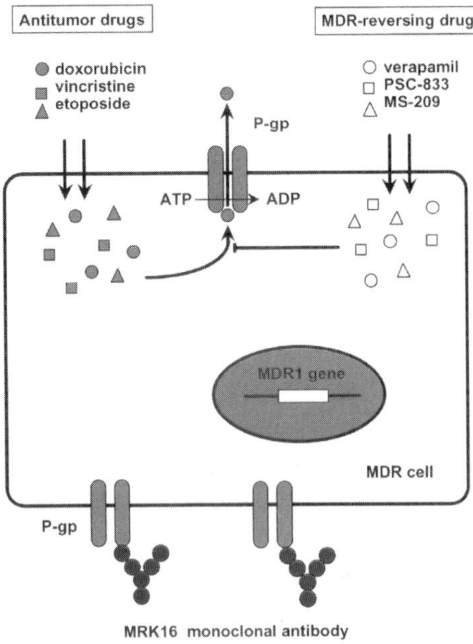

FIG. 1. P-Glycoprotein-mediated multidrug resistance and its reversal
P-Glycoprotein, encoded by the *MDR1* gene, transports various anticancer drugs from MDR cells in an energy-dependent manner. MDR-reversing agents, such as verapamil, PSC-833 and MS-209, inhibit P-glycoprotein-mediated drug transport. MRK16, a monoclonal antibody against P-glycoprotein is also useful to reverse MDR.

2. *Reversal of MDR*

Because P-gp appeared to be involved in both acquired and intrinsic MDR in human cancers, selective killing of tumor cells that express P-gp could be very important for cancer therapy. In 1981, we reported that the calcium channel blocker verapamil inhibited active drug efflux and restored drug sensitivity in MDR cells (*6*). Various compounds, including calcium channel blockers and calmodulin inhibitors, have been shown to enhance the cytotoxic activity of various agents (*7–10*). All of these agents antagonize MDR by increasing the drug accumulation in MDR cells, whereas they show little or no effect on drug-sensitive cells. Most of the reversing agents, such as verapamil, cyclosporin A, diltiazem and FK-506, are substrates for P-gp-mediated transport and competitively inhibit P-gp transport of antitumor drugs (*11*). A new generation of the MDR reversal agents has been developed and is in clinical trials. These include non-immunosuppressive cyclosporine PSC-833 and a quinoline derivative, MS-209. MS-209 was shown to inhibit both P-gp and MRP. In clinical trials, MDR-reversing agents have shown promising effects on drug-resistant hematologic malignancies.

It is important to note that any P-gp inhibitor could have deleterious effects *in vivo* because P-gp is also expressed in normal tissues, such as adrenal, gravid uterus, kidney, liver, colon and capillary endothelial cells in brain (*12*, *13*). P-gp expressed in normal tissues could prevent xenobiotic uptake, and therefore, many P-gp inhibitors affect the pharmacokinetics of antitumor drugs. To improve combined chemotherapy, the pharmacodynamic features of anti-cancer drugs and P-gp inhibitors should be carefully investigated.

In addition to small-molecular P-gp inhibitors, monoclonal antibodies to P-gp are useful to target this protein in drug-resistant cancers. Our research group has developed immunotherapeutic approaches for overcoming MDR using anti-P-gp monoclonal antibodies, MRK-16 and MRK-17 (*3*, *14*). The combination of anti-P-gp monoclonal antibodies with P-gp inhibitors may also be useful in reversing P-gp-mediated MDR. The combination of MRK-16 and PSC-833 synergistically reversed MDR *in vitro* and *in vivo* (*15*). Mechanistic analysis showed that PSC-833 increased MRK-16 binding to P-gp.

It may be possible to protect hematopoietic cells from toxic side effects of cancer chemotherapy by transducing the *MDR1* gene. Although this gene is expressed in various normal tissues as mentioned above, it is not widely expressed in bone marrow cells. Lack of protection by the drug transporter may be one of the reasons for severe bone marrow cell suppression by many chemotherapeutic agents. Therefore, successful introduction of the *MDR1* gene would allow hematopoietic cells to survive increased doses of chemotherapy. For this purpose, retrovirus-mediated gene transfer can be used, because of the potential for stable vector integration and expression (*16*). This therapeutic approach is interesting because it could be applied to a wide range of currently resistant solid tumors.

Proteasome as a Target against Drug Resistance

1. *Proteasome inhibition for reversal of stress-mediated resistance of solid tumors*

Resistance to chemotherapy is a principal problem in treating the most commonly seen solid tumors. Tumor cells, *in vivo*, are often exposed to such conditions as glucose deprivation, hypoxia, low pH, and other nutrient deprivation (*17*, *18*). These microenvironmental conditions are based upon inadequate vascularization in solid tumors, regardless of their origin or location. The microenvironment itself has been thought to be a major mechanism of drug resistance because it hinders drug access to tumor cells and reduces the oxygen radicals generated by antitumor drugs. The drug resistance can also be associated with decreased cell proliferation, cell-cell contact and adhesion of cancer cells to extracellular matrix. In addition, the microenvironmental stress conditions may select tumor cells that have decreased apoptotic potential through genetic alterations, thereby leading to resistance to apoptosis induction by antitumor drugs. Of further importance is that the stress conditions also induce drug resistance without such genetic alterations in tumor cells.

Pathophysiological stress conditions in culture commonly cause the glucose-regulated response of cancer cells, which is characterized by induction of endoplasmic reticulum (ER)-resident stress proteins, GRP78 and GRP94 (*19*). The stress response can be mediated by the unfolded protein response or ER stress response pathway that is induced following the accumulation of unfolded proteins in the ER. It is important to recall that overexpression of GRP78 is, indeed, observed in clinical settings. A possible link between glucose-regulated stress response and drug resistance was first reported by Shen *et al.* (*20*) They showed that GRP-inducing conditions caused significant resistance induction to doxorubicin in Chinese hamster ovary (CHO) cells. Subsequently, the stressed CHO cells were shown to become resistant to etoposide as well as to doxorubicin, both of which are antitumor topoisomerase (topo) II poisons. We also showed that such resistance induction occurred in human cancer cell lines (*21*). Thus, glucose-regulated stress response is associated with development of cellular resistance to topo II poisons.

Topo II poisons stabilize the cleavable complex, an intermediate product of the topo II-catalyzed reaction (*22*). Accumulation of cleavable complexes is thought to lead to eventual cell death, and a decrease in the number of cleavable complexes could confer drug resistance. In agreement with this, a decreased expression of topo IIα occurs under glucose-regulated stress conditions (*21*). We found that proteasome inhibition attenuated the inducible resistance by inhibiting the topo IIα depletion induced by glucose starvation and hypoxia as well as by the chemical stressor A23187 (*23, 24*). The topo IIα restoration was seen only at the protein level, indicating that topo IIα protein depletion occurred through a proteasome-mediated degradation mechanism. In agreement with this restoration, the stress-induced etoposide resistance was effectively prevented *in vitro* by the proteasome inhibitor lactacystin (*24*). Furthermore, lactacystin significantly enhanced the antitumor activity of etoposide in the refractory HT-29 xenograft. In this regard, a recently developed proteasome inhibitor, PS-341, which is now in phase I and II clinical trials (*25*), may also have potential for overcoming stress-induced resistance.

2. *Nuclear proteasome accumulation as a novel mechanism of drug resistance*

During the course of the above-described studies, we found that stress conditions stimulated nuclear accumulation of proteasome in HT-29 human colon cancer cells (*23, 26*). Accumulation under these conditions was also observed in A2780 ovarian cancer cells, suggesting that this response occurred regardless of the cell's origin. No changes were detected in the total expression levels of proteasome. Recently, we found that nuclear proteasome accumulation during glucose starvation was attenuated by stable expression of a mutant type of proteasome subunit, XAPC7, that lacked the nuclear localization signal (NLS) (*27*). It is important that the expression of NLS-defective XAPC7 also diminished the induction of resistance to the topo II-directed drugs etoposide and doxorubicin. Under normal conditions, however, the NLS-defective XAPC7 had little effect on either nuclear proteasome distribution or etoposide sensitivity. These results demonstrate that nuclear proteasome localization, possibly through up-regulation of the NLS-dependent transport, is involved in the development of drug resistance under stress conditions (Fig. 2).

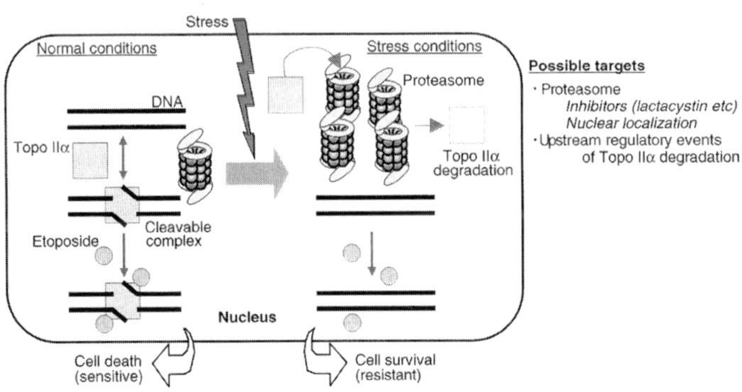

FIG. 2. Possible mechanisms of stress-induced topo II-directed drugs

We also demonstrated that XAPC7/dNLS-transfected cells showed slightly higher expression levels of topo IIα under glucose-starvation conditions than did XAPC7/WT-transfected cells (*27*). This observation raises the possibility that degradation of nuclear proteins, including topo IIα, is facilitated by nuclear proteasome accumulation under stress conditions. Although the exact mechanisms of drug resistance mediated by nuclear proteasome accumulation remain to be determined, our observations suggest that inhibiting nuclear distribution of proteasomes can be a selective approach to preventing stress-inducible drug resistance of solid tumors. Indeed, microenvironmental stresses are not observed in normal tissues, and the NLS-dependent pathway appears important particularly for stress-induced nuclear transport of proteasomes in cancer cells. Thus, further studies into the mechanisms of nuclear proteasome transport would provide tumor-selective strategies to circumvent the inducible resistance to topo II-directed drugs.

3. Other mechanisms of proteasome-mediated drug resistance

The proteasome is a major site for degradation of abnormal or irrelevant and regulatory proteins, such as transcription factors, oncoproteins and cyclins. Consequently, proteasome can be involved in various types of drug resistance (*25*). For example, NF-κB signaling is dependent on proteasome activity, and this pathway plays a role in protecting against drug-induced apoptosis in certain cell types. Indeed, PS-341 has been shown to block the protective response and to sensitize cancer cells to topo I inhibitors. The proteasome is also involved in a possible repair mechanism of camptothecin (CPT)-induced cleavable complexes through degrading topo I. Thus, proteasome inhibition may be useful for overcoming various types of drug resistance.

However, proteasomes are ubiquitously expressed in normal tissues and play essential roles in various cellular functions. Therefore, total inhibition of proteasome activities might have adverse effects. In this context, regulatory events upstream of the proteasome-mediated degradation, such as phosphorylation and ubiquitinylation of substrates, will be interesting to explore as potential targets. With respect to topoisomerase-targeted drug resistance, it will be especially important to elucidate the regulatory mechanisms of the stress-induced topo IIα and the CPT-induced topo I degradation (Fig. 2). Modification of topoisomerases with SUMO-1, a ubiquitin-like protein, may also be interesting. We recently identified the major sumoylation site of topo I and found that sumoylation enhances the cleavable complex formation and apoptosis induced by CPT (*28*). Thus, additional research on regulatory events upstream of the proteasome-mediated degradation could provide novel and specific strategies for overcoming drug resistance.

Glyoxalase I as a Target in Apoptosis Resistance

1. Apoptosis-resistant tumor cells

Apoptosis is an active cell death mechanism that plays a role in several biological processes. Various antitumor agents have been reported to elicit apoptosis in tumor cells (*29*). This implies that blocking the apoptosis signaling could be another mechanism for multidrug resistance to chemotherapy. Since tumor development is caused by an upset of balance between cell growth and death, abnormality in the machinery of apoptosis often occurs in tumors, causing a chemotherapy-resistant phenotype of the tumor cells. To determine the molecular basis of resistance to antitumor agent-induced apoptosis, we isolated and characterized several drug-resistant mutants that were also resistant to apoptosis induced by antitumor agents (*30*). To identify the factors responsible for the apoptosis resistance, we performed a cDNA subtractive hybridization with mRNA from human monocytic leukemia U937 and its variant UK711, which is resistant to apoptosis induced by antitumor agents (*31, 32*). We found that glyoxalase I was selectively overexpressed in the apoptosis-resistant UK711 cells.

2. *Glyoxalase I as an apoptosis resistance factor*

We observed an elevated expression of glyoxalase I in several apoptosis-resistant tumor cells. Glyoxalase I is an essential component in pathways leading to the detoxification of methylglyoxal, a side product of glycolysis (*33*). Methylglyoxal is a reactive dicarbonyl compound and is involved in a variety of detrimental processes, including advanced glycation end product (AGE) formation with protein and DNA modification (*34*). Methylglyoxal is hypothesized to be cytotoxic, owing to its protein- or DNA-modifying properties. In tumor cells, the high glycolytic activity caused by rapid deregulated growth increases the intracellular levels of methylglyoxal. To eliminate cytotoxicity, detoxification systems are required. The principal route for methylglyoxal catabolism is the glyoxalase pathway, which consists of two enzymes, glyoxalase I and glyoxalase II (*33*). The regulation of these enzymes in tumor cells and their involvement in drug resistance, however, have not been fully elucidated.

The mRNA expression of glyoxalase I as well as its enzyme activity was significantly elevated in several drug-resistant cells, including UK711, UK110, and K562/ADM, as compared with their parental cells. Since these mutant cell lines were populations that survived after treatment with etoposide or adriamycin, it is possible that the development of drug resistance is accompanied by this overexpression of the enzyme. When overexpressed in human leukemia cells, glyoxalase I inhibited etoposide- and adriamycin-induced apoptosis, indicating the direct involvement of the enzyme in apoptosis suppression caused by these drugs. The expression of glyoxalase I inhibited upstream signaling of apoptosis leading to caspase protease activation. Abnormalities in the glyoxalase system are also linked with human disease states including diabetes, malaria and muscular dystrophy, and several inhibitors of glyoxalase I have been designed from analogues of the hemithioacetal substrate based on glutathione derivatives (*35*). We tested the effect of the glyoxalase I inhibitors on the apoptosis resistance of human leukemia cells. We found that cotreatment with *S-p*-bromobenzylglutathione cyclopentyl diester (BBGC), a cell-permeable inhibitor of glyoxalase I, selectively enhanced etoposide-induced apoptosis in resistant UK711 cells, but not in parental U937 cells (*31*). These results indicate that glyoxalase I inhibitors are effective drug resistance-reversing agents in human leukemia cells.

3. *Glyoxalase I as a target in cancer chemotherapy*

We quantitatively measured glyoxalase I enzyme activity in 38 human solid tumor cell lines used in our anticancer drug-screening system (*32*). We found that glyoxalase I was not only overexpressed in prostate and colon cancers, but also its activity was higher in all of the cancer cell lines than in the normal tissue samples that we examined (Fig. 3). These observations suggest that the increase of glycolytic activity could be associated with tumorigenicity as well as the drug-resistant phenotype. Among several cancer cells, we found that glyoxalase I was frequently elevated in human lung carcinoma cells. We next examined the antiproliferative effect of the glyoxalase I inhibitor. A positive correlation between cellular glyoxalase I activity and BBGC sensitivity was observed in the lung cancer cell lines (*32*). Human lung cancer cells expressing higher glyoxalase I activity underwent apoptosis when treated with BBGC, but cells expressing lower activity did not. BBGC induced stress-activated protein kinase, c-Jun N-terminal kinase 1 (JNK1) and p38 mitogen-activated protein kinase (MAP kinase) activation, leading to caspase activation in glyoxalase I-overexpressing tumor cells. Moreover, the glyoxalase I inhibitor significantly inhibited xenografted human lung cancer and human prostate cancer growth (Fig. 4). We observed no decrease in the body weight of glyoxalase I inhibitor-treated mice throughout the experiments. Our results indicate that glyoxalase I is a tumor-specific target enzyme especially in human lung cancer cells, and glyoxalase I inhibitors are potent chemotherapeutic agents with minimal cytotoxicity. When we compared the glyoxalase I inhibitor with standard anticancer drugs, the pattern of drug sensitivity to BBGC in several human solid tumor cell lines differed from those of other antitu-

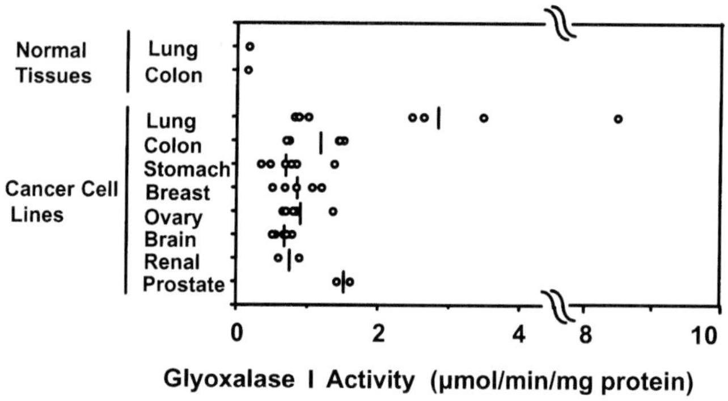

FIG. 3. Glyoxalase I activity in human solid tumor cell lines and human normal tissue samples
Cytosolic fractions were isolated, and glyoxalase 1 assays were performed. Bars, means for each cell line.

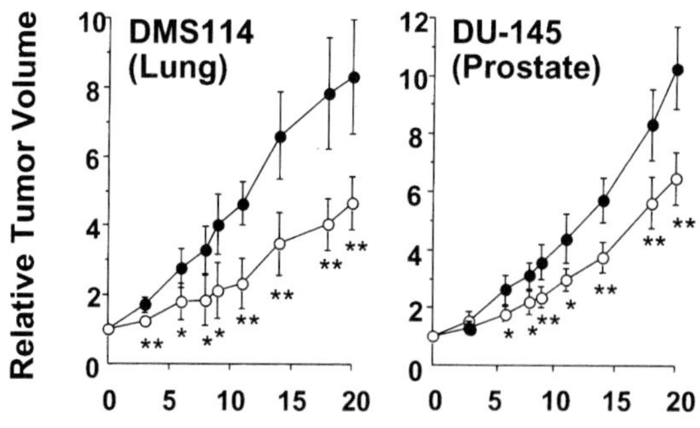

FIG. 4. Effect of BBGC on tumor growth in nude mice bearing human cancer xenografts
Tumor-bearing mice were treated with BBGC daily from days 0 to 8 at doses of 0 (● , control) and 100 mg/kg (○). The data shown are means±SD of five mice. Statistical evaluations were performed using Student's *t* test, comparing the group receiving BBGC treatment with the group receiving control treatment. * $P<0.05$, ** $P<0.01$.

mor drugs, such as DNA topoisomerase inhibitors, alkylating agents and antimitotic agents. These observations suggest that glyoxalase I inhibitors could be anticancer drugs with a novel mode of action.

4. Further insights in the mode of action of glyoxalase I-related factors in cells

Presently, the precise mechanism of apoptosis induced by glyoxalase I inhibitors is still unknown. Inhibition of glyoxalase I leads to the accumulation of methylglyoxal in cells. Since methylglyoxal is capable of inducing DNA modification and protein cross-links, DNA damage or inactivation of some antiapoptotic proteins by methylglyoxal could be an initial activator of apoptosis. Recently, several researchers have outlined the specific roles of intracellular methylglyoxal in apoptosis. Godbout *et al.* reported that methylglyoxal enhances cisplatin-induced apoptosis by activating protein kinase Cδ (*36*). It was also reported that tumor necrosis factor (TNF) induces a substantial increase in intracellular levels of methylglyoxal that leads to the formation of a specific methylglyoxal-derived advanced glycation end product (*37*). Methylglyoxal modification of proteins has also been detected in several human cancer cell lines. We recently identified heat-shock protein 27 (Hsp27) as a major methylglyoxal-modified protein in cancer cells (*38*). We showed that methylglyoxal modification was involved in Hsp27 oligomerization to prevent cytochrome *c*-mediated caspase activation during apoptosis. These data suggest that methylglyoxal modification of proteins could be a targeted process and that methylglyoxal may function as a signal molecule during the regulation of cell death. Further studies to clarify the role of intracellular methylglyoxal will give novel insights into the regulation of cell growth and provide rationale for glyoxalase-targeted chemotherapy.

Akt-Mediated Survival-Signaling Pathway

1. Akt as a promising target for cancer chemotherapy

The susceptibility of cells to apoptosis appears to be dependent on the balance between pro-apoptotic and survival (anti-apoptotic) signals. The fact that diverse chemotherapeutic drugs induce apoptosis, while engaging different intracellular targets, raises the possibility that anticancer drugs may induce apoptosis by decreasing survival signals, such as the Akt-mediated survival-signaling pathway.

The serine/threonine kinase Akt (also known as PKB or RAC-PK) is the cellular homologue of the retroviral oncogene product v-Akt (*39*). A number of reports indicate that growth factors and cytokines stimulate cell survival. After stimulation with growth factors and cytokines, phosphatidylinositide-3-OH kinase (PI3K) is activated and phosphorylates phosphoinositides. The interaction of the generated phospholipid second messenger molecule, phosphatidylinositol 3,4,5-trisphosphate (PIP_3), with the pleckstrin homology domain of Akt recruits Akt to the plasma membrane, where it is phosphorylated at two key regulatory sites, Thr^{308} (by 3-phosphoinositide-dependent protein kinase-1 (PDK1)) and Ser^{473} (by an as-yet-unidentified kinase PDK2) residues. Phosphorylation at both residues is necessary for full activation of Akt and the subsequent control of biological responses, including apoptosis inhibition (by phosphorylating the pro-apoptotic Bcl-2 family member Bad, the caspase family member caspase-9, the Forkhead transcription factor protein family, and IκB kinases) (*39*) and cell cycle progression (by phosphorylating $p21^{Waf1/Cip1}$, $p27^{Kip1}$, and

MDM2) (*39*, *40*). In this section, we document the regulation of the Akt signaling pathway by Hsp90 and the role of Akt-mediated survival-signaling pathway during chemotherapeutic drug-induced apoptosis.

2. *Identification of Akt and PDK1 as Hsp90 client proteins*

To find the molecules that interact with Akt, we performed immunoblot analysis after immunoprecipitation of Akt with an anti-Akt pAb. We could determine that Hsp90 was an Akt-binding protein (*41*). Hsp90 is an abundant and highly conserved protein involved in a diverse array of cellular processes. In contrast to other heat-shock proteins, Hsp90 is not required for maturation or maintenance of most proteins *in vivo*. Most of the identified cellular targets were signaling proteins and bound to Hsp90 via the NH_2-terminal ATP- and Hsp90-inhibitor geldanamycin-binding domain or the COOH-terminal oligomerization domain. Interestingly, Akt binds to Hsp90 through the middle domain of Hsp90 (amino acids 327–340 of Hsp90β). This result was supported by the fact that geldanamycin could not inhibit Akt binding to Hsp90. Hsp90 acts as a chaperone for unstable signal transducers and keeps them poised for activation until they are stabilized by conformational changes associated with signal transduction. Examination of the role of Hsp90 in Akt signaling by inhibiting Akt-Hsp90 binding with binding domain-containing Akt deletion mutants revealed that the blockade of Akt-Hsp90 binding inactivated Akt and increased the sensitivity of the cells to apoptosis-inducing stimuli, such as growth-factor withdrawal and chemotherapeutic drugs. We confirmed that Hsp90 binding to Akt was responsible for protection of Akt from protein phosphatase 2A (PP2A)-mediated dephosphorylation (*41*). Therefore, Akt-Hsp90 binding might play an important role in the stabilization of Akt kinase activity. Recently, we also reported that endothelial nitric oxide synthase (eNOS) formed a complex with Hsp90 through binding to Hsp90's middle domain (*42*). Because Akt-dependent phosphorylation of eNOS at Ser^{1179} was promoted by Hsp90, Hsp90 may function as a scaffold for Akt and its substrates.

Although Hsp90 inhibitors (e.g., geldanamycin, radicicol, and radicicol analogues) could not inhibit Akt-Hsp90 binding, treatment of the cells with Hsp90 inhibitors downregulated the phospho-Akt (Thr^{308}) level. Moreover, Hsp90 inhibitors did not directly affect Akt kinase activity *in vitro*. Therefore, Hsp90 inhibitors might suppress Akt signaling mainly by inhibiting upstream Akt kinases (e.g., PDK1, PI3K, PDK2). We recently showed that upstream Akt kinase PDK1 was a Hsp90 client protein (*43*). Treatment of the cells with Hsp90 inhibitors suppressed the PDK1-Hsp90 binding *in vivo* and decreased the amount of PDK1 without directly inhibiting PDK1 kinase activity. The proteasome was involved in the PDK1 degradation after inhibiting PDK1-Hsp90 binding. Treatment of proteasome inhibitors increased the amount of detergent-insoluble PDK1 in Hsp90 inhibitor-treated cells. Therefore, the association of PDK1 with Hsp90 regulates its stability, solubility, and signaling. These results indicate that Hsp90 plays an important role in the Akt signaling pathway by binding to both Akt and PDK1. Recently, 17-allylaminogeldanamycin (17-AAG) was reported to suppress Akt kinase activity by inhibiting PI3K activity in HER2-overexpressing breast cancer cells (*44*). Moreover, Akt was degraded by proteasome after 17-AAG treatment (*44*) in addition to the previously reported caspase-mediated cleavage (*45*, *46*). These results indicate that Hsp90 might be a promising target for developing new chemotherapeutic drugs to suppress the Akt-mediated survival-signaling pathway.

3. Upstream Akt kinase PDK1 is a molecular target of some chemotherapeutic drugs

Screening of chemotherapeutic drugs that possess direct effects on the Akt pathway revealed that staurosporine and a water-soluble CPT analogue, topotecan (10-hydroxy-9-dimethylaminomethyl-(*S*)-camptothecin), in addition to the above-mentioned Hsp90 inhibitors, possessed the ability to decrease the phospho-Akt (Thr^{308}) level in cells (Fig. 5).

Because the staurosporine analogue UCN-01 (7-hydroxystaurosporine) exhibited potent anti-tumor activity in *in vivo* and *in vitro* tumor models, its clinical usefulness has been investigated in the United States. UCN-01 was originally isolated as a selective protein kinase C (PKC) inhibitor from the culture broth of *Streptomyces* sp. The PKC family was thought to be a major target of UCN-01; however, it is still unclear whether PKC is the sole target of UCN-01 and how PKC inhibition is involved in its anti-tumor activity. Examining the effect of UCN-01 on the Akt signaling pathway revealed that UCN-01 directly suppressed upstream Akt kinase PDK1 with an IC_{50} value lower than 33 n*M* in *in vitro* and *in vivo* assays (*47*). UCN-01's inhibitory effect on PDK1 was also observed in xenografted murine NL-17 and human PC-3 tumors. By contrast, UCN-01 had marginal effects on Akt and PI3K activities. Overexpression of the active form of Akt diminished the cytotoxic effects of UCN-01, indicating that UCN-01 may exert its cytotoxicity in part by inhibiting the PDK1-Akt survival pathway. Because UCN-01 has already been proved to have potent anti-tumor activity *in vivo* and *in vitro*, the Akt-PDK1 pathway may be a promising target for tumor treatment.

We also tried to identify the molecular target(s) of topotecan on the Akt signaling pathway because topotecan decreased the Akt kinase activity in cells (*48*). Topotecan is a novel topoisomerase I inhibitor that has shown activity against numerous human tumor cell lines and xenografts. Topotecan has also shown clinical activity in small cell and non-small cell bronchogenic carcinoma, ovarian carcinoma and mye-

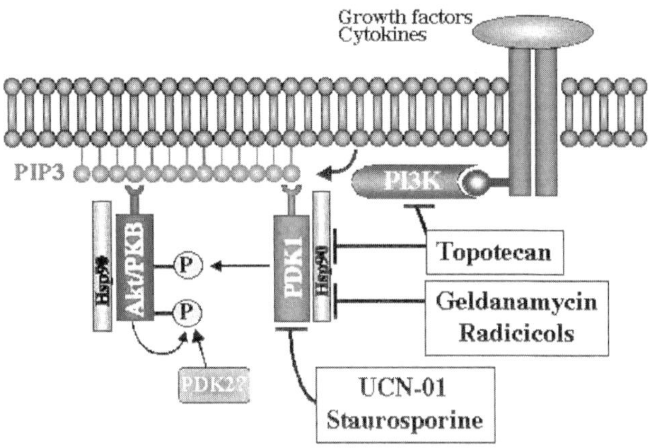

FIG. 5. Schematic representation of molecular targets of topotecan, UCN-01, and Hsp90 inhibitors (geldanamycin and radicicol and their analogues)

loid leukemia, and has been approved for the treatment of relapsed ovarian cancer and small cell lung cancer. Interestingly, Akt dephosphorylation could not be seen in topotecan-resistant A549/CPT cell line. This fact suggests that Akt inactivation plays an important role in the exhibition of topotecan-mediated cytotoxic effects. Topotecan was revealed to exert its cytotoxic effects in part by suppressing the kinase activities of upstream Akt kinases PI3K and PDK1. The PI3K-Akt signaling pathway appears to play an important role in angiogenesis. Examination of topotecan's effect on endothelial cells revealed that topotecan downregulated the *in vitro* migration of endothelial cells (*49*). Transfection of constitutively active *akt* cDNA restored topotecan's inhibitory effect on endothelial migration, indicating that topotecan might exert its antiangiogenic activity by downregulating the PI3K-Akt signaling pathway.

Because the Akt signaling pathway is also associated with metastasis formation of some tumor cells (*50*), the pathway (particularly upstream Akt kinase PDK1) is a promising new target for developing chemotherapeutic drugs to treat tumors (Fig. 5).

REFERENCES

1. Tsuruo T. Mechanisms of multidrug resistance and implications for therapy. *Jpn J Cancer Res* 1988; **79**: 285–96.
2. Sugimoto Y, Tsuruo T. DNA-mediated transfer and cloning of a human multidrug-resistant gene of Adriamycin-resistant myelogenous leukemia K562. *Cancer Res* 1987; **47**: 2620–5.
3. Hamada H, Tsuruo T. Functional role for the 170- to 180-kDa glycoprotein specific to drug-resistant tumor cells as revealed by monoclonal antibodies. *Proc Natl Acad Sci USA* 1986; **83**: 7785–9.
4. Hamada H, Tsuruo T. Purification of the 170- to 180-kilodalton membrane glycoprotein associated with multidrug resistance. *J Biol Chem* 1988; **263**: 1454–8.
5. Naito M, Hamada H, Tsuruo T. ATP/Mg^{2+}-dependent binding of vincristine to the plasma membrane of multidrug-resistant K562 cells. *J Biol Chem* 1988; **263**: 11887–91.
6. Tsuruo T, Iida H, Tsukagoshi S, Sakurai Y. Overcoming of vincristine resistance in P388 leukemia *in vivo* and *in vitro* through enhanced cytotoxicity of vincristine and vinblastine by verapamil. *Cancer Res* 1981; **41**: 1967–72.
7. Tsuruo T, Iida H, Tsukagoshi S, Sakurai Y. Increased accumulation of vincristine and adriamycin in drug resistant P388 tumor cells following incubation with calcium antagonists and calmodulin inhibitors. *Cancer Res* 1982; **42**: 4730–3.
8. Tsuruo T, Iida H, Tsukagoshi S, Sakurai Y. Potentiation of vincristine and adriamycin effects in human hemopoietic tumor cell lines by calcium antagonists and calmodulin inhibitors. *Cancer Res* 1983; **43**: 2267–72.
9. Tsuruo T, Iida H, Nojiri M, Tsukagoshi S, Sakurai Y. Circumvention of vincristine and adriamycin resistance *in vitro* and *in vivo* by calcium influx blockers. *Cancer Res* 1983; **43**: 2905–10.
10. Sato W, Fukazawa N, Nakanishi O, Baba M, Suzuki T, Yano O, Naito M, Tsuruo T. Reversal of multidrug resistance by a novel quinoline derivative, MS-209. *Cancer Chemother Pharmacol* 1995; **35**: 271–7.
11. Natio M, Tsuruo T. Competitive inhibition by verapamil of ATP-dependent high affinity vincristine binding to the plasma membrane of multidrug-resistant K562 cells

without calcium ion involvement. *Cancer Res* 1989; **49**: 1452–5.

12. Thiebaut F, Tsuruo T, Hamada H, Gottesman MM, Pastan I, Willingham MC. Cellular localization of the multidrug-resistance gene product P-glycoprotein in normal tissues. *Proc Natl Acad Sci USA* 1987; **84**: 7735–8.
13. Tatsuta T, Naito M, Oh-hara T, Sugawara I, Tsuruo T. Functional involvement of P-glycoprotein in blood-brain barrier. *J Biol Chem* 1992; **267**: 20383–91.
14. Hamada H, Miura K, Ariyoshi K, Heike Y, Sato S, Kameyama K, Kurosawa Y, Tsuruo T. Mouse-human chimeric antibody against the multidrug transporter P-glycoprotein. *Cancer Res* 1990; **50**: 3167–71.
15. Watanabe T, Naito M, Kokubo N, Tsuruo T. Regression of established tumors expressing P-glycoprotein by combinations of adriamycin, cyclosporin derivatives, and MRK-16 antibodies. *J Natl Cancer Inst* 1997; **89**: 512–8.
16. Sugimoto Y, Sato S, Tsukahara S, Suzuki M, Okochi E, Gottesman MM, Pastan I, Tsuruo T. Coexpression of a multidrug resistance gene (MDR1) and herpes simplex virus thymidine kinase gene in a bicistronic retroviral vector Ha-MDR-IRES-TK allows selective killing of MDR1-transduced human tumors transplanted in nude mice. *Cancer Gene Ther* 1997; **4**: 51–8.
17. Brown JM, Giaccia AJ. The unique physiology of solid tumors: opportunities (and problems) for cancer therapy. *Cancer Res* 1998; **58**: 1408–16.
18. Tomida A, Tsuruo T. Drug resistance mediated by cellular stress response to the microenvironment of solid tumors. *Anticancer Drug Des* 1999; **14**: 169–77.
19. Kaufman RJ, Scheuner D, Schroder M, Shen X, Lee K, Liu CY, Arnold SM. The unfolded protein response in nutrient sensing and differentiation. *Nat Rev Mol Cell Biol* 2002; **3**: 411–21.
20. Shen J, Hughes C, Chao C, Cai J, Bartels C, Gessner T, Subjeck J. Coinduction of glucose-regulated proteins and doxorubicin resistance in Chinese hamster cells. *Proc Natl Acad Sci USA* 1987; **84**: 3278–82.
21. Yun J, Tomida A, Nagata K, Tsuruo T. Glucose-regulated stresses confer resistance to VP-16 in human cancer cells through a decreased expression of DNA topoisomerase II. *Oncol Res* 1995; **7**: 583–90.
22. Rubin EH, Li TK, Duann P, Liu LF. Cellular resistance to topoisomerase poisons. *Cancer Treat Res* 1996; **87**: 243–60.
23. Kim HD, Tomida A, Ogiso Y, Tsuruo T. Glucose-regulated stresses cause degradation of DNA topoisomerase IIalpha by inducing nuclear proteasome during G1 cell cycle arrest in cancer cells. *J Cell Physiol* 1999; **180**: 97–104.
24. Ogiso Y, Tomida A, Lei S, Omura S, Tsuruo T. Proteasome inhibition circumvents solid tumor resistance to topoisomerase II-directed drugs. *Cancer Res* 2000; **60**: 2429–34.
25. Adams J. Proteasome inhibition: a novel approach to cancer therapy. *Trends Mol Med* 2002; **8**: S49–54.
26. Ogiso Y, Tomida A, Kim HD, Tsuruo T. Glucose starvation and hypoxia induce nuclear accumulation of proteasome in cancer cells. *Biochem Biophys Res Commun* 1999; **258**: 448–52.
27. Ogiso Y, Tomida A, Tsuruo T. Nuclear localization of proteasomes participates in stress-inducible resistance of solid tumor cells to topoisomerase II-directed drugs. *Can-*

cer Res 2002; **62**: 5008–12.
28. Horie K, Tomida A, Sugimoto Y, Yasugi T, Yoshikawa H, Taketani Y, Tsuruo T. SUMO-1 conjugation to intact DNA topoisomerase I amplifies cleavable complex formation induced by camptothecin. *Oncogene* 2002; **21**: 7913–22.
29. Kaufmann SH, Earnshaw WC. Induction of apoptosis by cancer chemotherapy. *Exp Cell Res* 2000; **256**: 42–9.
30. Kataoka S, Naito M, Tomida A, Tsuruo T. Resistance to antitumor agent-induced apoptosis in a mutant of human myeloid leukemia U937 cells. *Exp Cell Res* 1994; **215**: 199–205.
31. Sakamoto H, Mashima T, Kizaki A, Dan S, Hashimoto Y, Naito M, Tsuruo T. Glyoxalase I is involved in resistance of human leukemia cells to antitumor agent-induced apoptosis. *Blood* 2000; **95**: 3214–8.
32. Sakamoto H, Mashima T, Sato S, Hashimoto Y, Yamori T, Tsuruo T. Selective activation of apoptosis program by S-p-bromobenzylglutathione cyclopentyl diester in glyoxalase I-overexpressing human lung cancer cells. *Clin Cancer Res* 2001; **7**: 2513–8.
33. Thornalley PJ. The glyoxalase system: new developments towards functional characterization of a metabolic pathway fundamental to biological life. *Biochem J* 1990; **269**: 1–11.
34. Lo TW, Westwood ME, McLellan AC, Selwood T, Thornalley PJ. Binding and modification of proteins by methylglyoxal under physiological conditions. A kinetic and mechanistic study with N alpha-acetylarginine, N-alpha-acetylcysteine, and N-alpha-acetyllysine, and bovine serum albumin. *J Biol Chem* 1994; **269**: 32299–305.
35. Thornalley PK. Esterification of reduced glutathione. *Biochem J* 1991; **275**: 535–9.
36. Godbout JP, Pesavento J, Hartman ME, Manson SR, Freund GG. Methylglyoxal enhances cisplatin-induced cytotoxicity by activating protein kinase Cδ. *J Biol Chem* 2002; **277**: 2554–61.
37. Van Herreweghe F, Mao J, Chaplen FW, Grooten J, Gevaert K, Vandekerckhove J, Vancompernolle K. Tumor necrosis factor-induced modulation of glyoxalase I activities through phosphorylation by PKA results in cell death and is accompanied by the formation of a specific methylglyoxal-derived AGE. *Proc Natl Acad Sci USA* 2002; **99**: 949–54.
38. Sakamoto H, Mashima T, Yamamoto K, Tsuruo, T. Modulation of heat-shock protein 27 (Hsp27) anti-apoptotic activity by methylglyoxal-modification. *J Biol Chem* 2002; **277**: 45770–5.
39. Vanhaesebroeck B, Alessi DR. The PI3K-PDK1 connection: more than just a road to PKB. *Biochem J* 2000; **346**: 561–76.
40. Fujita N, Sato S, Katayama K, Tsuruo T. Akt-dependent phosphorylation of p27Kip1 promotes binding to 14-3-3 and cytoplasmic localization. *J Biol Chem* 2002; **277**: 28706–13.
41. Sato S, Fujita N, Tsuruo T. Modulation of Akt kinase activity by binding to Hsp90. *Proc Natl Acad Sci USA* 2000; **97**: 10832–7.
42. Fontana J, Fulton D, Chen Y, Fairchild TA, McCabe TJ, Fujita N, Tsuruo T, Sessa WC. Domain mapping studies reveal that the M domain of hsp90 serves as a molecular scaffold to regulate Akt-dependent phosphorylation of endothelial nitric oxide synthase and NO release. *Circ Res* 2002; **90**: 866–73.

43. Fujita N, Sato S, Ishida A, Tsuruo T. Involvement of Hsp90 in signaling and stability of 3-phosphoinositide-dependent kinase-1. *J Biol Chem* 2002; **277**: 10346–53.
44. Basso AD, Solit DB, Munster PN, Rosen N. Ansamycin antibiotics inhibit Akt activation and cyclin D expression in breast cancer cells that overexpress HER2. *Oncogene* 2002; **21**: 1159–66.
45. Bachelder RE, Wendt MA, Fujita N, Tsuruo T, Mercurio AM. The cleavage of Akt/PKB by death receptor signaling is an important event in detachment-induced apoptosis. *J Biol Chem* 2001; **276**: 34702–7.
46. Rokudai S, Fujita N, Hashimoto Y, Tsuruo T. Cleavage and inactivation of antiapoptotic Akt/PKB by caspases during apoptosis. *J Cell Physiol* 2000; **182**: 290–6.
47. Sato S, Fujita N, Tsuruo T. Interference with PDK1-Akt survival signaling pathway by UCN-01 (7-hydroxystaurosporine). *Oncogene* 2002; **21**: 1727–38.
48. Nakashio A, Fujita N, Rokudai S, Sato S, Tsuruo T. Prevention of phosphatidylinositol 3′-kinase-Akt survival-signaling pathway during topotecan-induced apoptosis. *Cancer Res* 2000; **60**: 5303–9.
49. Nakashio A, Fujita N, Tsuruo T. Topotecan inhibits VEGF- and bFGF-induced vascular endothelial cell migration via downregulation of PI3K-Akt signaling pathway. *Int J Cancer* 2002; **98**: 36–41.
50. Nakanishi K, Sakamoto M, Yasuda J, Takamura M, Fujita N, Tsuruo T, Toda S, Hirohashi S. Critical involvement of the phosphatidylinositol 3-kinase/Akt pathway in anchorage-independent growth and hematogenous intrahepatic metastasis of liver cancer. *Cancer Res* 2002; **62**: 2971–5.

Gann Monograph on Cancer Research 52, 2004

THE BASIC AND CLINICAL IMPLICATIONS OF ABC TRANSPORTERS, Y-BOX-BINDING PROTEIN-1 (YB-1) AND ANGIOGENESIS-RELATED FACTORS IN HUMAN MALIGNANCIES

Michihiko KUWANO[*1], Takeshi UCHIUMI[*2], Hiroshi HAYAKAWA[*2], Mayumi ONO[*2], Morimasa WADA[*2], Hiroto IZUMI[*3] and Kimitoshi KOHNO[*3]

*Research Center for Innovative Cancer Therapy, Kurume University[*1], Department of Medical Biochemistry, Graduate School of Medical Sciences, Kyushu University[*2] and Department of Molecular Biology, University of Occupational and Environmental Health[*3]*

In our laboratories, we have been studying molecular targets which might be advantageous for novel cancer therapeutics. In this review, we focus on how ATP-binding cassette (ABC) transporter superfamily genes, Y-box-binding protein-1 (YB-1), and tumor angiogenesis-associated factors could contribute to the development of novel strategies for molecular cancer therapeutics. ABC transporters such as P-glycoprotein/MDR1 and several MRP family proteins function to protect cells from xenobiotics, drugs and poisons, suggesting that ABC transporters are a double-edged sword. In this regard, P-glycoprotein/MDR1 is a representative ABC transporter which plays a critical role in the efflux of a wide range of drugs. We have reported that gene amplification, gene rearrangements, transcription factor YB-1 and CpG methylation on the promoter are involved in *MDR1* gene overexpression in cultured cancer cells. Among them, two mechanisms appear to be relevant to the up-regulation of *MDR1* gene in human malignancies. We first reported that *MDR1* gene promoter is activated in response to environmental stimuli, and is modulated by methylation/demethylation of CpG sites on the MDR1 promoter. We also demonstrated that YB-1 modulates not only transcription of various genes associated with cell growth, drug resistance and DNA synthesis, but also translation, mRNA stabilization and DNA repair/self-defense processes. Angiogenesis is also involved in tumor growth, invasion and metastasis of various malignancies, and so angiogenesis-related molecules also offer novel molecular targets for anticancer therapeutics.

A recent focus in cancer therapeutic strategy is the challenge to develop molecular cancer therapeutics. The American Association for Cancer Research has recently

*1 Kurume, Fukuoka 830-0011, Japan
*2 Fukuoka 812-8582, Japan
*3 Kitakyushu, Fukuoka 807-8555, Japan

This paper is dedicated to the memory of late Dr. Tomizo Yoshida on the occasion of the 100th anniversary of his birth. It was originally published in Cancer Science in January, 2003.

founded a new journal, "Molecular Cancer Therapeutics." The Japanese Association for Molecular Target Therapy of Cancer also focuses on molecular therapeutics. In our laboratories, we have studied how ATP-binding cassette (ABC) transporter superfamily genes, Y-box-binding protein-1 (YB-1), DNA topoisomerase IIα, glutathione *S*-transferases, thioredoxin and tumor angiogenesis-associated factors could contribute to novel strategies for molecular cancer therapeutics. By understanding how each molecular target is specifically expressed in cancer cells and normal cells, we can use evidence-based medicine to choose which anticancer agent is most suitable for each patient. Furthermore, some target-based drugs including Glivec targeting Bcr-Abl, Herceptin targeting Her2, Rituximab targeting CD20, and Iressa targeting EGF receptor are already in clinical use. In this review, we would like to discuss how ABC transporters and YB-1 are involved in limiting drug sensitivity to anticancer agents. We also refer to the development of novel anticancer agents targeting matrix metalloproteinases, vascular endothelial growth factor (VEGF) receptors and epidermal growth factor (EGF) receptor in association with angiogenesis. We will present a novel strategy for development of antiangiogenic drugs by targeting tumor stromal cells, including infiltrating monocyte/macrophages, based on an understanding at the molecular level of the cross-talk between cancer cells and stromal cells.

ABC Transporters: P-Glycoprotein/MDR1 and Several MRP Family Proteins Function to Protect Cells from Xenobiotics Including Drugs and Poisons

About 50 ABC transporter genes are thought to be present in the human chromosome (URL: 48 Human ATP-Binding Cassette Transporters, http://nutrigene.4t.com/humanabc.htm) (*1*). The acquisition of multidrug resistance in cancer cells is often associated with increased expression of various cell surface ABC transporters. ABC transporters are also known to recognize various physiological substances, as well as drugs, including anticancer agents (Table I).

Among the ABC transporters, P-glycoprotein encoded by the *MDR1* gene on 7q21.1 mediates drug resistance to the widest variety of anticancer agents, indicating that P-glycoprotein is one of the most important molecular targets in attempts to limit drug resistance/sensitivity in human malignancies (*2–4*). Expression of the *MDR1* gene is often augmented through gene amplification in human cancer cell lines selected *in vitro* for drug resistance to P-glycoprotein-targeting anticancer agents, and the gene amplification unit was estimated to be 800 kb to 1 Mb in size when the copy number was examined by using probes isolated from YAC contigs spanning the *MDR1* gene region (*5, 6*). A critical problem is how expression of the human *MDR1* gene is specifically modulated in human malignancies. Moreover, multidrug-resistant cell lines selected for resistance to taxol, doxorubicin or vincristine show gene rearrangements or retrovirus insertion in the 5′-flanking region (*7, 8*). However, gene amplification and rearrangements of the *MDR1* gene have not yet been reported in cancer patients.

Two mechanisms appeared be relevant to the up-regulation of the *MDR1* gene in human malignancies. Since the first report that the *MDR1* gene promoter is activated in response to environmental stimuli (*9*), many studies have consistently supported the idea that the *MDR1* gene is a stress-induced *SOS* gene (*10*). This up-regulation of the *MDR1* gene by anticancer agents or ultraviolet light irradiation is

TABLE I. Comparison of Chromosome Location, Expression in Normal Tissues and Tumors, and Substrates of Six ABC Transporter Family Genes

Gene	*MDR1/PGY1*	*MRP/MRP1*	*MRP2/cMOAT*	*MRP3*	*MRP4*	*MXR1/BCRP*
Protein	P-glycoprotein 1280 amino acids	multidrug resistance associated protein 1531 amino acids	canalicular multispecific organic anion transporter 1545 amino acids	MRP3 1527 amino acids	MRP4 1325 amino acids	MXR1/BCRP 655 amino acids
Chromosome	7q21	16p13.1	10q24	17q22	13q32	4q22
Expression in normal tissue	adrenal gland, kidney, liver (canalicular membrane),[a] colon, brain (endothelial cell), uterus (pregnancy)	placenta, testis, lung, skeletal muscle, heart, monocyte, liver (sinusoidal membrane)	liver (canalicular membrane), duodenum, kidney	liver, duodenum, colon, adrenal gland, pancreas, kidney	(pancreas, skeletal muscle, lung, kidney, bladder)[b]	placenta, breast, liver, intestine
Altered expression in human cancer	neuroblastoma, leukemia, lymphoma, breast, pancreas, colon, adrenal, liver, renal, ovarian, non-small-cell lung carcinoma	neuroblastoma, lymphoma, leukemia, non-small-cell lung, anaplastic thyroid, esophageal, gastric cancer	leukemia, colon cancer	colon cancer	NE[c]	breast cancer
Substrates	neutral and cationic organic compounds	glutathione and glucuronate conjugates, glutathione	glucuronate and glutathione conjugates, glutathione	glucuronate and sulfite conjugates, bile salts	nucleoside monophosphate analogues	NE
Anticancer drugs	**Vinca alkaloids** vincristine vinblastine **Anthracyclines** doxorubicin daunorubicin **Epipodophylotoxins** etoposide teniposide Pacritaxel Colchicine Actinomycin D	**Anthracyclines** doxorubicin daunorubicin **Epipodophylotoxins** etoposide teniposide **Vinca alkaloids** vincristine vinblastine **Antimetabolites** methotrexate	**Vinca alkaloids** vincristine vinblastine **Camptothecins** CPT-11 SN-38 cisplatin **Antimetabolites** methotrexate	**Epipodophylotoxins** etoposide teniposide **Anthracyclines** doxorubicin **Antimetabolites** methotrexate	**Antimetabolites** methotrexate thiopurines	**Anthracyclines** doxorubicin daunorubicin **Camptothecins** CPT-11 SN-38 topotecan **Antimetabolites** mitoxantrone

[a] Parentheses indicate precise subcellular location or cell type which expresses the mRNA in organs ("normal tissue" line) or the precise human cancer type ("human cancer" line).
[b] Low expression.
[c] Not established.

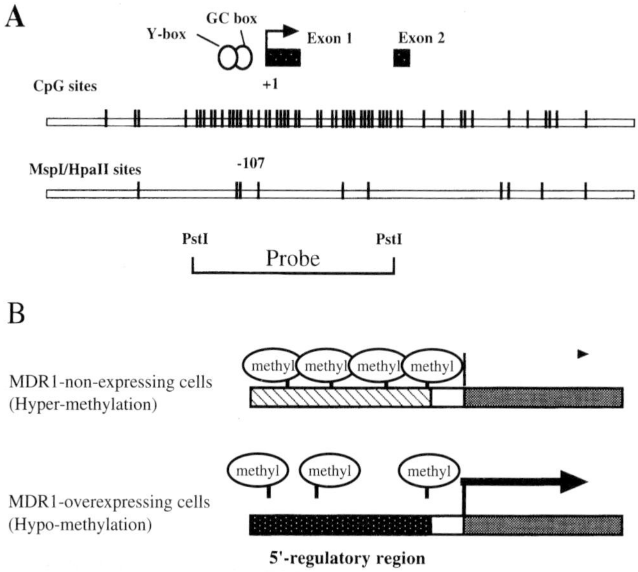

FIG. 1. Methylation status of CpG sites on the MDR1 promoter plays a key role in the switch-on of *MDR1* gene expression in human malignancies
(A) The MDR1 promoter region is rich in CpG sites. (B) The promoter region is hypomethylated in MDR1-overexpressing cells in cancerous tissues and hypermethylated in non-expressing cells.

mediated through activation of either YB-1 (*11–13*) or NF-Y. YB-1- or NF-Y-binding sites are localized at −70 to −100 bp on the human MDR1 promoter. Nuclear localization of YB-1 is significantly associated with expression of MDR1/P-glycoprotein in some tumor types, such as breast cancer (*14*) and osteosarcoma. (*15*)

Another key mechanism is methylation/demethylation of CpG sites on the MDR1 promoter. Three independent studies with drug-resistant cell lines in culture consistently support the idea that the methylation status of certain CpG sites on the MDR1 promoter plays a critical role in switch-on or -off of *MDR1* gene expression (Fig. 1). Introduction of YAC-human *MDR1* gene (800 kb) into mouse cells resulted in successful expression of the human *MDR1* gene and down-regulation of the mouse *mdr1a* gene, in concert with hypo- and hyper-methylation of CpG sites on the human MDR1 promoter and endogenous mouse *mdr1a* genes (*16*). Another line of evidence comes from the analysis of KB/CdR-1 and KB/CdR-2 cell lines, which were established after exposure of human epidermal cancer KB3-1 cells to 5-azacytidine; they show up-regulation of MDR1 mRNA and altered hypo-methylation status at CpG sites at −100 bp from the initiation site of transcription (*17*). Moreover, a multidrug-resistant cell line, KB/VJ300, which was isolated from human epidermal cancer KB3-1 cells shows a marked increase of MDR1 mRNA, but no amplification of the *MDR1* gene (*9*). Further study demonstrated a specific demethylation of CpG sites at around −100 bp on the MDR1 promoter in KB/VJ300 cells (*17*). Taken together, these experiments with cultured cell lines indicate a close linkage between methylation/demethylation status of CpG sites at −80 to −100 bp on the promoter and expression of the *MDR1* gene (Fig. 1).

One could next ask if the methylation status of the MDR1 promoter might also limit P-glycoprotein-mediated drug resistance in cancer patients. Analysis of the methylation status of the MDR1 promoter showed that methylation status is inversely correlated with the expression levels of MDR1 mRNA in myeloid leukemia and bladder cancers (*18*, *19*). Many studies have consistently reported that MDR1 mRNA or protein levels are increased in acute myeloid leukemia (AML) patients with refractory status. In bladder cancer, MDR1 mRNA levels are markedly increased by systemic or local treatment with anticancer agents (*19*). The methylation status of promoters of other genes besides the *MDR1* gene also closely affects recurrence in patients with bladder cancer (*20*). The underlying mechanism by which methylation status in the promoter regions of the *MDR1* gene and other genes is associated with malignancy in cancer patients remains unclear. However, the methylation status of the MDR1 promoter does appear to play a critical role in switch-on or -off of *MDR1* gene expression during therapeutic treatment (see Fig. 1). Further study is needed to examine why the methylation status of certain genes is altered in association with the pathological state of human malignancies, and also if methylation/demethylation status could be a molecular target for development of novel diagnosis and treatment strategies.

MRP1 was isolated as the first human MRP family protein by Cole *et al.* (*21*), and further *MRP* family genes such as human *MRP2* (*22*), *MRP3* (*23*) and *MRP4* (*24*) and others have been isolated. Various endogenous and exogenous substances, including drugs, are recognized and effluxed by MRP1 (*25*), MRP2 (*26–28*), MRP3 (*29*) and MRP4 (*30*), as established using various drug-resistant cell lines expressing ABC transporter cDNA and antisense cell lines or knock-out cell lines and mice (Table I). P-glycoprotein/MDR1 and MRP1 are expressed in various hematopoietic cancers and solid tumors, and their clinical significance in limiting drug sensitivity/resistance has often been discussed (*2*, *3*, *31*). Further study is required to understand if these ABC transporters play clinically significant roles in limiting the sensitivity of human malignancies to anticancer treatment.

YB-1: A Nucleic Acid-Binding Protein with Pleiotropic Functions in Cytoplasm and Nucleus

YB-1 is one of the most evolutionally conserved nucleic acid binding proteins. It possesses a wide variety of cellular functions, including transcriptional regulation, translational regulation, induction of repair systems for DNA damage, cell proliferation, and cellular SOS responses to environmental stress (*32*). YB-1 was first isolated as a transcription factor bound to the Y-box on the MHC class II promoter (*33*). The consensus binding site for YB-1 was defined as 5′-CTGATTGG-3′, identical to the CCAAT box on the promoter of the *MHC class II* gene and also *MDR1* (*11*, *12*) and *DNA topoisomerase II*α gene. Over the years, various identical or homologous human cDNA clones have been isolated (Fig. 2). The nucleic acid-binding domain of the vertebrate protein is ~40% identical to a cold-shock protein from bacteria. YB-1 is thus one of the superfamily of proteins that contain the cold-shock domain. We identified YB-1 interacting with Y-box on the MDR1 promoter, which is activated in response to environmental stimuli (*9*, *13*). YB-1 is now known to either positively or negatively regulate expression of various genes (Table II). YB-1 also shows pleiotropic modulation of not only transcription, but also translation or DNA repair/self-de-

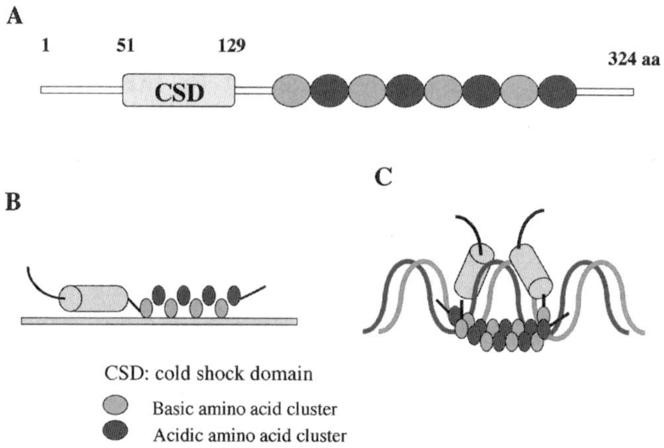

FIG. 2. Structure and functional domains of YB-1
(A) YB-1 protein (324 amino acids) consists of three domains: a variable N-terminal domain, a highly conserved nucleic acid-binding domain CSD (cold shock domain) and a C-terminal basic and acidic amino acid cluster domain. (B) The C-terminal region of YB-1 has strong affinity for single-stranded DNA/RNA *in vitro.* (C) The CSD of YB-1 has affinity for double-stranded DNA *in vitro* and the C-terminal region is involved in dimerization.

TABLE II. Summary of Genes Susceptible to YB-1-Dependent Regulation

Positive regulation	Negative regulation
MDR1	GM-CSF
$p21^{Cip1}$	Fas (CD95/Apo-1)
rat gelatinase A genes	MHC class II
HIV-1	grp 78
JCV early and late gene	thyrotropin receptor
rat alpha (1) procollagen gene	
matrix metalloproteinase 2	
myosin light chain 2v	
annexin I genes	

fense processes.

The structural and functional analysis of the human *YB-1* gene promoter shows multiple E-boxes and GC-boxes, and C-Myc binds to the E-boxes, resulting in transactivation of the *YB-1* gene through interaction with p73, a relative of p53 (*34*). Ohga *et al.* (*35*) have reported that introduction of antisense YB-1 results in altered drug sensitivity to cisplatin, mitomycin C and ultraviolet light irradiation. The two-hybrid system and protein affinity assay with YB-1 show not only that various protein synthesis-associated proteins, including ribosomal protein IRP2, interact with YB-1 (*36*), but also that cisplatin or ultraviolet light-modified DNA or 8-oxoguanine-containing RNA shows increased affinity for YB-1 (*37, 38*). Moreover, interaction of p53 or PCNA with YB-1 (*38, 39*) might be prerequisite for self-defense of cells exposed to DNA-damaging stimuli. Nuclear localization of YB-1 was found to be closely associated with the prognosis or survival of patients with ovarian cancer or with non-small cell lung cancer (*40*). YB-1 expression was also closely associated with drug resistance or patient outcome in breast cancers (*41*) and colon cancers (*42*). Expression of YB-1 thus appears to have prognostic and predictive significance in several human malignancies.

Angiogenesis: Role in Growth of Malignant Tumors

Angiogenesis is expected to be involved not only in tumor growth, invasion and metastasis of various malignancies, but also in switch-on of carcinogenesis in some animal models (*43*). Folkman proposed a kind of homeostasis of angiogenesis, and reported that protein fragments such as angiostatin and endostatin derived from physiological substances, plasminogen and type XVIII collagen, respectively, induce and sustain dormancy of tumors in mice (*44*).

Antiangiogenesis as a therapeutic strategy has been developed by targeting angiogenic factors and their cognate receptors, matrix metalloproteinases, integrins, aminopeptidases, and also by using antiangiogenic peptides themselves. Unfortunately, clinical trials of Marimastat, a matrix metalloproteinase-targeting agent, have resulted in side effects such as muscle and joint pains. We have performed a preclinical study on one metalloproteinase inhibitor with a similar chemical structure to Marimastat, and observed a marked inhibitory effect on angiogenesis *in vitro* as well as *in vivo*, and also on metastasis in an animal model (*45*). Drugs targeting VEGF/VEGF receptor may also be effective, because VEGF receptors are known to be mainly expressed in vascular endothelial cells, but not in cancer cells. A specific inhibitor of the VEGF receptor KDR/Flk-1, as well as Flt-1, shows specific and potent antiangiogenesis activity in various experimental model systems (*46*). However, VEGF/VEGF receptor targeting drugs has not yet been shown to have therapeutic efficacy in a clinical trial. We may need to understand the tumor-associated angiogenesis scenario in more detail at the molecular level.

To understand tumor angiogenesis, interaction of cancer cells with vessels and other many stroma cell types should be analyzed (*47*). For example, changes of cytokines, oxygen, glucose and pH, and also infiltration of monocytes/macrophages and other cell types are likely to be important. Oxygen stress and pH change apparently affect angiogenic switching in an angiogenesis model; hydrogen peroxide up-regulates an angiogenic factor, IL-8 (*48*), and acidic pH affects the production of a proteolytic fragment like angiostatin generated from plasminogen by cathepsins (*49*). We also reported that macrophage infiltration is closely associated with angiogenesis *in vitro* as well as *in vivo* (*50, 51*). Tumor necrosis factor (TNF)-α and interleukin (IL)-1, representative cytokines, enhance the production of potent angiogenic factors, VEGF, IL-8, basic fibroblast growth factor (bFGF), and metalloproteinase(s) from endothelial cells and cancer cells, resulting in switching-on of angiogenesis through autocrine and/or paracrine pathways. We found that treatment of macrophages with interferon-γ results in enhanced expression of *thymidine phosphorylase* gene through activation of the γ-activation sequence-like element (*52*), suggesting a possible involvement of interferon in macrophage activation in association with angiogenesis. Based on these results, we proposed a novel approach for development of antiangiogenic drugs by targeting tumor stromal cells, including infiltrating monocyte/macrophages, through an understanding of cross-talk between cancer cells and stromal cells at the molecular level (*47*).

A recent highlight is the development of drugs targeting the EGF receptor. Interaction of EGF/TGF (transforming growth factor) α with cell surface EGF recep-

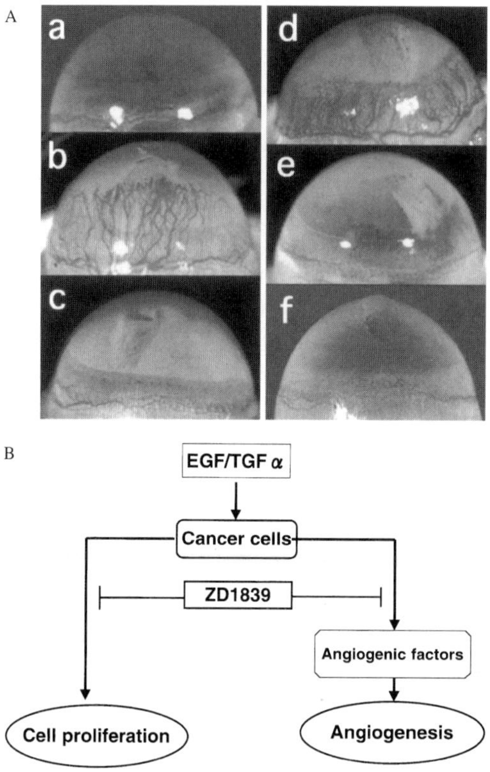

FIG. 3. Inhibition of angiogenesis by ZD1839 (Iressa)
(A) Effect of ZD1839 on angiogenesis *in vivo*. Angiogenesis induced in mouse corneas by EGF was inhibited by ZD1839 and partially inhibited by SU5416, an inhibitor of VEGF receptor KDR/Flk-1 tyrosine kinase. Angiogenesis induced by VEGF was inhibited by SU5416, but not by ZD1839. (a) Buffer alone, (b) EGF, (c) EGF with ZD1839, (d) VEGF, (e) VEGF with SU5416, (f) VEGF with ZD1839. (B) A model for dual inhibitory effects by ZD1839 on angiogenesis and cell proliferation. EGF/TGFα upregulates expression of angiogenic factors such as VEGF and IL-8 in cancer cells, and these angiogenesis-related factors induce angiogenesis by paracrine control. ZD1839 is also expected to inhibit cell proliferation and other EGF/TGFα-dependent processes promoting tumor growth.

tor induces various signals influencing cell survival, apoptosis, cell adhesion, proliferation and angiogenesis. We hypothesize that a specific inhibitor of EGF receptor tyrosine kinase can exert antiangiogenesis activity through the following mechanisms. Angiogenesis induced in corneas by EGF is almost completely blocked by a EGF receptor tyrosine kinase inhibitor, ZD1839 (Iressa), but not by a VEGF receptor tyrosine kinase inhibitor, SU5416 (Fig. 3A) (*46*). The former inhibitor could modulate production of various potent angiogenic factors such as VEGF, IL8, and others from cancer cells, resulting in inhibition of angiogenesis (Fig. 3B) (*53*). EGF receptor-targeting drugs could thus affect not only cell proliferation and the cell cycle, but also angiogenesis, and thus may modulate multiple biological functions associated with tumor growth and metastasis. Further efforts to understand the mechanisms of tumor angiogenesis should provide invaluable clues to facilitate the discovery of novel molecular targets for both diagnosis and therapeutic strategies against human malignant cancers.

Conclusion

Among various molecules which are closely associated with human malignancies, we have focused on ABC transporters and YB-1 in our laboratory. However, further work is still needed to establish how they are specifically expressed in human malignancies, and also to understand the structure-function relationships. We have also started basic studies on an antiangiogenesis strategy, which might circumvent drug resistance. It is necessary to understand at the molecular level how angiogenesis is specifically induced and progressed in human malignancies, and the effect of the tumor stroma and microenvironment.

Acknowledgments

We thank our colleagues who played invaluable roles in performing the studies mentioned in this review. This work was supported by cancer research funds from the Ministry of Education, Culture, Sports, Science and Technology of Japan, and by funds for the 2nd Term Comprehensive 10-Year Strategy for Cancer Control from the Ministry of Health, Labour and Welfare of Japan. One (M.K.) of authors is also supported by 21st Century COE Program for Medical Science, Kurume University.

REFERENCES

1. Allikmets R, Gerrard B, Hutchinson A, Dean M. Characterization of the human ABC superfamily: isolation and mapping of 21 new genes using the expressed sequence tags database. *Hum Mol Genet* 1996; **5**: 1649–55.
2. Alvarez M, Paull K, Monks A, Hose C, Lee JS, Weinstein J, Grever M, Bates S, Fojo T. Generation of a drug resistance profile by quantitation of mdr-1/P-glycoprotein in the cell lines of the National Cancer Institute Anticancer Drug Screen. *J Clin Invest* 1995; **95**: 2205–14.
3. Kuwano M, Toh S, Uchiumi T, Takano H, Kohno K, Wada M. Multidrug resistance-associated protein subfamily transporters and drug resistance. *Anticancer Drug Res* 1999; **14**: 123–31.
4. Scherf U, Ross DT, Waltham M, Smith LH, Lee JK, Tanabe L, Kohn KW, Reinhold WC, Myers TG, Andrews DT, Scudiero DA, Eisen MB, Sausville EA, Pommier Y, Botstein D, Brown PO, Weinstein JN. A gene expression database for the molecular pharmacology of cancer. *Nat Genet* 2000; **24**: 236–44.
5. Torigoe K, Harada T, Kusaba H, Uchiumi T, Kohno K, Green ED, Scherer SW, Tsui LC, Schlessinger D, Kuwano M, Wada M. Localization of 67 exons on a YAC contig spanning 1.5 Mb around the multidrug resistance gene region of human chromosome 7q21.1. *Genomics* 1998; **49**: 14–22.
6. Torigoe K, Sato S, Kusaba H, Kohno K, Kuwano M, Okumura K, Green ED, Tsui LC, Scherer SW, Schlessinger D, Wada M. A YAC-based contig of 1.5 Mb spanning the human multidrug resistance gene region and delineating the amplification unit in three human multidrug-resistant cell lines. *Genome Res* 1995; **5**: 233–44.
7. Harada T, Nagayama J, Kohno K, Mickley LA, Fojo T, Kuwano M, Wada M. Alu-associated interstitial deletions and chromosomal re-arrangement in 2 human multidrug-resistant cell lines. *Int J Cancer* 2000; **86**: 506–11.

8. Nagayama J, Iino M, Tada Y, Kusaba H, Kiue A, Ohshima K, Kuwano M, Wada M. Retrovirus insertion and transcriptional activation of the multidrug-resistance gene in leukemias treated by a chemotherapeutic agent *in vivo*. *Blood* 2001; **97**: 759–66.
9. Kohno K, Sato S, Takano H, Matsuo K, Kuwano M. The direct activation of human multidrug resistance gene (MDR1) by anticancer agents. *Biochem Biophys Res Commun* 1989; **165**: 1415–21.
10. Chaudhary PM, Roninson IB. Induction of multidrug resistance in human cells by transient exposure to different chemotherapeutic drugs. *J Natl Cancer Inst* 1993; **85**: 632–9.
11. Kohno K, Tanimura H, Sato S, Nakayama Y, Makino Y, Wada M, Fojo AT, Kuwano M. Cellular control of human multidrug resistance 1 (mdr-1) gene expression in absence and presence of gene amplification in human cancer cells. *J Biol Chem* 1994; **269**: 20503–8.
12. Ohga T, Uchiumi T, Makino Y, Koike K, Wada M, Kuwano M, Kohno K. Direct involvement of the Y-box binding protein YB-1 in genotoxic stress-induced activation of the human multidrug resistance 1 gene. *J Biol Chem* 1998; **273**: 5997–6000.
13. Uchiumi T, Kohno K, Tanimura H, Matsuo K, Sato S, Uchida Y, Kuwano M. Enhanced expression of the human multidrug resistance 1 gene in response to UV light irradiation. *Cell Growth Differ* 1993; **4**: 147–57.
14. Bargou RC, Jurchott K, Wagener C, Bergmann S, Metzner S, Bommert K, Mapara MY, Winzer KJ, Dietel M, Dorken B, Royer HD. Nuclear localization and increased levels of transcription factor YB-1 in primary human breast cancers are associated with intrinsic MDR1 gene expression. *Nat Med* 1997; **3**: 447–50.
15. Oda Y, Sakamoto A, Shinohara N, Ohga T, Uchiumi T, Kohno K, Tsuneyoshi M, Kuwano M, Iwamoto Y. Nuclear expression of YB-1 protein correlates with P-glycoprotein expression in human osteosarcoma. *Clin Cancer Res* 1998; **4**: 2273–7.
16. Kusaba H, Nakayama M, Harada T, Torigoe K, Green ED, Scherer SW, Kohno K, Kuwano M, Wada M. Maintenance of hypomethylation status and preferential expression of exogenous human MDR1/PGY1 gene in mouse L cells by YAC mediated transfer. *Somat Cell Mol Genet* 1997; **23**: 259–74.
17. Kusaba H, Nakayama M, Harada T, Nomoto M, Kohno K, Kuwano M, Wada, M. Association of 5′ CpG demethylation and altered chromatin structure in the promoter region with transcriptional activation of the multidrug resistance 1 gene in human cancer cells. *Eur J Biochem* 1999; **262**: 924–32.
18. Nakayama M, Wada M, Harada T, Nagayama J, Kusaba H, Ohshima K, Kozuru M, Komatsu H, Ueda R, Kuwano M. Hypomethylation status of CpG sites at the promoter region and overexpression of the human MDR1 gene in acute myeloid leukemias. *Blood* 1998; **92**: 4296–307.
19. Tada Y, Wada M, Kuroiwa K, Kinugawa N, Harada T, Nagayama J, Nakagawa M, Naito S, Kuwano M. MDR1 gene overexpression and altered degree of methylation at the promoter region in bladder cancer during chemotherapeutic treatment. *Clin Cancer Res* 2000; **6**: 4618–27.
20. Tada Y, Wada M, Taguchi K, Mochida Y, Kinugawa N, Tsuneyoshi M, Naito S, Kuwano M. The association of DAP-kinase hypermehylation with early recurrence in superficial bladder cancers. *Cancer Res* 2002; **62**: 4048–53.

21. Cole SP, Bhardwaj G, Gerlach JH, Mackie JE, Grant CE, Almquist KC, Stewart AJ, Kurz EU, Duncan AM, Deeley RG. Overexpression of a transporter gene in a multi-drug-resistant human lung cancer cell line. *Science* 1992; **258**: 1650–4.
22. Taniguchi K, Wada M, Kohno K, Nakamura T, Kawabe T, Kawakami M, Kagotani K, Okumura K, Akiyama S, Kuwano M. A human canalicular multispecific organic anion transporter (cMOAT) gene is overexpressed in cisplatin-resistant human cancer cell lines with decreased drug accumulation. *Cancer Res* 1996; **56**: 4124–9.
23. Uchiumi T, Hinoshita E, Haga S, Nakamura T, Tanaka T, Toh S, Furukawa M, Kawabe T, Wada M, Kagotani K, Okumura K, Kohno K, Akiyama S, Kuwano M. Isolation of a novel human canalicular multispecific organic anion transporter, cMOAT2/MRP3, and its expression in cisplatin-resistant cancer cells with decreased ATP-dependent drug transport. *Biochem Biophys Res Commun* 1998; **252**: 103–10.
24. Kool M, de Haas M, Scheffer GL, Scheper RJ, van Eijk MJ, Juijn JA, Baas F, Borst P. Analysis of expression of cMOAT (MRP2), MRP3, MRP4, and MRP5, homologues of the multidrug resistance-associated protein gene (MRP1), in human cancer cell lines. *Cancer Res* 1997; **57**: 3537–47.
25. Cole SP, Sparks KE, Fraser K, Loe DW, Grant CE, Wilson GM, Deeley RG. Pharmacological characterization of multidrug resistant MRP-transfected human tumor cells. *Cancer Res* 1994; **54**: 5902–10.
26. Chen ZS, Kawabe T, Ono M, Aoki S, Sumizawa T, Furukawa T, Uchiumi T, Wada M, Kuwano M, Akiyama SI. Effect of multidrug resistance-reversing agents on transporting activity of human canalicular multispecific organic anion transporter. *Mol Pharmacol* 1999; **56**: 1219–28.
27. Kawabe T, Chen ZS, Wada M, Uchiumi T, Ono M, Akiyama S, Kuwano M. Enhanced transport of anticancer agents and leukotriene C4 by the human canalicular multispecific organic anion transporter (cMOAT/MRP2). *FEBS Lett* 1999; **456**: 327–31.
28. Koike K, Kawabe T, Tanaka T, Toh S, Uchiumi T, Wada M, Akiyama S, Ono M, Kuwano M. A canalicular multispecific organic anion transporter (cMOAT) antisense cDNA enhances drug sensitivity in human hepatic cancer cells. *Cancer Res* 1997; **57**: 5475–9.
29. Haga S, Hinoshita E, Ikezaki K, Fukui M, Scheffer GL, Uchiumi T, Kuwano M. Involvement of the multidrug resistance protein 3 in drug sensitivity and its expression in human glioma. *Jpn J Cancer Res* 2001; **92**: 211–9.
30. Chen ZS, Lee K, Walther S, Raftogianis RB, Kuwano M, Zeng H, Kruh GD. Analysis of methotrexate and folate transport by multidrug resistance protein 4 (ABCC4): MRP4 is a component of the methotrexate efflux system. *Cancer Res* 2002; **62**: 3144–50.
31. Nooter K, Stoter G. Molecular mechanisms of multidrug resistance in cancer chemotherapy. *Pathol Res Pract* 1996; **192**: 768–80.
32. Wolffe AP. Structural and functional properties of the evolutionarily ancient Y-box family of nucleic acid binding proteins. *Bioessays* 1994; **16**: 245–51.
33. Didier DK, Schiffenbauer J, Woulfe SL, Zacheis M, Schwartz BD. Characterization of the cDNA encoding a protein binding to the major histocompatibility complex class II Y box. *Proc Natl Acad Sci USA* 1988; **85**: 7322–6.

34. Uramoto H, Izumi H, Ise T, Tada M, Uchiumi T, Kuwano M, Yasumoto K, Funa K, Kohno K. p73 interacts with c-Myc to regulate Y-box-binding protein-1 expression. *J Biol Chem* 2002; **277**: 31694–702.
35. Ohga T, Koike K, Ono M, Makino Y, Itagaki Y, Tanimoto M, Kuwano M, Kohno K. Role of the human Y box-binding protein YB-1 in cellular sensitivity to the DNA-damaging agents cisplatin, mitomycin C, and ultraviolet light. *Cancer Res* 1996; **56**: 4224–8.
36. Ashizuka M, Fukuda T, Nakamura T, Shirasuna K, Iwai K, Izumi H, Kohno K, Kuwano M, Uchiumi T. Novel translational control through an iron-responsive element by interaction of multifunctional protein YB-1 and IRP2. *Mol Cell Biol* 2002; **22**: 6375–83.
37. Hayakawa H, Uchiumi T, Fukuda T, Ashizuka M, Kuwano M, Sekiguchi M. Binding capacity of human YB-1 protein for RNA containing 8-oxoguanine. *Biochemistry* 2002; **41**: 12739–44.
38. Ise T, Nagatani G, Imamura T, Kato K, Takano H, Nomoto M, Izumi H, Ohmori H, Okamoto T, Ohga T, Uchiumi T, Kuwano M, Kohno K. Transcription factor Y-box binding protein 1 binds preferentially to cisplatin-modified DNA and interacts with proliferating cell nuclear antigen. *Cancer Res* 1999; **59**: 342–6.
39. Okamoto T, Izumi H, Imamura T, Takano H, Ise T, Uchiumi T, Kuwano M, Kohno K. Direct interaction of p53 with the Y-box binding protein, YB-1: a mechanism for regulation of human gene expression. *Oncogene* 2000; **19**: 6194–202.
40. Shibahara K, Sugio K, Osaki T, Uchiumi T, Maehara Y, Kohno K, Yasumoto K, Sugimachi K, Kuwano M. Nuclear expression of the Y-box binding protein, YB-1, as a novel marker of disease progression in non-small cell lung cancer. *Clin Cancer Res* 2001; **7**: 3151–5.
41. Janz M, Harbeck N, Dettmar P, Berger U, Schmidt A, Jurchott K, Schmitt M, Royer HD. Y-box factor YB-1 predicts drug resistance and patient outcome in breast cancer independent of clinically relevant tumor biologic factors HER2, uPA and PAI-1. *Int J Cancer* 2002; **97**: 278–82.
42. Shibao K, Takano H, Nakayama Y, Okazaki K, Nagata N, Izumi H, Uchiumi T, Kuwano M, Kohno K, Itoh H. Enhanced coexpression of YB-1 and DNA topoisomerase II alpha genes in human colorectal carcinomas. *Int J Cancer* 1999; **83**: 732–7.
43. Hanahan D, Folkman J. Patterns and emerging mechanisms of the angiogenic switch during tumorigenesis. *Cell* 1996; **86**: 353–64.
44. Folkman J. Angiogenesis in cancer, vascular, rheumatoid and other disease. *Nat Med* 1995; **1**: 27–31.
45. Shono T, Motoyama M, Tatsumi K, Ulbrich N, Iwamoto Y, Kuwano M, Ono M. A new synthetic matrix metalloproteinase inhibitor modulates both angiogenesis and urokinase type plasminogen activator activity. *Angiogenesis* 1998; **2**: 319–29.
46. Itokawa T, Nokihara H, Nishioka Y, Sone S, Iwamoto Y, Yamada Y, Cherrngton J, McMahon G, Shibuya M, Kuwano M, Mayumi O. Antiangiogenic effect by SU5416 is partly attributable to inhibition of Flt-1 receptor signaling. *Mol Cancer Ther* 2002; **1**: 295–302.
47. Kuwano M, Fukushi J, Okamoto M, Nishie A, Goto H, Ishibashi T, Ono M. Angiogenesis factors. *Intern Med* 2001; **40**: 565–72.

48. Shono T, Ono M, Izumi H, Jimi SI, Matsushima K, Okamoto T, Kohno K, Kuwano M. Involvement of the transcription factor NF-kappaB in tubular morphogenesis of human microvascular endothelial cells by oxidative stress. *Mol Cell Biol* 1996; **16**: 4231–9.
49. Morikawa W, Yamamoto K, Ishikawa S, Takemoto S, Ono M, Fukushi J, Naito S, Nozaki C, Iwanaga S, Kuwano M. Angiostatin generation by cathepsin D secreted by human prostate carcinoma cells. *J Biol Chem* 2000; **275**: 38912–20.
50. Torisu H, Ono M, Kiryu H, Furue M, Ohmoto Y, Nakayama J, Nishioka Y, Sone S, Kuwano M. Macrophage infiltration correlates with tumor stage and angiogenesis in human malignant melanoma: possible involvement of TNFalpha and IL-1alpha. *Int J Cancer* 2000; **85**: 182–8.
51. Yoshida S, Ono M, Shono T, Izumi H, Ishibashi T, Suzuki H, Kuwano M. Involvement of interleukin-8, vascular endothelial growth factor, and basic fibroblast growth factor in tumor necrosis factor alpha-dependent angiogenesis. *Mol Cell Biol* 1997; **17**: 4015–23.
52. Goto H, Kohno K, Sone S, Akiyama S, Kuwano M, Ono M. Interferon gamma-dependent induction of thymidine phosphorylase/platelet-derived endothelial growth factor through gamma-activated sequence-like element in human macrophages. *Cancer Res* 2001; **61**: 469–73.
53. Hirata A, Ogawa S, Kometani T, Kuwano T, Naito S, Kuwano M, Ono M. ZD1839 (Iressa) induces antiangiogenic effects through inhibition of epidermal growth factor receptor tyrosine kinase. *Cancer Res* 2002; **62**: 2554–60.

MOLECULAR MECHANISMS OF ANGIOGENESIS IN NON-SMALL CELL LUNG CANCER, AND THERAPEUTICS TARGETING RELATED MOLECULES

Seiji YANO, Yasuhiko NISHIOKA, Hisatsugu GOTO and Saburo SONE

*Department of Internal Medicine and Molecular Therapeutics, University of Tokushima School of Medicine**

Angiogenesis, neovascularization from pre-existing vasculature, is necessary to supply oxygen and nutrition for tumor growth in both primary and distant organs. It consists of sprouting and non-sprouting (the enlargement, splitting, and fusion of pre-existing vessels) processes, and both can occur concurrently. Growth of solid tumors, including non-small cell lung cancer (NSCLC), is usually dependent on angiogenesis, which is regulated by complex mechanisms involving various angiogenesis-related molecules. Vascular endothelial growth factor (VEGF), also known as vascular permeability factor (VPF), one of the most potent angiogenic molecules, regulates both angiogenesis and vascular permeability, and hence promotes tumor progression and development of malignant pleural effusions in NSCLC. Signals via epidermal growth factor receptor (EGFR) promote not only the tumor cell cycle, but also the process of angiogenesis. Therefore, these molecules are potential targets for anti-tumor vasculature therapy. Many agents targeting tumor vasculature have been developed, and several compounds have shown anti-tumor potential in preclinical studies. Their efficacy against NSCLC is currently being evaluated in clinical trials.

Lung cancer has been the leading cause of malignancy-related death in Japan since 1998, and more than 80% of cases are non-small cell lung cancer (NSCLC). Surgical resection is undoubtedly the first choice treatment for NSCLC patients in early stages (stage I and II). Over two-thirds of patients are, however, in advanced stages (*1*). Radiation therapy is generally preferred for patients with locoregionally advanced NSCLC (stage III), and chemotherapy for patients with disseminated disease (stage IV). Despite improvement of these therapeutic modalities, prolongation of survival of patients in advanced stages (especially stage IV) is not satisfactory. Therefore, novel and more effective therapeutic modalities are necessary for NSCLC in advanced stages.

It has been well established that the progression of tumors (growth of both primary and metastatic tumors) is critically dependent on angiogenesis (neovascularization) to supply oxygen and nutrition (*2*). Therefore, blockade of angiogenesis has

* 3-18-15 Kuramoto-cho, Tokushima 770-8503, Japan

This paper is dedicated to the memory of late Dr. Tomizo Yoshida on the occasion of the 100th anniversary of his birth. It was originally published in Cancer Science in June, 2003.

been expected to prevent the growth of tumor cells at both primary and metastatic sites, thereby preventing tumor progression, and thus improving the prognosis of patients with various types of malignant tumors, including NSCLC. From this point of view, dozens of compounds which target tumor vasculature have been developed, and many experimental studies have shown that anti-tumor vasculature agents are effective to control tumor-cell growth and metastases (*3*). In this article, the molecular mechanisms of angiogenesis in NSCLC are briefly reviewed and the strategy for control of NSCLC by anti-vasculature agents is discussed.

Molecular Mechanisms of Tumor Angiogenesis

1. *Types of angiogenesis*

Angiogenesis can occur through either sprouting or non-sprouting processes (*4*) (Fig. 1). Sprouting angiogenesis involves the branching (true sprouting) of new capillaries from pre-existing vessels. This type of angiogenesis begins with an angiogenic stimulus, followed by local degradation of the basement membrane surrounding the capillaries. Endothelial cell migration is then accompanied by the proliferation of cells at the leading edge of the migrating column. As they move, the endothelial cells begin to organize into three-dimensional structures to form new capillary tubes. All of these, then, require endothelial cell survival, mandating the interplay of numerous factors, which can act in a positive or negative fashion. These events are tightly regulated by various angiogenic factors, including vascular endothelial growth factor (VEGF), basic fibroblast growth factor (bFGF), angiopoietins, interleukin-8 (IL-8), and thymidine phosphorylase (TP) (*5*). These factors can be produced not only by tumor cells, but also by host stromal cells (*3*).

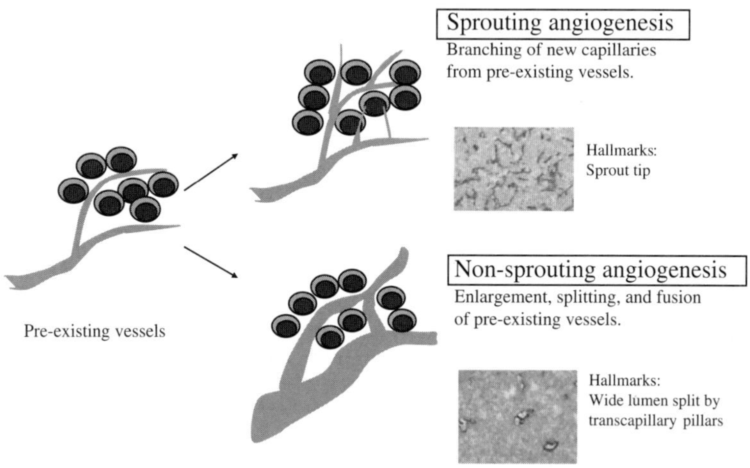

FIG. 1. Patterns of angiogenesis
Sprouting angiogenesis involves the branching (true sprouting) of new capillaries from pre-existing vessels. The hallmark of this type is sprout tips. Non-sprouting angiogenesis results from the enlargement, splitting, and fusion of pre-existing vessels produced by the proliferation of endothelial cells at the wall of a vessel. Transvascular bridges are sometimes observed in enlarged vessels produced by non-sprouting angiogenesis. Sprouting angiogenesis and non-sprouting angiogenesis can occur concurrently.

Non-sprouting angiogenesis results from the enlargement, splitting, and fusion of pre-existing vessels produced by the proliferation of endothelial cells within the wall of a vessel. Transvascular bridges are sometimes observed in enlarged vessels produced by non-sprouting angiogenesis. Non-sprouting angiogenesis can occur concurrently with sprouting angiogenesis not only in the vascularization of organs or tissues (lung, heart, yolk sac) during development, but also in tumor angiogenesis (*4*). We recently observed this type of angiogenesis in brain metastasis with progressive growth (*6*, *7*).

2. Angiogenesis as a poor prognosis factor of NSCLC

Tumors may be able to grow without neovascularization if a suitable vascular bed is available. Pezzella *et al.* reported non-angiogenic NSCLC tumors characterized by lack of parenchymal destruction and absence of both tumor-associated stroma and new vessels, though this type of tumor accounted for less than 20% of NSCLC (*8*). Several lines of evidence suggest that growth of solid tumors, including NSCLC, is usually dependent on angiogenesis (*9–11*). In fact, intratumoral microvessel density (IMD) was inversely correlated with survival of patients with surgically resected NSCLC (*9*, *10*). In addition, expression of several angiogenesis-related molecules, such as VEGF (*12*), matrix metalloproteinases (MMPs) (*13*), epidermal growth factor receptor (EGFR) (*14*), angiopoietin-2 (*15*), TP (*16*), cyclooxygenase 2 (Cox-2) (*17*), inversely correlated with prognosis of the patients with NSCLC. Among these molecules, we focused on VEGF, MMP, and EGFR, and explored the involvement of these molecules in the progression of NSCLC.

3. Involvement of angiogenesis-related molecules in NSCLC

VEGF

VEGF, the prototype of the VEGF family, which consists of VEGF, VEGF-B, VEGF-C, VEGF-D, and VEGF-E, is suggested to be the most potent and specific growth factor for endothelial cells and to play a very important role in angiogenesis (*3*, *18*). VEGF consists of at least 4 isoforms (VEGF121, VEGF165, VEGF189, VEGF206) which are regulated by splicing at the mRNA level, and VEGF165 is the most abundant isoform. VEGF binds with high affinity to two tyrosine kinase receptors, VEGFR-1 (Flt-1) and VEGFR-2 (Flk-1/KDR). Ligand binding causes receptor dimerization, autophosphorylation and signal transduction. Several studies have demonstrated that VEGF expression is directly correlated with IMD, and inversely correlated with the survival of patients with NSCLC (*12*). Yuan *et al.* further examined VEGF isoform expression in 57 surgically resected primary tumors from NSCLC patients using RT-PCR, and demonstrated that a high tumoral expression of VEGF189 was associated with a high IMD, shorter survival, and early postoperative relapse (*19*). Since VEGF189 is a membrane-associated form, unlike VEGF121 and VEGF165 (secreted form), VEGF189 might contribute more to local angiogenesis in NSCLC, while the amount of VEGF189 is less than 10% of the total VEGF expression.

Lung cancer frequently metastasizes to multiple organs, including the bone, lung, brain, and liver. We developed several metastasis models and determined the molecular mechanisms of multi-organ metastasis of lung cancer (*6*, *20–22*). Among multiple organ metastases, brain metastasis is one of the most serious problems, because it restricts the quality of life of the patient and is refractory to various anticancer modalities. We obtained a brain metastasis model by the injection of suitable cells into the internal carotid artery of nude mice (*6*) (Fig. 2A). As described above, we found that non-sprouting angiogenesis was predominantly observed, and that levels of VEGF production by NSCLC cells directly correlated with the potential to produce brain metastasis in this model (*6*). Brain metastases developed by VEGF high-producing cell lines progressed rapidly and had many enlarged vessels split by transcapillary pillars (a hallmark of non-sprouting angiogenesis). We further showed that the metastatic potential of VEGF low-producing cells was not augmented by transfection with *sense-VEGF165* or *-VEGF121* gene. However, the transfection of VEGF high-producing cells with *antisense-VEGF165* gene resulted in a decrease in brain metastasis formation (*6*) (Fig. 2B). These results suggest that VEGF is essential but not sufficient for promoting brain metastasis via angiogenesis, and that its inhibition could represent an important therapeutic target.

On the other hand, VEGF with multifunctional activities was recently found to be identical to vascular permeability factor (VPF) (*3*). Malignant pleural effusion (PE) is frequently associated with advanced lung cancer. One study showed that malignant PE fluid contained a high level of VEGF in lung cancer patients (*23*). We recently developed a valuable model for PE formation after i.v. injection of human lung adenocarcinoma cell lines (PC14 (*21*) and its metastatic variant PC14PE6) (*24*). Interestingly, VEGF was found to be responsible for the development of PE induced by

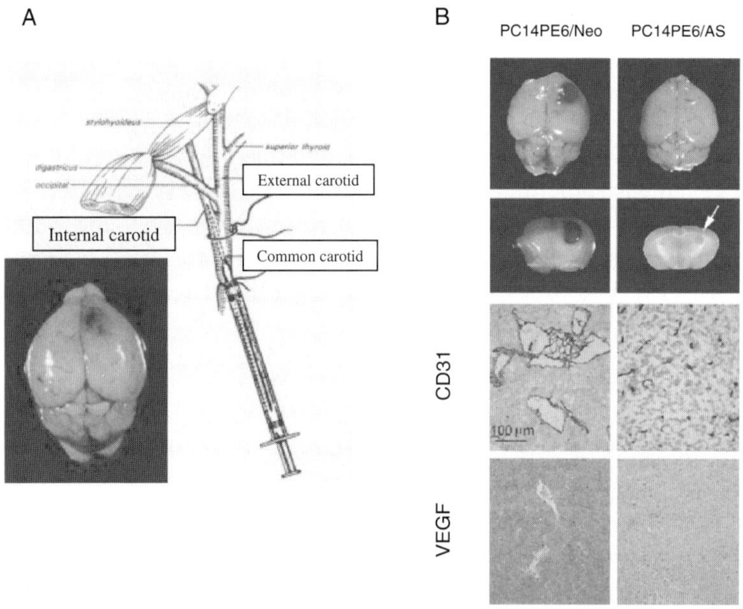

FIG. 2. Brain metastasis model and anti-metastatic effect by VEGF inhibition
A. Brain metastasis model based on internal carotid artery injection. B. Brain metastasis produced by lung cancer (PC14PE6) cells transfected with *antisense VEGF* gene. Note that PC14PE6 cells transfected with *antisense VEGF* gene (PC14PE6/AS) produced fewer brain metastases. VEGF expression and vascularization (determined by immunohistochemistry for CD31) were also decreased in brain tumors produced by PC14PE6/AS cells.

these lung adenocarcinoma cells (*24*). Thus, VEGF/VPF has been shown to be essential not only for angiogenesis, but also for PE formation in lung cancer, via the induction of vascular hyperpermeability. Since VEGF/VPF and its receptors can be therapeutically targeted, VEGF receptor inhibitors could be useful for the control of malignant PE in lung cancer patients.

There is currently much interest in the VEGF family because of its implication not only in angiogenesis, but also in lymphoangiogenesis (*18*). VEGF-C and VEGF-D have been shown to bind to VEGFR2 and VEGFR3 and to play pivotal roles in developmental and tumoral lymphoangiogenesis (*25*). In NSCLC, VEGF-C expression was reported to correlate with lymph-node metastasis, lymphatic invasion, and poor prognosis (*26*, *27*).

Collectively, these findings suggest that the VEGF family and its receptors may be potential therapeutic targets to block both angiogenesis and lymphoangiogenesis in NSCLC.

MMPs

MMPs are a family of zinc-dependent degradative enzymes of the extracellular matrix (ECM), and are important for tumor invasion (*28*). These enzymes have been classified into subgroups depending on their substrates (i.e., collagenases, gelatinases, stromelysins, membrane-type, and nonclassified). Since MMPs are necessary for blood vessel penetration, MMPs were suggested to play a crucial role not only in the process of tumor-cell invasion, but also in the process of angiogenesis. Several studies have demonstrated that MMPs, especially MMP-2 and MMP-9 (gelatinase A and B), membrane type 1 MMP (MT1-MMP), the activator of MMP-2, and stromelysin-3 are overexpressed in various types of tumors, and that their level of expression is correlated with tumor aggressiveness, as implied by increased histological grade, advanced clinical stage, and poor patient outcome (*13*, *29*). On the other hand, we assessed the expression of MMP-2 and MMP-9 at the mRNA level by means of *in situ* hybridization in 60 formalin-fixed paraffin-embedded samples of stage I NSCLC, and found that the levels of MMP-2 and MMP-9, as single factors, did not correlate with disease-free or overall survival (*30*). Thus, the prognostic significance of MMPs in NSCLC is still controversial. MMPs are known to be expressed by both cancer cells and stromal cells (*28*). We reported previously that MMP activity produced by human lung cancer cells varied among cell lines *in vitro* and *in vivo* (*31*). In addition, MMP activity (gelatinolytic activity assessed by film *in situ* zymography) derived from host-stroma cells also varies among organs (high in the liver and low in the lung) (Fig. 3A). We further demonstrated that MMP derived from the liver parenchyma facilitated the formation of liver metastasis by MMP-low-expressing lung cancer cell lines (*31*), suggesting that MMP could promote metastasis, presumably via invasion and angiogenesis, irrespective of its origin.

EGFR

EGFR is a 170-kDa transmembrane glycoprotein (*32*). Binding of specific ligands, such as EGF and transforming growth factor α (TGF-α), to EGFR results in the dimerization of EGFR and leads to autophosphorylation of the intracellular receptor tyrosine kinase. EGFR signaling (via ras–raf-1–MAPK, STAT, and PI3K–Akt) facilitates tumor-cell cycling, proliferation, invasion, and decreased apoptosis (*32*). In addition, since 1) EFGR is detected in the dividing tumor vasculature endothelial cells (*33*), 2) EGF induces neovascularization of mouse cornea (*34*), 3) block-

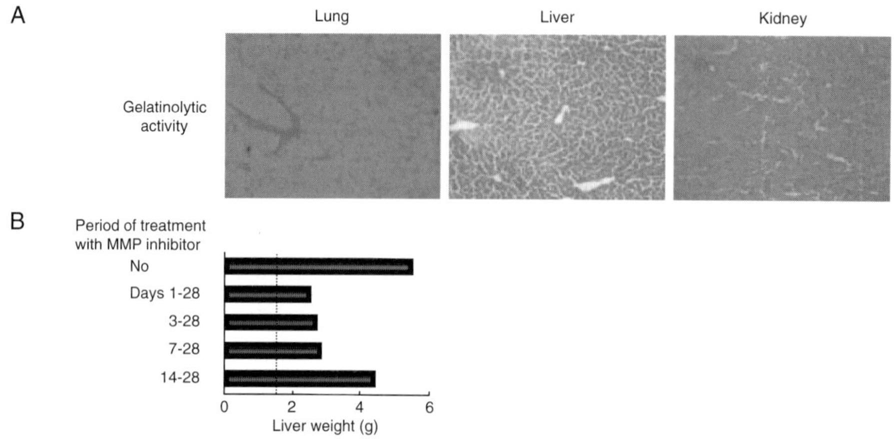

FIG. 3. Involvement of MMP in lung cancer progression
A. Heterogeneity of host-derived gelatinolytic activity determined by film *in situ* zymography. Note that high gelatinolytic activity was detected in the liver parenchyma, but gelatinolysis was not detected in the lung parenchyma. Gelatinolytic activity in the kidney was intermediate. B. Effect of treatment with MMP inhibitor for various periods on liver metastasis. SBC-3/DOX (1×10^6) cells were inoculated intravenously into NK-cell depleted SCID mice. The mice were given food with or without a MMP inhibitor (1% ONO-4817 content) for the indicated periods, and killed on day 28. Then, the formation of metastases was evaluated. Note that the anti-metastatic effect of MMP inhibitor was stronger when the drug was started by the time of establishment of micrometastasis (day 14).

ade of EGFR signaling down-regulates the production of proangiogenic cytokines, including VEGF and IL-8, by several tumor cell lines expressing EGFR (*34*), EGFR is likely to be involved, at least indirectly, in the regulation of angiogenic processes.

EGFR is commonly overexpressed in various types of malignancy, including NSCLC (*32*). Several studies showed an association between overexpression of EGFR and prognosis or histological grade of differentiation in NSCLC (*14, 32*). However, a recent meta-analysis study showed that EGFR expression was rarely (3/10 studies) related to patient outlook (*35*). Since activation (phosphorylation) of EGFR is essential for the signal transduction and hence progression of tumors, we hypothesized that activation of EGFR may more directly reflect the significance of this molecule in NSCLC, and thus evaluated the expression of phosphorylated EGFR, in addition to EGFR protein, in surgically resected tumors from NSCLC patients. We found that the expression of phosphorylated EGFR, but not overexpression of EGFR protein, inversely correlated with survival and time to tumor progression (*36*), suggesting that activation of EGFR, but not overexpression, may be an important prognostic factors for NSCLC patients. Further analysis to explore the correlation between vascularization and EGFR activation is ongoing.

Anti-Tumor Vasculature Therapy

The concept of targeting tumor vasculature was first advocated 30 years ago (*37*), and this concept has recently re-emerged because of the development of new anti-tumor vasculature agents. These agents have potential advantages, such as physical accessibility and genetic stability of target cells, over conventional cytotoxic chemotherapy (*3, 38*).

There are several strategies targeting tumor vasculature. The first is the modality selectively targeting angiogenesis (neovascularization) during the growth of small tumors (anti-angiogenic agents). Angiogenesis-related molecules, including VEGF, VEGF receptor 2, and MMP, were suggested as targets for this modality, and a large number of inhibitors have been developed. The second strategy is selective targeting of established tumor-associated vessels in large tumors (vascular-targeting agents), and tubulin in the dividing endothelial cells is one target of this type of modality. The third is long-term use of compounds which secondarily disrupt tumor vasculature, including anticancer drugs (taxans) and EGFR inhibitors.

1. Anti-angiogenic agents

VEGF inhibitors

Many compounds, including anti-VEGF antibody, anti-VEGF receptor 2 antibody, and phosphorylation inhibitors of VEGF receptor 2 tyrosine kinase, have been developed as VEGF inhibitors (*3, 38*). These compounds were reported to inhibit the growth of a wide variety of tumor cell lines in various animal models (*3, 38*). In addition, we demonstrated that a VEGF receptor tyrosine kinase inhibitor (PTK787) suppressed development of malignant PEs by VEGF high-producing PC14PE6 cells via inhibition of vascular hyperpermeability (*39*), suggesting that VEGF inhibitors may be useful for control of tumor growth and PEs.

Recently, neutralizing antibody for VEGF and inhibitors of VEGF receptor tyrosine kinase phosphorylation were evaluated for therapeutic potential in clinical trials. The early clinical trials showed that tumor regression was hardly observed when patients with solid tumors in advanced stages were treated with VEGF inhibitors alone. Based on these results, the therapeutic effect of anti-VEGF antibody in combination with cytotoxic chemotherapy was evaluated in recent trials. The combined use of anti-VEGF antibody (rhuMab VEGF) with chemotherapy (carboplatin+paclitaxel) improved the response rate and time to tumor progression in chemotherapy-naive advanced NSCLC patients (*40*). In addition, Langmuir reported the outcome of 28 patients with solid tumors who received anti-VEGF antibody (bevacizumab) for more than 1 year (*41*). In this particular population, the response rate was 50% (14/28 cases) and disease stabilization for more than 1 year was observed in an additional 13 cases, indicating the possibility of long-term disease stabilization by anti-VEGF antibody. Furthermore, in 16 patients with recurrent disease during the observation period, restarted bevacizumab treatment caused tumor regression in 2 cases and disease re-stabilization in 8 cases, suggesting that some patients who progress after long-term (6–12 months) bevacizumab+chemotherapy may have benefits from retreatment. Long-term treatment with VEGF inhibitors was reported to be well tolerated in the majority of the patients. Nevertheless, since adverse events, including deep venous thromboses and sudden and life-threatening hemoptysis, were reported in these studies, the potential toxicities of VEGF inhibitors must be considered in future trials.

MMP inhibitors

First-generation MMPIs, such as batimastat, have broad inhibitory activity against almost all MMPs and are not appropriate for oral administration. The second-generation inhibitors, such as marimastat, MMI270 (CGS27023A), and prinomastat, also have a broad spectrum, but can be orally administered. The third-generation inhibitors, such as BAY12-9566 and ONO-4817, were designed to have a selective spectrum of MMP inhibition, and many members of this generation do not inhibit MMP-1 (*28*). Many MMP inhibitors were reported to show promising anti-tumor efficiency against MMP-expressing tumor cells in preclinical studies (*28*). We recently reported that an MMP inhibitor (ONO-4817) could inhibit metastasis by MMP (gelatinases)-expressing lung cancer cell lines (PC14PE6, H226), and that the anti-metastatic effect of ONO-4817 could be augmented by the combined use of a cytotoxic anticancer drug (docetaxel) in our lung metastasis model (*42*). Interestingly, ONO-4817 also inhibited metastasis to the liver by MMP low-expressing cell lines (SBC-3/DOX, RERF-LC-AI) in our metastasis models. Film *in situ* zymography revealed that normal liver parenchyma expressed collagenase activity and facilitated metastasis by tumor cells without MMP expression in the liver (*31*). These results suggest that MMP inhibitors may inhibit metastasis if MMPs are expressed and involved in the growth of tumors, irrespective of their source (tumors or non-tumor parenchyma). However, the anti-metastatic effect of ONO-4817 was stronger when the drug was started by the time of establishment of micrometastasis (*31*) (Fig. 3B), suggesting limited value of this compound in the clinical treatment of malignant diseases.

MMP inhibitors are being evaluated for in the treatment of various malignant diseases and are at various stages of clinical trials. The major dose-limiting toxicity of broad-spectrum MMPIs is time- and dose-dependent musculoskeletal adverse events, including joint pain and stiffness, that limit both the dose level administered and the duration of therapy (*28*). These adverse events were suggested to be a toxicity associated with inhibition of MMP-1 (*28*). A phase III clinical trial showed that marimastat, a second-generation MMPI, prolonged progression-free survival of patients with inoperable gastric cancer, especially for patients who had previously received chemotherapy and did not have clinically detectable metastasis at the time of enrollment (*43*). Some phase III trials with MMP inhibitors, including marimastat, prinomastat (AG3340), and BAY-12-9566, were also performed for lung cancer patients in advanced stages, but no clinical efficacy has been reported (*44*, *45*). The insufficient effect of MMP inhibitors in these trials might be due to the heterogenous expression of MMP in tumors in lung cancer patients. In view of the preclinical findings, MMP inhibitors might affect tumor growth only at early stages, but not when the disease has progressed to advanced stages. It is also possible that immune-mediated effects on tumor cells are inhibited by MMP inhibitors, because of the inability of immune cells to invade tumors and destroy them. Therefore, the design of further clinical trials with MMP inhibitors should be carefully considered (e.g., enroll only patients with early-stage cancer with high expression of MMP).

2. *Vascular targeting agents*

Vascular targeting agents that damage established tumor vasculature are also of potential clinical use. Tubulin inhibitors (combretastatin A4 phosphate (*46*), ZD6126) (*47*) disrupt tubulin dimerization, damaged endothelial cells, and shut off blood flow. One report claimed that an anaplastic thyroid tumor completely disappeared after treatment with combretastatin (*46*).

We have shown that another vascular targeting agent, ZD6126 (ANG453), can shut-down blood flow, inducing tumor necrosis within 24 h (*48*). Importantly,

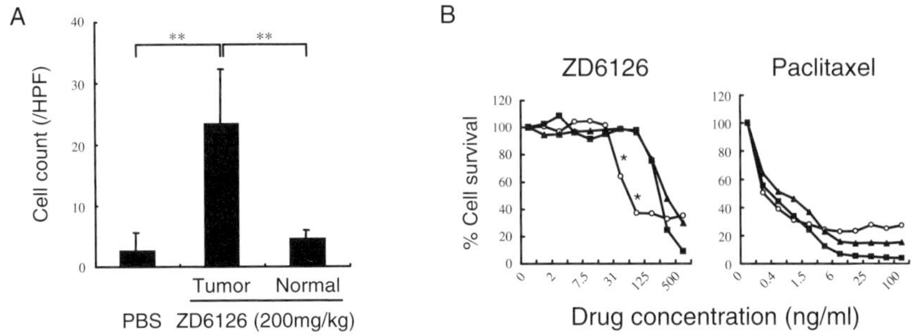

FIG. 4. Apoptosis induced by ZD6126 (tubulin inhibitor) is specific to tumor-associated vasculature endothelial cells

A. PC14PE6 (1×10^6) cells were inoculated intravenously into nude mice. Five weeks later, PBS or 200 mg/kg ZD6126 was administered intraperitoneally and the mice were killed after 24 h. Then, the lungs with metastatic colonies were harvested, frozen on dry ice, and sliced. The frozen sections were sequentially stained for TUNEL and CD31. Note that a single treatment with ZD6126 resulted in a 10-fold increase of apoptotic endothelial cells in the tumors compared with the control group. HPF, high power field; Normal, normal lung parenchyma. B. The effect of ZD6126 and paclitaxel on *in vitro* proliferation of human dermal endothelial cells (HMVEC (○)) and tumor cells (PC14PE6 (■) and H226 (▲)) was determined. The cells (2×10^3), plated in 96-well plates, were incubated overnight, and then different doses of ZD6126 or paclitaxel were added. The MTT dye reduction assay was performed after 72 h. Note that only ZD6126 selectively inhibited endothelial cell proliferation.

ZD6126 induced apoptosis of endothelial cells in tumors, but not in nontumor parenchyma, suggesting selectivity of this drug for tumor-associated endothelial cells (Fig. 4A). In addition, ZD6126 at higher concentrations (more than 125 ng/ml) could inhibit proliferation of both endothelial cells and tumor cells, but it inhibited only endothelial proliferation at lower concentrations (less than 30 ng/ml) (Fig. 4B), suggesting that ZD6126 inhibits the growth of endothelial cells more selectively than tumor cells. Although other tubulin binding inhibitors, such as docetaxel and paclitaxel, were also reported to have anti-angiogenic activity (*49*), their effect was not selective on endothelial cells (Fig. 4). The mechanism of the selectivity of ZD6126 against tumor endothelial cells remains unclear. Further examinations are warranted to clarify this mechanism.

On the other hand, monotherapy involving daily injection with ZD6126 inhibited lung metastasis of human NSCLC cell lines (*48*), and this effect could be further augmented by combined use of cisplatin (submitted for publication). The therapeutic efficacy of ZD6126 is being evaluated in clinical trials.

3. EGFR inhibitors

There are two strategies to target EGFR (*50*). The first is monoclonal antibody directed against the extracellular ligand-binding domain (e.g., IMC-C225 and ABX-EGF), and the other is synthetic small compounds which inhibit ATP binding to the tyrosine kinase domain, thereby shutting down the signal (*50*). ZD1839 and OSI-774 are selective, reversible inhibitors of EGFR tyrosine kinases, and CI-1033 is an irreversible inhibitor of all four EGF receptors (*50*). The EGFR inhibitor that is furthest along in clinical development is a small compound, ZD1839. In preclinical studies, ZD1839 was shown to induce apoptosis of EGFR-overexpressing tumor cells and it inhibited angiogenesis induced by EGF (*50*).

Phase I clinical trials with ZD1839 have shown excellent tolerance (with toxicity limited to mild rash and diarrhea) and efficacy in some advanced NSCLC patients (*51*). In a phase II trial (IDEAL 1: a multi-center, international study), 208 evaluable patients were randomized to either 250 or 500 mg oral daily administration of ZD1839 (*52*). The overall objective response rate at 250 or 500 mg was 18.4% and 19.0%, respectively. Disease control rate (complete response+partial response+stable disease) at 250 or 500 mg was 54.4% and 51.4%, respectively. Although multivariate analysis suggested that ethnicity was not a significant factor, Japanese patients showed better results in terms of response rate (27.5% for Japanese vs. 10.4% for non-Japanese) and disease control rate (65.7% for Japanese vs. 40.6% for non-Japanese). In addition, female sex and adenocarcinoma were found to be associated with a favorable response to ZD1839. Progression-free survival measured for 12 weeks was comparable with prior findings of second-line therapy in NSCLC: docetaxel gave a response rate of 7.1% and time to progression of 10.6 weeks. A provocative aspect of this trial was that symptom improvement was reported by a majority of patients after only 8 days of ZD1839 treatment (*52*). Based on these results, ZD1839 (250 mg/day) was approved in Japan in July, 2002 and has been widely used for NSCLC patients.

Bronchioloalveolar carcinoma (BAC), one of the subtypes of lung papillary adenocarcinoma, presents unique clinical features, such as endobronchial spread and bronchorrhea in advanced stages. The prognosis for BAC patients in advanced stages is extremely poor, similar to patients with other NSCLC types, because of the very low susceptibility to conventional chemotherapy and radiotherapy (*53*). Although alternative modalities, such as indomethacin, interferon α, and streptococcal preparation by inhalation, have been investigated in patients with extended BAC and bronchorrhea, the effect was quite unsatisfactory. Recently, we experienced two patients with chemotherapy-refractory BAC who were successfully treated with ZD1839 (*54*). In both cases (females), serous sputum production (greater than 200 ml/day before treatment) was markedly reduced within 3 days of starting the treatment with ZD1839, and hypoxia and radiographic signs of bilateral lung consolidation were visibly improved within 7 days. Following more than 10 months of treatment, no evidence of recurrence or severe adverse events were observed. Although large-scale studies are necessary to evaluate the efficiency of ZD1839 against BAC, these results suggest the presence of a population of BAC patients who show favorable response to ZD1839.

In Western countries, two phase III trials (INTACT 1 and 2) were recently performed to determine whether a combined use of cytotoxic chemotherapy could augment the efficacy of ZD1839 in chemotherapy-naive patients with advanced NSCLC (*55, 56*). More than 1000 patients were entered in each trial, and the patients underwent 6 cycles of chemotherapy (paclitaxel and carboplatin, or gemcitabine and cisplatin) in combination with daily ZD1839 (250 mg or 500 mg) or placebo. Although no major new adverse events were observed, ZD1839 did not improve survival, progression-free survival, or response rate. These results suggest no added benefit of concurrent use of ZD1839 with chemotherapy as the first line therapy.

While ZD1839 was reported to be well tolerated in clinical trials, pulmonary damage including life-threatening interstitial pneumonia was reported in more than 1% of the NSCLC patients treated with ZD1839 (*57*). Therefore, the safety of this drug should be carefully re-evaluated. In addition, since the response to EGFR inhibitors was not suggested to correlate with EGFR expression in tumor cells, the mechanism of the anti-tumor action needs to be clarified. It is also necessary to determine whether tumor vascularization is affected by treatment with EGFR inhibitors.

Future Directions

Since tumor angiogenesis is regulated by complex mechanisms, monotherapy with the majority of anti-vascular agents would be insufficient to obtain long-term disease control. Therefore, multi-agents or multi-modality therapy combined with other anticancer modalities may be necessary to obtain additional therapeutic benefit. There are at least three strategies. The first is the combined use of anti-angiogenic agents and vascular targeting agents focusing on tumor vasculature as a target. Since even vascular targeting agents induce extensive central necrosis in the tumor and the narrow peripheral rim of the tumor would re-grow in the presence of angiogenesis from the surrounding normal vessels, the addition of anti-angiogenic agents appears to be logical. The second is the use of anti-vascular agents as an adjuvant of surgical resection, because anti-tumor vasculature agents, especially anti-angiogenic agents, are expected to be more effective against residual tumors rather than bulky tumors. The third is the strategy which targets both tumor cells and tumor-associated endothelial cells. For this, anti-vasculature agents with cytotoxic agents or molecular-targeted drugs directed to tumor cells may be used in combination.

One impediment to the successful and rapid development of anti-tumor vasculature therapy is the lack of validated assays capable of measuring an anti-vascular effect directly in patients (*58*). Several techniques and assays (including dynamic magnetic resonance imaging (MRI) and $[^{15}O]H_2O$ positron emission tomography (PET) scanning to evaluate blood flow, $[^{17}F]$fluorodeoxyglucose PET scanning to evaluate metabolism, and detection of apoptotic endothelial cells in the tumors and peripheral blood) are currently being tested in ongoing clinical trials (*59*). Establishment of appropriate surrogate makers is required in the context of anti-tumor vasculature therapy.

Conclusions

Angiogenesis plays a critical role in the progression of the majority of NSCLC, and is regulated by complex mechanisms in the presence of various angiogenesis-related molecules. Anti-tumor vascular therapy is considered promising, and many compounds targeting tumor vasculature have been developed. Since several compounds have shown favorable anti-tumor potential in preclinical studies, their efficiency is currently being evaluated in clinical trials against various solid tumors, including NSCLC; these trials are expected to determine the optimal conditions, including optimal doses, optimal schedule, and optimal clinical setting, with establishment of appropriate surrogate markers. An optimal combined modality with anti-vascular therapy is probably necessary to obtain additional therapeutic benefits.

REFERENCES

1. Ries LAG, Eisner MP, Kosary CL. SEER cancer statistics review, 1973–1998. Bethesda, MD: National Cancer Institute; 2001.
2. Folkman J. Role of angiogenesis in tumor growth and metastasis. *Semin Oncol* 2002; **6** Suppl 16: 15–8.
3. Scappaticci FA. Mechanisms and future directions for angiogenesis-based cancer therapies. *J Clin Oncol* 2002; **20**: 3906–27.
4. Risau W. Mechanisms of angiogenesis. *Nature* 1997; **386**: 671–4.
5. Herbst RS, Fidler IJ. Angiogenesis and lung cancer: potential for therapy. *Clin Cancer Res* 2000; **6**: 4604–6.
6. Yano S, Shinohara H, Herbst RS, Kuniyasu H, Bucana CD, Ellis LM, Davis DW, McConkey DJ, Fidler IJ. Expression of vascular endothelial growth factor is essential but not sufficient for production and growth of brain metastasis. *Cancer Res* 2000; **60**: 4959–67.
7. Fidler IJ, Yano S, Zhang R, Fujimaki T, Bucana CD. The seed and soil hypothesis: vascularization and brain metastases. *Lancet Oncol* 2002; **3**: 53–7.
8. Pezzella F, Pastorino U, Tagliabue E, Andreola S, Sozzi G, Gasparini G, Menard S, Gatter KC, Harris AL, Fox S, Buyse M, Pilotti S, Pierotti M, Rilke F. Non-small-cell lung carcinoma tumor growth without morphological evidence of neo-angiogenesis. *Am J Pathol* 1997; **151**: 1417–23.
9. Fontanini G, Lucchi M, Vignati S, Mussi A, Ciardiello F, De Laurentiis M, De Placido S, Basolo F, Angeletti CA, Bevilacqua G. Angiogenesis as a prognostic indicator of survival in non-small-cell lung carcinoma: a prospective study. *J Natl Cancer Inst* 1997; **89**: 881–6.
10. Tanaka F, Otake Y, Yanagihara K, Kawano Y, Miyahara R, Li M, Yamada T, Hanaoka N, Inui K, Wada H. Evaluation of angiogenesis in non-small cell lung cancer: comparison between anti-CD34 antibody and anti-CD105 antibody. *Clin Cancer Res* 2001; **7**: 3410–5.
11. Meert AP, Paesmans M, Martin B, Delmotte P, Berghmans T, Verdebout JM, Lafitte JJ, Mascaux C, Sculier JP. The role of microvessel density on the survival of patients with lung cancer: a systematic review of the literature with meta-analysis. *Br J Cancer* 2002; **87**: 694–701.
12. Fontanini G, Vignati S, Boldrini L, Chine S, Silvestri V, Lucchi M, Mussi A, Angeletti CA, Bevilacqua G. Vascular endothelial growth factor is associated with neovascularization and influences progression of non-small cell lung carcinoma. *Clin Cancer Res* 1997; **3**: 861–5.
13. Brown PD, Bloxidge RE, Stuart NSE, Gatter KC, Carmichale J. Association between expression of activated 72-kilodalton gelatinase and tumor spread in non-small-cell lung carcinoma. *J Natl Cancer Inst* 1993; **85**: 574–8.
14. Fontanini G, De Laurentiis M, Vignati S, Chine S, Lucchi M, Silvestri V, Mussi A, De Placido S, Tortora G, Bianco AR, Gullick W, Angeletti CA, Bevilacqua G, Ciardiello F. Evaluation of epidermal growth factor-related growth factors and receptors and of neoangiogenesis in completely resected stage I-IIIA non-small-cell lung cancer: amphiregulin and microvessel count are independent prognostic indicators of survival. *Clin Cancer Res* 1998; **4**: 241–9.

15. Tanaka F, Ishikawa S, Yanagihara K, Miyahara R, Kawano Y, Li M, Otake Y, Wada H. Expression of angiopoietins and its clinical significance in non-small cell lung cancer. *Cancer Res* 2002; **62**: 7124–9.
16. Koukourakis MI, Giatromanolaki A, O'Byrne KJ, Comley M, Whitehouse RM, Talbot DC, Gatter KC, Harris AL. Platelet-derived endothelial cell growth factor expression correlates with tumour angiogenesis and prognosis in non-small-cell lung cancer. *Br J Cancer* 1997; **75**: 477–81.
17. Achiwa H, Yatabe Y, Hida T, Kuroishi T, Kozaki K, Nakamura S, Ogawa M, Sugiura T, Mitsudomi T, Takahashi T. Prognostic significance of elevated cyclooxygenase 2 expression in primary, resected lung adenocarcinomas. *Clin Cancer Res* 1999; **5**: 1001–5.
18. Dvorak HF. Vascular permeability factor/vascular endothelial growth factor: a critical cytokine in tumor angiogenesis and a potential target for diagnosis and therapy. *J Clin Oncol* 2002; **20**: 4368–80.
19. Yuan A, Yu CJ, Kuo SH, Chen WJ, Lin FY, Luh KT, Yang PC, Lee YC. Vascular endothelial growth factor 189 mRNA isoform expression specifically correlates with tumor angiogenesis, patient survival, and postoperative relapse in non-small-cell lung cancer. *J Clin Oncol* 2001; **19**: 432–41.
20. Yano S, Nishioka Y, Izumi K, Tsuruo T, Tanaka M, Miyasaka M, Sone S. Novel metastasis model of human lung cancer in SCID mice depleted of NK cells. *Int J Cancer* 1996; **67**: 211–7.
21. Yano S, Nokihara H, Hanibuchi M, Parajuli P, Shinohara T, Kawano T, Sone S. Model of malignant pleural effusion of human lung adenocarcinoma in SCID mice. *Oncol Res* 1997; **9**: 573–9.
22. Miki T, Yano S, Hanibuchi M, Sone S. Bone metastasis model with multiorgan dissemination of human small-cell lung cancer (SBC-5) cells in natural killer cell-depleted SCID mice. *Oncol Res* 2000; **12**: 209–17.
23. Yanagawa H, Takeuchi E, Suzuki Y, Ohmoto Y, Bando H, Sone S. Vascular endothelial growth factor in malignant pleural effusion associated with lung cancer. *Cancer Immunol Immunother* 1999; **48**: 396–400.
24. Yano S, Shinohara H, Herbst RS, Kuniyasu H, Bucana CD, Ellis LM, Fidler IJ. Production of experimental malignant pleural effusions is dependent on invasion of the pleura and expression of vascular endothelial growth factor/vascular permeability factor by human lung cancer cells. *Am J Pathol* 2000; **157**: 1893–903.
25. Plate KH. From angiogenesis to lymphangiogenesis. *Nat Med* 2001; **7**: 151–2.
26. Kajita T, Ohta Y, Kimura K, Tamura M, Tanaka Y, Tsunezuka Y, Oda M, Sasaki T, Watanabe G. The expression of vascular endothelial growth factor C and its receptors in non-small cell lung cancer. *Br J Cancer* 2001; **85**: 255–60.
27. Arinaga M, Noguchi T, Takeno S, Chujo M, Miura T, Uchida Y. Clinical significance of vascular endothelial growth factor C and vascular endothelial growth factor receptor 3 in patients with nonsmall cell lung carcinoma. *Cancer* 2003; **97**: 457–64.
28. Hidalgo M, Eckhardt SG. Development of matrix metalloproteinase inhibitors in cancer therapy. *J Natl Cancer Inst* 2001; **93**: 178–93.
29. Passlick B, Sienel W, Seen-Hibler R, Wockel W, Thetter O, Mutschler W, Pantel K. Overexpression of matrix metalloproteinase 2 predicts unfavorable outcome in early-stage non-small cell lung cancer. *Clin Cancer Res* 2000; **6**: 3944–8.

30. Herbst RS, Yano S, Kuniyasu H, Khuri FR, Bucana CD, Guo F, Liu D, Kemp B, Lee JJ, Hong WK, Fidler IJ. Differential expression of E-cadherin and type IV collagenase genes predicts outcome in patients with stage I non-small cell lung carcinoma. *Clin Cancer Res* 2000; **6**: 790–7.
31. Shiraga M, Yano S, Yamamoto A, Ogawa H, Goto H, Miki T, Miki K, Zhang H, Sone S. Organ heterogeneity of host-derived matrix metalloproteinase expression and its involvement in multiple-organ metastasis by lung cancer cell lines. *Cancer Res* 2002; **62**: 5967–73.
32. Klapper LN, Kirschbaum MH, Sela M, Yarden Y. Biochemical and clinical implications of the ErbB/HER signaling network of growth factor receptors. *Adv Cancer Res* 2000; **77**: 25–79.
33. Kim SJ, Uehara H, Karashima T, Shepherd DL, Killion JJ, Fidler IJ. Blockade of epidermal growth factor receptor signaling in tumor cells and tumor-associated endothelial cells for therapy of androgen-independent human prostate cancer growing in the bone of nude mice. *Clin Cancer Res* 2003; **9**: 1200–10.
34. Hirata A, Ogawa S, Kometani T, Kuwano T, Naito S, Kuwano M, Ono M. ZD1839 (Iressa) induces antiangiogenic effects through inhibition of epidermal growth factor receptor tyrosine kinase. *Cancer Res* 2002; **62**: 2554–60.
35. Meert AP, Martin B, Delmotte P, Berghmans T, Lafitte JJ, Mascaux C, Paesmans M, Steels E, Verdebout JM, Sculier JP. The role of EGF-R expression on patient survival in lung cancer: a systematic review with meta-analysis. *Eur Respir J* 2002; **20**: 975–81.
36. Kanematsu T, Yano S, Uehara H, Bando Y, Sone S. Phosphorylation, but not overexpression of epidermal growth factor receptor is associated with poor prognosis of non-small cell lung cancer patients. *Oncol Res* 2003; **13**: 289–98.
37. Folkman J. Tumor angiogenesis: therapeutic implications. *N Engl J Med* 1971; **285**: 1182–6.
38. Jain RK. Tumor angiogenesis and accessibility: role of vascular endothelial growth factor. *Semin Oncol* 2002; **6** Suppl 16: 3–9.
39. Yano S, Herbst RS, Shinohara S, Knighton B, Bucana CD, Killion JJ, Wood J, Fidler IJ. Treatment for malignant pleural effusion of human lung adenocarcinoma by inhibition of vascular endothelial growth factor receptor tyrosine kinase phosphorylation. *Clin Cancer Res* 2000; **6**: 957–65.
40. Johnson DH, DeVore R, Kabbinavar F, Herbst RS, Holmgren E, Novotny W. Carboplatin (C)+Paclitaxel (T)+RhuMab-VEGF (AVF) may prolong survival in advanced non-squamous lung cancer. *Proc Am Soc Clin Oncol* 2001; **20**: 1256a.
41. Langmuir VK, Cobleigh MA, Herbst RS, Holmgren E, Hurwitz H, Kabbinavar F, Miller K, Novotny W. Successful long-term therapy with bevacizumab (Avastin) in solid tumors. *Proc Am Soc Clin Oncol* 2002; **21**: 32a.
42. Yamamoto A, Yano S, Shiraga M, Ogawa H, Goto H, Miki T, Zhang H, Sone S. A third generation matrix metalloproteinase (MMP) inhibitor (ONO-4817) combined with docetaxel suppresses progression of lung-micrometastasis of MMP expressing tumor cells in nude mice. *Int J Cancer* 2003; **103**: 822–8.
43. Fielding J, Scholefield J, Stuart R, Hawkins R, McCulloch P, Maughan T, Seymour M, Van Cutsem E, Thorlacius-Ussing O, Hovendal C. A randomized double-blind placebo-controlled study of marimastat in patients with inoperable gastric adenocarci-

noma. *Proc Am Soc Clin Oncol* 2000; **19**: 929a.

44. Shepherd FA, Giaccone G, Debruyne C, Hirsh V, Smylie M, Rubin S, Martins H, Lamont A, Krzakowski M, Zee B, Sadura A, Seymour L. Randomized double-blind placebo-controlled trial of marimastat in patients with small cell lung cancer (SCLC) following response to first-line chemotherapy: an NCIC-CTG and EORTC study. *Proc Am Soc Clin Oncol* 2001; **20**: 11a.
45. Smylie M, Mercier R, Aboulafia D, Tucker R, Bonomi P, Collier M, Rose Keller M, Stuart-Smith J, Knowles M, Clendeninn NJ, Shepherd F. Phase III study of the matrix metalloprotease (MMP) inhibitor prinomastat in patients having advanced non-small cell lung cancer (NSCLC). *Proc Am Soc Clin Oncol* 2001; **20**: 1926a.
46. Randal J. Antiangiogenesis drugs target specific cancers, mechanisms. *J Natl Cancer Inst* 2000; **92**: 520–2.
47. Blakey DC, Westwood FR, Walker M, Hughes GD, Davis PD, Ashton SE, Ryan AJ. Antitumor activity of the novel vascular targeting agent ZD6126 in a panel of tumor models. *Clin Cancer Res* 2002; **8**: 1974–83.
48. Goto H, Yano S, Zhang H, Matsumori Y, Ogawa H, Blakey DC, Sone S. Activity of a new vascular targeting agent, ZD6126 in pulmonary metastases by human lung adenocarcinoma in nude mice. *Cancer Res* 2002; **62**: 3711–5.
49. Belotti D, Vergani V, Drudis T, Borsotti P, Pitelli MR, Viale G, Giavazzi R, Taraboletti G. The microtubule-affecting drug paclitaxel has antiangiogenic activity. *Clin Cancer Res* 1996; **2**: 1843–9.
50. Baselga J. Why the epidermal growth factor receptor? The rationale for cancer therapy. *Oncologist* 2002; **7** Suppl 4: 2–8.
51. Negoro S, Nakagawa K, Fukuoka M, Kudoh S, Tamura T, Yoshimura N, Takeda K, Tanigawara Y, Swaisland H. Final results of a phase I intermittent dose-escalation trial of ZD1839 ('Iressa') in Japanese patients with various solid tumors. *Proc Am Soc Clin Oncol* 2001; **20**: 324; 1292a.
52. Fukuoka M, Yano S, Giaccone G, Tamura T, Nakagawa K, Douillard JY, Nishiwaki Y, Vansteenkiste JF, Kudo S, Averbuch S, Macleod A Feyereislova A, Baselga J. Final results from a phase II trial of ZD1839 ('Iressa') for patients with advanced non-small-cell lung cancer (IDEAL 1). *Proc Am Soc Clin Oncol* 2002; **21**: 298a.
53. Barkley JE, Green MR. Bronchioloalveolar carcinoma. *J Clin Oncol* 1996; **14**: 2377–86.
54. Yano S, Kanematsu T, Miki T, Aono S, Azuma M, Yamamoto A, Uehara H, Sone S. A report of two bronchioloalveolar carcinoma cases which were rapidly improved by treatment with the epidermal growth factor receptor tyrosine kinase inhibitor ZD1839 ('Iressa'). *Cancer Sci* 2003; **94**: 453–8.
55. Giaccone G, Johnson DH, Manegold C, Scagliotti GV. A phase III clinical trial of ZD1839 (Iressa) in combination with gemcitabine and cisplatin in chemo-naive patients with advanced non-small cell lung cancer (INTACT 1). *Ann Oncol* 2002; **13** Suppl 5: 2–3.
56. Johnson DH, Herbst RS, Giaccone G, Schiller J. ZD1839 (Iressa) in combination with paclitaxel and carboplatin in chemotherapy-naive patients with advanced non-small cell lung cancer; results from a phase III clinical trial (INTACT 2). *Ann Oncol* 2002; **13** Suppl 5: 127–8.
57. Inoue A, Saijo Y, Maemondo M, Gomi K, Tokue Y, Kimura Y, Ebina M, Kikuchi T,

Moriya T, Nukiwa T. Severe acute interstitial pneumonia and gefitinib. *Lancet* 2003; **361**: 137–9.

58. Kerbel RS. Clinical trials of antiangiogenic drugs: opportunities, problems, and assessment of initial results. *J Clin Oncol* 2001; **19** Suppl 18: 45S–51S.
59. Herbst RS, Mullani NA, Davis DW, Hess KR, McConkey DJ, Charnsangavej C, O'Reilly MS, Kim HW, Baker C, Roach J, Ellis LM, Rashid A, Pluda J, Bucana C, Madden TL, Tran HT, Abbruzzese JL. Development of biologic markers of response and assessment of antiangiogenic activity in a clinical trial of human recombinant endostatin. *J Clin Oncol* 2002; **20**: 3804–14.

AUTHOR INDEX

SUBJECT INDEX

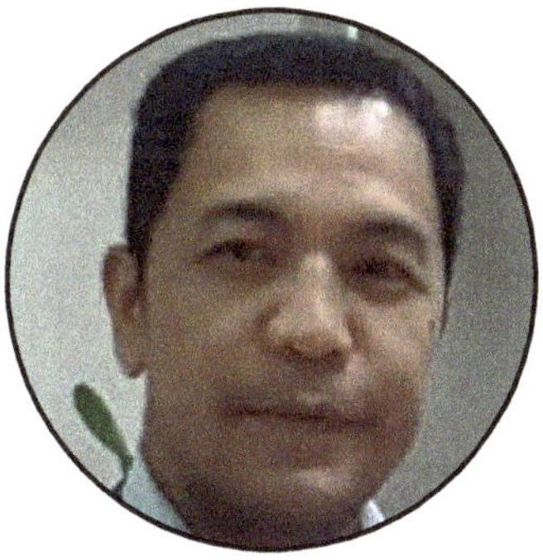

About the Editor

Jurex Cuenca Gallo

Dr. Jurex Gallo was conferred with his PhD degree in Chemical Engineering from De La Salle University – Manila in 2014. His expertise revolved in the fields of Material Science and Environmental Engineering focused on industrial and hazardous waste treatment and management. Presently, Dr. Gallo is affiliated as Senior Science Research Specialist of the Department of Science and Technology e-Asia Joint Research Program in the Philippines on developing functional carbon-based nanomaterials such as carbon nanotubes and graphene for energy and environmental applications.

Table of Contents

3 IMPACTS OF NANOTECHNOLOGY

4 APPLICATIONS OF NANOTECHNOLOGY

5 NANOMATERIALS: CORNERSTONES OF NANOSCIENCE AND NANOTECHNOLOGY

6 MOLECULAR SELF-ASSEMBLY

7 NANOELECTRONICS

8 NANOMETROLOGY CONCEPTS

List of Abbreviations

AFM	Atomic Force Microscopy
CMM	Coordinate Measuring Machine
CNT	Carbon Nanotubes
CSCNT	Cup Stacked Carbon Nanotubes
CVD	Chemical Vapor Deposition
DFT	Density Functional Theory
DSA	Directed Self Assembly
DWNT	Double Walled Carbon Nanotubes
FED	Field Emission Displays
FET	Field Effect Transistors
HOPG	Highly Oriented Pyrolitic Graphite
HPHT	High Pressure High Temperature
LEIS	Low Energy Ion Scattering
MWNT	Multi Walled Nanotubes
NEMS	Nanoelectromechanical Systems
NEXAFS	Near Edge X-ray Absorption Fine Structure
NIL	Nanoimprint Lithography
OPC	Optical Proximity Correction
PSM	Phase Shift Masks
RAIRS	Reflection Absorption Infrared Spectroscopy
RF	Radio Frequency
SAM	Scanning Acoustic Microscope
SAM	Self Assembled Monolayers

SEM	Scanning Electron Microscopy
SERS	Surface Enhanced Raman Scattering
SFG	Sum Frequency Generation
SHG	Second Harmonic Generation
SPL	Scanning Probe Lithography
STM	Scanning Tunneling Microscope
SWNT	Single Walled Nanotubes
TMR	Tunneling Magnetoresistance
TOFDRS	Time of Flight Direct Recoil Spectroscopy
TRPS	Tunable Resistive Pulse Sensing

Preface

Nanotechnology is the engineering of functional systems at the molecular scale. This covers both current work and concepts that are more advanced. "Nanotech" products that are on the market today are mostly gradually improved products where some form of nano-enabled material (such as carbon nanotubes, nanocomposite structures or nanoparticles of a particular substance) or nanotech process is used in the manufacturing process. In their ongoing quest to improve existing products by creating smaller components and better performance materials, all at a lower cost, the number of companies that will manufacture "nanoproducts" will grow very fast and soon make up the majority of all companies across many industries. Scientists have been studying and working with nanoparticles for centuries, but the effectiveness of their work has been hampered by their inability to see the structure of nanoparticles. In recent decades the development of microscopes capable of displaying particles as small as atoms has allowed scientists to see what they are working with. Researchers are developing customized nanoparticles; the size of molecules that can deliver drugs directly to diseased cells in your body. When it's perfected, this method should greatly reduce the damage treatment such as chemotherapy does to a patient's healthy cells. Nanotechnology holds some answers for how we might increase the capabilities of electronic devices while we reduce their weight and power consumption. Nanotechnology is having an impact on several aspects of food science, from how food is grown to how it is packaged. Companies are developing nanomaterials that will make a difference not only in the taste of food, but also in food safety, and the health benefits that food delivers. Nanotechnology is being used to reduce the cost of catalysts used in fuel cells to produce hydrogen ions from fuel such as methanol and to improve the efficiency of membranes used in fuel cells to separate hydrogen ions from other gases such as oxygen. Nanotechnology may hold the key to making space-flight more practical. Advancements in nanomaterials make lightweight spacecraft and a cable for the space elevator possible. By significantly reducing the amount of rocket fuel required, these advances could lower the cost of reaching orbit and traveling in space. Many benefits of nanotechnology depend on the fact that it is possible to tailor the structures of materials at extremely small scales to achieve specific properties, thus greatly extending the materials science toolkit. Using nanotechnology, materials can effectively be made stronger, lighter, more durable, more reactive, more sieve-like, or better electrical conductors, among many other traits.

Content Coverage

Chapters One and *Two* present fundamental concepts of nanotechnology and history of nanotechnology, respectively. The history of nanotechnology traces the development of the concepts and experimental work falling under the broad category of nanotechnology. Although nanotechnology is a relatively recent development in scientific research, the development of its central concepts happened over a longer period of time.

Chapters Three and *Four* present coverage of nanotechnology impacts and applications, separately. Nanotechnology is also being applied to or developed for application to a variety of industrial and purification processes.

Chapters Five and *Six* focus on nanomaterials and molecular self-assembly, correspondingly. Nanomaterials are slowly becoming commercialized and beginning to emerge as commodities.

Chapters Seven and *Eight* present about nanoelectronics which refer to the use of nanotechnology in electronic components, and nanometrology concerned with the science of measurement at the nanoscale level, separately.

CHAPTER 1

Nanotechnology: An overview

Chapter Contents

Nanotechnology is a field of research and innovation concerned with building 'things' - generally, materials and devices - on the scale of atoms and molecules. A nanometre is one-billionth of a metre: ten times the diameter of a hydrogen atom. The diameter of a human hair is, on average, 80,000 nanometres. At such scales, the ordinary rules of physics and chemistry no longer apply. For instance, materials' characteristics, such as their color, strength, conductivity and reactivity, can differ substantially between the nanoscale and the macro. Carbon 'nanotubes' are 100 times stronger than steel but six times lighter.

INTRODUCTION

Nanotechnology ("nanotech") is manipulation of matter on an atomic, molecular, and supramolecular scale. The earliest, widespread description of nanotechnology referred to the particular technological goal of precisely manipulating atoms and molecules for fabrication of macroscale products, also now referred to as molecular nanotechnology. A more generalized description of nanotechnology was subsequently established by the National Nanotechnology Initiative, which defines nanotechnology as the manipulation of matter with at least one dimension sized from 1 to 100 nanometers. This definition reflects the fact that quantum mechanical effects are important at this quantum-realm scale, and so the definition shifted from a particular technological goal to a research category inclusive of all types of research and technologies that deal with the special properties of matter which occur below the given size threshold. It is therefore common to see the plural form "nanotechnologies" as well as "nanoscale technologies" to refer to the broad range of research and applications whose common trait is size. Because of the variety of potential applications (including industrial and military), governments have invested billions of dollars in nanotechnology research. Until 2012, through its National Nanotechnology Initiative, the USA has invested 3.7 billion dollars, the European Union has invested 1.2 billion and Japan 750 million dollars.

Nanotechnology as defined by size is naturally very broad, including fields of science as diverse as surface science, organic chemistry, molecular biology, semiconductor physics, microfabrication, molecular engineering, etc. The associated research and applications are equally diverse, ranging from extensions of conventional device physics to completely new approaches based upon molecular self-assembly, from developing new materials with dimensions on the nanoscale to direct control of matter on the atomic scale.

Scientists currently debate the future implications of nanotechnology. Nanotechnology may be able to create many new materials and devices with a vast range of applications, such as in nanomedicine, nanoelectronics, biomaterials energy production, and consumer products. On the other hand, nanotechnology raises many of the same issues as any new technology, including concerns about the toxicity and environmental impact of nanomaterials, and their potential effects on global economics, as well as speculation about various doomsday scenarios. These concerns have led to a debate among advocacy groups and governments on whether special regulation of nanotechnology is warranted.

ORIGINS

The concepts that seeded nanotechnology were first discussed in 1959 by renowned physicist Richard Feynman in his talk *There's Plenty of Room at the Bottom*, in which he described the possibility of synthesis via direct manipulation of atoms. The term "nano-technology" was first used by Norio Taniguchi in 1974, though it was not widely known.

Inspired by Feynman's concepts, K. Eric Drexler used the term "nanotechnology" in his 1986 book *Engines of Creation: The Coming Era of Nanotechnology*, which proposed the idea of a nanoscale "assembler" which would be able to build a copy of itself and of other items of arbitrary complexity with atomic control. Also in 1986, Drexler co-founded The Foresight Institute (with which he is no longer affiliated) to help increase public awareness and understanding of nanotechnology concepts and implications.

Thus, emergence of nanotechnology as a field in the 1980s occurred through convergence of Drexler's theoretical and public work, which developed and popularized a conceptual framework for nanotechnology, and high-visibility experimental advances that drew additional wide-scale attention to the prospects of atomic control of matter. In the 1980s, two major breakthroughs sparked the growth of nanotechnology in modern era.

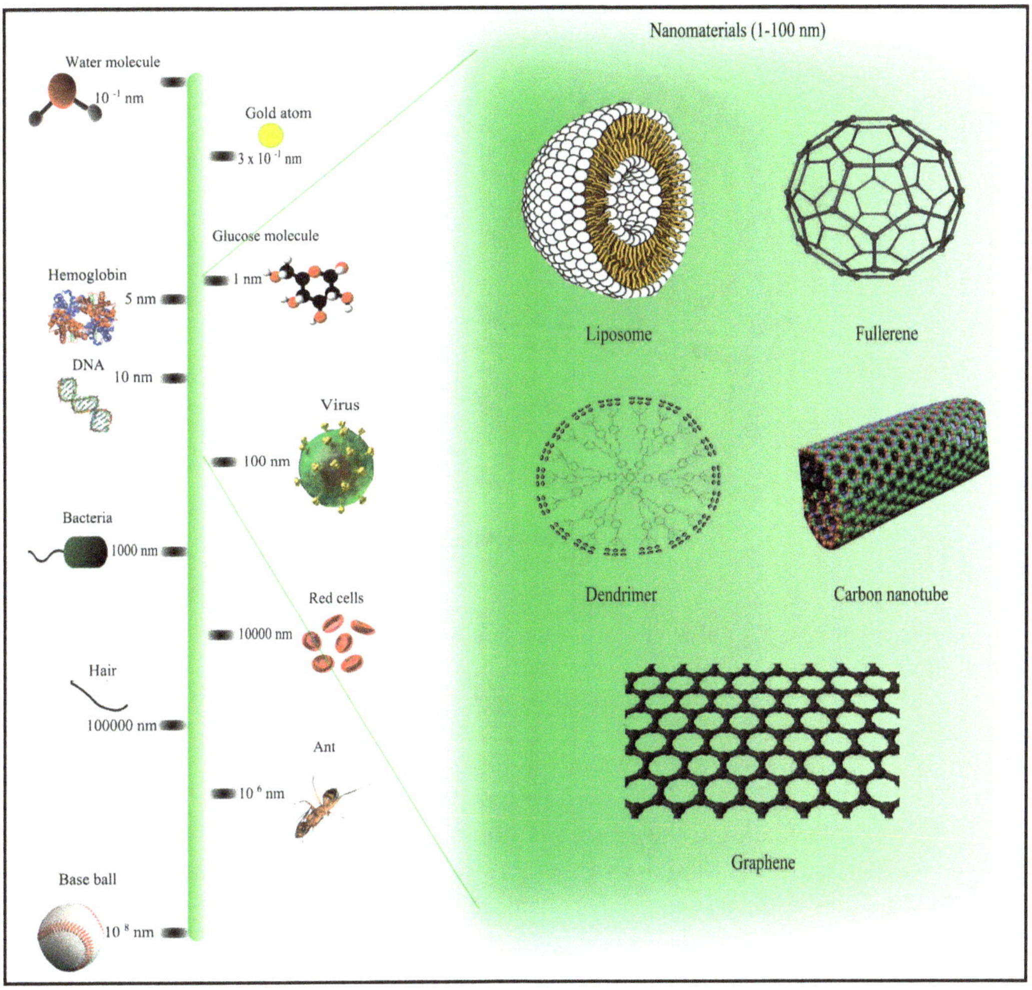

Comparison of Nanomaterials Sizes

First, the invention of the scanning tunneling microscope in 1981 which provided unprecedented visualization of individual atoms and bonds, and was successfully used to manipulate individual atoms in 1989. The microscope's developers Gerd Binnig and Heinrich Rohrer at IBM Zurich Research Laboratory received a Nobel Prize in Physics in 1986. Binnig, Quate and Gerber also invented the analogous atomic force microscope that year.

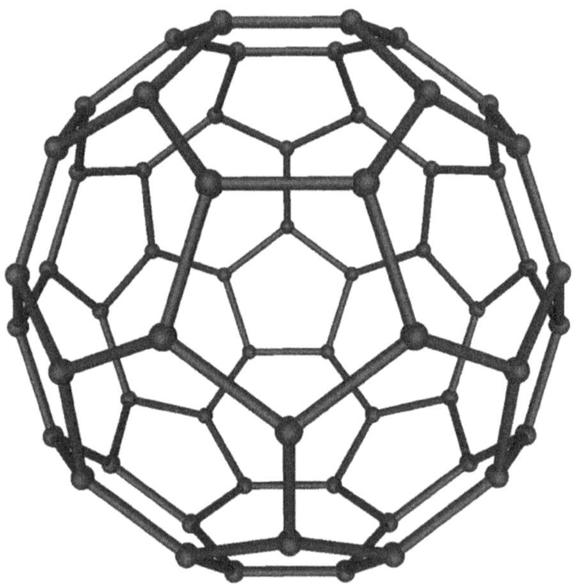

Buckminsterfullerene C_{60}, also known as the buckyball, is a representative member of the carbon structures known as fullerenes. Members of the fullerene family are a major subject of research falling under the nanotechnology umbrella.

Second, Fullerenes were discovered in 1985 by Harry Kroto, Richard Smalley, and Robert Curl, who together won the 1996 Nobel Prize in Chemistry. C_{60} was not initially described as nanotechnology; the term was used regarding subsequent work with related graphene tubes (called carbon nanotubes and sometimes called Bucky tubes) which suggested potential applications for nanoscale electronics and devices.

In the early 2000s, the field garnered increased scientific, political, and commercial attention that led to both controversy and progress. Controversies emerged regarding the definitions and potential implications of nanotechnologies, exemplified by the Royal Society's report on nanotechnology. Challenges were raised regarding the feasibility of applications envisioned by advocates of molecular nanotechnology, which culminated in a public debate between Drexler and Smalley in 2001 and 2003.

Meanwhile, commercialization of products based on advancements in nanoscale technologies began emerging. These products are limited to bulk applications of nanomaterials and do not involve atomic control of matter. Some examples include the Silver Nano platform for using silver nanoparticles as an antibacterial agent, nanoparticle-based transparent sunscreens, carbon fiber strengthening using silica nanoparticles, and carbon nanotubes for stain-resistant textiles.

Governments moved to promote and fund research into nanotechnology, such as in the U.S. with the National Nanotechnology Initiative, which formalized a size-based definition of nanotechnology and established funding for research on the nanoscale, and in Europe via the European Framework Programmes for Research and Technological Development.

By the mid-2000s new and serious scientific attention began to flourish. Projects emerged to produce nanotechnology roadmaps which center on atomically precise manipulation of matter and discuss existing and projected capabilities, goals, and applications.

FUNDAMENTAL CONCEPTS

Nanotechnology is the engineering of functional systems at the molecular scale. This covers both current work and concepts that are more advanced. In its original sense, nanotechnology refers to the projected ability to construct items from the bottom up, using techniques and tools being developed today to make complete, high performance products.

One nanometer (nm) is one billionth, or 10^{-9}, of a meter. By comparison, typical carbon-carbon bond lengths, or the spacing between these atoms in a molecule, are in the range 0.12–0.15 nm, and a DNA double-helix has a diameter around 2 nm. On the other hand, the smallest cellular life-forms, the bacteria of the genus Mycoplasma, are around 200 nm in length. By convention, nanotechnology is taken as the scale range 1 to 100 nm following the definition used by the National Nanotechnology Initiative in the US. The lower limit is set by the size of atoms (hydrogen has the smallest atoms, which are approximately a quarter of a nm diameter) since nanotechnology must build its devices from atoms and molecules. The upper limit is more or less arbitrary but is around the size below which phenomena not observed in larger structures start to become apparent and can be made use of in the nano device. These new phenomena make nanotechnology distinct from devices which are merely miniaturized versions of an equivalent macroscopic device; such devices are on a larger scale and come under the description of microtechnology.

To put that scale in another context, the comparative size of a nanometer to a meter is the same as that of a marble to the size of the earth. Or another way of putting it: a nanometer is the amount an average man's beard grows in the time it takes him to raise the razor to his face.

Two main approaches are used in nanotechnology. In the "bottom-up" approach, materials and devices are built from molecular components which assemble themselves chemically by principles of molecular recognition. In the "top-down" approach, nano-objects are constructed from larger entities without atomic-level control.

Areas of physics such as nanoelectronics, nanomechanics, nanophotonics and nanoionics have evolved during the last few decades to provide a basic scientific foundation of nanotechnology.

Larger to Smaller: A Materials Perspective

Several phenomena become pronounced as the size of the system decreases. These include statistical mechanical effects, as well as quantum mechanical effects, for example the "quantum size effect" where the electronic properties of solids are altered with great reductions in particle size. This effect does not come into play by going from macro to micro dimensions. However, quantum effects can become significant when the nanometer size range is reached, typically at distances of 100 nanometers or less, the so-called quantum realm. Additionally, a number of physical (mechanical, electrical, optical, etc.) properties change when compared to macroscopic systems. One example is the increase in surface area to volume ratio altering mechanical, thermal and catalytic properties of materials. Diffusion and reactions at nanoscale, nanostructures materials and nanodevices with fast ion transport are generally referred to nanoionics. *Mechanical* properties of nanosystems are of interest in the nanomechanics research. The catalytic activity of nanomaterials also opens potential risks in their interaction with biomaterials.

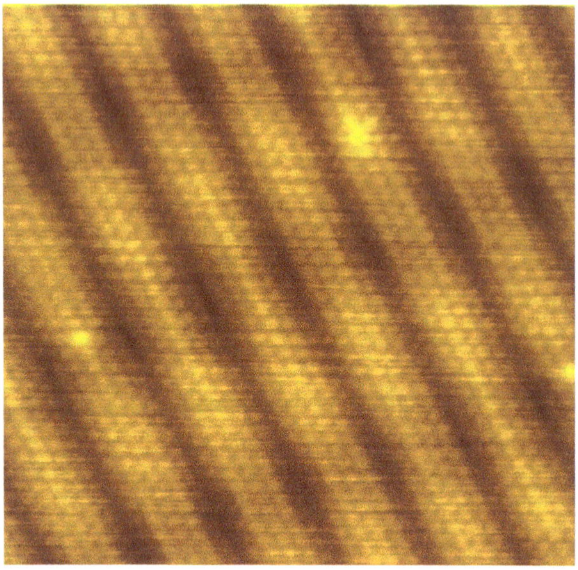

Image of reconstruction on a clean Gold(100) surface, as visualized using scanning tunneling microscopy. The positions of the individual atoms composing the surface are visible.

Materials reduced to the nanoscale can show different properties compared to what they exhibit on a macroscale, enabling unique applications. For instance, opaque substances can become transparent (copper); stable materials can turn combustible (aluminium); insoluble materials may become soluble (gold). A material such as gold, which is chemically inert at normal scales, can serve as a potent chemical catalyst at nanoscales. Much of the fascination with nanotechnology stems from these quantum and surface phenomena that matter exhibits at the nanoscale.

Simple to Complex: A Molecular Perspective

Modern synthetic chemistry has reached the point where it is possible to prepare small molecules to almost any structure. These methods are used today to manufacture a wide variety of useful chemicals such as pharmaceuticals or commercial polymers. This ability raises the question of extending this kind of control to the next-larger level, seeking methods to assemble these single molecules into supramolecular assemblies consisting of many molecules arranged in a well defined manner.

These approaches utilize the concepts of molecular self-assembly and/or supramolecular chemistry to automatically arrange themselves into some useful conformation through a bottom-up approach. The concept of molecular recognition is especially important: molecules can be designed so that a specific configuration or arrangement is favored due to non-covalent intermolecular forces. The Watson–Crick base pairing rules are a direct result of this, as is the specificity of an enzyme being targeted to a single substrate, or the specific folding of the protein itself. Thus, two or more components can be designed to be complementary and mutually attractive so that they make a more complex and useful whole.

Such bottom-up approaches should be capable of producing devices in parallel and be much cheaper than top-down methods, but could potentially be overwhelmed as the size and complexity of the desired assembly increases. Most useful structures require complex and thermodynamically unlikely arrangements of atoms. Nevertheless, there are many examples of self-assembly based on molecular recognition in biology, most notably Watson–Crick basepairing and enzyme-substrate interactions. The challenge for nanotechnology is whether these principles can be used to engineer new constructs in addition to natural ones.

Molecular Nanotechnology: A Long-Term View

Molecular nanotechnology, sometimes called molecular manufacturing, describes engineered nanosystems (nanoscale machines) operating on the molecular scale. Molecular nanotechnology is especially associated with the molecular assembler, a machine that can produce a desired structure or device atom-by-atom using the principles of mechanosynthesis. Manufacturing in the context of productive nanosystems is not related to, and should be clearly distinguished from, the conventional technologies used to manufacture nanomaterials such as carbon nanotubes and nanoparticles.

When the term "nanotechnology" was independently coined and popularized by Eric Drexler (who at the time was unaware of an earlier usage by Norio Taniguchi) it referred to a future manufacturing technology based on molecular machine systems. The premise was that molecular scale biological analogies of traditional machine components demonstrated molecular machines were possible: by the countless examples found in biology, it is known that sophisticated, stochastically optimised biological machines can be produced.

It is hoped that developments in nanotechnology will make possible their construction by some other means, perhaps using biomimetic principles. However, Drexler and other researchers have proposed that advanced nanotechnology, although perhaps initially implemented by biomimetic means, ultimately could be based on mechanical engineering principles, namely, a manufacturing technology based on the mechanical functionality of these components (such as gears, bearings, motors, and structural members) that would enable programmable, positional assembly to atomic specification. The physics and engineering performance of exemplar designs were analyzed in Drexler's book *Nanosystems*.

In general it is very difficult to assemble devices on the atomic scale, as one has to position atoms on other atoms of comparable size and stickiness. Another view, put forth by Carlo Montemagno, is that future nanosystems will be hybrids of silicon technology and biological molecular machines. Richard Smalley argued that mechanosynthesis are impossible due to the difficulties in mechanically manipulating individual molecules.

This led to an exchange of letters in the ACS publication Chemical & Engineering News in 2003. Though biology clearly demonstrates that molecular machine systems are possible, non-biological molecular machines are today only in their infancy. Leaders in research on non-biological molecular machines are Dr. Alex Zettl and his colleagues at Lawrence Berkeley Laboratories and UC Berkeley. They have constructed at least three distinct molecular devices whose motion is controlled from the desktop with changing voltage: a nanotube nanomotor, a molecular actuator, and a nanoelectromechanical relaxation oscillator.

An experiment indicating that positional molecular assembly is possible was performed by Ho and Lee at Cornell University in 1999. They used a scanning tunneling microscope to move an individual carbon monoxide molecule (CO) to an individual iron atom (Fe) sitting on a flat silver crystal, and chemically bound the CO to the Fe by applying a voltage.

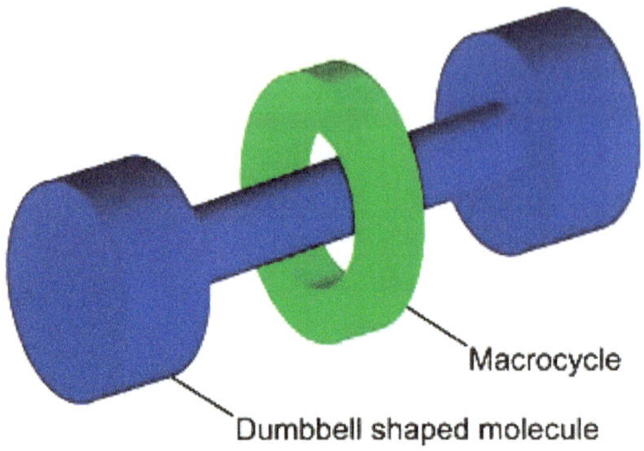

Graphical representation of a rotaxane, useful as a molecular switch.

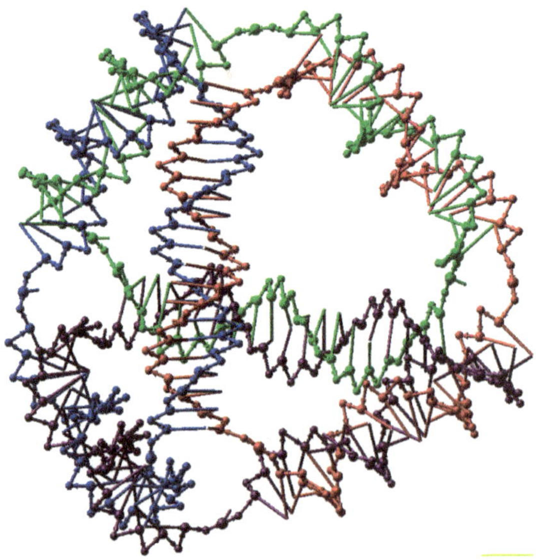

This DNA tetrahedron is an artificially designed nanostructure of the type made in the field of DNA nanotechnology. Each edge of the tetrahedron is a 20 base pair DNA double helix, and each vertex is a three-arm junction.

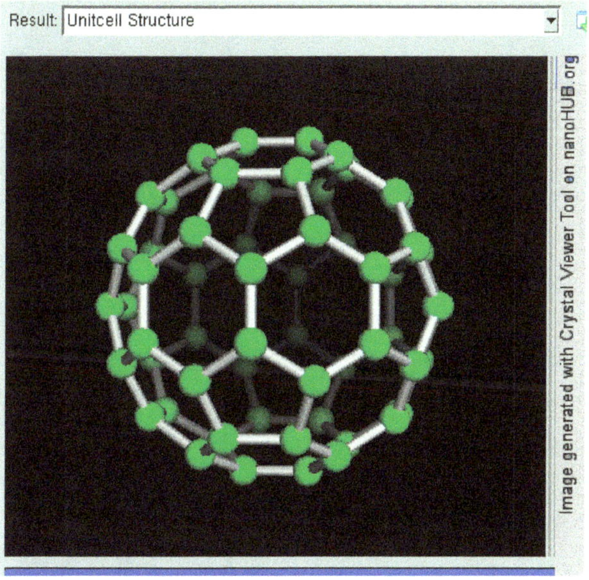

Rotating view of C_{60}, one kind of fullerene.

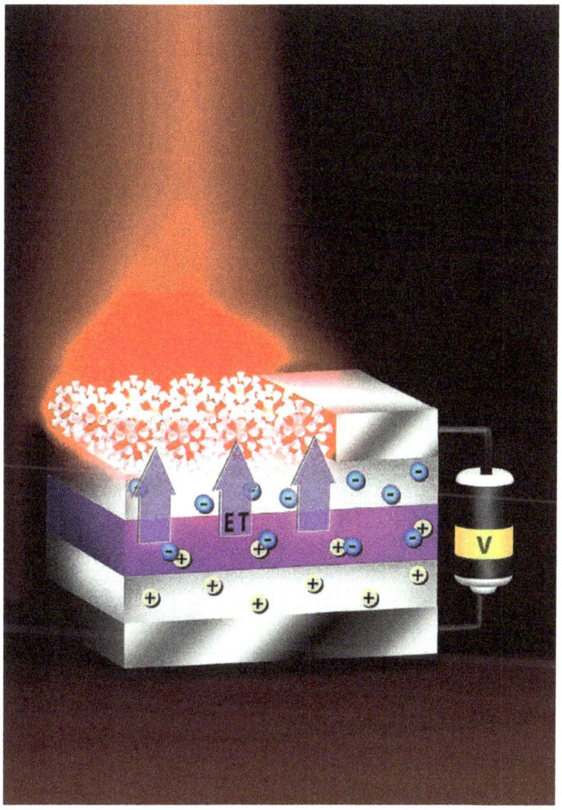

This device transfers energy from nano-thin layers of quantum wells to nanocrystals above them, causing the nanocrystals to emit visible light.

Nanomaterials

The nanomaterials field includes subfields which develop or study materials having unique properties arising from their nanoscale dimensions.

- Interface and colloid science has given rise to many materials which may be useful in nanotechnology, such as carbon nanotubes and other fullerenes, and various nanoparticles and nanorods. Nanomaterials with fast ion transport are related also to nanoionics and nanoelectronics.
- Nanoscale materials can also be used for bulk applications; most present commercial applications of nanotechnology are of this flavor.
- Progress has been made in using these materials for medical applications.
- Nanoscale materials such as nanopillars are sometimes used in solar cells which combats the cost of traditional Silicon solar cells.
- Development of applications incorporating semiconductor nanoparticles to be used in the next generation of products, such as display technology, lighting, solar cells and biological imaging.
- Recent application of nanomaterials include a range of biomedical applications, such as tissue engineering, drug delivery, and biosensors.

Bottom-up Approaches

These seek to arrange smaller components into more complex assemblies.

- DNA nanotechnology utilizes the specificity of Watson–Crick basepairing to construct well-defined structures out of DNA and other nucleic acids.
- Approaches from the field of "classical" chemical synthesis (Inorganic and organic synthesis) also aim at designing molecules with well-defined shape (e.g. bis-peptides).
- More generally, molecular self-assembly seeks to use concepts of supramolecular chemistry, and molecular recognition in particular, to cause single-molecule components to automatically arrange themselves into some useful conformation.
- Atomic force microscope tips can be used as a nanoscale "write head" to deposit a chemical upon a surface in a desired pattern in a process called dip pen nanolithography. This technique fits into the larger subfield of nanolithography.

Top-Down Approaches

These seek to create smaller devices by using larger ones to direct their assembly.

- Many technologies that descended from conventional solid-state silicon methods for fabricating microprocessors are now capable of creating features smaller than 100 nm, falling under the definition of nanotechnology. Giant magnetoresistance-based hard drives already on the market fit this description, as do atomic layer deposition (ALD) techniques. Peter Grünberg and Albert Fert received the Nobel

Prize in Physics in 2007 for their discovery of Giant magnetoresistance and contributions to the field of spintronics.

- Solid-state techniques can also be used to create devices known as nanoelectromechanical systems or NEMS, which are related to microelectromechanical systems or MEMS.
- Focused ion beams can directly remove material, or even deposit material when suitable precursor gasses are applied at the same time. For example, this technique is used routinely to create sub-100 nm sections of material for analysis in Transmission electron microscopy.
- Atomic force microscope tips can be used as a nanoscale "write head" to deposit a resist, which is then followed by an etching process to remove material in a top-down method.

Functional Approaches

These seek to develop components of a desired functionality without regard to how they might be assembled.

- Magnetic assembly for the synthesis of anisotropic superparamagnetic materials such as recently presented magnetic nanochains.
- Molecular scale electronics seeks to develop molecules with useful electronic properties. These could then be used as single-molecule components in a nanoelectronic device. For an example see rotaxane.
- Synthetic chemical methods can also be used to create synthetic molecular motors, such as in a so-called nanocar.

Biomimetic Approaches

- Bionics or biomimicry seeks to apply biological methods and systems found in nature, to the study and design of engineering systems and modern technology. Biomineralization is one example of the systems studied.
- Bionanotechnology is the use of biomolecules for applications in nanotechnology, including use of viruses and lipid assemblies. Nanocellulose is a potential bulk-scale application.

Speculative

These subfields seek to anticipate what inventions nanotechnology might yield, or attempt to propose an agenda along which inquiry might progress. These often take a big-picture view of nanotechnology, with more emphasis on its societal implications than the details of how such inventions could actually be created.

- Molecular nanotechnology is a proposed approach which involves manipulating single molecules in finely controlled, deterministic ways. This is more theoretical than the other subfields, and many of its proposed techniques are beyond current capabilities.

- Nanorobotics centers on self-sufficient machines of some functionality operating at the nanoscale. There are hopes for applying nanorobots in medicine, but it may not be easy to do such a thing because of several drawbacks of such devices. Nevertheless, progress on innovative materials and methodologies has been demonstrated with some patents granted about new nanomanufacturing devices for future commercial applications, which also progressively helps in the development towards nanorobots with the use of embedded nanobioelectronics concepts.
- Productive nanosystems are "systems of nanosystems" which will be complex nanosystems that produce atomically precise parts for other nanosystems, not necessarily using novel nanoscale-emergent properties, but well-understood fundamentals of manufacturing. Because of the discrete (i.e. atomic) nature of matter and the possibility of exponential growth, this stage is seen as the basis of another industrial revolution. Mihail Roco, one of the architects of the USA's National Nanotechnology Initiative, has proposed four states of nanotechnology that seem to parallel the technical progress of the Industrial Revolution, progressing from passive nanostructures to active nanodevices to complex nanomachines and ultimately to productive nanosystems.
- Programmable matter seeks to design materials whose properties can be easily, reversibly and externally controlled though a fusion of information science and materials science.
- Due to the popularity and media exposure of the term nanotechnology, the words picotechnology and femtotechnology have been coined in analogy to it, although these are only used rarely and informally.

Dimensionality in Nanomaterials

Nanomaterials can be classified in 0D, 1D, 2D and 3D nanomaterials. The dimensionality play a major role in determining the characteristic of nanomaterials including physical, chemical and biological characteristics. With the decrease in dimensionality, an increase in surface-to-volume ratio is observed. This indicate that smaller dimensional nanomaterials have higher surface area compared to 3D nanomaterials. Recently, two dimensional (2D) nanomaterials are extensively investigated for electronic, biomedical, drug delivery and biosensor applications.

TOOLS AND TECHNIQUES

There are several important modern developments. The atomic force microscope (AFM) and the Scanning Tunneling Microscope (STM) are two early versions of scanning probes that launched nanotechnology. There are other types of scanning probe microscopy. Although conceptually similar to the scanning confocal microscope developed by Marvin Minsky in 1961 and the scanning acoustic microscope (SAM) developed by Calvin Quate and coworkers in the 1970s, newer scanning probe microscopes have much higher resolution, since they are not limited by the wavelength of sound or light.

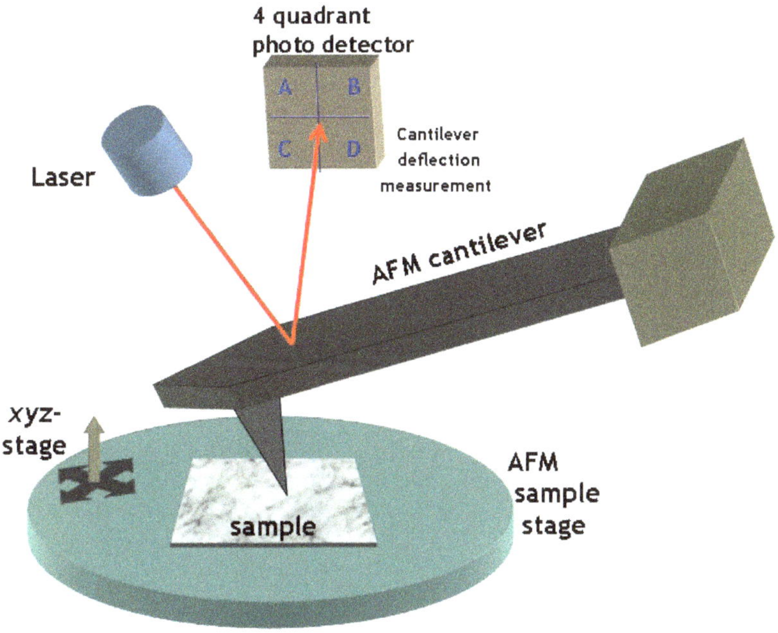

Typical AFM setup. A microfabricated cantilever with a sharp tip is deflected by features on a sample surface, much like in a phonograph but on a much smaller scale. A laser beam reflects off the backside of the cantilever into a set of photodetectors, allowing the deflection to be measured and assembled into an image of the surface.

The tip of a scanning probe can also be used to manipulate nanostructures (a process called positional assembly). Feature-oriented scanning methodology may be a promising way to implement these nanomanipulations in automatic mode. However, this is still a slow process because of low scanning velocity of the microscope.

Various techniques of nanolithography such as optical lithography, X-ray lithography dip pen nanolithography, electron beam lithography or nanoimprint lithography were also developed. Lithography is a top-down fabrication technique where a bulk material is reduced in size to nanoscale pattern.

Another group of nanotechnological techniques include those used for fabrication of nanotubes and nanowires, those used in semiconductor fabrication such as deep ultraviolet lithography, electron beam lithography, focused ion beam machining, nanoimprint lithography, atomic layer deposition, and molecular vapor deposition, and further including molecular self-assembly techniques such as those employing di-block copolymers. The precursors of these techniques preceded the nanotech era, and are extensions in the development of scientific advancements rather than techniques which were devised with the sole purpose of creating nanotechnology and which were results of nanotechnology research.

The top-down approach anticipates nanodevices that must be built piece by piece in stages, much as manufactured items are made. Scanning probe microscopy is an important technique both for characterization and synthesis of nanomaterials. Atomic force microscopes and scanning tunneling microscopes can be used to look at surfaces and to move atoms around. By designing different tips for these microscopes, they can be used for carving out structures on surfaces and to help guide self-assembling structures. By using, for example, feature-oriented scanning approach, atoms or molecules can be moved around on a surface with scanning probe microscopy techniques. At present, it is expensive and time-consuming for mass production but very suitable for laboratory experimentation.

In contrast, bottom-up techniques build or grow larger structures atom by atom or molecule by molecule. These techniques include chemical synthesis, self-assembly and positional assembly. Dual polarization interferometry is one tool suitable for characterization of self-assembled thin films. Another variation of the bottom-up approach is molecular beam epitaxy or MBE. Researchers at Bell Telephone Laboratories like John R. Arthur. Alfred Y. Cho, and Art C. Gossard developed and implemented MBE as a research tool in the late 1960s and 1970s. Samples made by MBE were key to the discovery of the fractional quantum Hall effect for which the 1998 Nobel Prize in Physics was awarded. MBE allows scientists to lay down atomically precise layers of atoms and, in the process, build up complex structures. Important for research on semiconductors, MBE is also widely used to make samples and devices for the newly emerging field of spintronics.

However, new therapeutic products, based on responsive nanomaterials, such as the ultradeformable, stress-sensitive Transfersome vesicles, are under development and already approved for human use in some countries.

APPLICATIONS

As of August 21, 2008, the Project on Emerging Nanotechnologies estimates that over 800 manufacturer-identified nanotech products are publicly available, with new ones hitting the market at a pace of 3–4 per week. The project lists all of the products in a publicly accessible online database. Most applications are limited to the use of "first generation" passive nanomaterials which includes titanium dioxide in sunscreen, cosmetics, surface coatings, and some food products; Carbon allotropes used to produce gecko tape; silver in food packaging, clothing, disinfectants and household appliances; zinc oxide in sunscreens and cosmetics, surface coatings, paints and outdoor furniture varnishes; and cerium oxide as a fuel catalyst.

Further applications allow tennis balls to last longer, golf balls to fly straighter, and even bowling balls to become more durable and have a harder surface. Trousers and socks have been infused with nanotechnology so that they will last longer and keep people cool in the summer. Bandages are being infused with silver nanoparticles to heal cuts faster. Video game consoles and personal computers may become cheaper, faster, and contain more memory thanks to nanotechnology. Nanotechnology may have the ability to make existing medical applications cheaper and easier to use in places like the general practitioner's office and at home. Cars are being manufactured with nanomaterials so they may need fewer metals and less fuel to operate in the future.

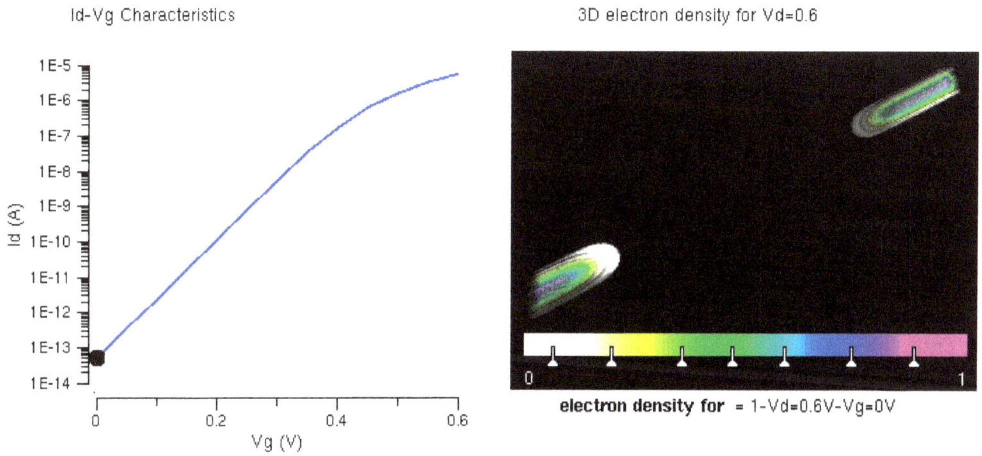

One of the major applications of nanotechnology is in the area of nanoelectronics with MOSFET's being made of small nanowires ~10 nm in length. Here is a simulation of such a nanowire.

Scientists are now turning to nanotechnology in an attempt to develop diesel engines with cleaner exhaust fumes. Platinum is currently used as the diesel engine catalyst in these engines. The catalyst is what cleans the exhaust fume particles. First a reduction catalyst is employed to take nitrogen atoms from NOx molecules in order to free oxygen. Next the oxidation catalyst oxidizes the hydrocarbons and carbon monoxide to form carbon dioxide and water. Platinum is used in both the reduction and the oxidation catalysts. Using platinum though, is inefficient in that it is expensive and unsustainable. Danish company InnovationsFonden invested DKK 15 million in a search for new catalyst substitutes using nanotechnology. The goal of the project, launched in the autumn of 2014, is to maximize surface area and minimize the amount of material required. Objects tend to minimize their surface energy; two drops of water, for example, will join to form one drop and decrease surface area. If the catalyst's surface area that is exposed to the exhaust fumes is maximized, efficiency of the catalyst is maximized. The team working on this project aims to create nanoparticles that will not merge. Every time the surface is optimized, material is saved. Thus, creating these nanoparticles will increase the effectiveness of the resulting diesel engine catalyst—in turn leading to cleaner exhaust fumes—and will decrease cost. If successful, the team hopes to reduce platinum use by 25%.

Nanotechnology also has a prominent role in the fast developing field of Tissue Engineering. When designing scaffolds, researchers attempt to the mimic the nanoscale features of a Cell's microenvironment to direct its differentiation down a suitable lineage. For example, when creating scaffolds to support the growth of bone, researchers may mimic osteoclast resorption pits.

Researchers have successfully used DNA origami-based nanobots capable of carrying out logic functions to achieve targeted drug delivery in cockroaches. It is said that the computational power of these nanobots can be scaled up to that of a Commodore 64.

IMPLICATIONS

An area of concern is the effect that industrial-scale manufacturing and use of nanomaterials would have on human health and the environment, as suggested by nanotoxicology research. For these reasons, some groups advocate that nanotechnology be regulated by governments. Others counter that overregulation would stifle scientific research and the development of beneficial innovations. Public health research agencies, such as the National Institute for Occupational Safety and Health are actively conducting research on potential health effects stemming from exposures to nanoparticles.

Some nanoparticle products may have unintended consequences. Researchers have discovered that bacteriostatic silver nanoparticles used in socks to reduce foot odor are being released in the wash. These particles are then flushed into the waste water stream and may destroy bacteria which are critical components of natural ecosystems, farms, and waste treatment processes.

Public deliberations on risk perception in the US and UK carried out by the Center for Nanotechnology in Society found that participants were more positive about nanotechnologies for energy applications than for health applications, with health applications raising moral and ethical dilemmas such as cost and availability.

Experts, including director of the Woodrow Wilson Center's Project on Emerging Nanotechnologies David Rejeski, have testified that successful commercialization depends on adequate oversight, risk research strategy, and public engagement. Berkeley, California is currently the only city in the United States to regulate nanotechnology; Cambridge, Massachusetts in 2008 considered enacting a similar law, but ultimately rejected it. Relevant for both research on and application of nanotechnologies, the insurability of nanotechnology is contested. Without state regulation of nanotechnology, the availability of private insurance for potential damages is seen as necessary to ensure that burdens are not socialized implicitly.

Health and Environmental Concerns

Nanofibers are used in several areas and in different products, in everything from aircraft wings to tennis rackets. Inhaling airborne nanoparticles and nanofibers may lead to a number of pulmonary diseases, e.g. fibrosis. Researchers have found that when rats breathed in nanoparticles, the particles settled in the brain and lungs, which led to significant increases in biomarkers for inflammation and stress response and that nanoparticles induce skin aging through oxidative stress in hairless mice.

A two-year study at UCLA's School of Public Health found lab mice consuming nano-titanium dioxide showed DNA and chromosome damage to a degree "linked to all the big killers of man, namely cancer, heart disease, neurological disease and aging".

A major study published more recently in Nature Nanotechnology suggests some forms of carbon nanotubes – a poster child for the "nanotechnology revolution" – could be as harmful as asbestos if inhaled in sufficient quantities. Anthony Seaton of the Institute of Occupational Medicine in Edinburgh, Scotland, who contributed to the article on carbon nanotubes said "We know that some of them probably have the potential to cause mesothelioma. So those sorts of materials need to be handled very carefully." In the absence of specific regulation forthcoming from governments, Paull and Lyons (2008) have called for an exclusion of engineered nanoparticles in food. A newspaper article reports that workers in a paint factory developed serious lung disease and nanoparticles were found in their lungs.

REGULATION

Calls for tighter regulation of nanotechnology have occurred alongside a growing debate related to the human health and safety risks of nanotechnology. There is significant debate about who is responsible for the regulation of nanotechnology. Some regulatory agencies currently cover some nanotechnology products and processes (to varying degrees) – by "bolting on" nanotechnology to existing regulations – there are clear gaps in these regimes. Davies (2008) has proposed a regulatory road map describing steps to deal with these shortcomings.

Stakeholders concerned by the lack of a regulatory framework to assess and control risks associated with the release of nanoparticles and nanotubes have drawn parallels with bovine spongiform encephalopathy ("mad cow" disease), thalidomide, genetically modified food, nuclear energy, reproductive technologies, biotechnology, and asbestosis. Dr. Andrew Maynard, chief science advisor to the Woodrow Wilson Center's Project on Emerging Nanotechnologies, concludes that there is insufficient funding for human health and safety research, and as a result there is currently limited understanding of the human health and safety risks associated with nanotechnology. As a result, some academics have called for stricter application of the precautionary principle, with delayed marketing approval, enhanced labelling and additional safety data development requirements in relation to certain forms of nanotechnology.

The Royal Society report identified a risk of nanoparticles or nanotubes being released during disposal, destruction and recycling, and recommended that "manufacturers of products that fall under extended producer responsibility regimes such as end-of-life regulations publish procedures outlining how these materials will be managed to minimize possible human and environmental exposure" (p. xiii).

The Center for Nanotechnology in Society has found that people respond to nanotechnologies differently, depending on application – with participants in public deliberations more positive about nanotechnologies for energy than health applications – suggesting that any public calls for nano regulations may differ by technology sector.

REFERENCES

1. Drexler, K. Eric (1986). Engines of Creation: The Coming Era of Nanotechnology. Doubleday. ISBN 0-385-19973-2.
2. Drexler, K. Eric (1992). Nanosystems: Molecular Machinery, Manufacturing, and Computation. New York: John Wiley & Sons. ISBN 0-471-57547-X.
3. Apply nanotech to up industrial, agri output, The Daily Star (Bangladesh), 17 April 2012.
4. Saini, Rajiv; Saini, Santosh; Sharma, Sugandha (2010). "Nanotechnology: The

Future Medicine". Journal of Cutaneous and Aesthetic Surgery. 3 (1): 32–33. doi:10.4103/0974-2077.63301. PMC 2890134Freely accessible. PMID 20606992.

5. Buzea, C.; Pacheco, I. I.; Robbie, K. (2007). "Nanomaterials and nanoparticles: Sources and toxicity". Biointerphases. 2 (4): MR17–MR71. doi:10.1116/1.2815690. PMID 20419892.
6. Binnig, G.; Rohrer, H. (1986). "Scanning tunneling microscopy". IBM Journal of Research and Development. 30 (4): 355–69.
7. "Press Release: the 1986 Nobel Prize in Physics". Nobelprize.org. 15 October 1986. Retrieved 12 May 2011.
8. Kroto, H. W.; Heath, J. R.; O'Brien, S. C.; Curl, R. F.; Smalley, R. E. (1985). "C60: Buckminsterfullerene". Nature. 318 (6042): 162–163. Bibcode:1985Natur.318..162K. doi:10.1038/318162a0.
9. Adams, W. W.; Baughman, R. H. (2005). "RETROSPECTIVE: Richard E. Smalley (1943-2005)". Science. 310 (5756): 1916. doi:10.1126/science.1122120. PMID 16373566.
10. "Nanoscience and nanotechnologies: opportunities and uncertainties". Royal Society and Royal Academy of Engineering. July 2004. Retrieved 13 May 2011.
11. "Nanotechnology: Drexler and Smalley make the case for and against 'molecular assemblers'". Chemical & Engineering News. American Chemical Society. 81 (48): 37–42. 1 December 2003. doi:10.1021/cen-v081n036.p037. Retrieved 9 May 2010.
12. "Nanotechnology Information Center: Properties, Applications, Research, and Safety Guidelines". American Elements. Retrieved 13 May 2011.
13. "Analysis: This is the first publicly available on-line inventory of nanotechnology-based consumer products". The Project on Emerging Nanotechnologies. 2008. Retrieved 13 May 2011.
14. "Productive Nanosystems Technology Roadmap" (PDF).
15. "NASA Draft Nanotechnology Roadmap" (PDF).
16. Allhoff, Fritz; Lin, Patrick; Moore, Daniel (2010). What is nanotechnology and why does it matter?: from science to ethics. John Wiley and Sons. pp. 3–5. ISBN 1-4051-7545-1.
17. Prasad, S. K. (2008). Modern Concepts in Nanotechnology. Discovery Publishing House. pp. 31–32. ISBN 81-8356-296-5.
18. Kahn, Jennifer (2006). "Nanotechnology". National Geographic. 2006 (June): 98–119.
19. Kralj, Slavko; Makovec, Darko (27 October 2015). "Magnetic Assembly of Superparamagnetic Iron Oxide Nanoparticle Clusters into Nanochains and Nanobundles". ACS Nano. 9 (10): 9700–9707. doi:10.1021/acsnano.5b02328.
20. Rodgers, P. (2006). "Nanoelectronics: Single file". Nature Nanotechnology. doi:10.1038/nnano.2006.5.

21. Lubick N; Betts, Kellyn (2008). "Silver socks have cloudy lining". Environ Sci Technol. 42 (11): 3910. Bibcode:2008EnST...42.3910L. doi:10.1021/es0871199. PMID 18589943.

22. Phoenix, Chris (March 2005) Nanotechnology: Developing Molecular Manufacturing. crnano.org

23. "Some papers by K. Eric Drexler". imm.org.

24. Carlo Montemagno, Ph.D. California NanoSystems Institute

25. "Cover Story – Nanotechnology". Chemical and Engineering News. 81 (48): 37–42. December 1, 2003.

26. Regan, BC; Aloni, S; Jensen, K; Ritchie, RO; Zettl, A (2005). "Nanocrystal-powered nanomotor" (PDF). Nano letters. 5 (9): 1730–3. Bibcode:2005NanoL...5.1730R. doi:10.1021/nl0510659. PMID 16159214.

27. Regan, B. C.; Aloni, S.; Jensen, K.; Zettl, A. (2005). "Surface-tension-driven nanoelectromechanical relaxation oscillator" (PDF). Applied Physics Letters. 86 (12): 123119. Bibcode:2005ApPhL..86l3119R. doi:10.1063/1.1887827.

28. Goodman, R.P.; Schaap, I.A.T.; Tardin, C.F.; Erben, C.M.; Berry, R.M.; Schmidt, C.F.; Turberfield, A.J. (9 December 2005). "Rapid chiral assembly of rigid DNA building blocks for molecular nanofabrication". Science. 310 (5754): 1661–1665. Bibcode:2005Sci...310.1661G. doi:10.1126/science.1120367. ISSN 0036-8075. PMID 16339440.

29. "Wireless Nanocrystals Efficiently Radiate Visible Light". Retrieved 5 August 2015.

30. Narayan, R. J.; Kumta, P. N.; Sfeir, Ch.; Lee, D-H; Choi, D.; Olton, D. (2004). "Nanostructured Ceramics in Medical Devices: Applications and Prospects". JOM. 56 (10): 38–43. Bibcode:2004JOM....56j..38N. doi:10.1007/s11837-004-0289-x.

31. Cho, Hongsik; Pinkhassik, Eugene; David, Valentin; Stuart, John; Hasty, Karen (31 May 2015). "Detection of early cartilage damage using targeted nanosomes in a post-traumatic osteoarthritis mouse model". Nanomedicine: Nanotechnology, Biology and Medicine. Elsevier. 11 (4): 939–946. doi:10.1016/j.nano.2015.01.011. Retrieved 25 July 2015.

32. Kerativitayanan, Punyavee; Carrow, James K.; Gaharwar, Akhilesh K. (May 2015). "Nanomaterials for Engineering Stem Cell Responses". Advanced Healthcare Materials. 4: n/a–n/a. doi:10.1002/adhm.201500272. PMID 26010739.

33. Gaharwar, A.K. [et al., edited by] (2013). Nanomaterials in tissue engineering : fabrication and applications. Oxford: Woodhead Publishing. ISBN 978-0-85709-596-1.

34. Gaharwar, AK; Peppas, NA; Khademhosseini, A (March 2014). "Nanocomposite hydrogels for biomedical applications.". Biotechnology and Bioengineering. 111 (3): 441–53. doi:10.1002/bit.25160. PMC 3924876Freely accessible. PMID 24264728.

35. Levins, Christopher G.; Schafmeister, Christian E. (2006). "The Synthesis of Curved and Linear Structures from a Minimal Set of Monomers". ChemInform. 37 (5). doi:10.1002/chin.200605222.

36. "Applications/Products". National Nanotechnology Initiative. Archived from the original on 2010-11-20. Retrieved 2007-10-19.

37. "The Nobel Prize in Physics 2007". Nobelprize.org. Retrieved 2007-10-19.

38. Das S, Gates AJ, Abdu HA, Rose GS, Picconatto CA, Ellenbogen JC (2007). "Designs for Ultra-Tiny, Special-Purpose Nanoelectronic Circuits". IEEE Transactions on Circuits and Systems I. 54 (11): 2528–2540. doi:10.1109/TCSI.2007.907864.

39. Mashaghi, S.; Jadidi, T.; Koenderink, G.; Mashaghi, A. "Lipid Nanotechnology". Int. J. Mol. Sci. 2013 (14): 4242–4282.

40. Hogan, C. Michael (2010) "Virus" in Encyclopedia of Earth. National Council for Science and the Environment. eds. S. Draggan and C. Cleveland

41. Ghalanbor Z, Marashi SA, Ranjbar B (2005). "Nanotechnology helps medicine: nanoscale swimmers and their future applications". Med Hypotheses. 65 (1): 198–199. doi:10.1016/j.mehy.2005.01.023. PMID 15893147.

42. Kubik T, Bogunia-Kubik K, Sugisaka M (2005). "Nanotechnology on duty in medical applications". Curr Pharm Biotechnol. 6 (1): 17–33. PMID 15727553.

43. Leary, SP; Liu, CY; Apuzzo, ML (2006). "Toward the Emergence of Nanoneurosurgery: Part III-Nanomedicine: Targeted Nanotherapy, Nanosurgery, and Progress Toward the Realization of Nanoneurosurgery". Neurosurgery. 58 (6): 1009–1026. doi:10.1227/01.NEU.0000217016.79256.16. PMID 16723880.

44. Shetty RC (2005). "Potential pitfalls of nanotechnology in its applications to medicine: immune incompatibility of nanodevices". Med Hypotheses. 65 (5): 998–9. doi:10.1016/j.mehy.2005.05.022. PMID 16023299.

45. Cavalcanti, A.; Shirinzadeh, B.; Freitas, R.; Kretly, L. (2007). "Medical Nanorobot Architecture Based on Nanobioelectronics". Recent Patents on Nanotechnology. 1: 1–10. doi:10.2174/187221007779814745. PMID 19076015.

46. Boukallel M, Gauthier M, Dauge M, Piat E, Abadie J (2007). "Smart microrobots for mechanical cell characterization and cell convoying". IEEE Trans. Biomed. Eng. 54 (8): 1536–40. doi:10.1109/TBME.2007.891171. PMID 17694877.

47. "International Perspective on Government Nanotechnology Funding in 2005" (PDF).

48. Lapshin, R. V. (2004). "Feature-oriented scanning methodology for probe microscopy and nanotechnology" (PDF). Nanotechnology. UK: IOP. 15 (9): 1135–1151. Bibcode:2004Nanot..15.1135L. doi:10.1088/0957-4484/15/9/006. ISSN 0957-4484.

49. Lapshin, R. V. (2011). "Feature-oriented scanning probe microscopy". In H. S. Nalwa. Encyclopedia of Nanoscience and Nanotechnology (PDF). 14. USA: American Scientific Publishers. pp. 105–115. ISBN 1-58883-163-9.

50. Kafshgari MH, Voelcker NH, Harding FJ (2015) Applications of zero-valent silicon nanostructures in biomedicine. Nanomedicine (Lond) 10 (16):2553-71. doi:10.2217/nnm.15.91 PMID 26295171
51. Rajan, Reshmy; Jose, Shoma; Mukund, V. P. Biju; Vasudevan, Deepa T. (2011-01-01). "Transferosomes - A vesicular transdermal delivery system for enhanced drug permeation". Journal of Advanced Pharmaceutical Technology & Research. 2 (3): 138–143. doi:10.4103/2231-4040.85524. ISSN 2231-4040. PMC 3217704Freely accessible. PMID 22171309.
52. Kurtoglu M. E.; Longenbach T.; Reddington P.; Gogotsi Y. (2011). "Effect of Calcination Temperature and Environment on Photocatalytic and Mechanical Properties of Ultrathin Sol–Gel Titanium Dioxide Films". Journal of the American Ceramic Society. 94 (4): 1101–1108. doi:10.1111/j.1551-2916.2010.04218.x.
53. "Nanotechnology Consumer Products". nnin.org. 2010. Retrieved November 23, 2011.
54. Nano in computing and electronics at NanoandMe.org
55. Nano in medicine at NanoandMe.org
56. Nano in transport at NanoandMe.org
57. Catalytic Converter at Wikipedia.org
58. How Catalytic Converters Work at howstuffworks.com
59. Nanotechnology to provide cleaner diesel engines. RDmag.com. September 2014
60. Cassidy (2014). "Nanotechnology in the Regeneration of Complex Tissues". Bone and Tissue Regeneration Insights: 25. doi:10.4137/BTRI.S12331.
61. Cassidy, J. W.; Roberts, J. N.; Smith, C. A.; Robertson, M.; White, K.; Biggs, M. J.; Oreffo, R. O. C.; Dalby, M. J. (2014). "Osteogenic lineage restriction by osteoprogenitors cultured on nanometric grooved surfaces: The role of focal adhesion maturation". Acta Biomaterialia. 10 (2): 651–660. doi:10.1016/j.actbio.2013.11.008.
62. Amir, Y.; Ben-Ishay, E.; Levner, D.; Ittah, S.; Abu-Horowitz, A.; Bachelet, I. (2014). "Universal computing by DNA origami robots in a living animal". Nature Nanotechnology. 9 (5): 353–357. Bibcode:2014NatNa...9..353A. doi:10.1038/nnano.2014.58.
63. "CDC – Nanotechnology – NIOSH Workplace Safety and Health Topic". National Institute for Occupational Safety and Health. June 15, 2012. Retrieved 2012-08-24.
64. "CDC – NIOSH Publications and Products – Filling the Knowledge Gaps for Safe Nanotechnology in the Workplace". National Institute for Occupational Safety and Health. November 7, 2012. Retrieved 2012-11-08.
65. Lubick, N; Betts, Kellyn (2008). "Silver socks have cloudy lining". Environmental Science & Technology. 42 (11): 3910. Bibcode:2008EnST...42.3910L. doi:10.1021/es0871199. PMID 18589943.
66. Murray R.G.E. (1993) Advances in Bacterial Paracrystalline Surface Layers. T. J. Beveridge, S. F. Koval (Eds.). Plenum Press. ISBN 978-0-306-44582-8. pp. 3–9.

67. Harthorn, Barbara Herr (January 23, 2009) "People in the US and the UK show strong similarities in their attitudes toward nanotechnologies". Nanotechnology Today.
68. Testimony of David Rejeski for U.S. Senate Committee on Commerce, Science and Transportation Project on Emerging Nanotechnologies. Retrieved on 2008-3-7.
69. DelVecchio, Rick (November 24, 2006) Berkeley considering need for nano safety. sfgate.com
70. Bray, Hiawatha (January 26, 2007) Cambridge considers nanotech curbs – City may mimic Berkeley bylaws. boston.com
71. Recommendations for a Municipal Health & Safety Policy for Nanomaterials: A Report to the Cambridge City Manager. nanolawreport.com. July 2008.
72. Encyclopedia of Nanoscience and Society, edited by David H. Guston, Sage Publications, 2010; see Articles on Insurance and Reinsurance (by I. Lippert).
73. Byrne, J. D.; Baugh, J. A. (2008). "The significance of nanoparticles in particle-induced pulmonary fibrosis". McGill journal of medicine : MJM : an international forum for the advancement of medical sciences by students. 11 (1): 43–50. PMC 2322933Freely accessible. PMID 18523535.
74. Elder, A. (2006). Tiny Inhaled Particles Take Easy Route from Nose to Brain. urmc.rochester.edu Archived September 21, 2006, at the Wayback Machine.
75. Wu, J; Liu, W; Xue, C; Zhou, S; Lan, F; Bi, L; Xu, H; Yang, X; Zeng, FD (2009). "Toxicity and penetration of TiO2 nanoparticles in hairless mice and porcine skin after subchronic dermal exposure". Toxicology letters. 191 (1): 1–8. doi:10.1016/j.toxlet.2009.05.020. PMID 19501137.
76. Jonaitis, TS; Card, JW; Magnuson, B (2010). "Concerns regarding nano-sized titanium dioxide dermal penetration and toxicity study". Toxicology letters. 192 (2): 268–9. doi:10.1016/j.toxlet.2009.10.007. PMID 19836437.
77. Schneider, Andrew (March 24, 2010) "Amid Nanotech's Dazzling Promise, Health Risks Grow". AOL News
78. Weiss, R. (2008). Effects of Nanotubes May Lead to Cancer, Study Says.
79. Paull, J. & Lyons, K. (2008). "Nanotechnology: The Next Challenge for Organics" (PDF). Journal of Organic Systems. 3: 3–22.
80. Smith, Rebecca (August 19, 2009). "Nanoparticles used in paint could kill, research suggests". London: Telegraph. Retrieved May 19, 2010.
81. Nanofibres 'may pose health risk'. BBC. 2012-08-24
82. Schinwald, A.; Murphy, F. A.; Prina-Mello, A.; Poland, C. A.; Byrne, F.; Movia, D.; Glass, J. R.; Dickerson, J. C.; Schultz, D. A.; Jeffree, C. E.; MacNee, W.; Donaldson, K. (2012). "The Threshold Length for Fiber-Induced Acute Pleural Inflammation: Shedding Light on the Early Events in Asbestos-Induced Mesothelioma". Toxicological Sciences. 128 (2): 461–470. doi:10.1093/toxsci/kfs171.
83. Is Chronic Inflammation the Key to Unlocking the Mysteries of Cancer? Acientific American. 2008-11-09

84. Kevin Rollins (Nems Mems Works, LLC). "Nanobiotechnology Regulation: A Proposal for Self-Regulation with Limited Oversight". Volume 6 – Issue 2. Retrieved 2 September 2010.
85. Bowman D, Hodge G (2006). "Nanotechnology: Mapping the Wild Regulatory Frontier". Futures. 38 (9): 1060–1073. doi:10.1016/j.futures.2006.02.017.
86. Davies, J. C. (2008). Nanotechnology Oversight: An Agenda for the Next Administration.
87. Rowe, G. (2005). "Difficulties in evaluating public engagement initiatives: Reflections on an evaluation of the UK GM Nation? Public debate about transgenic crops". Public Understanding of Science. 14 (4): 331–352. doi:10.1177/0963662505056611.
88. Maynard, A.Testimony by Dr. Andrew Maynard for the U.S. House Committee on Science and Technology. (2008-4-16). Retrieved on 2008-11-24. Archived May 29, 2008, at the Wayback Machine.
89. Faunce, T.; Murray, K.; Nasu, H.; Bowman, D. (2008). "Sunscreen Safety: The Precautionary Principle, the Australian Therapeutic Goods Administration and Nanoparticles in Sunscreens". NanoEthics. 2 (3): 231–240. doi:10.1007/s11569-008-0041-z.
90. Thomas Faunce; Katherine Murray; Hitoshi Nasu & Diana Bowman (24 July 2008). "Sunscreen Safety: The Precautionary Principle, The Australian Therapeutic Goods Administration and Nanoparticles in Sunscreens" (PDF). Springer Science + Business Media B.V. Retrieved 18 June 2009.

CHAPTER 2

History of Nanotechnology

Chapter Contents

The history of nanotechnology, in some sense dates back to prehistoric times when early humans/hominoids made use of naturally-occurring, nanoscale elements. Depicted in the header above, nano-sized carbon molecules integrate nicely with the more porous rock surface of the cave walls to remain embedded for thousands of years.

The process and appreciation of miniaturization, the entire principle of nanotechnology, is also not new to the electronic or even the post-industrial eras. For thousands of years prior, the east has regarded small as superior and aesthetically pleasing.

INTRODUCTION

The history of nanotechnology traces the development of the concepts and experimental work falling under the broad category of nanotechnology. Although nanotechnology is a relatively recent development in scientific research, the development of its central concepts happened over a longer period of time. The emergence of nanotechnology in the 1980s was caused by the convergence of experimental advances such as the invention of the scanning tunneling microscope in 1981 and the discovery of fullerenes in 1985, with the elucidation and popularization of a conceptual framework for the goals of nanotechnology beginning with the 1986 publication of the book *Engines of Creation*. The field was subject to growing public awareness and controversy in the early 2000s, with prominent debates about both its potential implications as well as the feasibility of the applications envisioned by advocates of molecular nanotechnology, and with governments moving to promote and fund research into nanotechnology. The early 2000s also saw the beginnings of commercial applications of nanotechnology, although these were limited to bulk applications of nanomaterials rather than the transformative applications envisioned by the field.

EARLY USES OF NANOMATERIALS

The earliest evidence of the use and applications of nanotechnology can be traced back to carbon nanotubes, cementite nanowires found in the microstructure of wootz steel manufactured in ancient india from the time period of 600 BC and exported globally.

Although nanoparticles are associated with modern science, they were used by artisans as far back as the ninth century in Mesopotamia for creating a glittering effect on the surface of pots.

In modern times, pottery from the Middle Ages and Renaissance often retains a distinct gold- or copper-colored metallic glitter. This luster is caused by a metallic film that was applied to the transparent surface of a glazing, which containes silver and copper nanoparticles dispersed homogeneously in the glassy matrix of the ceramic glaze. These nanoparticles are created by the artisans by adding copper and silver salts and oxides together with vinegar, ochre, and clay on the surface of previously-glazed pottery. The technique originated in the Muslim world. As Muslims were not allowed to use gold in artistic representations, they sought a way to create a similar effect without using real gold. The solution they found was using luster.

CONCEPTUAL ORIGINS

Richard Feynman

The American physicist Richard Feynman lectured, “There’s Plenty of Room at the Bottom,” at an American Physical Society meeting at Caltech on December 29, 1959, which is often held to have provided inspiration for the field of nanotechnology. Feynman had described a process by which the ability to manipulate individual atoms and molecules might be developed, using one set of precise tools to build and operate another proportionally smaller set, so on down to the needed scale. In the course of this, he noted, scaling issues would arise from the changing magnitude of various physical phenomena: gravity would become less important, surface tension and Van der Waals attraction would become more important.

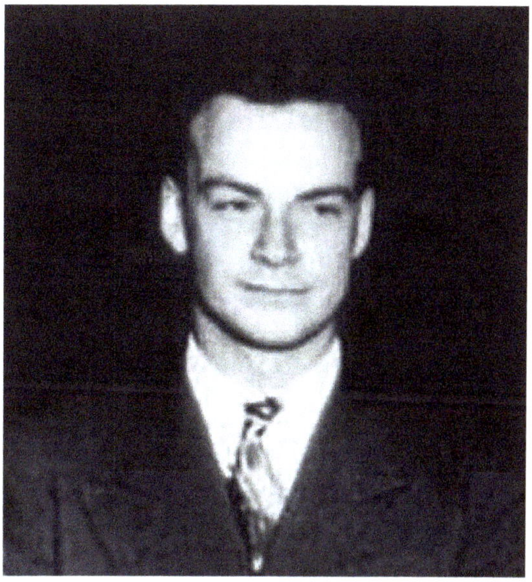

Richard Feynman gave a 1959 talk which many years later inspired the conceptual foundations of nanotechnology.

After Feynman's death, scholars studying the historical development of nanotechnology have concluded that his actual role in catalyzing nanotechnology research was limited, based on recollections from many of the people active in the nascent field in the 1980s and 1990s. Chris Toumey, a cultural anthropologist at the University of South Carolina, found that the published versions of Feynman's talk had a negligible influence in the twenty years after it was first published, as measured by citations in the scientific literature, and not much more influence in the decade after the Scanning Tunneling Microscope was invented in 1981. Subsequently, interest in "Plenty of Room" in the scientific literature greatly increased in the early 1990s. This is probably because the term "nanotechnology" gained serious attention just before that time, following its use by K. Eric Drexler in his 1986 book, *Engines of Creation: The Coming Era of Nanotechnology*, which took the Feynman concept of a billion tiny factories and added the idea that they could make more copies of themselves via computer control instead of control by a human operator; and in a cover article headlined "Nanotechnology", published later that year in a mass-circulation science-oriented magazine, *OMNI*. Toumey's analysis also includes comments from distinguished scientists in nanotechnology who say that "Plenty of Room" did not influence their early work, and in fact most of them had not read it until a later date.

These and other developments hint that the retroactive rediscovery of Feynman's "Plenty of Room" gave nanotechnology a packaged history that provided an early date of December 1959, plus a connection to the charisma and genius of Richard Feynman. Feynman's stature as a Nobel laureate and as an iconic figure in 20th century science surely helped advocates of nanotechnology and provided a valuable intellectual link to the past.

Norio Taniguchi

The Japanese scientist called Norio Taniguchi of the Tokyo University of Science was the first to use the term "nano-technology" in a 1974 conference, to describe semiconductor processes such as thin film deposition and ion beam milling exhibiting characteristic control on the order of a nanometer. His definition was, "'Nano-technology' mainly consists of the processing of, separation, consolidation, and deformation of materials by one atom or one molecule." However, the term was not used again until 1981 when Eric Drexler, who was unaware of Taniguchi's prior use of the term, published his first paper on nanotechnology in 1981.

K. Eric Drexler

In the 1980s the idea of nanotechnology as a deterministic, rather than stochastic, handling of individual atoms and molecules was conceptually explored in depth by K. Eric Drexler, who promoted the technological significance of nano-scale phenomena and devices through speeches and two influential books.

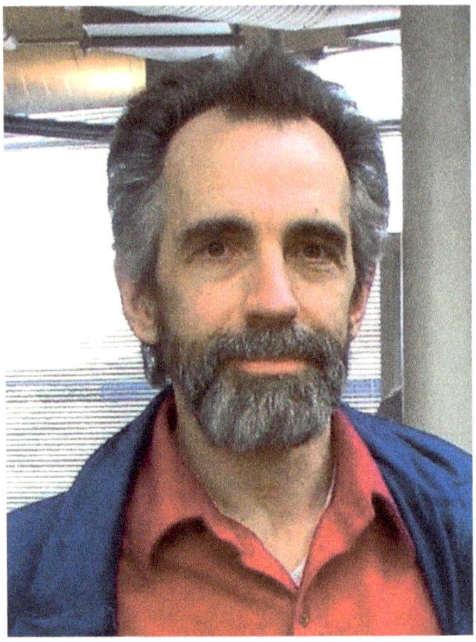

K. Eric Drexler developed and popularized the concept of nanotechnology and founded the field of molecular nanotechnology.

In 1980, Drexler encountered Feynman's provocative 1959 talk "There's Plenty of Room at the Bottom" while preparing his initial scientific paper on the subject, "Molecular Engineering: An approach to the development of general capabilities for molecular manipulation," published in the *Proceedings of the National Academy of Sciences* in 1981. The term "nanotechnology" (which paralleled Taniguchi's "nano-technology") was independently applied by Drexler in his 1986 book *Engines of Creation: The Coming Era of Nanotechnology*, which proposed the idea of a nanoscale "assembler" which would be able to build a copy of itself and of other items of arbitrary complexity. He also first published the term "grey goo" to describe what might happen if a hypothetical self-replicating machine, capable of independent operation, were constructed and released. Drexler's vision of nanotechnology is often called "Molecular Nanotechnology" (MNT) or "molecular manufacturing."

His 1991 Ph.D. work at the MIT Media Lab was the first doctoral degree on the topic of molecular nanotechnology and (after some editing) his thesis, "Molecular Machinery and Manufacturing with Applications to Computation," was published as *Nanosystems: Molecular Machinery, Manufacturing, and Computation,* which received the Association of American Publishers award for Best Computer Science Book of 1992. Drexler founded the Foresight Institute in 1986 with the mission of "Preparing for nanotechnology." Drexler is no longer a member of the Foresight Institute.

EXPERIMENTAL ADVANCES

Nanotechnology and nanoscience got a boost in the early 1980s with two major developments: the birth of cluster science and the invention of the scanning tunneling microscope (STM). These developments led to the discovery of fullerenes in 1985 and the structural assignment of carbon nanotubes a few years later

Invention of Scanning Probe Microscopy

The scanning tunneling microscope, an instrument for imaging surfaces at the atomic level, was developed in 1981 by Gerd Binnig and Heinrich Rohrer at IBM Zurich Research Laboratory, for which they were awarded the Nobel Prize in Physics in 1986. Binnig, Calvin Quate and Christoph Gerber invented the first atomic force microscope in 1986. The first commercially available atomic force microscope was introduced in 1989.

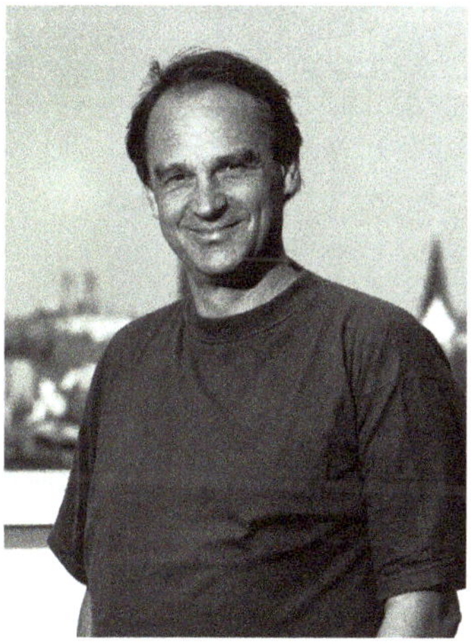
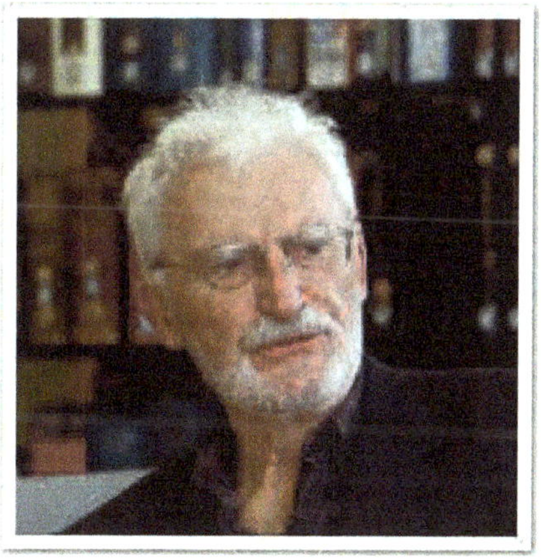

Gerd Binnig (left) and Heinrich Rohrer (right) won the 1986 Nobel Prize in Physics for their 1981 invention of the scanning tunneling microscope.

IBM researcher Don Eigler was the first to manipulate atoms using a scanning tunneling microscope in 1989. He used 35 Xenon atoms to spell out the IBM logo. He shared the 2010 Kavli Prize in Nanoscience for this work.

Advances in Interface and Colloid Science

Interface and colloid science had existed for nearly a century before they became associated with nanotechnology. The first observations and size measurements of nanoparticles had been made during the first decade of the 20th century by Richard Adolf Zsigmondy, winner of the 1925 Nobel Prize in Chemistry, who made a detailed study of gold sols and other nanomaterials with sizes down to 10 nm using an ultramicroscope which was capable of visualizing particles much smaller than the light wavelength. Zsigmondy was also the first to use the term "nanometer" explicitly for characterizing particle size. In the 1920s, Irving Langmuir, winner of the 1932 Nobel Prize in Chemistry, and Katharine B. Blodgett introduced the concept of a monolayer, a layer of material one molecule thick. In the early 1950s, Derjaguin and Abrikosova conducted the first measurement of surface forces.

In 1974 the process of atomic layer deposition for depositing uniform thin films one atomic layer at a time was developed and patented by Tuomo Suntola and co-workers in Finland.

In another development, the synthesis and properties of semiconductor nanocrystals were studied. This led to a fast increasing number of semiconductor nanoparticles of quantum dots.

Discovery of Fullerenes

Fullerenes were discovered in 1985 by Harry Kroto, Richard Smalley, and Robert Curl, who together won the 1996 Nobel Prize in Chemistry. Smalley's research in physical chemistry investigated formation of inorganic and semiconductor clusters using pulsed molecular beams and time of flight mass spectrometry. As a consequence of this expertise, Curl introduced him to Kroto in order to investigate a question about the constituents of astronomical dust. These are carbon rich grains expelled by old stars such as R Corona Borealis. The result of this collaboration was the discovery of C_{60} and the fullerenes as the third allotropic form of carbon. Subsequent discoveries included the endohedral fullerenes, and the larger family of fullerenes the following year.

The discovery of carbon nanotubes is largely attributed to Sumio Iijima of NEC in 1991, although carbon nanotubes have been produced and observed under a variety of conditions prior to 1991. Iijima's discovery of multi-walled carbon nanotubes in the insoluble material of arc-burned graphite rods in 1991 and Mintmire, Dunlap, and White's independent prediction that if single-walled carbon nanotubes could be made, then they would exhibit remarkable conducting properties helped create the initial buzz that is now associated with carbon nanotubes. Nanotube research accelerated greatly following the independent discoveries by Bethune at IBM and Iijima at NEC of *single-walled* carbon nanotubes and methods to specifically produce them by adding transition-metal catalysts to the carbon in an arc discharge.

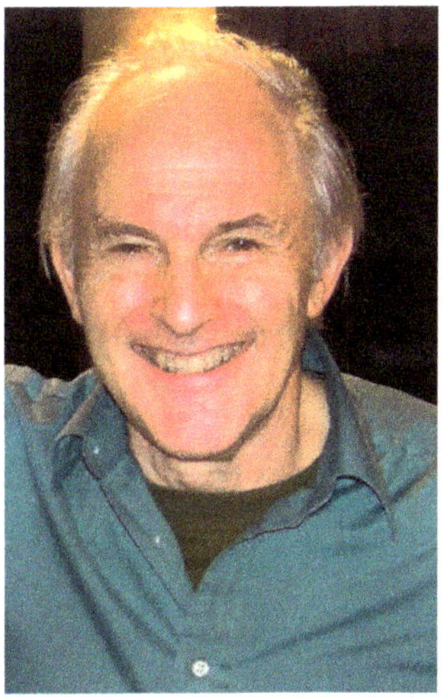 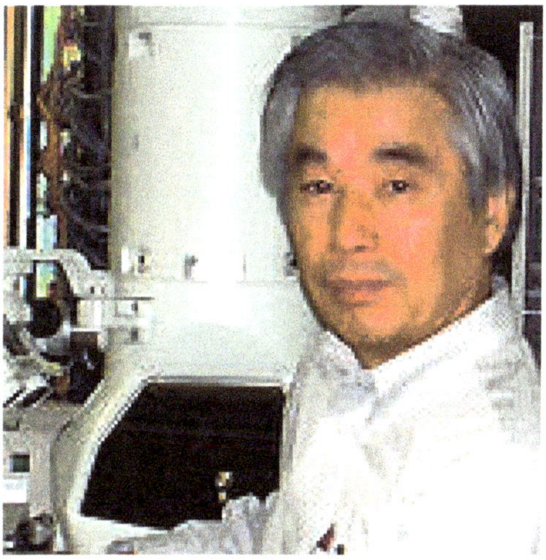

Harry Kroto (left) won the 1996 Nobel Prize in Chemistry along with Richard Smalley (pictured below) and Robert Curl for their 1985 discovery of buckminsterfullerene, while Sumio Iijima (right) won the inaugural 2008 Kavli Prize in Nanoscience for his 1991 discovery of carbon nanotubes.

In the early 1990s Huffman and Kraetschmer, of the University of Arizona, discovered how to synthesize and purify large quantities of fullerenes. This opened the door to their characterization and functionalization by hundreds of investigators in government and industrial laboratories. Shortly after, rubidium doped C_{60} was found to be a mid temperature (Tc = 32 K) superconductor. At a meeting of the Materials Research Society in 1992, Dr. T. Ebbesen (NEC) described to a spellbound audience his discovery and characterization of carbon nanotubes. This event sent those in attendance and others downwind of his presentation into their laboratories to reproduce and push those discoveries forward. Using the same or similar tools as those used by Huffman and Kratschmer, hundreds of researchers further developed the field of nanotube-based nanotechnology.

Government Support

National Nanotechnology Initiative

The National Nanotechnology Initiative is a United States federal nanotechnology research and development program. "The NNI serves as the central point of communication, cooperation, and collaboration for all Federal agencies engaged in nanotechnology research, bringing together the expertise needed to advance this broad and complex field." Its goals are to advance a world-class nanotechnology research and development (R&D) program, foster the transfer of new technologies into products for commercial and public benefit, develop and sustain educational resources, a skilled workforce, and the supporting infrastructure and tools to advance nanotechnology, and support responsible development of nanotechnology. The initiative was spearheaded by Mihail Roco, who formally proposed the National Nanotechnology Initiative to the Office of Science and

Technology Policy during the Clinton administration in 1999, and was a key architect in its development. He is currently the Senior Advisor for Nanotechnology at the National Science Foundation, as well as the founding chair of the National Science and Technology Council subcommittee on Nanoscale Science, Engineering and Technology.

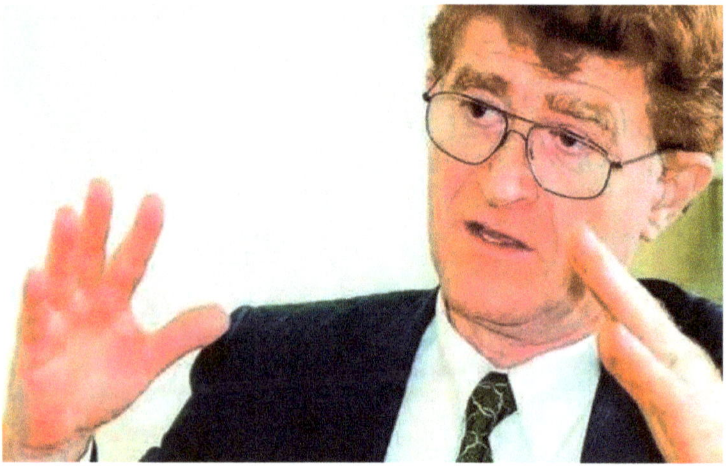

Mihail Roco of the National Science Foundation formally proposed the National Nanotechnology Initiative to the White House, and was a key architect in its initial development.

President Bill Clinton advocated nanotechnology development. In a 21 January 2000 speech at the California Institute of Technology, Clinton said, "Some of our research goals may take twenty or more years to achieve, but that is precisely why there is an important role for the federal government." Feynman's stature and concept of atomically precise fabrication played a role in securing funding for nanotechnology research, as mentioned in President Clinton's speech:

My budget supports a major new National Nanotechnology Initiative, worth $500 million. Caltech is no stranger to the idea of nanotechnology the ability to manipulate matter at the atomic and molecular level. Over 40 years ago, Caltech's own Richard Feynman asked, "What would happen if we could arrange the atoms one by one the way we want them?"

President George W. Bush further increased funding for nanotechnology. On December 3, 2003 Bush signed into law the 21st Century Nanotechnology Research and Development Act, which authorizes expenditures for five of the participating agencies totaling US$3.63 billion over four years. The NNI budget supplement for Fiscal Year 2009 provides $1.5 billion to the NNI, reflecting steady growth in the nanotechnology investment.

"Why the future doesn't need us"

"Why the future doesn't need us" is an article written by Bill Joy, then Chief Scientist at Sun Microsystems, in the April 2000 issue of *Wired* magazine. In the article, he argues that "Our most powerful 21st-century technologies — robotics, genetic engineering, and nanotech — are threatening to make humans an endangered species." Joy argues that developing technologies provide a much greater danger to humanity than any technology before it has ever presented. In particular, he focuses on genetics, nanotechnology and robotics. He argues that 20th-century technologies of destruction, such as the nuclear bomb, were limited to large governments, due to the complexity and cost of such devices, as well as the difficulty in acquiring the required materials. He also voices concern about increasing computer power. His worry is that computers will eventually become more intelligent than we are, leading to such dystopian scenarios as robot rebellion. He notably quotes the Unabomber on this topic. After the publication of the article, Bill Joy suggested assessing technologies to gauge their implicit dangers, as well as having scientists refuse to work on technologies that have the potential to cause harm.

In the AAAS Science and Technology Policy Yearbook 2001 article titled *A Response to Bill Joy and the Doom-and-Gloom Technofuturists*, Bill Joy was criticized for having technological tunnel vision on his prediction, by failing to consider social factors. In Ray Kurzweil's *The Singularity Is Near*, he questioned the regulation of potentially dangerous technology, asking "Should we tell the millions of people afflicted with cancer and other devastating conditions that we are canceling the development of all bioengineered treatments because there is a risk that these same technologies may someday be used for malevolent purposes?".

Prey

Prey is a 2002 novel by Michael Crichton which features an artificial swarm of nanorobots which develop intelligence and threaten their human inventors. The novel generated concern within the nanotechnology community that the novel could negatively affect public perception of nanotechnology by creating fear of a similar scenario in real life.

Drexler–Smalley Debate

Richard Smalley, best known for co-discovering the soccer ball-shaped "buckyball" molecule and a leading advocate of nanotechnology and its many applications, was an outspoken critic of the idea of molecular assemblers, as advocated by Eric Drexler. In 2001 he introduced scientific objections to them attacking the notion of universal assemblers in a 2001 *Scientific American* article, leading to a rebuttal later that year from Drexler and colleagues, and eventually to an exchange of open letters in 2003.

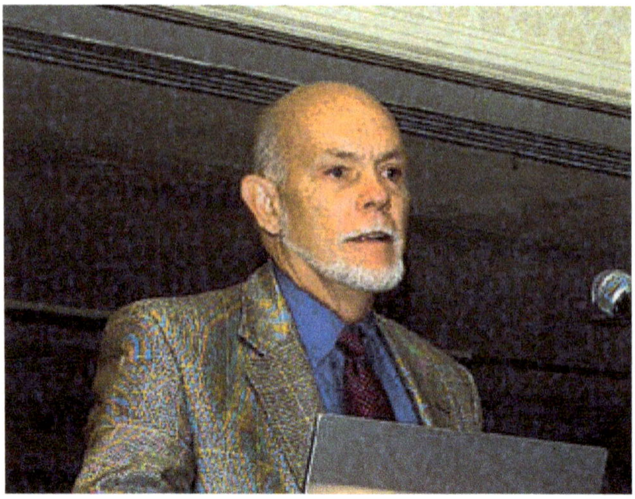

Richard Smalley, a co-discoverer of the fullerenes, was involved in a public debate with Eric Drexler about the feasibility of molecular assemblers.

Smalley criticized Drexler's work on nanotechnology as naive, arguing that chemistry is extremely complicated, reactions are hard to control, and that a universal assembler is science fiction. Smalley believed that such assemblers were not physically possible and introduced scientific objections to them. His two principal technical objections, which he had termed the "fat fingers problem" and the "sticky fingers problem", argued against the feasibility of molecular assemblers being able to precisely select and place individual atoms. He also believed that Drexler's speculations about apocalyptic dangers of molecular assemblers threaten the public support for development of nanotechnology.

Smalley first argued that "fat fingers" made MNT impossible. He later argued that nanomachines would have to resemble chemical enzymes more than Drexler's assemblers and could only work in water. He believed these would exclude the possibility of "molecular assemblers" that worked by precision picking and placing of individual atoms. Also, Smalley argued that nearly all of modern chemistry involves reactions that take place in a solvent (usually water), because the small molecules of a solvent contribute many things, such as lowering binding energies for transition states. Since nearly all known chemistry requires a solvent, Smalley felt that Drexler's proposal to use a high vacuum environment was not feasible.

Smalley also believed that Drexler's speculations about apocalyptic dangers of self-replicating machines that have been equated with "molecular assemblers" would threaten the public support for development of nanotechnology. To address the debate between Drexler and Smalley regarding molecular assemblers *Chemical & Engineering News* published a point-counterpoint consisting of an exchange of letters that addressed the issues.

Drexler and coworkers responded to these two issues in a 2001 publication. Drexler and colleagues noted that Drexler never proposed universal assemblers able to make absolutely anything, but instead proposed more limited assemblers able to make a very wide variety of things. They challenged the relevance of Smalley's arguments to the more specific proposals advanced in *Nanosystems*. Drexler maintained that both were straw man arguments, and in the case of enzymes, Prof. Klibanov wrote in 1994, "...using an enzyme in organic solvents eliminates several obstacles..." Drexler also addresses this in Nanosystems by showing mathematically that well-designed catalysts can provide the effects of a solvent and can fundamentally be made even more efficient than a solvent/ enzyme reaction could ever be. Drexler had difficulty in getting Smalley to respond, but in December 2003, *Chemical & Engineering News* carried a 4-part debate.

Ray Kurzweil spends four pages in his book 'The Singularity Is Near' to showing that Richard Smalley's arguments are not valid, and disputing them point by point. Kurzweil ends by stating that Drexler's visions are very practicable and even happening already.

Royal Society Report on the Implications of Nanotechnology

The Royal Society and Royal Academy of Engineering's 2004 report on the implications of nanoscience and nanotechnologies was inspired by Prince Charles' concerns about nanotechnology, including molecular manufacturing. However, the report spent almost no time on molecular manufacturing. In fact, the word "Drexler" appears only once in the body of the report (in passing), and "molecular manufacturing" or "molecular nanotechnology" not at all. The report covers various risks of nanoscale technologies, such as nanoparticle toxicology. It also provides a useful overview of several nanoscale fields. The report contains an annex (appendix) on grey goo, which cites a weaker variation of Richard Smalley's contested argument against molecular manufacturing. It concludes that there is no evidence that autonomous, self-replicating nanomachines will be developed in the foreseeable future, and suggests that regulators should be more concerned with issues of nanoparticle toxicology.

INITIAL COMMERCIAL APPLICATIONS

The early 2000s saw the beginnings of the use of nanotechnology in commercial products, although most applications are limited to the bulk use of passive nanomaterials. Examples include titanium dioxide and zinc oxide nanoparticles in sunscreen, cosmetics and some food products; silver nanoparticles in food packaging, clothing, disinfectants and household appliances such as Silver Nano; carbon nanotubes for stain-resistant textiles; and cerium oxide as a fuel catalyst. As of March 10, 2011, the Project on Emerging Nanotechnologies estimated that over 1300 manufacturer-identified nanotech products are publicly available, with new ones hitting the market at a pace of 3–4 per week.

The National Science Foundation funded researcher David Berube to study the field of nanotechnology. His findings are published in the monograph Nano-Hype: The Truth Behind the Nanotechnology Buzz. This study concludes that much of what is sold as "nanotechnology" is in fact a recasting of straightforward materials science, which is leading to a "nanotech industry built solely on selling nanotubes, nanowires, and the like" which will "end up with a few suppliers selling low margin products in huge volumes." Further applications which require actual manipulation or arrangement of nanoscale components await further research. Though technologies branded with the term 'nano' are sometimes little related to and fall far short of the most ambitious and transformative technological goals of the sort in molecular manufacturing proposals, the term still connotes such ideas. According to Berube, there may be a danger that a "nano bubble" will form, or is forming already, from the use of the term by scientists and entrepreneurs to garner funding, regardless of interest in the transformative possibilities of more ambitious and far-sighted work.

REFERENCES

1. http://www.nature.com/news/2006/061113/full/news061113-11.html
2. Reiss, Gunter; Hutten, Andreas (2010). "Magnetic Nanoparticles". In Sattler, Klaus D. Handbook of Nanophysics: Nanoparticles and Quantum Dots. CRC Press. pp. 2–1. ISBN 9781420075458.
3. Khan, Firdos Alam (2012). Biotechnology Fundamentals. CRC Press. p. 328. ISBN 9781439820094.
4. Rawson, Philip S. (1984). Ceramics. University of Pennsylvania Press. ISBN 0-8122-1156-1.
5. Gribbin, John; Gribbin, Mary (1997). Richard Feynman: A Life in Science. Dutton. p. 170. ISBN 0-452-27631-4.
6. Hapgood, Fred (November 1986). ""Nanotechnology" / "Tinytech"". Omni: 56.
7. Drexler, Eric (15 December 2009). "The promise that launched the field of nanotechnology". Metamodern: The Trajectory of Technology. Retrieved 13 May 2011.
8. Toumey, Chris (2005). "Apostolic Succession". Engineering & Science. 1/2: 16–23.
9. Toumey, Chris (2008). "Reading Feynman into Nanotechnology: A Text for a New Science" (PDF). Techné. 13 (3): 133–168.
10. Milburn, Colin (2008). Nanovision: Engineering the Future. Duke University Press. ISBN 0-8223-4265-0.
11. Taniguchi, Norio (1974). "On the Basic Concept of 'Nano-Technology'". Proceedings of the International Conference on Production Engineering, Tokyo, 1974, Part II. Japan Society of Precision Engineering.
12. Bassett, Deborah R. (2010). "Taniguchi, Norio". In Guston, David H. Encyclopedia of nanoscience and society. London: SAGE. p. 747. ISBN 9781452266176. Retrieved 3 August 2014.
13. Koodali, Ranjit T.; Klabunde, Kenneth J. (2012). "Nanotechnology: Fandamental Principles and Applications". In Kent, James A. Handbook of industrial chemistry and biotechnology, volume 1 (12th ed.). New York: Springer. p. 250. ISBN 9781461442592. Retrieved 3 August 2014.
14. Maynard, edited by Graeme A. Hodge, Diana M. Bowman, Andrew D. (2010). "Tracing and disputing the story of nanotechnology". In Hodge, Graeme A.; Bowman, Diana M.; Maynard, Andrew D. International handbook on regulating

nanotechnologies. Cheltenham, UK: Edward Elgar. p. 54. ISBN 9781849808125. Retrieved 4 August 2014.

15. Drexler, K. Eric. Molecular Machinery and Manufacturing with Applications to Computation (PDF) (Ph.D. thesis). Massachusetts Institute of Technology.
16. Drexler, K. Eric (1992). Nanosystems: Molecular Machinery, Manufacturing, and Computation. Wiley. ISBN 0-471-57518-6. Retrieved 14 May 2011.
17. Binnig, G.; Rohrer, H. (1986). "Scanning tunneling microscopy". IBM Journal of Research and Development. 30 (4): 355–69.
18. "Press Release: the 1996 Nobel Prize in Physics". Nobelprize.org. 15 October 1986. Retrieved 12 May 2011.
19. Shankland, Stephen (28 September 2009). "IBM's 35 atoms and the rise of nanotech". CNET. Retrieved 12 May 2011.
20. "The Kavli Prize Laureates 2010". The Norwegian Academy of Science and Letters. Retrieved 13 May 2011.
21. Efremov, I.F. (1976). "Periodic Colloidal Structures". In Matijevic, E. Surface and Colloid Science. 8. New York: Wiley.
22. Lyklema, J. (2000). Fundamentals of Interface and Colloid Science. Academic Press. ISBN 978-0-12-460523-7.
23. Zsigmondy, R. (1914). Colloids and the Ultramicroscope. New York: J.Wiley and Sons. Retrieved 10 May 2011.
24. Derjaguin, B. V.; Titijevskaia, A. S.; Abricossova, I. I.; Malkina, A. D. (1954). "Investigations of the forces of interaction of surfaces in different media and their application to the problem of colloid stability". Discussions of the Faraday Society. 18: 24. doi:10.1039/DF9541800024.
25. "History of Atomic Layer Deposition". Finnish Micro & Nano Technology Network. Archived from the original on 18 September 2007.
26. Kroto, H. W.; Heath, J. R.; O'Brien, S. C.; Curl, R. F.; Smalley, R. E. (1985). "C60: Buckminsterfullerene". Nature. 318 (6042): 162–163. Bibcode:1985Natur.318..162K. doi:10.1038/318162a0.
27. Adams, W Wade; Baughman, Ray H (2005). "Retrospective: Richard E. Smalley (1943-2005)". Science. 310 (5756) (published Dec 23, 2005). p. 1916. doi:10.1126/science.1122120. PMID 16373566
28. Monthioux, Marc; Kuznetsov, V (2006). "Who should be given the credit for the discovery of carbon nanotubes?" (PDF). Carbon. 44 (9): 1621–1623. doi:10.1016/j.carbon.2006.03.019.
29. Iijima, Sumio (7 November 1991). "Helical microtubules of graphitic carbon". Nature. 354 (6348): 56–58. Bibcode:1991Natur.354...56I. doi:10.1038/354056a0.
30. Mintmire, J.W.; Dunlap, BI; White, CT (1992). "Are Fullerene Tubules Metallic?". Physical Review Letters. 68 (5): 631–634. Bibcode:1992PhRvL..68..631M. doi:10.1103/PhysRevLett.68.631. PMID 10045950.

31. Bethune, D. S.; Klang, C. H.; De Vries, M. S.; Gorman, G.; Savoy, R.; Vazquez, J.; Beyers, R. (1993). "Cobalt-catalyzed growth of carbon nanotubes with single-atomic-layer walls". Nature. 363 (6430): 605–607. Bibcode:1993Natur.363..605B. doi:10.1038/363605a0.
32. Iijima, Sumio; Ichihashi, Toshinari (1993). "Single-shell carbon nanotubes of 1-nm diameter". Nature. 363 (6430): 603–605. Bibcode:1993Natur.363..603I. doi:10.1038/363603a0.
33. "The Discovery of Single-Wall Carbon Nanotubes at IBM". IBM.
34. "About the NNI | Nano".
35. "Dr. Mihail C. Roco, Senior Advisor for Nanotechnology, National Science Foundation". National Science Foundation. Retrieved 8 November 2009.
36. "President Clinton's Address to Caltech on Science and Technology". California Institute of Technology. Retrieved 13 May 2011.
37. Jones, Richard M. (21 January 2000). "President Requests Significant Increase in FY 2001 Research Budget". FYI: The AIP Bulletin of Science Policy News. American Institute of Physics. Retrieved 13 May 2011.
38. "21st Century Nanotechnology Research and Development Act (Public Law 108-153)". United States Government Printing Office. Retrieved 12 May 2011.
39. "Remarks Prepared for Delivery: National Nanotechnology Initiative Conference, Senator George Allen, Thursday, April 1, 2004". United States National Nanotechnology Initiative. Archived from the original on 27 September 2007.
40. "National Nanotechnology Initiative: FY 2009 Budget & Highlights" (PDF). United States National Nanotechnology Initiative. Archived from the original (PDF) on 27 May 2010.
41. "Brown, John Seely and Duguid, Paul" (13 April 2000). "A Response to Bill Joy and the Doom-and-Gloom Technofuturists" (PDF). Retrieved 12 May 2011.
42. Edwards, Steven A. (2006). The Nanotech Pioneers: Where Are They Taking Us?. Weinheim: Wiley-VCH. pp. 22–23.
43. Smalley, Richard E. (September 2001). "Of Chemistry, Love and Nanobots". Scientific American. 285 (3): 76–7. doi:10.1038/scientificamerican0901-76. PMID 11524973.
44. Drexler, K. Eric; Forrest, David; Freitas, Robert A.; Hall, J. Storrs; Jacobstein, Neil; McKendree, Tom; Merkle, Ralph; Peterson, Christine (2001). "Debate About Assemblers — Smalley Rebuttal". Institute for Molecular Manufacturing. Retrieved 9 May 2010.
45. "Nanotechnology: Drexler and Smalley make the case for and against 'molecular assemblers'". Chemical & Engineering News. American Chemical Society. 81 (48): 37–42. 1 December 2003. doi:10.1021/cen-v081n036.p037. Retrieved 9 May 2010.
46. Phoenix, Chris (December 2003). "Of Chemistry, Nanobots, and Policy". Center for Responsible Nanotechnology. Retrieved 12 May 2011.
47. Kurzweil, Ray (2005). The Singularity Is Near. pp. 193–196. ISBN 0-670-03384-7.

48. "Nanoscience and nanotechnologies: opportunities and uncertainties". Royal Society and Royal Academy of Engineering. July 2004. Retrieved 13 May 2011.
49. "Royal Society in Denial". Center for Responsible Nanotechnology. 31 July 2004. Retrieved 13 May 2011.
50. "Nanotechnology Information Center: Properties, Applications, Research, and Safety Guidelines". American Elements. Retrieved 13 May 2011.
51. "Analysis: This is the first publicly available on-line inventory of nanotechnology-based consumer products". The Project on Emerging Nanotechnologies. 2008. Retrieved 13 May 2011.
52. Berube, David (2006). Nano-Hype: The Truth Behind the Nanotechnology Buzz. Amherst, NY: Prometheus Books.

CHAPTER 3

Impacts of Nanotechnology

Chapter Contents

Nanotechnology is often described as an emerging technology—one that not only holds promise for society, but also is capable of revolutionizing our approaches to common problems. Nanotechnology is not a completely new field; however, it is only recently that discoveries in this field have advanced so far as to warrant examination of their impact upon the world around us.

Nanotechnology has direct beneficial applications for medicine and the environment, but like all technologies it may have unintended effects that can adversely impact the environment, both within the human body and within the natural ecosystem. While taking advantage of this new technology for health, environmental, and sustainability benefits, science needs to examine the environmental and health implications.

INTRODUCTION

The impact of nanotechnology extends from its medical, ethical, mental, legal and environmental applications, to fields such as engineering, biology, chemistry, computing, materials science, and communications.

Major benefits of nanotechnology include improved manufacturing methods, water purification systems, energy systems, physical enhancement, nanomedicine, better food production methods, nutrition and large-scale infrastructure auto-fabrication. Nanotechnology's reduced size may allow for automation of tasks which were previously inaccessible due to physical restrictions, which in turn may reduce labor, land, or maintenance requirements placed on humans.

Potential risks include environmental, health, and safety issues; transitional effects such as displacement of traditional industries as the products of nanotechnology become dominant, which are of concern to privacy rights advocates. These may be particularly important if potential negative effects of nanoparticles are overlooked.

Whether nanotechnology merits special government regulation is a controversial issue. Regulatory bodies such as the United States Environmental Protection Agency and the Health and Consumer Protection Directorate of the European Commission have started dealing with the potential risks of nanoparticles. The organic food sector has been the first to act with the regulated exclusion of engineered nanoparticles from certified organic produce, firstly in Australia and the UK, and more recently in Canada, as well as for all food certified to Demeter International standards

OVERVIEW

The presence of nanomaterials (materials that contain nanoparticles) is not in itself a threat. It is only certain aspects that can make them risky, in particular their mobility and their increased reactivity. Only if certain properties of certain nanoparticles were harmful to living beings or the environment would we be faced with a genuine hazard. In this case it can be called nanopollution.

In addressing the health and environmental impact of nanomaterials we need to differentiate between two types of nanostructures: (1) Nanocomposites, nanostructured surfaces and nanocomponents (electronic, optical, sensors etc.), where nanoscale particles are incorporated into a substance, material or device ("fixed" nano-particles); and (2) "free" nanoparticles, where at some stage in production or use individual nanoparticles of a substance are present. These free nanoparticles could be nanoscale species of elements, or simple compounds, but also complex compounds where for instance a nanoparticle of a particular element is coated with another substance ("coated" nanoparticle or "core-shell" nanoparticle).

There seems to be consensus that, although one should be aware of materials containing fixed nanoparticles, the immediate concern is with free nanoparticles.

Nanoparticles are very different from their everyday counterparts, so their adverse effects cannot be derived from the known toxicity of the macro-sized material. This poses significant issues for addressing the health and environmental impact of free nanoparticles.

To complicate things further, in talking about nanoparticles it is important that a powder or liquid containing nanoparticles almost never be monodisperse, but contain instead a range of particle sizes. This complicates the experimental analysis as larger nanoparticles might have different properties from smaller ones. Also, nanoparticles show a tendency to aggregate, and such aggregates often behave differently from individual nanoparticles.

HEALTH IMPACT

The health impacts of nanotechnology are the possible effects that the use of nanotechnological materials and devices will have on human health. As nanotechnology is an emerging field, there is great debate regarding to what extent nanotechnology will benefit or pose risks for human health. Nanotechnology's health impacts can be split into two aspects: the potential for nanotechnological innovations to have medical applications to cure disease, and the potential health hazards posed by exposure to nanomaterials.

Medical Applications

Nanomedicine is the medical application of nanotechnology. The approaches to nanomedicine range from the medical use of nanomaterials, to nanoelectronic biosensors, and even possible future applications of molecular nanotechnology. Nanomedicine seeks to deliver a valuable set of research tools and clinically helpful devices in the near future. The National Nanotechnology Initiative expects new commercial applications in the pharmaceutical industry that may include advanced drug delivery systems, new therapies, and in vivo imaging. Neuro-electronic interfaces and other nanoelectronics-based sensors are another active goal of research. Further down the line, the speculative field of molecular nanotechnology believes that cell repair machines could revolutionize medicine and the medical field.

Nanomedicine research is directly funded, with the US National Institutes of Health in 2005 funding a five-year plan to set up four nanomedicine centers. In April 2006, the journal Nature Materials estimated that 130 nanotech-based drugs and delivery systems were being developed worldwide. Nanomedicine is a large industry, with nanomedicine sales reaching $6.8 billion in 2004. With over 200 companies and 38 products worldwide, a minimum of $3.8 billion in nanotechnology R&D is being invested every year. As the nanomedicine industry continues to grow, it is expected to have a significant impact on the economy.

Health Hazards

Nanotoxicology is the field which studies potential health risks of nanomaterials. The extremely small size of nanomaterials means that they are much more readily taken up by the human body than larger sized particles. How these nanoparticles behave inside the organism is one of the significant issues that needs to be resolved. The behavior of nanoparticles is a function of their size, shape and surface reactivity with the surrounding tissue. Apart from what happens if non-degradable or slowly degradable nanoparticles accumulate in organs, another concern is their potential interaction with biological processes inside the body: because of their large surface, nanoparticles on exposure to tissue and fluids will immediately adsorb onto their surface some of the macromolecules they encounter. The large number of variables influencing toxicity means that it is difficult to generalize about health risks associated with exposure to nanomaterials – each new nanomaterial must be assessed individually and all material properties must be taken into account. Health and environmental issues combine in the workplace of companies engaged in producing or using nanomaterials and in the laboratories engaged in nanoscience and nanotechnology research. It is safe to say that current workplace exposure standards for dusts cannot be applied directly to nanoparticle dusts.

The extremely small size of nanomaterials also means that they are much more readily taken up by the human body than larger sized particles. How these nanoparticles behave inside the body is one of the issues that needs to be resolved. The behavior of nanoparticles is a function of their size, shape and surface reactivity with the surrounding tissue. They could cause overload on phagocytes, cells that ingest and destroy foreign matter, thereby triggering stress reactions that lead to inflammation and weaken the body's defense against other pathogens. Apart from what happens if non-degradable or slowly degradable nanoparticles accumulate in organs, another concern is their potential interaction with biological processes inside the body: because of their large surface, nanoparticles on exposure to tissue and fluids will immediately adsorb onto their surface some of the macromolecules they encounter. This may, for instance, affect the regulatory mechanisms of enzymes and other proteins.

The National Institute for Occupational Safety and Health has conducted initial research on how nanoparticles interact with the body's systems and how workers might be exposed to nano-sized particles in the manufacturing or industrial use of nanomaterials. NIOSH currently offers interim guidelines for working with nanomaterials consistent with the best scientific knowledge. At The National Personal Protective Technology Laboratory of NIOSH, studies investigating the filter penetration of nanoparticles on NIOSH-certified and EU marked respirators, as well as non-certified dust masks have been conducted. These studies found that the most penetrating particle size range was between 30 and 100 nanometers, and leak size was the largest factor in the number of nanoparticles found inside the respirators of the test dummies.

Other properties of nanomaterials that influence toxicity include: chemical composition, shape, surface structure, surface charge, aggregation and solubility, and the presence or absence of functional groups of other chemicals. The large number of variables influencing toxicity means that it is difficult to generalize about health risks associated with exposure to nanomaterials – each new nanomaterial must be assessed individually and all material properties must be taken into account.

Literature reviews have been showing that release of engineered nanoparticles and incurred personal exposure can happen during different work activities. The situation alerts regulatory bodies to necessitate prevention strategies and regulations at nanotechnology workplaces.

ENVIRONMENTAL IMPACT

The environmental impact of nanotechnology is the possible effects that the use of nanotechnological materials and devices will have on the environment. As nanotechnology is an emerging field, there is great debate regarding to what extent industrial and commercial use of nanomaterials will affect organisms and ecosystems.

Nanotechnology's environmental impact can be split into two aspects: the potential for nanotechnological innovations to help improve the environment, and the possibly novel type of pollution that nanotechnological materials might cause if released into the environment.

Environmental Applications

Green nanotechnology refers to the use of nanotechnology to enhance the environmental sustainability of processes producing negative externalities. It also refers to the use of the products of nanotechnology to enhance sustainability. It includes making green nano-products and using nano-products in support of sustainability. Green nanotechnology has been described as the development of clean technologies, "to minimize potential environmental and human health risks associated with the manufacture and use of nanotechnology products, and to encourage replacement of existing products with new nano-products that are more environmentally friendly throughout their lifecycle."

Green nanotechnology has two goals: producing nanomaterials and products without harming the environment or human health, and producing nano-products that provide solutions to environmental problems. It uses existing principles of green chemistry and green engineering to make nanomaterials and nano-products without toxic ingredients, at low temperatures using less energy and renewable inputs wherever possible, and using lifecycle thinking in all design and engineering stages.

Pollution

Nanopollution is a generic name for all waste generated by nanodevices or during the nanomaterials manufacturing process. Nanowaste is mainly the group of particles that are released into the environment, or the particles that are thrown away when still on their products.

SOCIAL IMPACT

Beyond the toxicity risks to human health and the environment which are associated with first-generation nanomaterials, nanotechnology has broader societal impact and poses broader social challenges. Social scientists have suggested that nanotechnology's social issues should be understood and assessed not simply as "downstream" risks or impacts. Rather, the challenges should be factored into "upstream" research and decision-making in order to ensure technology development that meets social objectives

Many social scientists and organizations in civil society suggest that technology assessment and governance should also involve public participation

Over 800 nano-related patents were granted in 2003, with numbers increasing to nearly 19,000 internationally by 2012. Corporations are already taking out broad-ranging patents on nanoscale discoveries and inventions. For example, two corporations, NEC and IBM, hold the basic patents on carbon nanotubes, one of the current cornerstones of nanotechnology. Carbon nanotubes have a wide range of uses, and look set to become crucial to several industries from electronics and computers, to strengthened materials to drug delivery and diagnostics. Carbon nanotubes are poised to become a major traded commodity with the potential to replace major conventional raw materials.

Nanotechnologies may provide new solutions for the millions of people in developing countries who lack access to basic services, such as safe water, reliable energy, health care, and education. The 2004 UN Task Force on Science, Technology and Innovation noted that some of the advantages of nanotechnology include production using little labor, land, or maintenance, high productivity, low cost, and modest requirements for materials and energy. However, concerns are frequently raised that the claimed benefits of nanotechnology will not be evenly distributed, and that any benefits (including technical and/or economic) associated with nanotechnology will only reach affluent nations.

Longer-term concerns center on the impact that new technologies will have for society at large, and whether these could possibly lead to either a post-scarcity economy, or alternatively exacerbate the wealth gap between developed and developing nations. The effects of nanotechnology on the society as a whole, on human health and the environment, on trade, on security, on food systems and even on the definition of "human", have not been characterized or politicized.

REGULATION

Significant debate exists relating to the question of whether nanotechnology or nanotechnology-based products merit special government regulation. This debate is related to the circumstances in which it is necessary and appropriate to assess new substances prior to their release into the market, community and environment.

Regulatory bodies such as the United States Environmental Protection Agency and the Food and Drug Administration in the U.S. or the Health & Consumer Protection Directorate of the European Commission have started dealing with the potential risks posed by nanoparticles. So far, neither engineered nanoparticles nor the products and materials that contain them are subject to any special regulation regarding production, handling or labelling. The Material Safety Data Sheet that must be issued for some materials often does not differentiate between bulk and nanoscale size of the material in question and even when it does these MSDS are advisory only.

Limited nanotechnology labeling and regulation may exacerbate potential human and environmental health and safety issues associated with nanotechnology. It has been argued that the development of comprehensive regulation of nanotechnology will be vital to ensure that the potential risks associated with the research and commercial application of nanotechnology do not overshadow its potential benefits. Regulation may also be required to meet community expectations about responsible development of nanotechnology, as well as ensuring that public interests are included in shaping the development of nanotechnology.

In "The Consumer Product Safety Commission and Nanotechnology," E. Marla Felcher suggests that the Consumer Product Safety Commission, which is charged with protecting the public against unreasonable risks of injury or death associated with consumer products, is ill-equipped to oversee the safety of complex, high-tech products made using nanotechnology.

FAIL-SAFES IN NANOTECHNOLOGY

Fail-safes in nanotechnology are devices or features integrated with nanotechnology which, in the event of failure, respond in a way that will cause no harm, or at least a minimum of harm, to other devices or personnel. Fail-safe principles are governed by national standards and engineering practices, and are widely used in conventional engineering design. It is possible to scale down macro-scale fail-safe principles and devices for similar applications at the nano-scale. The use of fail-safes in nanotechnology applications supports social acceptance of those applications by reducing the risks to users; as of 2009, there are both theoretical and practical ways to implement fail-safe designs in nanotechnology.

A predominant challenge to the social acceptance of nanotechnology is concerned with the medical use of nanostructures in the human body. While any structure for medical use would be developed to be bio-compatible and harmless, sound engineering design must take into account all possibilities of failure. Thus, the design would include ways to manipulate the structures in the body in the event of failure.

Ferrous Nanoparticles

Many researchers are looking into creating nano-scale robots ("nanobots"), for the purpose of undertaking tasks where only robots on the nano scale can be used, such as inside the human body. These robots would have the ability to construct other nanostructures or perform medical procedures, and will be introduced into the body via an injection. The robots' shells and circuits would be made of ferrous nanoparticles so that a magnetic field could be used to prevent or manipulate their movement. In case of failure or malfunction, a small EMP or an MRI could be used to deactivate the nanobots. Both techniques induce an electromagnetic field, corrupting the memory and shorting out the circuitry of any electronic device within range.

Amino Acids

Researchers are pursuing the building of nanostructures using amino acids. Nanostructures that are created using amino acids are constructed using only synthetic types of amino acids, which tags these structures with unique molecules. These engineered amino acids essentially form synthetic proteins that differ from the naturally occurring proteins in the human body. This difference in the engineered amino acids makes these proteins easy to isolate and target. In case of failure or malfunction, it is possible to identify these proteins using the specifically targeted molecules, which act as a flag to indicate the location of the target. Then, another mechanism would be used to isolate them and deactivate them.

DNA

DNA within our bodies naturally breaks down, replicates itself, and rebuilds itself every time a cell divides. These processes are all controlled and completed by various enzymes. DNA molecules are composed of corresponding base pair nucleotides in a double-helix formation, which makes these processes very efficient, accurate, and predictable. Due to the ease with which DNA molecules can be fashioned, many publications in the academic society are geared towards creating nanostructures using DNA. With a DNA-based nano-device, synthetic proteins could be created, designed to deactivate a nano-device. These synthetic proteins would be injected into the body to break down the DNA and render a nano-device harmless in the event of a malfunction.

Biological proteins within the human body serve three main functions: they are structural building blocks, enzymes, and facilitate cellular signaling. Synthetic proteins could be developed as a form of indicator and attached to a DNA-based nano-device. This indicator would then be used for the purpose of monitoring nano-devices in the human body. If all DNA-based nano-devices were closely monitored in the human body, they could be controlled quickly in the event of a malfunction.

Programming

In nanotechnology, particularly in nanobots, the need for a sound programming architecture is very important due to a potentially higher risk of damage in the event of a malfunction. A two-layer approach can be used to control nano-devices: (1) by providing a preprogrammed fail-safe functionality in case of anticipated failures; and (2) a remote-controlled override for use in unforeseen situations. The "remote"-controlled nano-device would require a specialist in the room, to guide the nanobot throughout the procedure.

Cellular Engineering

Many researchers are developing methods that use bacteria to deliver drugs. These bacteria can be "programmed" to perform a specific task, and can be directed to go to targeted locations in the body. However, the bacteria may damage healthy organs or fail to deliver the medicine to the sick organ in the case of a malfunction. In such cases, a fail-safe mechanism is required to neutralize the bacteria and prevent damage. An antibiotic is generally suitable as the fail-safe agent.

REFERENCES

1. "About the National Nanotechnology Initiative". United States National Nanotechnology Initiative. 2016. Retrieved 4 June 2016.
2. Paull, John (2010) , Nanotechnology: No Free Lunch, Platter, 1(1) 8-17
3. Paull, John (2011) "Nanomaterials in food and agriculture: The big issue of small matter for organic food and farming", In: Neuhoff, Daniel; Halberg, Niels; Rasmussen, I.A.; Hermansen, J.E.; Ssekyewa, Charles and Sohn, Sang Mok (Eds.) Proceedings of the Third Scientific Conference of ISOFAR, ISOFAR, Bonn, 2, pp. 96-99.
4. Nanomedicine, Volume I: Basic Capabilities, by Robert A. Freitas Jr. 1999, ISBN 1-57059-645-X
5. Wagner V, Dullaart A, Bock AK, Zweck A (2006). "The emerging nanomedicine landscape". Nat. Biotechnol. 24 (10): 1211–1217. doi:10.1038/nbt1006-1211.

PMID 17033654.

6. Freitas RA Jr. (2005). "What is Nanomedicine?" (PDF). Nanomedicine: Nanotechnology, Biology and Medicine. 1 (1): 2–9. doi:10.1016/j.nano.2004.11.003. PMID 17292052.
7. Nanotechnology in Medicine and the Biosciences, by Coombs RRH, Robinson DW. 1996, ISBN 2-88449-080-9
8. Editorial. (2006). "Nanomedicine: A matter of rhetoric?". Nat Materials. 5 (4): 243. doi:10.1038/nmat1625. PMID 16582920.
9. Nanotechnology: A Gentle Introduction to the Next Big Idea, by MA Ratner, D Ratner. 2002, ISBN 0-13-101400-5
10. "Current Intelligence Bulletin 63: Occupational Exposure to Titanium Dioxide" (PDF). United States National Institute for Occupational Safety and Health. Retrieved 2012-02-19.
11. Zhuang Z, Viscusi D (December 7, 2011). "CDC - NIOSH Science Blog - Respiratory Protection for Workers Handling Engineering Nanoparticles". National Institute for Occupational Safety and Health. Retrieved 2012-08-24.
12. Shaffer RE, Rengasamy S (2009). "Respiratory protection against airborne nanoparticles: a review". J Nanopart Res. 11: 1661–1672. doi:10.1007/s11051-009-9649-3.
13. Rengasamy S, Eimer BC (2011). "Total inward leakage of nanoparticles through filtering facepiece respirators". Ann Occup Hyg. 55: 253–263. doi:10.1093/annhyg/meq096.
14. Nel, Andre; et al. (3 February 2006). "Toxic Potential of Materials at the Nanolevel". Science. 311 (5761): 622–627. doi:10.1126/science.1114397. PMID 16456071.
15. Magrez, Arnaud; et al. (2006). "Cellular Toxicity of Carbon-Based Nanomaterials". Nano Letters. 6 (6): 1121–1125. doi:10.1021/nl060162e. PMID 16771565.
16. Ding Y, et al. (2016). "Airborne engineered nanomaterials in the workplace—a review of release and worker exposure during nanomaterial production and handling processes". J. Hazard. Mater. doi:10.1016/j.jhazmat.2016.04.075.
17. Kuhlbusch T, et al. (2011). "Nanoparticle exposure at nanotechnology workplaces: a review". Part. Fibre Toxicol. 8 (1): 22. doi:10.1186/1743-8977-8-22.
18. Pietroiusti A, Magrini A (2014). "Engineered nanoparticles at the workplace: currentknowledge about workers' risk". Occup. Med. (Lond.). 64 (5): 319–330. doi:10.1093/occmed/kqu051.
19. "Environment and Green Nano - Topics - Nanotechnology Project". Retrieved 11 September 2011.
20. What is Green Engineering, US Environmental Protection Agency
21. Kearnes, Matthew; Grove-White, Robin; Macnaghten, Phil; Wilsdon, James; Wynne, Brian (2006). "From Bio to Nano: Learning Lessons from the UK Agricultural Biotechnology Controversy". Science as Culture. Science as Culture. Routledge

(published December 2006). 15 (4): 291–307. doi:10.1080/09505430601022619. Retrieved 2007-10-19.

22. http://csec.lancs.ac.uk/docs/nano%20project%20sci%20com%20proofs%20nov05.pdf
23. .Nanotechnology Law & Business http://www.nanolabweb.com/index.cfm/action/main.default.viewArticle/articleID/135/CFID/60255/CFTOKEN/45212442/. Missing or empty |title= (help)
24. http://www.wmin.ac.uk/sshl/pdf/CSDBUlletinMohr.pdf
25. Demos | Publications | Governing at the Nanoscale Archived December 14, 2007, at the Wayback Machine.
26. Smith, Erin Geiger (14 February 2013). "U.S.-based inventors lead world in nanotechnology patents: study". Technology. Reuters. Retrieved 4 June 2016.
27. Prigg, Mark (2 October 2015). "The end of silicon? IBM reveals carbon nanotube breakthrough that could revolutionise computing and lead to ultrafast artificial intelligence 'brain chips'". Associated Newspapers Ltd, The Daily Mail. Retrieved 4 June 2016.
28. Invernizzi N, Foladori G, Maclurcan D (2008). "Nanotechnology's Controversial Role for the South". Science Technology and Society. 13 (1): 123–148. doi:10.1177/097172180701300105.
29. Bowman D, Hodge G (2007). "A Small Matter of Regulation: An International Review of Nanotechnology Regulation". Columbia Science and Technology Law Review. 8: 1–32.
30. Bowman D; Fitzharris, M (2007). "Too Small for Concern? Public Health and Nanotechnology". Australian and New Zealand Journal of Public Health. 31 (4): 382–384. doi:10.1111/j.1753-6405.2007.00092.x. PMID 17725022.
31. Bowman D, Hodge G (2006). "Nanotechnology: Mapping the Wild Regulatory Frontier". Futures. 38 (9): 1060–1073. doi:10.1016/j.futures.2006.02.017.
32. Felcher, EM. (2008). The Consumer Product Safety Commission and Nanotechnology
33. Whitesides, George M. and J Christopher Love. "The Art of Building Small." Scientific American Reports Sep. 2007: 13-21.
34. Šafařík, Ivo, and Mirka Šafaříková. "Magnetic Nanoparticles and Biosciences." Chemical Monthly 133.6 (2002): 737-759.
35. Schafmeister, Christian E. "Molecular Lego." Scientific American Reports Sep 2007: 22-29.
36. Seeman, Nadrian C. "Nanotechnology and the Double Helix." Scientific American Reports. Sep. 2007: 30-39.
37. May, Mike. "Nanotechnology: Thinking Small." Environmental Health Perspectives, Vol. 107, No. 9 (Sep., 1999), pp. A450-A451 Published by: The National Institute of Environmental Health Sciences (NIEHS) Stable URL: <http://www.jstor.org/stable/3434647>.

38. Shapiro, Ehud, and Beneson, Yaakov. "Bringing DNA Computers to Life." Scientific American Reports Sep 2007: 41-47.

39. Knapp, Louise. "Bad Bacteria Key to Drug Delivery." Wired. 28 Feb. 2003. CondéNet, Inc. 10 Oct. 2008. <http://www.wired.com/medtech/health/news/2003/02/57547>.

40. Cao, Guozhong. Nanostructures & Nanomaterials: Synthesis, Properties & Applications. London, UK: Imperial College Press, 2004.

CHAPTER 4

Applications of Nanotechnology

Chapter Contents

- **Introduction**
- **Applications By Type**
- **Nano-Tech Catalyst**

Nanotechnology involves the understanding, manipulation, and control of matter at dimensions of roughly 1 to 100 nanometers. Nanotechnology encompasses science, engineering and technology and involves imaging, measuring, modeling, and manipulating matter at the nanoscale. The development of unique nanoscale structures has the potential to revolutionize industry, including electronics, medicine, and consumer products.

INTRODUCTION

The 2000s have seen the beginnings of the applications of nanotechnology in commercial products, although most applications are limited to the bulk use of passive nanomaterials. Examples include titanium dioxide and zinc oxide nanoparticles in sunscreen, cosmetics and some food products; silver nanoparticles in food packaging, clothing, disinfectants and household appliances such as Silver Nano; carbon nanotubes for stain-resistant textiles; and cerium oxide as a fuel catalyst. As of March 10, 2011, the Project on Emerging Nanotechnologies estimated that over 1300 manufacturer-identified nanotech products are publicly available, with new ones hitting the market at a pace of 3–4 per week.

Nanotechnology is being used in developing countries to help treat disease and prevent health issues. The umbrella term for this kind of nanotechnology is Nanomedicine.

Nanotechnology is also being applied to or developed for application to a variety of industrial and purification processes. Purification and environmental cleanup applications include the desalination of water, water filtration, wastewater treatment, groundwater treatment, and other nanoremediation. In industry, applications may include construction materials, military goods, and nano-machining of nano-wires, nano-rods, few layers of graphene, etc. Also, recently a new field arisen from the root of Nanotechnology is called Nanobiotechnology. Nanobiotechnology is the biology-based, application-oriented frontier area of research in the hybrid discipline of Nanoscience and biotechnology with an equivalent contribution.

APPLICATIONS BY TYPE

- Nanomedicine
- Nanobiotechnology
- Green nanotechnology
- Energy applications of nanotechnology
- Industrial applications of nanotechnology
- Potential applications of carbon nanotubes
- Nanoart

Nanomedicine

Nanomedicine is the medical application of nanotechnology. Nanomedicine ranges from the medical applications of nanomaterials and biological devices, to nanoelectronic biosensors, and even possible future applications of molecular nanotechnology such as biological machines. Current problems for nanomedicine involve understanding the issues related to toxicity and environmental impact of nanoscale materials (materials whose structure is on the scale of nanometers, i.e. billionths of a meter).

Functionalities can be added to nanomaterials by interfacing them with biological molecules or structures. The size of nanomaterials is similar to that of most biological molecules and structures; therefore, nanomaterials can be useful for both in vivo and in vitro biomedical research and applications. Thus far, the integration of nanomaterials with biology has led to the development of diagnostic devices, contrast agents, analytical tools, physical therapy applications, and drug delivery vehicles.

Nanomedicine seeks to deliver a valuable set of research tools and clinically useful devices in the near future. The National Nanotechnology Initiative expects new commercial applications in the pharmaceutical industry that may include advanced drug delivery systems, new therapies, and in vivo imaging. Nanomedicine research is receiving funding from the US National Institutes of Health, including the funding in 2005 of a five-year plan to set up four nanomedicine centers.

Nanomedicine sales reached $16 billion in 2015, with a minimum of $3.8 billion in nanotechnology R&D being invested every year. Global funding for emerging nanotechnology increased by 45% per year in recent years, with product sales exceeding

$1 trillion in 2013. As the nanomedicine industry continues to grow, it is expected to have a significant impact on the economy.

Drug Delivery

Nanotechnology has provided the possibility of delivering drugs to specific cells using nanoparticles.

The overall drug consumption and side-effects may be lowered significantly by depositing the active agent in the morbid region only and in no higher dose than needed. Targeted drug delivery is intended to reduce the side effects of drugs with concomitant decreases in consumption and treatment expenses. Drug delivery focuses on maximizing bioavailability both at specific places in the body and over a period of time. This can potentially be achieved by molecular targeting by nanoengineered devices. More than $65 billion are wasted each year due to poor bioavailability. A benefit of using nanoscale for medical technologies is that smaller devices are less invasive and can possibly be implanted inside the body, plus biochemical reaction times are much shorter. These devices are faster and more sensitive than typical drug delivery. The efficacy of drug delivery through nanomedicine is largely based upon: a) efficient encapsulation of the drugs, b) successful delivery of drug to the targeted region of the body, and c) successful release of the drug.

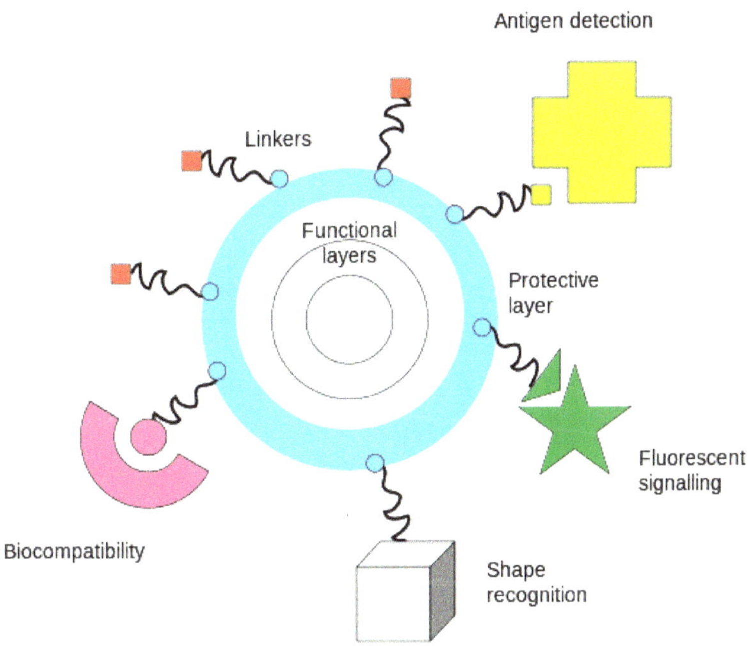

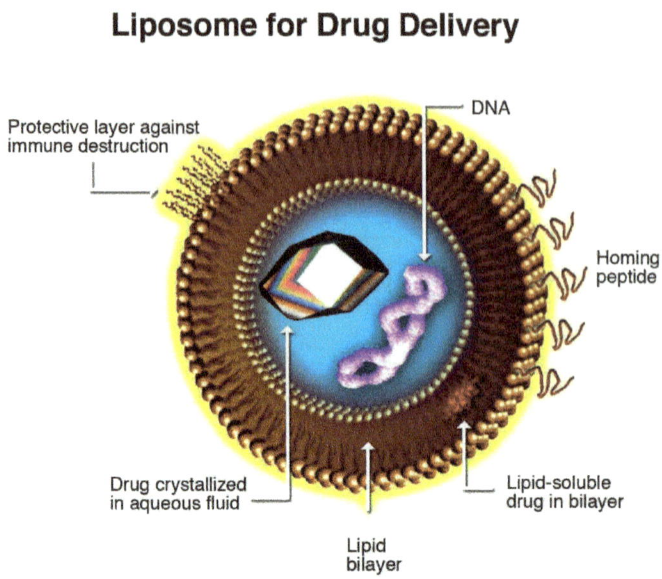

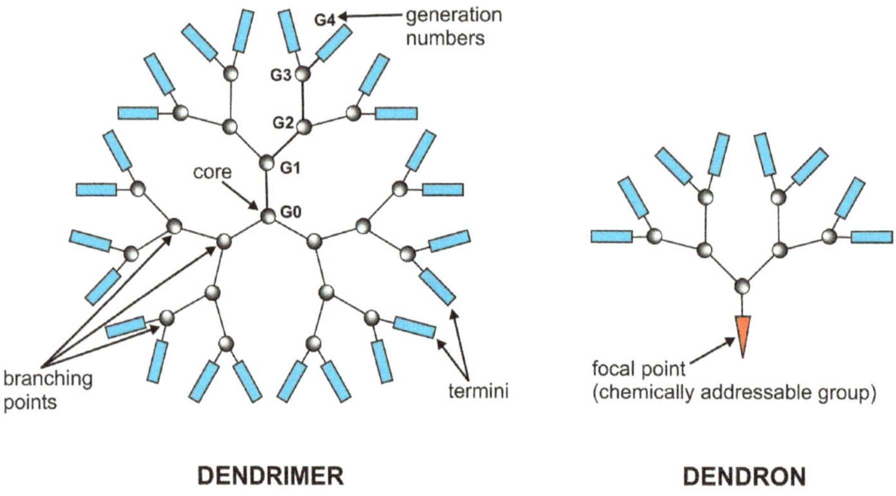

Nanoparticles *(top)*, liposomes*(middle)*, and dendrimers *(bottom)* are some nanomaterials being investigated for use in nanomedicine.

Drug delivery systems, lipid- or polymer-based nanoparticles, can be designed to improve the pharmacokinetics and biodistribution of the drug. However, the pharmacokinetics and pharmacodynamics of nanomedicine is highly variable among different patients. When designed to avoid the body's defence mechanisms, nanoparticles have beneficial properties that can be used to improve drug delivery. Complex drug delivery mechanisms are being developed, including the ability to get drugs through cell membranes and into cell cytoplasm. Triggered response is one way for drug molecules to be used more efficiently. Drugs are placed in the body and only activate on encountering a particular signal. For example, a drug with poor solubility will be replaced by a drug delivery system where both hydrophilic and hydrophobic environments exist, improving the solubility. Drug delivery systems may also be able to prevent tissue damage through regulated drug release; reduce drug clearance rates; or lower the volume of distribution and reduce the effect on non-target tissue. However, the biodistribution of these nanoparticles is still imperfect due to the complex host's reactions to nano- and microsized materials and the difficulty in targeting specific organs in the body. Nevertheless, a lot of work is still ongoing to optimize and better understand the potential and limitations of nanoparticulate systems. While advancement of research proves that targeting and distribution can be augmented by nanoparticles, the dangers of nanotoxicity become an important next step in further understanding of their medical uses.

Nanoparticles can be used in combination therapy for decreasing antibiotic resistance or for their antimicrobial properties. Nanoparticles might also used to circumvent multidrug resistance (MDR) mechanisms.

Types of Systems Used

Two forms of nanomedicine that have already been tested in mice and are awaiting human trials that will be using gold nanoshells to help diagnose and treat cancer, and using liposomes as vaccine adjuvants and as vehicles for drug transport. Similarly, drug detoxification is also another application for nanomedicine which has shown promising results in rats. Advances in Lipid nanotechnology was also instrumental in engineering medical nanodevices and novel drug delivery systems as well as in developing sensing applications. Another example can be found in dendrimers and nanoporous materials. Another example is to use block co-polymers, which form micelles for drug encapsulation.

Polymeric nano-particles are a competing technology to lipidic (based mainly on Phospholipids) nano-particles. There is an additional risk of toxicity associated with polymers not widely studied or understood. The major advantages of polymers is stability, lower cost and predictable characterisation. However, in the patient's body this very stability (slow degradation) is a negative factor. Phospholipids on the other hand are membrane lipids (already present in the body and surrounding each cell), have a GRAS (Generally Recognised As Safe) status from FDA and are derived from natural sources without any complex chemistry involved. They are not metabolised but rather absorbed by the body and the degradation products are themselves nutrients (fats or micronutrients).

Protein and peptides exert multiple biological actions in the human body and they have been identified as showing great promise for treatment of various diseases and disorders. These macromolecules are called biopharmaceuticals. Targeted and/or controlled delivery of these biopharmaceuticals using nanomaterials like nanoparticles and Dendrimers is an emerging field called nanobiopharmaceutics, and these products are called nanobiopharmaceuticals.

Another highly efficient system for microRNA delivery for example are nanoparticles formed by the self-assembly of two different microRNAs deregulated in cancer.

Another vision is based on small electromechanical systems; nanoelectromechanical systems are being investigated for the active release of drugs. Some potentially important applications include cancer treatment with iron nanoparticles or gold shells. Nanotechnology is also opening up new opportunities in implantable delivery systems, which are often preferable to the use of injectable drugs, because the latter frequently display first-order kinetics (the blood concentration goes up rapidly, but drops exponentially over time). This rapid rise may cause difficulties with toxicity, and drug efficacy can diminish as the drug concentration falls below the targeted range.

Applications

Some nanotechnology-based drugs that are commercially available or in human clinical trials include:

- Abraxane, approved by the U.S. Food and Drug Administration (FDA) to treat breast cancer, non-small- cell lung cancer (NSCLC) and pancreatic cancer, is the nanoparticle albumin bound paclitaxel.
- Doxil was originally approved by the FDA for the use on HIV-related Kaposi's sarcoma. It is now being used to also treat ovarian cancer and multiple myeloma. The drug is encased in liposomes, which helps to extend the life of the drug that is being distributed. Liposomes are self-assembling, spherical, closed colloidal structures that are composed of lipid bilayers that surround an aqueous space. The liposomes also help to increase the functionality and it helps to decrease the damage that the drug does to the heart muscles specifically.
- Onivyde, liposome encapsulated irinotecan to treat metastatic pancreatic cancer, was approved by FDA in October 2015.
- C-dots (Cornell dots) are the smallest silica-based nanoparticles with the size <10 nm. The particles are infused with organic dye which will light up with fluorescence. Clinical trial is underway since 2011 to use the C-dots as diagnostic tool to assist surgeons to identify the location of tumor cells.
- An early phase clinical trial using the platform of 'Minicell' nanoparticle for drug delivery have been tested on patients with advanced and untreatable cancer. Built from the membranes of mutant bacteria, the minicells were loaded with paclitaxel and coated with cetuximab, antibodies that bind the epidermal growth factor receptor (EGFR) which is often overexpressed in a number of cancers, as a 'homing' device to the tumor cells. The tumor cells recognize the bacteria from which the minicells have been derived, regard it as invading microorganism and engulf it. Once inside, the payload of anti-cancer drug kills the tumor cells. Measured at 400 nanometers, the minicell is bigger than synthetic particles developed for drug delivery. The researchers indicated that this larger size gives the minicells a better profile in side-effects because the minicells will preferentially leak out of the porous blood vessels around the tumor cells and do not reach the liver, digestive system and skin. This Phase 1 clinical trial demonstrated that this treatment is well tolerated by the patients. As a platform technology, the minicell drug delivery system can be used to treat a number of different cancers with different anti-cancer drugs with the benefit of lower dose and less side-effects.

- In 2014, a Phase 3 clinical trial for treating inflammation and pain after cataract surgery, and a Phase 2 trial for treating dry eye disease were initiated using nanoparticle loteprednol etabonate. In 2015, the product, KPI-121 was found to produce statistically significant positive results for the post-surgery treatment.

Cancer

Existing and potential drug nanocarriers have been reviewed.

Nanoparticles have high surface area to volume ratio. This allows for many functional groups to be attached to a nanoparticle, which can seek out and bind to certain tumor cells. Additionally, the small size of nanoparticles (10 to 100 nanometers), allows them to preferentially accumulate at tumor sites (because tumors lack an effective lymphatic drainage system). Limitations to conventional cancer chemotherapy include drug resistance, lack of selectivity, and lack of solubility. Nanoparticles have the potential to overcome these problems.

In photodynamic therapy, a particle is placed within the body and is illuminated with light from the outside. The light gets absorbed by the particle and if the particle is metal, energy from the light will heat the particle and surrounding tissue. Light may also be used to produce high energy oxygen molecules which will chemically react with and destroy most organic molecules that are next to them (like tumors). This therapy is appealing for many reasons. It does not leave a "toxic trail" of reactive molecules throughout the body (chemotherapy) because it is directed where only the light is shined and the particles exist. Photodynamic therapy has potential for a noninvasive procedure for dealing with diseases, growth and tumors. Kanzius RF therapy is one example of such therapy (nanoparticle hyperthermia) . Also, gold nanoparticles have the potential to join numerous therapeutic functions into a single platform, by targeting specific tumor cells, tissues and organs.

Visualization

In vivo imaging is another area where tools and devices are being developed. Using nanoparticle contrast agents, images such as ultrasound and MRI have a favorable distribution and improved contrast. This might be accomplished by self assembled biocompatible nanodevices that will detect, evaluate, treat and report to the clinical doctor automatically.

The small size of nanoparticles endows them with properties that can be very useful in oncology, particularly in imaging. Quantum dots (nanoparticles with quantum confinement properties, such as size-tunable light emission), when used in conjunction with MRI (magnetic resonance imaging), can produce exceptional images of tumor sites. Nanoparticles of cadmium selenide (quantum dots) glow when exposed to ultraviolet light. When injected, they seep into cancer tumors. The surgeon can see the glowing tumor, and use it as a guide for more accurate tumor removal.These nanoparticles are much brighter than organic dyes and only need one light source for excitation. This means that the use of fluorescent quantum dots could produce a higher contrast image and at a lower cost than today's organic dyes used as contrast media. The downside, however, is that quantum dots are usually made of quite toxic elements.

Tracking movement can help determine how well drugs are being distributed or how substances are metabolized. It is difficult to track a small group of cells throughout the body, so scientists used to dye the cells. These dyes needed to be excited by light of a certain wavelength in order for them to light up. While different color dyes absorb different frequencies of light, there was a need for as many light sources as cells. A way around this problem is with luminescent tags. These tags are quantum dots attached to proteins that penetrate cell membranes. The dots can be random in size, can be made of bio-inert material, and they demonstrate the nanoscale property that color is size-dependent. As a result, sizes are selected so that the frequency of light used to make a group of quantum dots fluoresce is an even multiple of the frequency required to make another group incandesce. Then both groups can be lit with a single light source. They have also found a way to insert nanoparticles into the affected parts of the body so that those parts of the body will glow showing the tumor growth or shrinkage or also organ trouble.

Sensing

Nanotechnology-on-a-chip is one more dimension of lab-on-a-chip technology. Magnetic nanoparticles, bound to a suitable antibody, are used to label specific molecules, structures or microorganisms. Gold nanoparticles tagged with short segments of DNA can be used for detection of genetic sequence in a sample. Multicolor optical coding for biological assays has been achieved by embedding different-sized quantum dots into polymeric microbeads. Nanopore technology for analysis of nucleic acids converts strings of nucleotides directly into electronic signatures.

Sensor test chips containing thousands of nanowires, able to detect proteins and other biomarkers left behind by cancer cells, could enable the detection and diagnosis of cancer in the early stages from a few drops of a patient's blood. Nanotechnology is helping to advance the use of arthroscopes, which are pencil-sized devices that are used in surgeries with lights and cameras so surgeons can do the surgeries with smaller incisions. The smaller the incisions the faster the healing time which is better for the patients. It is also helping to find a way to make an arthroscope smaller than a strand of hair.

Research on nanoelectronics-based cancer diagnostics could lead to tests that can be done in pharmacies. The results promise to be highly accurate and the product promises to be inexpensive. They could take a very small amount of blood and detect cancer anywhere in the body in about five minutes, with a sensitivity that is a thousand times better than in a conventional laboratory test. These devices that are built with nanowires to detect cancer proteins; each nanowire detector is primed to be sensitive to a different cancer marker. The biggest advantage of the nanowire detectors is that they could test for anywhere from ten to one hundred similar medical conditions without adding cost to the testing device. Nanotechnology has also helped to personalize oncology for the detection, diagnosis, and treatment of cancer. It is now able to be tailored to each individual's tumor for better performance. They have found ways that they will be able to target a specific part of the body that is being affected by cancer.

Blood Purification

Magnetic micro particles are proven research instruments for the separation of cells and proteins from complex media. The technology is available under the name Magnetic-activated cell sorting or Dynabeads among others. More recently it was shown in animal models that magnetic nanoparticles can be used for the removal of various noxious compounds including toxins, pathogens, and proteins from whole blood in an extracorporeal circuit similar to dialysis. In contrast to dialysis, which works on the principle of the size related diffusion of solutes and ultrafiltration of fluid across a semi-permeable membrane, the purification with nanoparticles allows specific targeting of substances. Additionally larger compounds which are commonly not dialyzable can be removed.

The purification process is based on functionalized iron oxide or carbon coated metal nanoparticles with ferromagnetic or superparamagnetic properties. Binding agents such as proteins, antibodies, antibiotics, or synthetic ligands are covalently linked to the particle surface. These binding agents are able to interact with target species forming an agglomerate. Applying an external magnetic field gradient allows exerting a force on the nanoparticles. Hence the particles can be separated from the bulk fluid, thereby cleaning it from the contaminants.

The small size (< 100 nm) and large surface area of functionalized nanomagnets leads to advantageous properties compared to hemoperfusion, which is a clinically used technique for the purification of blood and is based on surface adsorption. These advantages are high loading and accessibility of the binding agents, high selectivity towards the target compound, fast diffusion, small hydrodynamic resistance, and low dosage.

This approach offers new therapeutic possibilities for the treatment of systemic infections such as sepsis by directly removing the pathogen. It can also be used to selectively remove cytokines or endotoxins or for the dialysis of compounds which are not accessible by traditional dialysis methods. However the technology is still in a preclinical phase and first clinical trials are not expected before 2017.

Tissue Engineering

Nanotechnology may be used as part of tissue engineering to help reproduce or repair or reshape damaged tissue using suitable nanomaterial-based scaffolds and growth factors. Tissue engineering if successful may replace conventional treatments like organ transplants or artificial implants. Nanoparticles such as graphene, carbon nanotubes, molybdenum disulfide and tungsten disulfide are being used as reinforcing agents to fabricate mechanically strong biodegradable polymeric nanocomposites for bone tissue engineering applications. The addition of these nanoparticles in the polymer matrix at low concentrations (~0.2 weight %) leads to significant improvements in the compressive and flexural mechanical properties of polymeric nanocomposites. Potentially, these nanocomposites may be used as a novel, mechanically strong, light weight composite as bone implants.

For example, a flesh welder was demonstrated to fuse two pieces of chicken meat into a single piece using a suspension of gold-coated nanoshells activated by an infrared laser. This could be used to weld arteries during surgery. Another example is nanonephrology, the use of nanomedicine on the kidney.

Medical Devices

Neuro-electronic interfacing is a visionary goal dealing with the construction of nanodevices that will permit computers to be joined and linked to the nervous system. This idea requires the building of a molecular structure that will permit control and detection of nerve impulses by an external computer. A refuelable strategy implies energy is refilled continuously or periodically with external sonic, chemical, tethered, magnetic, or biological electrical sources, while a nonrefuelable strategy implies that all power is drawn from internal energy storage which would stop when all energy is drained. A nanoscale enzymatic biofuel cell for self-powered nanodevices have been developed that uses glucose from biofluids including human blood and watermelons. One limitation to this innovation is the fact that electrical interference or leakage or overheating from power consumption is possible. The wiring of the structure is extremely difficult because they must be positioned precisely in the nervous system. The structures that will provide the interface must also be compatible with the body's immune system.

Molecular nanotechnology is a speculative subfield of nanotechnology regarding the possibility of engineering molecular assemblers, machines which could re-order matter at a molecular or atomic scale. Nanomedicine would make use of these nanorobots, introduced into the body, to repair or detect damages and infections. Molecular nanotechnology is highly theoretical, seeking to anticipate what inventions nanotechnology might yield and to propose an agenda for future inquiry. The proposed elements of molecular nanotechnology, such as molecular assemblers and nanorobots are far beyond current capabilities. Future advances in nanomedicine could give rise to life extension through the repair of many processes thought to be responsible for aging. K. Eric Drexler, one of the founders of nanotechnology, postulated cell repair machines, including ones operating within cells and utilizing as yet hypothetical molecular machines, in his 1986 book Engines of Creation, with the first technical discussion of medical nanorobots by Robert Freitas appearing in 1999. Raymond Kurzweil, a futurist and transhumanist, stated in his book *The Singularity Is Near* that he believes that advanced medical nanorobotics could completely remedy the effects of aging by 2030.According to Richard Feynman, it was his former graduate student and collaborator Albert Hibbs who originally suggested to him (circa 1959) the idea of a *medical* use for Feynman's theoretical micromachines. Hibbs suggested that certain repair machines might one day be reduced in size to the point that it would, in theory, be possible to (as Feynman put it) "swallow the doctor". The idea was incorporated into Feynman's 1959 essay *There's Plenty of Room at the Bottom.*

Nanobiotechnology

Nanobiotechnology, bionanotechnology, and nanobiology are terms that refer to the intersection of nanotechnology and biology. Given that the subject is one that has only emerged very recently, bionanotechnology and nanobiotechnology serve as blanket terms for various related technologies.

This discipline helps to indicate the merger of biological research with various fields of nanotechnology. Concepts that are enhanced through nanobiology include: nanodevices (such as biological machines), nanoparticles, and nanoscale phenomena that occurs within the discipline of nanotechnology. This technical approach to biology allows scientists to imagine and create systems that can be used for biological research. Biologically inspired nanotechnology uses biological systems as the inspirations for technologies not yet created. However, as with nanotechnology and biotechnology, bionanotechnology does have many potential ethical issues associated with it.

The most important objectives that are frequently found in nanobiology involve applying nanotools to relevant medical/biological problems and refining these applications. Developing new tools, such as peptoid nanosheets, for medical and biological purposes is another primary objective in nanotechnology. New nanotools are often made by refining the applications of the nanotools that are already being used. The imaging of native biomolecules, biological membranes, and tissues is also a major topic for the nanobiology researchers. Other topics concerning nanobiology include the use of cantilever array sensors and the application of nanophotonics for manipulating molecular processes in living cells.

Recently, the use of microorganisms to synthesize functional nanoparticles has been of great interest. Microorganisms can change the oxidation state of metals. These microbial processes have opened up new opportunities for us to explore novel applications, for example, the biosynthesis of metal nanomaterials. In contrast to chemical and physical methods, microbial processes for synthesizing nanomaterials can be achieved in aqueous phase under gentle and environmentally benign conditions. This approach has become an attractive focus in current green bionanotechnology research towards sustainable development.

Terminology

The terms are often used interchangeably. When a distinction is intended, though, it is based on whether the focus is on applying biological ideas or on studying biology with nanotechnology. Bionanotechnology generally refers to the study of how the goals of nanotechnology can be guided by studying how biological "machines" work and adapting these biological motifs into improving existing nanotechnologies or creating new ones. Nanobiotechnology, on the other hand, refers to the ways that nanotechnology is used to create devices to study biological systems.

In other words, nanobiotechnology is essentially miniaturized biotechnology, whereas bionanotechnology is a specific application of nanotechnology. For example, DNA nanotechnology or cellular engineering would be classified as bionanotechnology because they involve working with biomolecules on the nanoscale. Conversely, many new medical technologies involving nanoparticles as delivery systems or as sensors would be examples of nanobiotechnology since they involve using nanotechnology to advance the goals of biology.

The definitions enumerated above will be utilized whenever a distinction between nanobio and bionano is made in this article. However, given the overlapping usage of the terms in modern parlance, individual technologies may need to be evaluated to determine which term is more fitting. As such, they are best discussed in parallel.

Concepts

Most of the scientific concepts in bionanotechnology are derived from other fields. Biochemical principles that are used to understand the material properties of biological systems are central in bionanotechnology because those same principles are to be used to create new technologies. Material properties and applications studied in bionanoscience include mechanical properties(e.g. deformation, adhesion, failure), electrical/electronic (e.g. electromechanical stimulation, capacitors, energy storage/batteries), optical (e.g. absorption, luminescence, photochemistry), thermal (e.g. thermomutability, thermal management), biological (e.g. how cells interact with nanomaterials, molecular flaws/defects, biosensing, biological mechanisms s.a. mechanosensing), nanoscience of disease (e.g. genetic disease, cancer, organ/tissue failure), as well as computing (e.g. DNA computing) and agriculture(target delivery of pesticides, hormones and fertilizers. The impact of bionanoscience, achieved through structural and mechanistic analyses of biological processes at nanoscale, is their translation into synthetic and technological applications through nanotechnology. Nano-biotechnology takes most of its fundamentals from nanotechnology. Most of the devices designed for nano-biotechnological use are directly based on other existing nanotechnologies. Nano-biotechnology is often used to describe the overlapping multidisciplinary activities associated with biosensors, particularly where photonics, chemistry, biology, biophysics, nano-medicine, and engineering converge. Measurement in biology using wave guide techniques, such as dual polarization interferometry, are another example.

Applications

Applications of bionanotechnology are extremely widespread. Insofar as the distinction holds, nanobiotechnology is much more commonplace in that it simply provides more tools for the study of biology. Bionanotechnology, on the other hand, promises to recreate biological mechanisms and pathways in a form that is useful in other ways.

Nanomedicine

Nanomedicine is a field of medical science whose applications are increasing more and more thanks to nanorobots and biological machines, which constitute a very useful tool to develop this area of knowledge. In the past years, researchers have done many improvements in the different devices and systems required to develop nanorobots. This supposes a new way of treating and dealing with diseases such as cancer; thanks to nanorobots, side effects of chemotherapy have been controlled, reduced and even eliminated, so some years from now, cancer patients will be offered an alternative to treat this disease instead of chemotherapy, which causes secondary effects such as hair loss, fatigue or nausea killing not only cancerous cells but also the healthy ones. At a clinical level, cancer treatment with nanomedicine will consist on the supply of nanorobots to the patient through an injection that will seek for cancerous cells leaving untouched the healthy ones. Patients that will be treated through nanomedicine will not notice the presence of this nanomachines inside them; the only thing that is going to be noticeable is the progressive improvement of their health.

Nanobiotechnology

Nanobiotechnology (sometimes referred to as nanobiology) is best described as helping modern medicine progress from treating symptoms to generating cures and regenerating biological tissues. Three American patients have received whole cultured bladders with the help of doctors who use nanobiology techniques in their practice. Also, it has been demonstrated in animal studies that a uterus can be grown outside the body and then placed in the body in order to produce a baby. Stem cell treatments have been used to fix diseases that are found in the human heart and are in clinical trials in the United States. There is also funding for research into allowing people to have new limbs without having to resort to prosthesis. Artificial proteins might also become available to manufacture without the need for harsh chemicals and expensive machines. It has even been surmised that by the year 2055, computers may be made out of biochemicals and organic salts.

Another example of current nanobiotechnological research involves nanospheres coated with fluorescent polymers. Researchers are seeking to design polymers whose fluorescence is quenched when they encounter specific molecules. Different polymers would detect different metabolites. The polymer-coated spheres could become part of new biological assays, and the technology might someday lead to particles which could be introduced into the human body to track down metabolites associated with tumors and other health problems. Another example, from a different perspective, would be evaluation and therapy at the nanoscopic level, i.e. the treatment of Nanobacteria (25-200 nm sized) as is done by NanoBiotech Pharma.

While nanobiology is in its infancy, there are a lot of promising methods that will rely on nanobiology in the future. Biological systems are inherently nano in scale; nanoscience must merge with biology in order to deliver biomacromolecules and molecular machines that are similar to nature. Controlling and mimicking the devices and processes that are constructed from molecules is a tremendous challenge to face the converging disciplines of nanotechnology. All living things, including humans, can be considered to be nanofoundries. Natural evolution has optimized the "natural" form of nanobiology over millions of years. In the 21st century, humans have developed the technology to artificially tap into nanobiology. This process is best described as "organic merging with synthetic." Colonies of live neurons can live together on a biochip device; according to research from Dr. Gunther Gross at the University of North Texas. Self-assembling nanotubes have the ability to be used as a structural system. They would be composed together with rhodopsins; which would facilitate the optical computing process and help with the storage of biological materials. DNA (as the software for all living things) can be used as a structural proteomic system - a logical component for molecular computing. Ned Seeman - a researcher at New York University - along with other researchers are currently researching concepts that are similar to each other.

Bionanotechnology

DNA nanotechnology is one important example of bionanotechnology. The utilization of the inherent properties of nucleic acids like DNA to create useful materials is a promising area of modern research. Another important area of research involves taking advantage of membrane properties to generate synthetic membranes. Proteins that self-assemble to generate functional materials could be used as a novel approach for the large-scale production of programmable nanomaterials. One example is the development of amyloids found in bacterial biofilms as engineered nanomaterials that can be programmed genetically to have different properties. Protein folding studies provide a third important avenue of research, but one that has been largely inhibited by our inability to predict protein folding with a sufficiently high degree of accuracy. Given the myriad uses that biological systems have for proteins, though, research into understanding protein folding is of high importance and could prove fruitful for bionanotechnology in the future.

Lipid nanotechnology is another major area of research in bionanotechnology, where physico-chemical properties of lipids such as their antifouling and self-assembly is exploited to build nanodevices with applications in medicine and engineering.

Nanobiotechnology Applications in Agriculture

Meanwhile, nanotechnology application to biotechnology will also leave no field untouched by its groundbreaking scientific innovations for human wellness; the agricultural industry is no exception. Basically, nanomaterials are distinguished depending on the origin: natural, incidental and engineered nanoparticles. Among these, engineered nanoparticles have received wide attention in all fields of science, including medical, materials and agriculture technology with significant socio-economical growth. In the agriculture industry, engineered nanoparticles have been serving as nano carrier, containing herbicides, chemicals, or genes, which target particular plant parts to release their content. Previously nanocapsules containing herbicides have been reported to effectively penetrate through cuticles and tissues, allowing the slow and constant release of the active substances. Likewise, other literature describes that nano-encapsulated slow release of fertilizers has also become a trend to save fertilizer consumption and to minimize environmental pollution through precision farming. These are only a few examples from numerous research works which might open up exciting opportunities for nanobiotechnology application in agriculture. Also, application of this kind of engineered nanoparticles to plants should be considered the level of amicability before it is employed in agriculture practices. Based on a thorough literature survey, it was understood that there is only limited authentic information available to explain the biological consequence of engineered nanoparticles on treated plants. Certain reports underline the phytotoxicity of various origin of engineered nanoparticles to the plant caused by the subject of concentrations and sizes . At the same time, however, an equal number of studies were reported with a positive outcome of nanoparticles, which facilitate growth promoting nature to treat plant. In particular, compared to other nanoparticles, silver and gold nanoparticles based applications elicited beneficial results on various plant species with less and/or no toxicity. Silver nanoparticles (AgNPs) treated leaves of Asparagus showed the increased content of ascorbate and chlorophyll. Similarly, AgNPs-treated common bean and corn has increased shoot and root length, leaf surface area, chlorophyll, carbohydrate and protein contents reported earlier. The gold nanoparticle has been used to induce growth and seed yield in Brassica juncea.

Tools

This field relies on a variety of research methods, including experimental tools (e.g. imaging, characterization via AFM/optical tweezers etc.), x-ray diffraction based tools, synthesis via self-assembly, characterization of self-assembly (using e.g. MP-SPR, DPI, recombinant DNA methods, etc.), theory (e.g. statistical mechanics, nanomechanics, etc.), as well as computational approaches (bottom-up multi-scale simulation, supercomputing).

Green Nanotechnology

Green nanotechnology refers to the use of nanotechnology to enhance the environmental sustainability of processes producing negative externalities. It also refers to the use of the products of nanotechnology to enhance sustainability. It includes making green nano-products and using nano-products in support of sustainability.

Green nanotechnology has been described as the development of clean technologies, "to minimize potential environmental and human health risks associated with the manufacture and use of nanotechnology products, and to encourage replacement of existing products with new nano-products that are more environmentally friendly throughout their lifecycle."

Goals

Green nanotechnology has two goals: producing nanomaterials and products without harming the environment or human health, and producing nano-products that provide solutions to environmental problems. It uses existing principles of green chemistry and green engineering to make nanomaterials and nano-products without toxic ingredients, at low temperatures using less energy and renewable inputs wherever possible, and using lifecycle thinking in all design and engineering stages.

In addition to making nanomaterials and products with less impact to the environment, green nanotechnology also means using nanotechnology to make current manufacturing processes for non-nano materials and products more environmentally friendly. For example, nanoscale membranes can help separate desired chemical reaction products from waste materials. Nanoscale catalysts can make chemical reactions more efficient and less wasteful. Sensors at the nanoscale can form a part of process control systems, working with nano-enabled information systems. Using alternative energy systems, made possible by nanotechnology, is another way to "green" manufacturing processes.

The second goal of green nanotechnology involves developing products that benefit the environment either directly or indirectly. Nanomaterials or products directly can clean hazardous waste sites, desalinate water, treat pollutants, or sense and monitor environmental pollutants. Indirectly, lightweight nanocomposites for automobiles and other means of transportation could save fuel and reduce materials used for production; nanotechnology-enabled fuel cells and light-emitting diodes (LEDs) could reduce pollution from energy generation and help conserve fossil fuels; self-cleaning nanoscale surface coatings could reduce or eliminate many cleaning chemicals used in regular maintenance routines; and enhanced battery life could lead to less material use and less waste. Green Nanotechnology takes a broad systems view of nanomaterials and products, ensuring that unforeseen consequences are minimized and that impacts are anticipated throughout the full life cycle.

Current Research

Solar cells

Research is underway to use nanomaterials for purposes including more efficient solar cells, practical fuel cells, and environmentally friendly batteries. The most advanced nanotechnology projects related to energy are: storage, conversion, manufacturing improvements by reducing materials and process rates, energy saving (by better thermal insulation for example), and enhanced renewable energy sources.

One major project that is being worked on is the development of nanotechnology in solar cells. Solar cells are more efficient as they get tinier and solar energy is a renewable resource. The price per watt of solar energy is lower than one dollar.

Research is ongoing to use nanowires and other nanostructured materials with the hope of to create cheaper and more efficient solar cells than are possible with conventional planar silicon solar cells. Another example is the use of fuel cells powered by hydrogen, potentially using a catalyst consisting of carbon supported noble metal particles with diameters of 1-5 nm. Materials with small nanosized pores may be suitable for hydrogen storage. Nanotechnology may also find applications in batteries, where the use of nanomaterials may enable batteries with higher energy content or supercapacitors with a higher rate of recharging.

Nanotechnology is already used to provide improved performance coatings for photovoltaic (PV) and solar thermal panels. Hydrophobic and self-cleaning properties combine to create more efficient solar panels, especially during inclement weather. PV covered with nanotechnology coatings are said to stay cleaner for longer to ensure maximum energy efficiency is maintained.

Nanoremediation and Water Treatment

Nanotechnology offers the potential of novel nanomaterials for the treatment of surface water, groundwater, wastewater, and other environmental materials contaminated by toxic metal ions, organic and inorganic solutes, and microorganisms. Due to their unique activity toward recalcitrant contaminants, many nanomaterials are under active research and development for use in the treatment of water and contaminated sites.

The present market of nanotech-based technologies applied in water treatment consists of reverse osmosis, nanofiltration, ultrafiltration membranes. Indeed, among emerging products one can name nanofiber filters, carbon nanotubes and various nanoparticles. Nanotechnology is expected to deal more efficiently with contaminants which convectional water treatment systems struggle to treat, including bacteria, viruses and heavy metals. This efficiency generally stems from the very high specific surface area of nanomaterials which increases dissolution, reactivity and sorption of contaminants.

Some potential applications include:

- To maintain public health, pathogens in water need to be identified rapidly and reliably. Unfortunately, traditional laboratory culture tests take days to complete. Faster methods involving enzymes, immunological or genetic tests are under development.
- Water filtration may be improved with the use of nanofiber membranes and the use of nanobiocides, which appear promisingly effective.
- Biofilms are mats of bacteria wrapped in natural polymers. These can be difficult to treat with antimicrobials or other chemicals. They can be cleaned up mechanically, but at the cost of substantial down-time and labour. Work is in progress to develop enzyme treatments that may be able to break down such biofilms.

Environmental Remediation

Nanoremediation is the use of nanoparticles for environmental remediation. Nanoremediation has been most widely used for groundwater treatment, with additional extensive research in wastewater treatment. Nanoremediation has also been tested for soil and sediment cleanup. Even more preliminary research is exploring the use of nanoparticles to remove toxic materials from gases.

Some nanoremediation methods, particularly the use of nano zero-valent iron for groundwater cleanup, have been deployed at full-scale cleanup sites. Nanoremediation is an emerging industry; by 2009, nanoremediation technologies had been documented in at least 44 cleanup sites around the world, predominantly in the United States. During nanoremediation, a nanoparticle agent must be brought into contact with the target contaminant under conditions that allow a detoxifying or immobilizing reaction. This process typically involves a pump-and-treat process or *in situ* application. Other methods remain in research phases.

Scientists have been researching the capabilities of buckminsterfullerene in controlling pollution, as it may be able to control certain chemical reactions. Buckminsterfullerene has been demonstrated as having the ability of inducing the protection of reactive oxygen species and causing lipid peroxidation. This material may allow for hydrogen fuel to be more accessible to consumers.

Water Filtration

Nanofiltration is a relatively recent membrane filtration process used most often with low total dissolved solids water such as surface water and fresh groundwater, with the purpose of softening (polyvalent cation removal) and removal of disinfection by-product precursors such as natural organic matter and synthetic organic matter. Nanofiltration is also becoming more widely used in food processing applications such as dairy, for simultaneous concentration and partial (monovalent ion) demineralisation.

Nanofiltration is a membrane filtration based method that uses nanometer sized cylindrical through-pores that pass through the membrane at a 90°. Nanofiltration membranes have pore sizes from 1-10 Angstrom, smaller than that used in microfiltration and ultrafiltration, but just larger than that in reverse osmosis. Membranes used are predominantly created from polymer thin films. Materials that are commonly used include polyethylene terephthalate or metals such as aluminum. Pore dimensions are controlled by pH, temperature and time during development with pore densities ranging from 1 to 106 pores per cm^2. Membranes made from polyethylene terephthalate and other similar materials, are referred to as "track-etch" membranes, named after the way the pores on the membranes are made. "Tracking" involves bombarding the polymer thin film with high energy particles. This results in making tracks that are chemically developed into the membrane, or "etched" into the membrane, which are the pores. Membranes created from metal such as alumina membranes, are made by electrochemically growing a thin layer of aluminum oxide from aluminum metal in an acidic medium.

Some water-treatment devices incorporating nanotechnology are already on the market, with more in development. Low-cost nanostructured separation membranes methods have been shown to be effective in producing potable water in a recent study.

Energy Applications of Nanotechnology

Over the past few decades, the fields of science and engineering have been seeking to develop new and improved types of energy technologies that have the capability of improving life all over the world. In order to make the next leap forward from the current generation of technology, scientists and engineers have been developing energy applications of nanotechnology. Nanotechnology, a new field in science, is any technology that contains components smaller than 100 nanometers. For scale, a single virus particle is about 100 nanometers in width.

An important subfield of nanotechnology related to energy is nanofabrication. Nanofabrication is the process of designing and creating devices on the nanoscale. Creating devices smaller than 100 nanometers opens many doors for the development of new ways to capture, store, and transfer energy. The inherent level of control that nanofabrication could give scientists and engineers would be critical in providing the capability of solving many of the problems that the world is facing today related to the current generation of energy technologies.

People in the fields of science and engineering have already begun developing ways of utilizing nanotechnology for the development of consumer products. Benefits already observed from the design of these products are an increased efficiency of lighting and heating, increased electrical storage capacity, and a decrease in the amount of pollution from the use of energy. Benefits such as these make the investment of capital in the research and development of nanotechnology a top priority.

Consumer Products

Recently, previously established and entirely new companies such as BetaBatt, Inc. and Oxane Materials are focusing on nanomaterials as a way to develop and improve upon older methods for the capture, transfer, and storage of energy for the development of consumer products.

ConsERV, a product developed by the Dais Analytic Corporation, uses nanoscale polymer membranes to increase the efficiency of heating and cooling systems and has already proven to be a lucrative design. The polymer membrane was specifically configured for this application by selectively engineering the size of the pores in the membrane to prevent air from passing, while allowing moisture to pass through the membrane. ConsERV's value is demonstrated in the form of an energy recovery a device which pretreats the incoming fresh air to a building using the energy found in the exhaust air steam using no moving parts to lower the energy and carbon footprint of existing forms of heating and cooling equipment Polymer membranes can be designed to selectively allow particles of one size and shape to pass through while preventing other. This makes for a powerful tool that can be used in all markets - consumer, commercial, industrial, and government products from biological weapons protection to industrial chemical separations. Dais's near term uses of this 'family' of selectively engineered nanotechnology materials, aside from ConsERV, include (a.) a completely new cooling cycle capable of replacing the refrigerant based cooling cycle the world has known for the past 100 plus years. This product, under development, is named NanoAir. NanoAir uses only water and this selectively engineered membrane material to cool (or heat) and dehumidify (or humidify) air. There are no fluorocarbon producing gasses used, and the energy required to cool a space drops as thermodynamics does the actual cooling. The company was awarded an Advanced Research Program Administration - Energy award in 2010, and a United States Department of Defense (DoD) grant in 2011 both designed to accelerate this newer, energy efficient technology closer to commercialization, and (b.) a novel way to clean most all contaminated forms of water called NanoClear. By using the selectivity of this hermetic, engineered composite material it can transfer only a water molecule from one face of the membrane to the other leaving behind the contaminants. It should also be noted Dais received a US Patent (Patent Number 7,990,679) in October 2011 titled "Nanoparticle Ultracapacitor". This patented item again uses the selectively engineered material to create an energy storage mechanism projected to have performance and cost advantages over existing storage technologies. The company has used this patent's concepts to create a functional energy storage prototype device named NanoCap. NanoCap is a form of ultra-capacitor potentially useful to power a broad range of applications including most forms of transportation, energy storage (especially useful as a storage media for renewable energy technologies), telecommunication infrastructure, transistor gate dielectrics, and consumer battery applications (cell phones, computers, etc.).

A New York-based company called Applied NanoWorks, Inc. has been developing a consumer product that utilizes LED technology to generate light. Light-emitting diodes or LEDs, use only about 10% of the energy that a typical incandescent or fluorescent light bulb uses and typically last much longer, which makes them a viable alternative to traditional light bulbs. While LEDs have been around for decades, this company and others like it have been developing a special variant of LED called the white LED. White LEDs consist of semi-conducting organic layers that are only about 100 nanometers in distance from each other and are placed between two electrodes, which create an anode, and a cathode. When voltage is applied to the system, light is generated when electricity passes through the two organic layers. This is called electroluminescence. The semiconductor properties of the organic layers are what allow for the minimal amount of energy necessary to generate light. In traditional light bulbs, a metal filament is used to generate light when electricity is run through the filament. Using metal generates a great deal of heat and therefore lowers efficiency.

Research for longer lasting batteries has been an ongoing process for years. Researchers have now begun to utilize nanotechnology for battery technology. mPhase Technologies in conglomeration with Rutgers University and Bell Laboratories have utilized nanomaterials to alter the wetting behavior of the surface where the liquid in the battery lies to spread the liquid droplets over a greater area on the surface and therefore have greater control over the movement of the droplets. This gives more control to the designer of the battery. This control prevents reactions in the battery by separating the electrolytic liquid from the anode and the cathode when the battery is not in use and joining them when the battery is in need of use.

Thermal applications also are a future applications of nanothechonlogy creating low cost system of heating, ventilation, and air conditioning, changing molecular structure for better management of temperature

Reduction of Energy Consumption

A reduction of energy consumption can be reached by better insulation systems, by the use of more efficient lighting or combustion systems, and by use of lighter and stronger materials in the transportation sector. Currently used light bulbs only convert approximately 5% of the electrical energy into light. Nanotechnological approaches like or quantum caged atoms (QCAs) could lead to a strong reduction of energy consumption for illumination.

Increasing the Efficiency of Energy Production

Today's best solar cells have layers of several different semiconductors stacked together to absorb light at different energies but they still only manage to use 40 percent of the Sun's energy. Commercially available solar cells have much lower efficiencies (15-20%). Nanostructuring has been used to improve the efficiencies of established photovoltaic tehcnologies, for example by improving current collection in amorphous silicon devices, plasmonic enhancement in dye-sensitized solar cells, and improved light trapping in crystalline silicon. Furthermore, nanotechnology could help increase the efficiency of light conversion by using nanostructures with a continuum of bandgaps, or by controlling the directivity and photon escape probability of photovoltaic devices.

The degree of efficiency of the internal combustion engine is about 30-40% at present. Nanotechnology could improve combustion by designing specific catalysts with maximized surface area. In 2005, scientists at the University of Toronto developed a spray-on nanoparticle substance that, when applied to a surface, instantly transforms it into a solar collector.

Nuclear Accident Cleanup and Waste Storage

Nanomaterials deployed by swarm robotics may be helpful for decontaminating a site of a nuclear accident which poses hazards to humans because of high levels of radiation and radioactive particles. Hot nuclear compounds such as corium or melting fuel rods may be contained in "bubbles" made from nanomaterials that are designed to isolate the harmful effects of nuclear activity occurring inside of them from the outside environment that organisms inhabit.

Economic Benefits

The relatively recent shift toward using nanotechnology with respect to the capture, transfer, and storage of energy has and will continue to have many positive economic impacts on society. The control of materials that nanotechnology offers to scientists and engineers of consumer products is one of the most important aspects of nanotechnology. This allows for an improved efficiency of products across the board.

A major issue with current energy generation is the loss of efficiency from the generation of heat as a by-product of the process. A common example of this is the heat generated by the internal combustion engine. The internal combustion engine loses about 64% of the energy from gasoline as heat and an improvement of this alone could have a significant economic impact. However, improving the internal combustion engine in this respect has proven to be extremely difficult without sacrificing performance. Improving the efficiency of fuel cells through the use of nanotechnology appears to be more plausible by using molecularly tailored catalysts, polymer membranes, and improved fuel storage.

In order for a fuel cell to operate, particularly of the hydrogen variant, a noble-metal catalyst (usually platinum, which is very expensive) is needed to separate the electrons from the protons of the hydrogen atoms. However, catalysts of this type are extremely sensitive to carbon monoxide reactions. In order to combat this, alcohols or hydrocarbons compounds are used to lower the carbon monoxide concentration in the system. This adds an additional cost to the device. Using nanotechnology, catalysts can be designed through nanofabrication that are much more resistant to carbon monoxide reactions, which improves the efficiency of the process and may be designed with cheaper materials to additionally lower costs.

Fuel cells that are currently designed for transportation need rapid start-up periods for the practicality of consumer use. This process puts a lot of strain on the traditional polymer electrolyte membranes, which decreases the life of the membrane requiring frequent replacement. Using nanotechnology, engineers have the ability to create a much more durable polymer membrane, which addresses this problem. Nanoscale polymer membranes are also much more efficient in ionic conductivity. This improves the efficiency of the system and decreases the time between replacements, which lowers costs.

Another problem with contemporary fuel cells is the storage of the fuel. In the case of hydrogen fuel cells, storing the hydrogen in gaseous rather than liquid form improves the efficiency by 5%. However, the materials that we currently have available to us significantly limit fuel storage due to low stress tolerance and costs. Scientists have come up with an answer to this by using a nanoporous styrene material (which is a relatively inexpensive material) that when super-cooled to around -196°C, naturally holds on to hydrogen atoms and when heated again releases the hydrogen for use.

Capacitors: Then and Now

For decades, scientists and engineers have been attempting to make computers smaller and more efficient. A crucial component of computers are capacitors. A capacitor is a device that is made of a pair of electrodes separated by an insulator that each stores an opposite charge. A capacitor stores a charge when it is removed from the circuit that it is connected to; the charge is released when it is replaced back into the circuit. Capacitors have an advantage over batteries in that they release their charge much more quickly than a battery.

Traditional or foil capacitors are composed of thin metal conducting plates separated by an electrical insulator, which are then stacked or rolled and placed in a casing. The problem with a traditional capacitor such as this is that they limit how small an engineer can design a computer. Scientists and engineers have since turned to nanotechnology for a solution to the problem.

Using nanotechnology, researchers developed what they call "ultracapacitors." An ultracapacitor is a general term that describes a capacitor that contains nanocomponents. Ultracapacitors are being researched heavily because of their high density interior, compact size, reliability, and high capacitance. This decrease in size makes it increasingly possible to develop much smaller circuits and computers. Ultracapacitors also have the capability to supplement batteries in hybrid vehicles by providing a large amount of energy during peak acceleration and allowing the battery to supply energy over longer periods of time, such as during a constant driving speed. This could decrease the size and weight of the large batteries needed in hybrid vehicles as well as take additional stress off the battery. However, the combination of ultracapacitors and a battery is not cost effective due to the need of additional DC/DC electronics to coordinate the two.

Nanoporous carbon aerogel is one type of material that is being utilized for the design of ultracapacitors. These aerogels have a very large interior surface area and can have its properties altered by changing the pore diameter and distribution along with adding nanosized alkali metals to alter its conductivity.

Carbon nanotubes are another possible material for use in an ultracapacitor. Carbon nanotubes are created by vaporizing carbon and allowing it to condense on a surface. When the carbon condenses, it forms a nanosized tube composed of carbon atoms. This tube has a high surface area, which increases the amount of charge that can be stored. The low reliability and high cost of using carbon nanotubes for ultracapacitors is currently an issue of research.

In a study concerning ultracapacitors or supercapacitors, researchers at the Sungkyunkwan University in the Republic of Korea explored the possibility of increasing the capacitance of electrodes through the addition of fluorine atoms to the walls of carbon nanotubes. As briefly mentioned before, carbon nanotubes are an increasing form of capacitors due to their superb chemical stability, high conductivity, light mass, and their large surface area. These researchers fluorinated single-walled carbon nanotubes (SWCNTs) at high temperatures to bind fluorine atoms to the walls. The attached fluorine atoms changed the non-polar nanotubes to become polar molecules. This can be attributed to the charge transfer from the fluorine. This created dipole-dipole layers along the carbon nanotube walls. Testing of these fluorinated SWCNTs against normal state SWCNTs showed a difference in capacitance. It was determined that the fluorinated SWCNTs are advantageous in fabricating electrodes for capacitors and improve the wettability with aqueous electrolytes, which promotes the overall performance of supercapacitors. While this study brought to knowledge a more efficient example of capacitors, little is known about this new supercapacitor, large scale synthesis is lacking and is necessary for any massive production, and preparation conditions are quite tedious in achieving the final product.

Theory of Capacitance

Understanding the concept of capacitance can be helpful in understanding why nanotechnology is such a powerful tool for the design of higher energy storing capacitors. A capacitor's capacitance (C) or amount of energy stored is equal to the amount of charge (Q) stored on each plate divided by the voltage (V) between the plates. Another representation of capacitance is that capacitance (C) is approximately equal to the permittivity (ε) of the dielectric times the area (A) of the plates divided by the distance (d) between them. Therefore, capacitance is proportional to the surface area of the conducting plate and inversely proportional to the distance between the plates.

Using carbon nanotubes as an example, a property of carbon nanotubes is that they have a very high surface area to store a charge. Using the above proportionality that capacitance (C) is proportional to the surface area (A) of the conducting plate; it becomes obvious that using nanoscaled materials with high surface area would be great for increasing capacitance. The other proportionality described above is that capacitance (C) is inversely proportional to the distance (d) between the plates. Using nanoscaled plates such as carbon nanotubes with nanofabrication techniques, gives the capability of decreasing the space between plates which again increases capacitance.

Industrial Applications of Nanotechnology

Nanotechnology is impacting the field of consumer goods, several products that incorporate nanomaterials are already in a variety of items; many of which people do not even realize contain nanoparticles, products with novel functions ranging from easy-to-clean to scratch-resistant. Examples of that car bumpers are made lighter, clothing is more stain repellant, sunscreen is more radiation resistant, synthetic bones are stronger, cell phone screens are lighter weight, glass packaging for drinks leads to a longer shelf-life, and balls for various sports are made more durable.Using nanotech, in the mid-term modern textiles will become "smart", through embedded "wearable electronics", such novel products have also a promising potential especially in the field of cosmetics, and has numerous potential applications in heavy industry. Nanotechnology is predicted to be a main driver of technology and business in this century and holds the promise of higher performance materials, intelligent systems and new production methods with significant impact for all aspects of society.

Foods

A complex set of engineering and scientific challenges in the food and bioprocessing industry for manufacturing high quality and safe food through efficient and sustainable means can be solved through nanotechnology. Bacteria identification and food quality monitoring using biosensors; intelligent, active, and smart food packaging systems; nanoencapsulation of bioactive food compounds are few examples of emerging applications of nanotechnology for the food industry. Nanotechnology can be applied in the production, processing, safety and packaging of food. A nanocomposite coating process could improve food packaging by placing anti-microbial agents directly on the surface of the coated film. Nanocomposites could increase or decrease gas permeability of different fillers as is needed for different products. They can also improve the mechanical and heat-resistance properties and lower the oxygen transmission rate. Research is being performed to apply nanotechnology to the detection of chemical and biological substances for sensanges in foods.

In general, food substances are not allowed to be adulterated, according to the Food, Drug and Cosmetic Act (section 402). Additives to food must conform to all regulations in the food additives amendment of 1958 as well as the FDA Modernization Act of 1997. In addition, color additives are obliged to comply with all regulations stipulated by the Color Additive Amendments of 1960. A safety assessment must be performed on all food substances for submission and approval by the US FDA. The mandatory information in this assessment includes the identity, technical effects, self-limiting levels of use, dietary exposure and safety studies for the manufacturing processes used, including the use of nanotechnology. Food manufacturers are obliged to assess whether the identity, safety or regulatory status of a food substance is affected by significant changes in manufacturing processes, such as the use of nanotechnology. In their guidance document published in April 2012, the US FDA discusses what considerations and recommendations may apply to such an assessment.

Nano-foods

New foods are among the nanotechnology-created consumer products coming onto the market at the rate of 3 to 4 per week, according to the Project on Emerging Nanotechnologies (PEN), based on an inventory it has drawn up of 609 known or claimed nano-products. On PEN's list are three foods—a brand of canola cooking oil called Canola Active Oil, a tea called Nanotea and a chocolate diet shake called Nanoceuticals Slim Shake Chocolate. According to company information posted on PEN's Web site, the canola oil, by Shemen Industries of Israel, contains an additive called "nanodrops" designed to carry vitamins, minerals and phytochemicals through the digestive system and urea. The shake, according to U.S. manufacturer RBC Life Sciences Inc., uses cocoa infused "NanoClusters" to enhance the taste and health benefits of cocoa without the need for extra sugar.

Consumer Goods

Surfaces and Coatings

The most prominent application of nanotechnology in the household is self-cleaning or "easy-to-clean" surfaces on ceramics or glasses. Nano ceramic particles have improved the smoothness and heat resistance of common household equipment such as the flat iron.

The first sunglasses using protective and anti-reflective ultrathin polymer coatings are on the market. For optics, nanotechnology also offers scratch resistant surface coatings based on nanocomposites. Nano-optics could allow for an increase in precision of pupil repair and other types of laser eye surgery.

Textiles

The use of engineered nanofibers already makes clothes water- and stain-repellent or wrinkle-free. Textiles with a nanotechnological finish can be washed less frequently and at lower temperatures. Nanotechnology has been used to integrate tiny carbon particles membrane and guarantee full-surface protection from electrostatic charges for the wearer. Many other applications have been developed by research institutions such as the Textiles Nanotechnology Laboratory at Cornell University, and the UK's Dstl and its spin out company P2i.

Cosmetics

One field of application is in sunscreens. The traditional chemical UV protection approach suffers from its poor long-term stability. A sunscreen based on mineral nanoparticles such as titanium oxide offer several advantages. Titanium oxide nanoparticles have a comparable UV protection property as the bulk material, but lose the cosmetically undesirable whitening as the particle size is decreased.

Sports

Nanotechnology may also play a role in sports such as soccer, football, and baseball. Materials for new athletic shoes may be made in order to make the shoe lighter (and the athlete faster). Baseball bats already on the market are made with carbon nanotubes that reinforce the resin, which is said to improve its performance by making it lighter. Other items such as sport towels, yoga mats, exercise mats are on the market and used by players in the National Football League, which use antimicrobial nanotechnology to prevent parasuram from illnesses caused by bacteria such as Methicillin-resistant Staphylococcus aureus (commonly known as MRSA).

Aerospace and Vehicle Manufacturers

Lighter and stronger materials will be of immense use to aircraft manufacturers, leading to increased performance. Spacecraft will also benefit, where weight is a major factor. Nanotechnology might thus help to reduce the size of equipment and thereby decrease fuel-consumption required to get it airborne. Hang gliders may be able to halve their weight while increasing their strength and toughness through the use of nanotech materials. Nanotech is lowering the mass of supercapacitors that will increasingly be used to give power to assistive electrical motors for launching hang gliders off flatland to thermal-chasing altitudes.

Much like aerospace, lighter and stronger materials would be useful for creating vehicles that are both faster and safer. Combustion engines might also benefit from parts that are more hard-wearing and more heat-resistant.

Military

Biological Sensors

Nanotechnology can improve the military's ability to detect biological agents. By using nanotechnology, the military would be able to create sensor systems that could detect biological agents. The sensor systems are already well developed and will be one of the first forms of nanotechnology that the military will start to use.

Uniform Material

Nanoparticles can be injected into the material on soldiers' uniforms to not only make the material more durable, but also to protect soldiers from many different dangers such as high temperatures, impacts and chemicals. The nanoparticles in the material protect soldiers from these dangers by grouping together when something strikes the armor and stiffening the area of impact. This stiffness helps lessen the impact of whatever hit the armor, whether it was extreme heat or a blunt force. By reducing the force of the impact, the nanoparticles protect the soldier wearing the uniform from any injury the impact could have caused.

Another way nanotechnology can improve soldiers' uniforms is by creating a better form of camouflage. Mobile pigment nanoparticles injected into the material can produce a better form of camouflage. These mobile pigment particles would be able to change the color of the uniforms depending upon the area that the soldiers are in. There is still much research being done on this self-changing camouflage.

Nanotechnology can improve thermal camouflage. Thermal camouflage helps protect soldiers from people who are using night vision technology. Surfaces of many different military items can be designed in a way that electromagnetic radiation can help lower the infrared signatures of the object that the surface is on. Surfaces of soldiers' uniforms and surfaces of military vehicle are a few surfaces that can be designed in this way. By lowering the infrared signature of both the soldiers and the military vehicles the soldiers are using, it will provide better protection from infrared guided weapons or infrared surveillance sensors.

Communication Method

There is a way to use nanoparticles to create coated polymer threads that can be woven into soldiers' uniforms. These polymer threads could be used as a form of communication between the soldiers. The system of threads in the uniforms could be set to different light wavelengths, eliminating the ability for anyone else to listen in. This would lower the risk of having anything intercepted by unwanted listeners.

Medical System

A medical surveillance system for soldiers to wear can be made using nanotechnology. This system would be able to watch over their health and stress levels. The systems would be able to react to medical situations by releasing drugs or compressing wounds as necessary. This means that if the system detected an injury that was bleeding, it would be able to compress around the wound until further medical treatment could be received. The system would also be able to release drugs into the soldier's body for health reasons, such as pain killers for an injury. The system would be able to inform the medics at base of the soldier's health status at all times that the soldier is wearing the system. The energy needed to communicate this information back to base would be produced through the soldier's body movements.

Weapons

Nanoweapon is the name given to military technology currently under development which seeks to exploit the power of nanotechnology in the modern battlefield.

Risks in Military

- People such as state agencies, criminals and enterprises could use nano-robots to eavesdrop on conversations held in private.
- Grey goo: an uncontrollable, self-replicating nano-machine or robot.
- Nanoparticles used in different military materials could potentially be a hazard to the soldiers that are wearing the material, if the material is allowed to get worn out. As the uniforms wear down it is possible for nanomaterial to break off and enter the soldiers' bodies. Having nanoparticles entering the soldiers' bodies would be very unhealthy and could seriously harm them. There is not a lot of information on what the actual damage to the soldiers would be, but there have been studies on the effect of nanoparticles entering a fish through its skin. The studies showed that the different fish in the study suffered from varying degrees of brain damage. Although brain damage would be a serious negative effect, the studies also say that the results cannot be taken as an accurate example of what would happen to soldiers if nanoparticles entered their bodies. There are very strict regulations on the scientists that manufacture products with nanoparticles. With these strict regulations, they are able to largely decrease the danger of nanoparticles wearing off of materials and entering the soldiers' systems.

Catalysis

Chemical catalysis benefits especially from nanoparticles, due to the extremely large surface to volume ratio. The application potential of nanoparticles in catalysis ranges from fuel cell to catalytic converters and photocatalytic devices. Catalysis is also important for the production of chemicals. For example, nanoparticles with a distinct chemical surrounding (ligands), or specific optical properties.

Platinum nanoparticle are now being considered in the next generation of automotive catalytic converters because the very high surface area of nanoparticles could reduce the amount of platinum required. However, some concerns have been raised due to experiments demonstrating that they will spontaneously combust if methane is mixed with the ambient air. Ongoing research at the Centre National de la Recherche Scientifique (CNRS) in France may resolve their true usefulness for catalytic applications. Nanofiltration may come to be an important application, although future research must be careful to investigate possible toxicity.

Construction

Nanotechnology has the potential to make construction faster, cheaper, safer, and more varied. Automation of nanotechnology construction can allow for the creation of structures from advanced homes to massive skyscrapers much more quickly and at much lower cost. In the near future, Nanotechnology can be used to sense cracks in foundations of architecture and can send nanobots to repair them.

Nanotechnology is an active research area that encompasses a number of disciplines such as electronics, bio-mechanics and coatings. These disciplines assist in the areas of civil engineering and construction materials. If nanotechnology is implemented in the construction of homes and infrastructure, such structures will be stronger. If buildings are stronger, then fewer of them will require reconstruction and less waste will be produced.

Nanotechnology in construction involves using nanoparticles such as alumina and silica. Manufacturers are also investigating the methods of producing nano-cement. If cement with nano-size particles can be manufactured and processed, it will open up a large number of opportunities in the fields of ceramics, high strength composites and electronic applications.

Nanomaterials still have a high cost relative to conventional materials, meaning that they are not likely to feature in high-volume building materials. The day when this technology slashes the consumption of structural steel has not yet been contemplated.

Cement

Much analysis of concrete is being done at the nano-level in order to understand its structure. Such analysis uses various techniques developed for study at that scale such as Atomic Force Microscopy (AFM), Scanning Electron Microscopy (SEM) and Focused Ion Beam (FIB). This has come about as a side benefit of the development of these instruments to study the nanoscale in general, but the understanding of the structure and behavior of concrete at the fundamental level is an important and very appropriate use of nanotechnology. One of the fundamental aspects of nanotechnology is its interdisciplinary nature and there has already been cross over research between the mechanical modeling of bones for medical engineering to that of concrete which has enabled the study of chloride diffusion in concrete (which causes corrosion of reinforcement). Concrete is, after all, a macro-material strongly influenced by its nano-properties and understanding it at this new level is yielding new avenues for improvement of strength, durability and monitoring as outlined in the following paragraphs

Silica (SiO2) is present in conventional concrete as part of the normal mix. However, one of the advancements made by the study of concrete at the nanoscale is that particle packing in concrete can be improved by using nano-silica which leads to a densifying of the micro and nanostructure resulting in improved mechanical properties. Nano-silica addition to cement based materials can also control the degradation of the fundamental C-S-H (calcium-silicatehydrate) reaction of concrete caused by calcium leaching in water as well as block water penetration and therefore lead to improvements in durability. Related to improved particle packing, high energy milling of ordinary Portland cement (OPC) clinker and standard sand, produces a greater particle size diminution with respect to conventional OPC and, as a result, the compressive strength of the refined material is also 3 to 6 times higher (at different ages).

Steel

Steel is a widely available material that has a major role in the construction industry. The use of nanotechnology in steel helps to improve the physical properties of steel. Fatigue, or the structural failure of steel, is due to cyclic loading. Current steel designs are based on the reduction in the allowable stress, service life or regular inspection regime. This has a significant impact on the life-cycle costs of structures and limits the effective use of resources. Stress risers are responsible for initiating cracks from which fatigue failure results. The addition of copper nanoparticles reduces the surface un-evenness of steel, which then limits the number of stress risers and hence fatigue cracking. Advancements in this technology through the use of nanoparticles would lead to increased safety, less need for regular inspection, and more efficient materials free from fatigue issues for construction.

Steel cables can be strengthened using carbon nanotubes. Stronger cables reduce the costs and period of construction, especially in suspension bridges, as the cables are run from end to end of the span.

The use of vanadium and molybdenum nanoparticles improves the delayed fracture problems associated with high strength bolts. This reduces the effects of hydrogen embrittlement and improves steel micro-structure by reducing the effects of the inter-granular cementite phase.

Welds and the Heat Affected Zone (HAZ) adjacent to welds can be brittle and fail without warning when subjected to sudden dynamic loading. The addition of nanoparticles such as magnesium and calcium makes the HAZ grains finer in plate steel. This nanoparticle addition leads to an increase in weld strength. The increase in strength results in a smaller resource requirement because less material is required in order to keep stresses within allowable limits.

Wood

Nanotechnology represents a major opportunity for the wood industry to develop new products, substantially reduce processing costs, and open new markets for biobased materials.

Wood is also composed of nanotubes or "nanofibrils"; namely, lignocellulosic (woody tissue) elements which are twice as strong as steel. Harvesting these nanofibrils would lead to a new paradigm in sustainable construction as both the production and use would be part of a renewable cycle. Some developers have speculated that building functionality onto lignocellulosic surfaces at the nanoscale could open new opportunities for such things as self-sterilizing surfaces, internal self-repair, and electronic lignocellulosic devices. These non-obtrusive active or passive nanoscale sensors would provide feedback on product performance and environmental conditions during service by monitoring structural loads, temperatures, moisture content, decay fungi, heat losses or gains, and loss of conditioned air. Currently, however, research in these areas appears limited.

Due to its natural origins, wood is leading the way in cross-disciplinary research and modelling techniques. BASF have developed a highly water repellent coating based on the actions of the lotus leaf as a result of the incorporation of silica and alumina nanoparticles and hydrophobic polymers. Mechanical studies of bones have been adapted to model wood, for instance in the drying process.

Glass

Research is being carried out on the application of nanotechnology to glass, another important material in construction. Titanium dioxide (TiO_2) nanoparticles are used to coat glazing since it has sterilizing and anti-fouling properties. The particles catalyze powerful reactions that break down organic pollutants, volatile organic compounds and bacterial membranes. TiO_2 is hydrophilic (attraction to water), which can attract rain drops that then wash off the dirt particles. Thus the introduction of nanotechnology in the Glass industry, incorporates the self-cleaning property of glass.

Fire-protective glass is another application of nanotechnology. This is achieved by using a clear intumescent layer sandwiched between glass panels (an interlayer) formed of silica nanoparticles (SiO_2), which turns into a rigid and opaque fire shield when heated. Most of glass in construction is on the exterior surface of buildings. So the light and heat entering the building through glass has to be prevented. The nanotechnology can provide a better solution to block light and heat coming through windows.

Coatings

Coatings is an important area in construction coatings are extensively use to paint the walls, doors, and windows. Coatings should provide a protective layer bound to the base material to produce a surface of the desired protective or functional properties. The coatings should have self healing capabilities through a process of "self-assembly". Nanotechnology is being applied to paints to obtained the coatings having self healing capabilities and corrosion protection under insulation. Since these coatings are hydrophobic and repels water from the metal pipe and can also protect metal from salt water attack.

Nanoparticle based systems can provide better adhesion and transparency. The TiO_2 coating captures and breaks down organic and inorganic air pollutants by a photocatalytic process, which leads to putting roads to good environmental use.

Fire Protection and Detection

Fire resistance of steel structures is often provided by a coating produced by a spray-on-cementitious process. The nano-cement has the potential to create a new paradigm in this area of application because the resulting material can be used as a tough, durable, high temperature coating. It provides a good method of increasing fire resistance and this is a cheaper option than conventional insulation.

Risks in Construction

In building construction nanomaterials are widely used from self-cleaning windows to flexible solar panels to wi-fi blocking paint. The self-healing concrete, materials to block ultraviolet and infrared radiation, smog-eating coatings and light-emitting walls and ceilings are the new nanomaterials in construction. Nanotechnology is a promise for making the "smart home" a reality. Nanotech-enabled sensors can monitor temperature, humidity, and airborne toxins, which needs nanotech-based improved batteries. The building components will be intelligent and interactive since the sensor uses wireless components, it can collect the wide range of data.

If nanosensors and nanomaterials become an everyday part of the buildings, as with smart homes, what are the consequences of these materials on human beings?

- Effect of nanoparticles on health and environment: Nanoparticles may also enter the body if building water supplies are filtered through commercially available nanofilters. Airborne and waterborne nanoparticles enter from building ventilation and wastewater systems.
- Effect of nanoparticles on societal issues: As sensors become commonplace, a loss of privacy and autonomy may result from users interacting with increasingly intelligent building components.

Potential Applications of Carbon Nanotubes

Carbon nanotubes (CNTs) are cylinders of one or more layers of graphene (lattice). Diameters of single-walled carbon nanotubes (SWNTs) and multi-walled carbon nanotubes (MWNTs) are typically 0.8 to 2 nm and 5 to 20 nm, respectively, although MWNT diameters can exceed 100 nm. CNT lengths range from less than 100 nm to 0.5 m.

Individual CNT walls can be metallic or semiconducting depending on the orientation of the lattice with respect to the tube axis, which is called chirality. MWNT's cross-sectional area offers an elastic modulus approaching 1 TPa and a tensile strength of 100 GPa, over 10-fold higher than any industrial fiber. MWNTs are typically metallic and can carry currents of up to 10^9 A cm^{-2}. SWNTs can display thermal conductivity of 3500 W m^{-1} K^{-1}, exceeding that of diamond.

As of 2013, carbon nanotube production exceeded several thousand tons per year, used for applications in energy storage, automotive parts, boat hulls, sporting goods, water filters, thin-film electronics, coatings, actuators and electromagnetic shields. CNT-related publications more than tripled in the prior decade, while rates of patent issuance also increased. Most output was of unorganized architecture. Organized CNT architectures such as "forests", yarns and regular sheets were produced in much smaller volumes. CNTs have even been proposed as the tether for a purported space elevator.

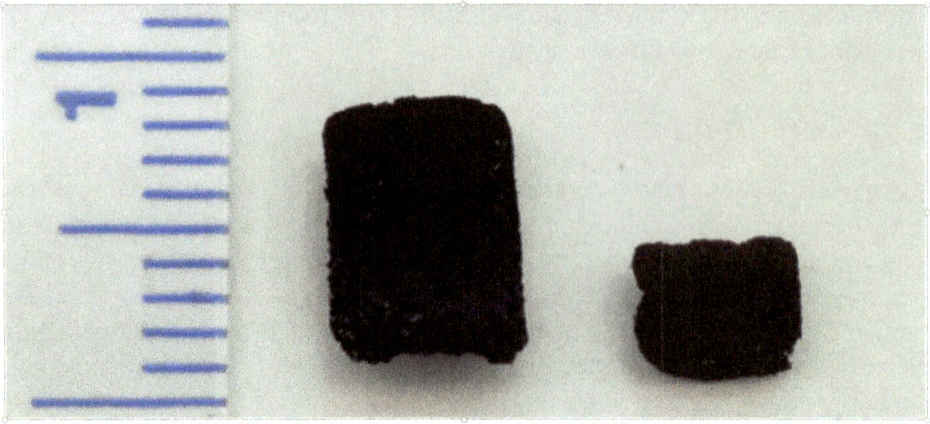

3D carbon nanotube scaffolds.

Recently, several studies have highlighted the prospect of using carbon nanotubes as building blocks to fabricate three-dimensional macroscopic (>1mm in all three dimensions) all-carbon devices. Lalwani et al. have reported a novel radical initiated thermal crosslinking method to fabricated macroscopic, free-standing, porous, all-carbon scaffolds using single- and multi-walled carbon nanotubes as building blocks. These scaffolds possess macro-, micro-, and nano- structured pores and the porosity can be tailored for specific applications. These 3D all-carbon scaffolds/architectures may be used for the fabrication of the next generation of energy storage, supercapacitors, field emission transistors, high-performance catalysis, photovoltaics, and biomedical devices and implants.

Composite Materials

Because of the carbon nanotube's superior mechanical properties, many structures have been proposed ranging from everyday items like clothes and sports gear to combat jackets and space elevators. However, the space elevator will require further efforts in refining carbon nanotube technology, as the practical tensile strength of carbon nanotubes must be greatly improved.

For perspective, outstanding breakthroughs have already been made. Pioneering work led by Ray H. Baughman at the NanoTech Institute has shown that single and multi-walled nanotubes can produce materials with toughness unmatched in the man-made and natural worlds.

Carbon nanotubes are also a promising material as building blocks in hierarchical composite materials given their exceptional mechanical properties (~1 TPa in modulus, and ~100 GPa in strength). Initial attempts to incorporate CNTs into hierarchical structures (such as yarns, fibres or films) has led to mechanical properties that were significantly lower than these potential limits. Windle *et al.* have used an *in situ* chemical vapor deposition (CVD) spinning method to produce continuous CNT yarns from CVD-grown CNT aerogels. CNT yarns can also be manufactured by drawing out CNT bundles from a CNT forest and subsequently twisting to form the fibre (draw-twist method). The Windle group have fabricated CNT yarns with strengths as high as ~9 GPa at small gage lengths of ~1 mm, however, strengths of only about ~1 GPa were reported at the longer gage length of 20 mm. The reason why fibre strengths have been low compared to the strength of individual CNTs is due to a failure to effectively transfer load to the constituent (discontinuous) CNTs within the fibre. One potential route for alleviating this problem is via irradiation (or deposition) induced covalent inter-bundle and inter-CNT cross-linking to effectively 'join up' the CNTs, with higher dosage levels leading to the possibility of amorphous carbon/carbon nanotube composite fibres. Espinosa *et al.* developed high performance DWNT-polymer composite yarns by twisting and stretching ribbons of randomly oriented bundles of DWNTs thinly coated with polymeric organic compounds. These DWNT-polymer yarns exhibited an unusually high energy to failure of ~100 $J \cdot g^{-1}$ (comparable to one of the toughest natural materials – spider silk), and strength as high as ~1.4 GPa. Effort is ongoing to produce CNT composites that incorporate tougher matrix materials, such as Kevlar, to further improve on the mechanical properties toward those of individual CNTs.

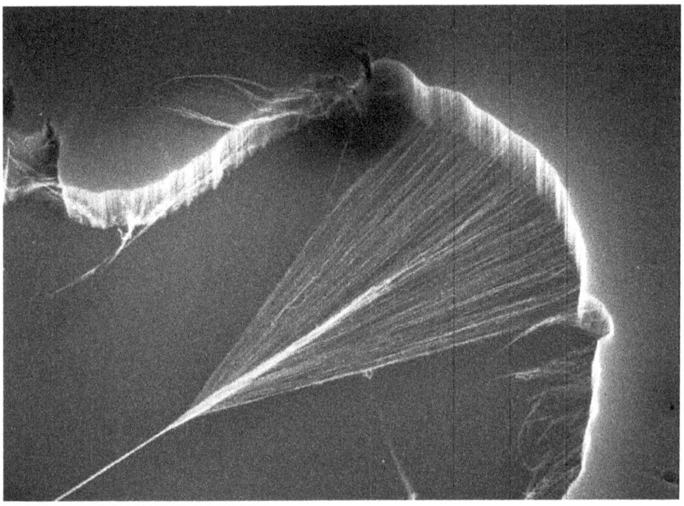

Carbon nanotubes being spun to form a yarn, CSIRO

Because of the high mechanical strength of carbon nanotubes, research is being made into weaving them into clothes to create stab-proof and bulletproof clothing. The nanotubes would effectively stop the bullet from penetrating the body, although the bullet's kinetic energy would likely cause broken bones and internal bleeding.

Mixtures

MWNTs were first used as electrically conductive fillers in metals, at concentrations as high as 83.78 percent by weight (wt%). MWNT-polymer composites reach conductivities as high as 10,000 S m^{-1} at 10 wt % loading. In the automotive industry, CNT plastics are used in electrostatic-assisted painting of mirror housings, as well as fuel lines and filters that dissipate electrostatic charge. Other products include electromagnetic interference (EMI)–shielding packages and silicon wafer carriers.

For load-bearing applications, CNT powders are mixed with polymers or precursor resins to increase stiffness, strength and toughness. These enhancements depend on CNT diameter, aspect ratio, alignment, dispersion and interfacial interaction. Premixed resins and master batches employ CNT loadings from 0.1 to 20 wt%. Nanoscale stick-slip among CNTs and CNT-polymer contacts can increase material damping, enhancing sporting goods, including tennis racquets, baseball bats and bicycle frames.

CNT resins enhance fiber composites, including wind turbine blades and hulls for maritime security boats that are made by enhancing carbon fiber composites with CNT-enhanced resin. CNTs are deployed as additives in the organic precursors of stronger 1-μm diameter carbon fibers. CNTs influence the arrangement of carbon in pyrolyzed fiber.

Toward the challenge of organizing CNTs at larger scales, hierarchical fiber composites are created by growing aligned forests onto glass, silicon carbide (SiC), alumina and carbon fibers, creating so-called "fuzzy" fibers. Fuzzy epoxy CNT-SiC and CNT-alumina fabric showed 69% improved crack-opening (mode I) and/or in-plane shear interlaminar (mode II) toughness. Applications under investigation include lightning-strike protection, deicing, and structural health monitoring for aircraft.

MWNTs can be used as a flame-retardant additive to plastics due to changes in rheology by nanotube loading. Such additives can replace halogenated flame retardants, which face environmental restrictions.

CNT/Concrete blends offer increased tensile strength and reduced crack propagation.

Buckypaper (nanotube aggregate) can significantly improve fire resistance due to efficient heat reflection.

Textiles

The previous studies on the use of CNTs for textile functionalization were focused on fiber spinning for improving physical and mechanical properties. Recently a great deal of attention has been focused on coating CNTs on textile fabrics. Various methods have been employed for modifying fabrics using CNTs. Shim et al. produced intelligent e-textiles for Human Biomonitoring using a polyelectrolyte-based coating with CNTs. Additionally, Panhuis et al. dyed textile material by immersion in either a poly (2-methoxy aniline-5-sulfonic acid) PMAS polymer solution or PMAS-SWNT dispersion with enhanced conductivity and capacitance with a durable behavior. In another study, Hu and coworkers coated single-walled carbon nanotubes with a simple "dipping and drying" process for wearable electronics and energy storage applications. In the recent study, Li and coworkers using elastomeric separator and almost achieved a fully stretchable supercapacitor based on buckled single-walled carbon nanotube macrofilms. The electrospun polyurethane was used and provided sound mechanical stretchability and the whole cell achieve excellent charge-discharge cycling stability. CNTs have an aligned nanotube structure and a negative surface charge. Therefore, they have similar structures to direct dyes, so the exhaustion method is applied for coating and absorbing CNTs on the fiber surface for preparing multifunctional fabric including antibacterial, electric conductive, flame retardant and electromagnetic absorbance properties.

Later, CNT yarns and laminated sheets made by direct chemical vapor deposition (CVD) or forest spinning or drawing methods may compete with carbon fiber for high-end uses, especially in weight-sensitive applications requiring combined electrical and mechanical functionality. Research yarns made from few-walled CNTs have reached a stiffness of 357 GPa and a strength of 8.8 GPa for a gauge length comparable to the millimeter-long CNTs within the yarn. Centimeter-scale gauge lengths offer only 2-GPa gravimetric strengths, matching that of Kevlar.

Because the probability of a critical flaw increases with volume, yarns may never achieve the strength of individual CNTs. However, CNT's high surface area may provide interfacial coupling that mitigates these deficiencies. CNT yarns can be knotted without loss of strength. Coating forest-drawn CNT sheets with functional powder before inserting twist yields weavable, braidable and sewable yarns containing up to 95 wt % powder. Uses include superconducting wires, battery and fuel cell electrodes and self-cleaning textiles.

As yet impractical fibers of aligned SWNTs can be made by coagulation-based spinning of CNT suspensions. Cheaper SWNTs or spun MWNTs are necessary for commercialization. Carbon nanotubes can be dissolved in superacids such as fluorosulfuric acid and drawn into fibers in dry jet-wet spinning.

DWNT-polymer composite yarns have been made by twisting and stretching ribbons of randomly oriented bundles of DWNTs thinly coated with polymeric organic compounds.

Body armor—combat jackets Cambridge University developed the fibres and licensed a company to make them. In comparison, the bullet-resistant fiber Kevlar fails at 27–33 J/g.

Synthetic muscles offer high contraction/extension ratio given an electric current

SWNT are in use as an experimental material for removable, structural bridge panels.

In 2015 researchers incorporated CNTs and graphene into spider silk, increasing its strength and toughness to a new record. They sprayed 15 Pholcidae spiders with water containing the nanotubes or flakes.The resulting silk had a fracture strength up to 5.4 GPa, a Young's modulus up to 47.8 GPa and a toughness modulus up to 2.1 GPa, surpassing both synthetic polymeric high performance fibres (e.g. Kevlar49) and knotted fibers.

Carbon Nanotube Springs

"Forests" of stretched, aligned MWNT springs can achieve an energy density 10 times greater than that of steel springs, offering cycling durability, temperature insensitivity, no spontaneous discharge and arbitrary discharge rate. SWNT forests are expected to be able to store far more than MWNTs.

Alloys

Adding small amounts of CNTs to metals increases tensile strength and modulus with potential in aerospace and automotive structures. Commercial aluminum-MWNT composites have strengths comparable to stainless steel (0.7 to 1 GPa) at one-third the density (2.6 g cm^{-3}), comparable to more expensive aluminium-lithium alloys.

Coatings and Films

CNTs can serve as a multifunctional coating material. For example, paint/MWNT mixtures can reduce biofouling of ship hulls by discouraging attachment of algae and barnacles. They are a possible alternative to environmentally hazardous biocide-containing paints.

Mixing CNTs into anticorrosion coatings for metals can enhance coating stiffness and strength and provide a path for cathodic protection.

CNTs provide a less expensive alternative to ITO for a range of consumer devices. Besides cost, CNT's flexible, transparent conductors offer an advantage over brittle ITO coatings for flexible displays. CNT conductors can be deposited from solution and patterned by methods such as screen printing. SWNT films offer 90% transparency and a sheet resistivity of 100 ohm per square. Such films are under development for thin-film heaters, such as for defrosting windows or sidewalks.

Carbon nanotubes forests and foams can also be coated with a variety of different materials to change their functionality and performance. Examples include silicon coated CNTs to create flexible energy-dense batteries, graphene coatings to create highly elastic aerogels and silicon carbide coatings to create a strong structural material for robust high-aspect-ratio 3D-micro architectures.

Optical Power Detectors

A spray-on mixture of carbon nanotubes and ceramic demonstrates unprecedented ability to resist damage while absorbing laser light. Such coatings that absorb as the energy of high-powered lasers without breaking down are essential for optical power detectors that measure the output of such lasers. These are used, for example, in military equipment for defusing unexploded mines. The composite consists of multiwall carbon nanotubes and a ceramic made of silicon, carbon and nitrogen. Including boron boosts the breakdown temperature. The nanotubes and graphene-like carbon transmit heat well, while the oxidation-resistant ceramic boosts damage resistance. Creating the coating involves dispersing the nanotubes in toluene, to which a clear liquid polymer containing boron was added. The mixture was heated to 1,100 °C (2,010 °F). The result is crushed into a fine powder, dispersed again in toluene and sprayed in a thin coat on a copper surface. The coating absorbed 97.5 percent of the light from a far-infrared laser and tolerated 15 kilowatts per square centimeter for 10 seconds. Damage tolerance is about 50 percent higher than for similar coatings, e.g., nanotubes alone and carbon paint.

Radar Absorption

Radars work in the microwave frequency range, which can be absorbed by MWNTs. Applying the MWNTs to the aircraft would cause the radar to be absorbed and therefore seem to have a smaller radar cross-section. One such application could be to paint the nanotubes onto the plane. Recently there has been some work done at the University of Michigan regarding carbon nanotubes usefulness as stealth technology on aircraft. It has been found that in addition to the radar absorbing properties, the nanotubes neither reflect nor scatter visible light, making it essentially invisible at night, much like painting current stealth aircraft black except much more effective. Current limitations in manufacturing, however, mean that current production of nanotube-coated aircraft is not possible. One theory to overcome these current limitations is to cover small particles with the nanotubes and suspend the nanotube-covered particles in a medium such as paint, which can then be applied to a surface, like a stealth aircraft.

Microelectronics

Nanotube-based transistors, also known as carbon nanotube field-effect transistors (CNTFETs), have been made that operate at room temperature and that are capable of digital switching using a single electron. However, one major obstacle to realization of nanotubes has been the lack of technology for mass production. In 2001 IBM researchers demonstrated how metallic nanotubes can be destroyed, leaving semiconducting ones behind for use as transistors. Their process is called "constructive destruction," which includes the automatic destruction of defective nanotubes on the wafer. This process, however, only gives control over the electrical properties on a statistical scale.

SWNTs are attractive for transistors because of their low electron scattering and their bandgap. SWNTs are compatible with field-effect transistor (FET) architectures and high-k dielectrics. Despite progress following the CNT transistor's appearance in 1998, including a tunneling FET with a subthreshold swing of <60 mV per decade (2004), a radio (2007) and an FET with sub-10-nm channel length and a normalized current density of 2.41 mA μm^{-1} at 0.5 V, greater than those obtained for silicon devices.

However, control of diameter, chirality, density and placement remains insufficient for commercial production. Less demanding devices of tens to thousands of SWNTs are more immediately practical. The use of CNT arrays/transistor increases output current and compensates for defects and chirality differences, improving device uniformity and reproducibility. For example, transistors using horizontally aligned CNT arrays achieved mobilities of 80 $cm^2\ V^{-1}\ s^{-1}$, subthreshold slopes of 140 mV per decade and on/off ratios as high as 10^5. CNT film deposition methods enable conventional semiconductor fabrication of more than 10,000 CNT devices per chip.

Printed CNT thin-film transistors (TFTs) are attractive for driving organic light-emitting diode displays, showing higher mobility than amorphous silicon (~1 $cm^2\ V^{-1}\ s^{-1}$) and can be deposited by low-temperature, nonvacuum methods. Flexible CNT TFTs with a mobility of 35 $cm^2\ V^{-1}\ s^{-1}$ and an on/off ratio of 6×10^6 were demonstrated. A vertical CNT FET showed sufficient current output to drive OLEDs at low voltage, enabling red-green-blue emission through a transparent CNT network. CNTs are under consideration for radio-frequency identification tags. Selective retention of semiconducting SWNTs during spin-coating and reduced sensitivity to adsorbates were demonstrated.

The International Technology Roadmap for Semiconductors suggests that CNTs could replace Cu in microelectronic interconnects, owing to their low scattering, high current-carrying capacity, and resistance to electromigration. For this, vias comprising tightly packed (>10^{13} cm^{-2}) metallic CNTs with low defect density and low contact resistance are needed. Recently, complementary metal oxide semiconductor (CMOS)–compatible 150-nm-diameter interconnects with a single CNT–contact hole resistance of 2.8 kOhm were demonstrated on full 200-mm-diameter wafers. Also, as a replacement for solder bumps, CNTs can function both as electrical leads and heat dissipaters for use in high-power amplifiers.

Last, a concept for a nonvolatile memory based on individual CNT crossbar electromechanical switches has been adapted for commercialization by patterning tangled CNT thin films as the functional elements. This required development of ultrapure CNT suspensions that can be spin-coated and processed in industrial clean room environments and are therefore compatible with CMOS processing standards.

Transistors

Carbon nanotube field-effect transistors (CNTFETs) can operate at room temperature and are capable of digital switching using a single electron. In 2013, a CNT logic circuit was demonstrated that could perform useful work. Major obstacles to nanotube-based microelectronics include the absence of technology for mass production, circuit density, positioning of individual electrical contacts, sample purity, control over length, chirality and desired alignment, thermal budget and contact resistance.

One of the main challenges was regulating conductivity. Depending on subtle surface features, a nanotube may act as a conductor or as a semiconductor.

Another way to make carbon nanotube transistors has been to use random networks of them. By doing so one averages all of their electrical differences and one can produce devices in large scale at the wafer level. This approach was first patented by Nanomix Inc. (date of original application June 2002). It was first published in the academic literature by the United States Naval Research Laboratory in 2003 through independent research work. This approach also enabled Nanomix to make the first transistor on a flexible and transparent substrate.

Since the electron mean free path in SWCNTs can exceed 1 micrometer, long channel CNTFETs exhibit near-ballistic transport characteristics, resulting in high speeds. CNT devices are projected to operate in the frequency range of hundreds of gigahertz.

Nanotubes can be grown on nanoparticles of magnetic metal (Fe, Co) that facilitates production of electronic (spintronic) devices. In particular control of current through a field-effect transistor by magnetic field has been demonstrated in such a single-tube nanostructure.

History

In 2001 IBM researchers demonstrated how metallic nanotubes can be destroyed, leaving semiconducting nanotubes for use as components. Using “constructive destruction”, they destroyed defective nanotubes on the wafer. This process, however, only gives control over the electrical properties on a statistical scale. In 2003 room-temperature ballistic transistors with ohmic metal contacts and high-k gate dielectric were reported, showing 20–30x more current than state-of-the-art siliconMOSFETs. Palladium is a high-work function metal that was shown to exhibit Schottky barrier-free contacts to semiconducting nanotubes with diameters >1.7 nm.

The potential of carbon nanotubes was demonstrated in 2003 when room-temperature ballistic transistors with ohmic metal contacts and high-k gate dielectric were reported, showing 20–30x higher ON current than state-of-the-art Si MOSFETs. This presented an important advance in the field as CNT was shown to potentially outperform Si. At the time, a major challenge was ohmic metal contact formation. In this regard, palladium, which is a high-work function metal was shown to exhibit Schottky barrier-free contacts to semiconducting nanotubes with diameters >1.7 nm.

The first nanotube integrated memory circuit was made in 2004. One of the main challenges has been regulating the conductivity of nanotubes. Depending on subtle surface features a nanotube may act as a plain conductor or as a semiconductor. A fully automated method has however been developed to remove non-semiconductor tubes.

In 2013, researchers demonstrated a Turing-complete prototype micrometer-scale computer. Carbon nanotube transistors as logic-gate circuits with densities comparable to modern CMOS technology has not yet been demonstrated.

In 2014 networks of purified semiconducting carbon nanotubes were used as the active material in p-type thin film transistors. They were created using 3-D printers using inkjet or gravure methods on flexible substrates, including polyimide and polyethylene (PET) and transparent substrates such as glass. These transistors reliably exhibit high-mobilities ($> 10\ cm^2\ V^{-1}\ s^{-1}$) and ON/OFF ratios ($> 1000$) as well as threshold voltages below 5 V. They offer current density and low power consumption as well as environmental stability and mechanical flexibility. Hysterisis in the current-voltage curses as well as variability in the threshold voltage remain to be solved.

In 2015 researchers announced a new way to connect wires to SWNTs that make it possible to continue shrinking the width of the wires without increasing electrical resistance. The advance was expected to shrink the contact point between the two materials to just 40 atoms in width and later less. They tubes align in regularly spaced rows on silicon wafers. Simluations indicated that designs could be optimized either for high performance or for low power consumption. Commercial devices were not expected until the 2020s.

Thermal Management

Large structures of carbon nanotubes can be used for thermal management of electronic circuits. An approximately 1 mm–thick carbon nanotube layer was used as a special material to fabricate coolers, this material has very low density, ~20 times lower weight than a similar copper structure, while the cooling properties are similar for the two materials.

Buckypaper has characteristics appropriate for use as a heat sink for chipboards, a backlight for LCD screens or as a faraday cage.

Solar Cells

One of the promising applications of single-walled carbon nanotubes (SWNTs) is their use in solar panels, due to their strong UV/Vis-NIR absorption characteristics. Research has shown that they can provide a sizable increase in efficiency, even at their current unoptimized state. Solar cells developed at the New Jersey Institute of Technology use a carbon nanotube complex, formed by a mixture of carbon nanotubes and carbon buckyballs (known as fullerenes) to form snake-like structures. Buckyballs trap electrons, but they can't make electrons flow. Add sunlight to excite the polymers, and the buckyballs will grab the electrons. Nanotubes, behaving like copper wires, will then be able to make the electrons or current flow.

Additional research has been conducted on creating SWNT hybrid solar panels to increase the efficiency further. These hybrids are created by combining SWNT's with photo-excitable electron donors to increase the number of electrons generated. It has been found that the interaction between the photo-excited porphyrin and SWNT generates electro-hole pairs at the SWNT surfaces. This phenomenon has been observed experimentally, and contributes practically to an increase in efficiency up to 8.5%.

Nanotubes can potentially replace indium tin oxide in solar cells as a transparent conductive film in solar cells to allow light to pass to the active layers and generate photocurrent.

CNTs in organic solar cells help reduce energy loss (carrier recombination) and enhance resistance to photooxidation. Photovoltaic technologies may someday incorporate CNT-Silicon heterojunctions to leverage efficient multiple-exciton generation at p-n junctions formed within individual CNTs. In the nearer term, commercial photovoltaics may incorporate transparent SWNT electrodes.

Hydrogen Storage

In addition to being able to store electrical energy, there has been some research in using carbon nanotubes to store hydrogen to be used as a fuel source. By taking advantage of the capillary effects of the small carbon nanotubes, it is possible to condense gases in high density inside single-walled nanotubes. This allows for gases, most notably hydrogen (H_2), to be stored at high densities without being condensed into a liquid. Potentially, this storage method could be used on vehicles in place of gas fuel tanks for a hydrogen-powered car. A current issue regarding hydrogen-powered vehicles is the on-board storage of the fuel. Current storage methods involve cooling and condensing the H_2 gas to a liquid state for storage which causes a loss of potential energy (25–45%) when compared to the energy associated with the gaseous state. Storage using SWNTs would allow one to keep the H2 in its gaseous state, thereby increasing the storage efficiency. This method allows for a volume to energy ratio slightly smaller to that of current gas powered vehicles, allowing for a slightly lower but comparable range.

An area of controversy and frequent experimentation regarding the storage of hydrogen by adsorption in carbon nanotubes is the efficiency by which this process occurs. The effectiveness of hydrogen storage is integral to its use as a primary fuel source since hydrogen only contains about one fourth the energy per unit volume as gasoline. Studies however show that what is the most important is the surface area of the materials used. Hence activated carbon with surface area of 2600 m2/g can store up to 5,8% w/w. In all these carbonaceous materials, hydrogen is stored by physisorption at 70-90K.

Experimental Capacity

One experiment sought to determine the amount of hydrogen stored in CNTs by utilizing elastic recoil detection analysis (ERDA). CNTs (primarily SWNTs) were synthesized via chemical vapor disposition (CVD) and subjected to a two-stage purification process including air oxidation and acid treatment, then formed into flat, uniform discs and exposed to pure, pressurized hydrogen at various temperatures. When the data was analyzed, it was found that the ability of CNTs to store hydrogen decreased as temperature increased. Moreover, the highest hydrogen concentration measured was ~0.18%; significantly lower than commercially viable hydrogen storage needs to be. A separate experimental work performed by using a gravimetric method also revealed the maximum hydrogen uptake capacity of CNTs to be as low as 0.2%.

Carbon nanotubes are also a promising material as building blocks in hierarchical composite materials given their exceptional mechanical properties (~1 TPa in modulus, and ~100 GPa in strength). Initial attempts to incorporate CNTs into hierarchical structures (such as yarns, fibres or films) has led to mechanical properties that were significantly lower than these potential limits. Windle et al. have used an in situ chemical vapor deposition (CVD) spinning method to produce continuous CNT yarns from CVD-grown CNT aerogels. CNT yarns can also be manufactured by drawing out CNT bundles from a CNT forest and subsequently twisting to form the fibre (draw-twist method). The Windle group have fabricated CNT yarns with strengths as high as ~9 GPa at small gage lengths of ~1 mm, however, strengths of only about ~1 GPa were reported at the longer gage length of 20 mm. The reason why fibre strengths have been low compared to the strength of individual CNTs is due to a failure to effectively transfer load to the constituent (discontinuous) CNTs within the fibre. One potential route for alleviating this problem is via irradiation (or deposition) induced covalent inter-bundle and inter-CNT cross-linking to effectively 'join up' the CNTs, with higher dosage levels leading to the possibility of amorphous carbon/carbon nanotube composite fibres. Espinosa et al. developed high performance DWNT-polymer composite yarns by twisting and stretching ribbons of randomly oriented bundles of DWNTs thinly coated with polymeric organic compounds. These DWNT-polymer yarns exhibited an unusually high energy to failure of ~100 J·g−1 (comparable to one of the toughest natural materials – spider silk), and strength as high as ~1.4 GPa. Effort is ongoing to produce CNT composites that incorporate tougher matrix materials, such as Kevlar, to further improve on the mechanical properties toward those of individual CNTs. In another experiment, CNTs were synthesized via CVD and their structure was characterized using Raman spectroscopy. Utilizing microwave digestion, the samples were exposed to different acid concentrations and different temperatures for various amounts of time in an attempt to find the optimum purification method for SWNTs of the diameter determined earlier. The purified samples were then exposed to hydrogen gas at various high pressures, and their adsorption by weight percent was plotted. The data showed that hydrogen adsorption levels of up to 3.7% are possible with a very pure sample and under the proper conditions. It is thought that microwave digestion helps improve the hydrogen adsorption capacity of the CNTs by opening up the ends, allowing access to the inner cavities of the nanotubes.

Limitations on Efficient Hydrogen Adsorption

The biggest obstacle to efficient hydrogen storage using CNTs is the purity of the nanotubes. To achieve maximum hydrogen adsorption, there must be minimum graphene, amorphous carbon, and metallic deposits in the nanotube sample. Current methods of CNT synthesis require a purification step. However, even with pure nanotubes, the adsorption capacity is only maximized under high pressures, which are undesirable in commercial fuel tanks.

Electronic Components

Various companies are developing transparent, electrically conductive CNT films and nanobuds to replace indium tin oxide (ITO) in LCDs, touch screens and photovoltaic devices. Nanotube films show promise for use in displays for computers, cell phones, Personal digital assistants, and automated teller machines. CNT diodes display a photovoltaic effect.

Multi-walled nanotubes (MWNT coated with magnetite) can generate strong magnetic fields. Recent advances show that MWNT decorated with maghemite nanoparticles can be oriented in a magnetic field and enhance the electrical properties of the composite material in the direction of the field for use in electric motor brushes.

A layer of 29% iron enriched single-walled nanotubes (SWNT) placed on top of a layer of explosive material such as PETN can be ignited with a regular camera flash.

CNTs can be used as electron guns in miniature cathode ray tubes (CRT) in high-brightness, low-energy, low-weight displays. A display would consist of a group of tiny CRTs, each providing the electrons to illuminate the phosphor of one pixel, instead of having one CRT whose electrons are aimed using electric and magnetic fields. These displays are known as field emission displays (FEDs).

CNTs can act as antennas for radios and other electromagnetic devices.

Conductive CNTs are used in brushes for commercial electric motors. They replace traditional carbon black. The nanotubes improve electrical and thermal conductivity because they stretch through the plastic matrix of the brush. This permits the carbon filler to be reduced from 30% down to 3.6%, so that more matrix is present in the brush. Nanotube composite motor brushes are better-lubricated (from the matrix), cooler-running (both from better lubrication and superior thermal conductivity), less brittle (more matrix, and fiber reinforcement), stronger and more accurately moldable (more matrix). Since brushes are a critical failure point in electric motors, and also don't need much material, they became economical before almost any other application.

Wires for carrying electric current may be fabricated from nanotubes and nanotube-polymer composites. Small wires have been fabricated with specific conductivity exceeding copper and aluminum; the highest conductivity non-metallic cables.

CNT are under investigation as an alternative to tungsten filaments in incandescent light bulbs.

Interconnects

Metallic carbon nanotubes have aroused research interest for their applicability as very-large-scale integration (VLSI) interconnects because of their high thermal stability, high thermal conductivity and large current carrying capacity. An isolated CNT can carry current densities in excess of 1000 MA/sq-cm without damage even at an elevated temperature of 250 °C (482 °F), eliminating electromigration reliability concerns that plague Cu interconnects. Recent modeling work comparing the two has shown that CNT bundle interconnects can potentially offer advantages over copper. Recent experiments demonstrated resistances as low as 20 Ohms using different architectures, detailed conductance measurements over a wide temperature range were shown to agree with theory for a strongly disordered quasi-one-dimensional conductor.

Hybrid interconnects that employ CNT vias in tandem with copper interconnects may offer advantages from a reliability/thermal-management perspective. In 2016, the European Union has funded a four million euro project over three years to evaluate manufacturability and performance of composite interconnects employing both CNT and copper interconnects. The project named CONNECT (CarbON Nanotube compositE InterconneCTs) involves the joint efforts of seven European research and industry partners on fabrication techniques and processes to enable reliable Carbon NanoTubes for on-chip interconnects in ULSI microchip production.

Electrical Cables and W ires

Wires for carrying Electric current may be fabricated from pure nanotubes and nanotube-polymer composites. It has already been demonstrated that carbon nanotube wires can successfully be used for power or data transmission. Recently small wires have been fabricated with specific conductivity exceeding copper and aluminum; these cables are the highest conductivity carbon nanotube and also highest conductivity non-metal cables. Recently, composite of carbon nanotube and copper have been shown to exhibit nearly one hundred times higher current-carrying-capacity than pure copper or gold. Significantly, the electrical conductivity of such a composite is similar to pure Cu. Thus, this Carbon nanotube-copper (CNT-Cu) composite possesses the highest observed current-carrying capacity among electrical conductors. Thus for a given cross-section of electrical conductor, the CNT-Cu composite can withstand and transport one hundred times higher current compared to metals such as copper and gold.

Energy Storage

The use of CNTs as a catalyst support in fuel cells can potentially reduce platinum usage by 60% compared with carbon black. Doped CNTs may enable the complete elimination of Pt.

Supercapacitor

MIT Research Laboratory of Electronics uses nanotubes to improve supercapacitors. The activated charcoal used in conventional ultracapacitors has many small hollow spaces of various size, which create together a large surface to store electric charge. But as charge is quantized into elementary charges, i.e. electrons, and each such elementary charge needs a minimum space, a significant fraction of the electrode surface is not available for storage because the hollow spaces are not compatible with the charge's requirements. With a nanotube electrode the spaces may be tailored to size—few too large or too small—and consequently the capacity should be increased considerably.

A 40-F supercapacitor with a maximum voltage of 3.5 V that employed forest-grown SWNTs that are binder- and additive-free achieved an energy density of 15.6 Wh kg^{-1} and a power density of 37 kW kg^{-1}. CNTs can be bound to the charge plates of capacitors to dramatically increase the surface area and therefore energy density.

Batteries

Carbon nanotubes' (CNTs) exciting electronic properties have shown promise in the field of batteries, where typically they are being experimented as a new electrode material, particularly the anode for lithium ion batteries. This is due to the fact that the anode requires a relatively high reversible capacity at a potential close to metallic lithium, and a moderate irreversible capacity, observed thus far only by graphite-based composites, such as CNTs. They have shown to greatly improve capacity and cyclability of lithium-ion batteries, as well as the capability to be very effective buffering components, alleviating the degradation of the batteries that is typically due to repeated charging and discharging. Further, electronic transport in the anode can be greatly improved using highly metallic CNTs.

More specifically, CNTs have shown reversible capacities from 300 to 600 $mAhg^{-1}$, with some treatments to them showing these numbers rise to up to 1000 $mAhg^{-1}$. Meanwhile, graphite, which is most widely used as an anode material for these lithium batteries, has shown capacities of only 320 $mAhg^{-1}$. By creating composites out of the CNTs, scientists see much potential in taking advantage of these exceptional capacities, as well as their excellent mechanical strength, conductivities, and low densities.

MWNTs are used in lithium ion batteries. In these batteries, small amounts of MWNT powder are blended with active materials and a polymer binder, such as 1 wt % CNT loading in LiCoO2 cathodes and graphite anodes. CNTs provide increased electrical connectivity and mechanical integrity, which enhances rate capability and cycle life.

Paper Batteries

A paper battery is a battery engineered to use a paper-thin sheet of cellulose (which is the major constituent of regular paper, among other things) infused with aligned carbon nanotubes. The potential for these devices is great, as they may be manufactured via a roll-to-roll process, which would make it very low-cost, and they would be lightweight, flexible, and thin. In order to productively use paper electronics (or any thin electronic devices), the power source must be equally thin, thus indicating the need for paper batteries. Recently, it has been shown that surfaces coated with CNTs can be used to replace heavy metals in batteries. More recently, functional paper batteries have been demonstrated, where a lithium-ion battery is integrated on a single sheet of paper through a lamination process as a composite with $Li^4Ti^5O^{12}$ (LTO) or $LiCoO^2$ (LCO). The paper substrate would function well as the separator for the battery, where the CNT films function as the current collectors for both the anode *and* the cathode. These rechargeable energy devices show potential in RFID tags, functional packaging, or new disposable electronic applications.

Improvements have also been shown in lead-acid batteries, based on research performed by Bar-Ilan University using high quality SWCNT manufactured by OCSiAl. The study demonstrated an increase in the lifetime of lead acid batteries by 4.5 times and a capacity increase of 30% on average and up to 200% at high discharge rates.

Chemical

CNT can be used for desalination. Water molecules can be separated from salt by forcing them through electrochemically robust nanotube networks with controlled nanoscale porosity. This process requires far lower pressures than conventional reverse osmosis methods. Compared to a plain membrane, it operates at a 20 °C lower temperature, and at a 6x greater flow rate. Membranes using aligned, encapsulated CNTs with open ends permit flow through the CNTs› interiors. Very-small-diameter SWNTs are needed to reject salt at seawater concentrations. Portable filters containing CNT meshes can purify contaminated drinking water. Such networks can electrochemically oxidize organic contaminants, bacteria and viruses.

CNT membranes can filter carbon dioxide from power plant emissions.

CNT can be filled with biological molecules, aiding biotechnology.

CNT have the potential to store between 4.2 and 65% hydrogen by weight. If they can be mass-produced economically, 13.2 litres (2.9 imp gal; 3.5 US gal) of CNT could contain the same amount of energy as a 50 litres (11 imp gal; 13 US gal) gasoline tank.

CNTs can be used to produce nanowires of other elements/molecules, such as gold or zinc oxide. Nanowires in turn can be used to cast nanotubes of other materials, such as gallium nitride. These can have very different properties from CNTs—for example, gallium nitride nanotubes are hydrophilic, while CNTs are hydrophobic, giving them possible uses in organic chemistry.

Mechanical

Oscillators based on CNT have achieved speeds of > 50 GHz.

CNT electrical and mechanical properties suggest them as alternatives to traditional electrical actuators.

Actuators

The exceptional electrical and mechanical properties of carbon nanotubes have made them alternatives to the traditional electrical actuators for both microscopic and macroscopic applications. Carbon nanotubes are very good conductors of both electricity and heat, and they are also very strong and elastic molecules in certain directions.

Loudspeaker

Carbon nanotubes have also been applied in the acoustics (such as loudspeaker and earphone). In 2008, it was shown that a sheet of nanotubes can operate as a loudspeaker if an alternating current is applied. The sound is not produced through vibration but thermoacoustically. In 2013, a carbon nanotube (CNT) thin yarn thermoacoustic earphone together with CNT thin yarn thermoacoustic chip was demonstrated by a research group of Tsinghua-Foxconn Nanotechnology Research Center in Tsinghua University, using a Si-based semi-conducting technology compatible fabrication process.

Near-term commercial uses include replacing piezoelectric speakers in greeting cards.

Optical

- Carbon nanotube photoluminescence (fluorescence) can be used to observe semiconducting single-walled carbon nanotube species. Photoluminescence maps, made by acquiring the emission and scanning the excitation energy, can facilitate sample characterization.
- Nanotube fluorescence is under investigation for biomedical imaging and sensors.
- The reflectivity of buckypaper produced with "super-growth" chemical vapor deposition is 0.03 or less, potentially enabling performance gains for pyroelectric infrared detectors.

Environmental

Environmental Remediation

A CNT nano-structured sponge (nanosponge) containing sulfur and iron is more effective at soaking up water contaminants such as oil, fertilizers, pesticides and pharmaceuticals. Their magnetic properties make them easier to retrieve once the clean-up job is done. The sulfur and iron increases sponge size to around 2 centimetres (0.79 in). It also increases porosity due to beneficial defects, creating buoyancy and reusability. Iron, in the form of ferrocene makes the structure easier to control and enables recovery using magnets. Such nanosponges increase the absorption of the toxic organic solvent dichlorobenzene from water by 3.5 times. The sponges can absorb vegetable oil up to 150 times their initial weight and can absorb engine oil as well.

Earlier, a magnetic boron-doped MWNT nanosponge that could absorb oil from water. The sponge was grown as a forest on a substrate via chemical vapor disposition. Boron puts kinks and elbows into the tubes as they grow and promotes the formation of covalent bonds. The nanosponges retain their elastic property after 10,000 compressions in the lab. The sponges are both superhydrophobic, forcing them to remain at the water's surface and oleophilic, drawing oil to them.

Water Treatment

It has been shown that carbon nanotubes exhibit strong adsorption affinities to a wide range of aromatic and aliphatic contaminants in water, due to their large and hydrophobic surface areas. They also showed similar adsorption capacities as activated carbons in the presence of natural organic matter. As a result, they have been suggested as promising adsorbents for removal of contaminant in water and wastewater treatment systems.

Moreover, membranes made out of carbon nanotube arrays have been suggested as switchable molecular sieves, with sieving and permeation features that can be dynamically activated/deactivated by either pore size distribution (passive control) or external electrostatic fields (active control).

Other Applications

Carbon nanotubes have been implemented in nanoelectromechanical systems, including mechanical memory elements (NRAM being developed by Nantero Inc.) and nanoscale electric motors.

Carboxyl-modified single-walled carbon nanotubes (so called zig-zag, armchair type) can act as sensors of atoms and ions of alkali metals Na, Li, K. In May 2005, Nanomix Inc. placed on the market a hydrogen sensor that integrated carbon nanotubes on a silicon platform. Since then, Nanomix has been patenting many such sensor applications, such as in the field of carbon dioxide, nitrous oxide, glucose, DNA detection, etc. End of 2014, Tulane University researchers have tested Nanomix's fast and fully automated point of care diagnostic system in Sierra Leone to help for rapid testing for Ebola. Nanomix announced that a product could be launched within three to six months.

Eikos Inc of Franklin, Massachusetts and Unidym Inc. of Silicon Valley, California are developing transparent, electrically conductive films of carbon nanotubes to replace indium tin oxide (ITO). Carbon nanotube films are substantially more mechanically robust than ITO films, making them ideal for high-reliability touchscreens and flexible displays. Printable water-based inks of carbon nanotubes are desired to enable the production of these films to replace ITO. Nanotube films show promise for use in displays for computers, cell phones, PDAs, and ATMs.

A nanoradio, a radio receiver consisting of a single nanotube, was demonstrated in 2007.

A flywheel made of carbon nanotubes could be spun at extremely high velocity on a floating magnetic axis in a vacuum, and potentially store energy at a density approaching that of conventional fossil fuels. Since energy can be added to and removed from flywheels very efficiently in the form of electricity, this might offer a way of storing electricity, making the electrical grid more efficient and variable power suppliers (like wind turbines) more useful in meeting energy needs. The practicality of this depends heavily upon the cost of making massive, unbroken nanotube structures, and their failure rate under stress.

Carbon nanotube springs have the potential to indefinitely store elastic potential energy at ten times the density of lithium-ion batteries with flexible charge and discharge rates and extremely high cycling durability.

Ultra-short SWNTs (US-tubes) have been used as nanoscaled capsules for delivering MRI contrast agents in vivo.

Carbon nanotubes provide a certain potential for metal-free catalysis of inorganic and organic reactions. For instance, oxygen groups attached to the surface of carbon nanotubes have the potential to catalyze oxidative dehydrogenations or selective oxidations. Nitrogen-doped carbon nanotubes may replace platinum catalysts used to reduce oxygen in fuel cells. A forest of vertically aligned nanotubes can reduce oxygen in alkaline solution more effectively than platinum, which has been used in such applications since the 1960s. Here, the nanotubes have the added benefit of not being subject to carbon monoxide poisoning.

Wake Forest University engineers are using multiwalled carbon nanotubes to enhance the brightness of field-induced polymer electroluminescent technology, potentially offering a step forward in the search for safe, pleasing, high-efficiency lighting. In this technology, moldable polymer matrix emits light when exposed to an electric current. It could eventually yield high-efficiency lights without the mercury vapor of compact fluorescent lamps or the bluish tint of some fluorescents and LEDs, which has been linked with circadian rhythm disruption.

Candida albicans has been used in combination with carbon nanotubes (CNT) to produce stable electrically conductive bio-nano-composite tissue materials that have been used as temperature sensing elements.

The SWNT production company OCSiAl developed a series of masterbatches for industrial use of single-wall CNTs in multiple types of rubber blends and tires, with initial trials showing increases in hardness, viscosity, tensile strain resistance and resistance to abrasion while reducing elongation and compression In tires the three primary characteristics of durability, fuel efficiency and traction were improved using SWNTs. The development of rubber masterbatches built on earlier work by the Japanese National Institute of Advanced Industrial Science & Technology showing rubber to be a viable candidate for improvement with SWNTs.

Introducing MWNTs to polymers can improve flame retardancy and retard thermal degradation of polymer. The results confirmed that combination of MWNTs and ammonium polyphosphates show a synergistic effect for improving flame retardancy.

Nanoart

NanoArt is a novel art discipline related to science and technology. It depicts natural or synthetic structures with features sized at the nanometer scale, which are observed by electron or scanning probe microscopy techniques in scientific laboratories. The recorded two or three dimensional images and movies are processed for artistic appeal and presented to the general audience.

One of the aims of NanoArt is to familiarize people with nanoscale objects and advances in their synthesis and manipulation. NanoArt has been presented at traditional art exhibitions around the world. Besides, online competitions have been launched in the 2000s such as the "NANO" 2003 show at Los Angeles County Museum of Art and "Nanomandala", the 2004 and 2005 installations in New York and Rome by Victoria Vesna and James Gimzewski, and the regular "Science as Art" section launched at the 2006 Materials Research Society Meeting.

A characteristic example of nanoart is *A Boy and His Atom*, a one-minute stop-motion animated film created in 2012 by IBM Research from 242 images sized by 45×25 nm, which were recorded with a scanning tunneling microscope. The movie tells the story of a boy and a wayward atom who meet and become friends. The film was accepted into the Tribeca Online Film Festival and shown at the New York Tech Meet-up and the World Science Festival.

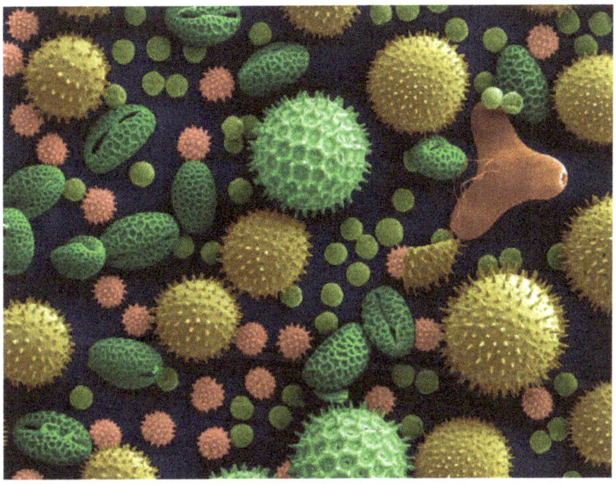

Colorized scanning electron microscopy (SEM) image of pollen from a variety of common plants: sunflower, morning glory, hollyhock, lily, primrose and castor bean

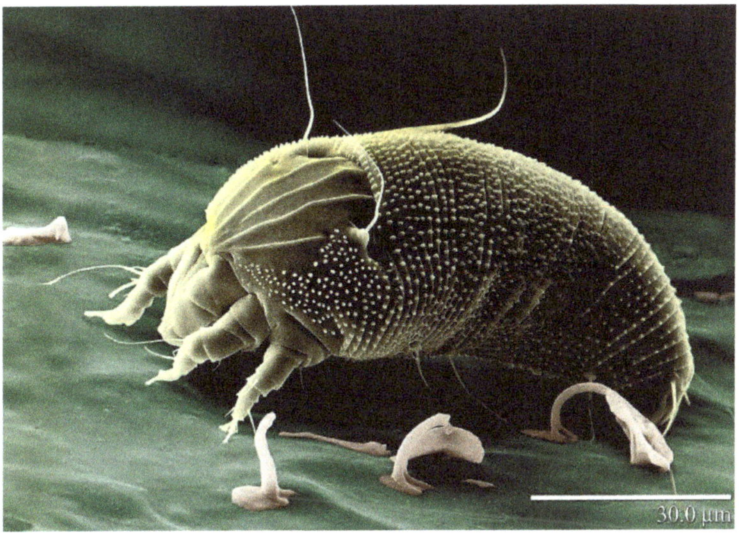

Colorized SEM image of a rust mite

Earlier in 2007 a book *Teeny Ted from Turnip Town* was created at the Simon Fraser University in Canada using a gallium-ion beam with a diameter of ~7 nanometers. The book contains 30 silicon-based pages sized by 0.07×0.10 mm; it was published in 100 copies and has an ISBN number.

In 2015, Jonty Hurwitz pioneered a new technique for creating nanosculpture using multiphoton lithography and photogrammetry. His work *Trust* was prepared in collaboration with Karlsruhe Institute of Technology and set a Guinness World Record as the "Smallest Sculpture of a Human Form".

NANO-TECH CATALYST

Scientists at the Department of Energy's Oak Ridge National Laboratory while attempting to create a nanotechnology based catalyst-mediated series of chemical reactions to turn CO2 into a usable fuel have discovered a process to turn the Carbon dioxide into ethanol, which will serve as a way forward to climate change by both decreasing CO_2 in the atmosphere and using the ethanol (CH_3CH_2OH) as an additive to fuels to increase efficiency and thereby decrease consumption. Reportedly it is also related that the process is cheap in cost and efficient in functioning.

REFERENCES

1. "Nanotechnology Information Center: Properties, Applications, Research, and Safety Guidelines". American Elements. Retrieved 13 May 2011.
2. "Analysis: This is the first publicly available on-line inventory of nanotechnology-based consumer products". The Project on Emerging Nanotechnologies. 2008. Retrieved 13 May 2011.
3. Jayasena, Buddhika; Subbiah Sathyan (2011). "A novel mechanical cleavage method for synthesizing few-layer graphenes". Nanoscale Research Letters. 6 (95). Bibcode:2011NRL.....6...95J. doi:10.1186/1556-276X-6-95. PMC 3212245Freely accessible. PMID 21711598.
4. Raja muthuramalingam thangavelu et al (2016) Nanobiotechnological approach using plant rooting hormones synthesized silver nanoparticle as a "nanobullets" for the dynamic applications in horticulture -An in vitro and ex vitro study, Arabian Journal of chemistry,http://dx.doi.org/10.1016/j.arabjc.2016.09.022
5. Avery Thompson (October 17, 2016). "Scientists Accidentally Discover Efficient Process to Turn CO2 Into Ethano". Popular Mechanics. Retrieved October 18, 2016.
6. Morgan McCorkle, Communications (October 12, 2016). "Nano-spike catalysts convert carbon dioxide directly into ethanol". Oak Pridge National Laboratory. Retrieved October 18, 2016.
7. Nanomedicine, Volume I: Basic Capabilities, by Robert A. Freitas Jr. 1999, ISBN 1-57059-645-X
8. Wagner V; Dullaart A; Bock AK; Zweck A. (2006). "The emerging nanomedicine landscape". Nat. Biotechnol. 24 (10): 1211–1217. doi:10.1038/nbt1006-1211. PMID 17033654.
9. Freitas RA Jr. (2005). "What is Nanomedicine?" (PDF). Nanomedicine: Nanotechnology, Biology and Medicine. 1 (1): 2–9. doi:10.1016/j.nano.2004.11.003. PMID 17292052.
10. Nanotechnology in Medicine and the Biosciences, by Coombs RRH, Robinson DW. 1996, ISBN 2-88449-080-9
11. "Market report on emerging nanotechnology now available". Market Report. US National Science Foundation. 25 February 2014. Retrieved 7 June 2016.

12. LaVan DA; McGuire T; Langer R. (2003). "Small-scale systems for in vivo drug delivery". Nat. Biotechnol. 21 (10): 1184–1191. doi:10.1038/nbt876. PMID 14520404.

13. Cavalcanti A; Shirinzadeh B; Freitas RA Jr.; Hogg T. (2008). "Nanorobot architecture for medical target identification". Nanotechnology. 19 (1): 015103(15pp). Bibcode:2008Nanot..19a5103C. doi:10.1088/0957-4484/19/01/015103.

14. Boisseau, P.; Loubaton, B. (2011). "Nanomedicine, nanotechnology in medicine". Comptes Rendus Physique. 12 (7): 620–636. doi:10.1016/j.crhy.2011.06.001.

15. Rao, Shasha; Tan, Angel; Thomas, Nicky; Prestidge, Clive. "Perspective and potential of oral lipid-based delivery to optimize pharmacological therapies against cardiovascular diseases". Journal of Controlled Release. 193: 174–187. doi:10.1016/j.jconrel.2014.05.013.

16. University of Waterloo, Nanotechnology in Targeted Cancer Therapy, https://www.youtube.com/watch?v=RBjWwlnq3cA 15 January 2010

17. Allen TM; Cullis PR (2004). "Drug Delivery Systems: Entering the Mainstream". Science. 303 (5665): 1818–1822. Bibcode:2004Sci...303.1818A. doi:10.1126/science.1095833. PMID 15031496.

18. Walsh MD; Hanna SK; Sen J; Rawal S; Cabral CB; Yurkovetskiy AV; Fram RJ; Lowinger TB; et al. (2012). "Pharmacokinetics and antitumor efficacy of XMT-1001, a novel, polymeric topoisomerase I inhibitor, in mice bearing HT-29 human colon carcinoma xenografts". Clin. Cancer Res. 18 (9): 2591–602. doi:10.1158/1078-0432.CCR-11-1554. PMID 22392910.

19. Chu KS; Hasan W; Rawal S; Walsh MD; Enlow EM; Luft JC; Bridges AS; Kuijer JL; et al. (Jul 2013). "Plasma, tumor and tissue pharmacokinetics of Docetaxel delivered via nanoparticles of different sizes and shapes in mice bearing SKOV-3 human ovarian carcinoma xenograft". Nanomedicine. 9 (5): 686–93. doi:10.1016/j.nano.2012.11.008. PMID 23219874.

20. Caron WP; Song G; Kumar P; Rawal S; Zamboni WC (2012). "Interpatient pharmacokinetic and pharmacodynamic variability of carrier-mediated anticancer agents". Clin. Pharmacol. Ther. 91 (5): 802–12. doi:10.1038/clpt.2012.12. PMID 22472987.

21. Bertrand N; Leroux JC (2011). "The journey of a drug carrier in the body: an anatomo-physiological perspective". Journal of Controlled Release. 161 (2): 152–63. doi:10.1016/j.jconrel.2011.09.098. PMID 22001607.

22. Nagy ZK, Zsombor K.; Balogh A; Vajna B; Farkas A; Patyi G; Kramarics A; Marosi G (2011). "Comparison of Electrospun and Extruded Soluplus-Based Solid Dosage Forms of Improved Dissolution". Journal of Pharmaceutical Sciences. 101 (1): n/a. doi:10.1002/jps.22731. PMID 21918982.

23. Minchin, Rod (2008). "Sizing up targets with nanoparticles". Nature Nanotechnology. 3 (1): 12–13. Bibcode:2008NatNa...3...12M. doi:10.1038/nnano.2007.433. PMID 18654442.

24. Banoee, M.; Seif, S.; Nazari, Z. E.; Jafari-Fesharaki, P.; Shahverdi, H. R.; Moballegh, A.; Moghaddam, K. M.; Shahverdi, A. R. (2010). "ZnO nanoparticles

enhanced antibacterial activity of ciprofloxacin against Staphylococcus aureus and Escherichia coli". J Biomed Mater Res B Appl Biomater. 93 (2): 557–61. doi:10.1002/jbm.b.31615. PMID 20225250.

25. Seil JT; Webster TJ (2012). "Antimicrobial applications of nanotechnology: methods and literature". Int J Nanomedicine. 7: 2767–81. doi:10.2147/IJN.S24805. PMID 22745541.
26. Borzabadi-Farahani A; Borzabadi E; Lynch E. (2013). "Nanoparticles in orthodontics, a review of antimicrobial and anti-caries applications". Acta Odontol Scand. 72 (6): 413–417. doi:10.3109/00016357.2013.859728. PMID 24325608.
27. Conde, J.; de la Fuente, JM; Baptista, PV. "Nanomaterials for reversion of multidrug resistance in cancer: a new hope for an old idea?." Front. Pharmacol.2013. Vol 4 No 134.
28. Sanjeev Soni, Himanshu Tyagi, Robert A. Taylor, Amod Kumar, Role of optical coefficients and healthy tissue-sparing characteristics in gold nanorod-assisted thermal therapy, International Journal of Hyperthermia, 2013, Vol. 29, No. 1 , Pages 87-97
29. Nanospectra Biosciences, Inc. – Publications (http://www.nanospectra.com/clinicians/spublications.html)
30. Mozafari, M.R. (ed), (2006) Nanocarrier Technologies: Frontiers of Nanotherapy (Chapters 1 and 2) pages 10–11, 25–34
31. Bertrand N; Bouvet C; Moreau P & Leroux JC (2010). "Transmembrane pH-Gradient Liposomes To Treat Cardiovascular Drug Intoxication". ACS Nano. 4 (12): 7552–7558. doi:10.1021/nn101924a. PMID 21067150.
32. Mashaghi S.; Jadidi T.; Koenderink G.; Mashaghi A. (2013). "Lipid Nanotechnology". Int. J. Mol. Sci. 2013 (14): 4242–4282. doi:10.3390/ijms14024242. PMC 3588097Freely accessible. PMID 23429269.
33. Conde, J; Oliva, N; Atilano, M; Song, HS; Artzi, N (2015). "Self-assembled RNA-triple-helix hydrogel scaffold for microRNA modulation in the tumour microenvironment". Nat Mater. doi:10.1038/nmat4497.
34. FDA (October 2012). "Highlights of Prescribing Information, Abraxane for Injectable Suspension" (PDF).
35. "Paclitaxel (Abraxane)". U.S. Food and Drug Administration. 11 October 2012. Retrieved 10 December 2012.
36. FDA Press Announcements (6 September 2013). "FDA approves Abraxane for late-stage pancreatic cancer". FDA.
37. Martis, Elvis A.; Badve, Rewa R.; Degwekar, Mukta D. (January 2012). "Nanotechnology based devices and applications in medicine: An overview". Chronicles of Young Scientists. 3 (1): 68–73. doi:10.4103/2229-5186.94320.
38. News Release (22 October 2015). "FDA approves new treatment for advanced pancreatic cancer". FDA.
39. Gibney, Michael (18 April 2013). "Cornell nanosized 'dots' for diagnostics may now deliver drugs". fiercedrugdelivery.com. Retrieved 17 June 2013.

40. Elvidge, Suzanne (11 November 2012). "Bacterial 'minicells' deliver cancer drugs straight to the target". fiercedrugdelivery.com. Retrieved 10 December 2012.
41. "First trial in humans of 'minicells': a completely new way of delivering anti-cancer drugs". fiercedrugdelivery.com. 12 November 2012. Retrieved 10 December 2012.
42. Press Release (19 June 2014). "Kala Pharmaceuticals Initiates Phase3 Clinical Trial for Treatment of Post-Surgical Ocular Inflammation and Phase 2 Clinical Trial in Dry Eye Disease" (PDF). Kala Pharmaceuticals.
43. Press Release (1 April 2015). "Kala Pharmaceuticals Announces Positive Results from Phase 3 Trial of KPI-121 in Cataract Surgery" (PDF). Kala Pharmaceuticals.
44. Wang AZ, Langer R, Farokhzad OC (2012). "Nanoparticle delivery of cancer drugs". Annu. Rev. Med. 63: 185–98. doi:10.1146/annurev-med-040210-162544. PMID 21888516.
45. Pérez-Herrero E, Fernández-Medarde A (2015). "Advanced targeted therapies in cancer: Drug nanocarriers, the future of chemotherapy". Eur J Pharm Biopharm. 93: 52–79. doi:10.1016/j.ejpb.2015.03.018. PMID 25813885.
46. Nguyen-Ngoc T, Raymond E (2015). "Reinvention of chemotherapy: drug conjugates and nanoparticles". Curr Opin Oncol. 27: 232–42. doi:10.1097/CCO.0000000000000183. PMID 25783982.
47. Ghaz-Jahanian MA, Abbaspour-Aghdam F, Anarjan N, Berenjian A, Jafarizadeh-Malmiri H (2015). "Application of chitosan-based nanocarriers in tumor-targeted drug delivery". Mol. Biotechnol. 57 (3): 201–18. doi:10.1007/s12033-014-9816-3. PMID 25385004.
48. Nie, Shuming; Yun Xing; Gloria J. Kim & Jonathan W. Simmons (2007). "Nanotechnology Applications in Cancer". Annual Review of Biomedical Engineering. 9 (1): 257–88. doi:10.1146/annurev.bioeng.9.060906.152025. PMID 17439359.
49. Chidambaram, M.; Manavalan, R.; Kathiresan, K. (2011). "Nanotherapeutics to overcome conventional cancer chemotherapy limitations". Journal of pharmacy & pharmaceutical sciences : a publication of the Canadian Society for Pharmaceutical Sciences, Societe canadienne des sciences pharmaceutiques. 14 (1): 67–77. PMID 21501554.
50. Loo C; Lin A; Hirsch L; Lee MH; Barton J; Halas N; West J; Drezek R. (2004). "Nanoshell-enabled photonics-based imaging and therapy of cancer". Technol Cancer Res Treat. 3 (1): 33–40. doi:10.1177/153303460400300104. PMID 14750891.
51. Conde J, Tian F, Hernández Y, Bao C, Cui D, Janssen KP, Ibarra MR, Baptista PV, Stoeger T, de la Fuente JM. In vivo tumor targeting via nanoparticle-mediated therapeutic siRNA coupled to inflammatory response in lung cancer mouse models. Biomaterials. 2013;34(31):7744-53. doi:10.1016/j.biomaterials.2013.06.041
52. Yasitha L Hewakuruppu et al., Plasmonic " pump – probe " method to study semi-transparent nanofluids, Applied Optics, 52(24) 6041-6050.

53. Coffey, Rebecca (August 2010). "20 Things You Didn't Know About Nanotechnology". Discover. 31 (6): 96.
54. Zheng G; Patolsky F; Cui Y; Wang WU; Lieber CM (2005). "Multiplexed electrical detection of cancer markers with nanowire sensor arrays". Nat. Biotechnol. 23 (10): 1294–1301. doi:10.1038/nbt1138. PMID 16170313.
55. Hall, J. Storrs (2005). Nanofuture : what's next for nanotechnology. Amherst, NY: Prometheus Books. ISBN 978-1591022879.
56. "Drug Store Cancer Tests". Technology Review. 2005-10-31. Retrieved 2009-10-08.
57. Keller, John (2013). "Nanotechnology has also helped to personalize oncology for the detection, diagnosis, and treatment of cancer. It is now able to be tailored to each individual's tumor for better performance". Military & Aerospace Electronics. 23 (6): 27.
58. Herrmann, I. K. et al. Nanomagnet-based removal of lead and digoxin from living rats. Nanoscale 5, 8718–8723 (2013).
59. Kang J. H.; et al. (2014). "An extracorporeal blood-cleansing device for sepsis therapy". Nat. Med. 20: 1211–1216. doi:10.1038/nm.3640.
60. Berry C. C.; Curtis A. S. G. (2003). "Functionalisation of magnetic nanoparticles for applications in biomedicine". J. Phys. Appl. Phys. 36: R198. doi:10.1088/0022-3727/36/13/203.
61. Herrmann I. K.; et al. (2013). "Endotoxin Removal by Magnetic Separation-Based Blood Purification". Adv. Healthcare Mater. 2: 829–835. doi:10.1002/adhm.201200358.
62. Lee J.-J.; et al. (2014). "Synthetic Ligand-Coated Magnetic Nanoparticles for Microfluidic Bacterial Separation from Blood". Nano Lett. 14: 1–5. doi:10.1021/nl3047305.
63. Schumacher C. M.; et al. (2013). "Quantitative Recovery of Magnetic Nanoparticles from Flowing Blood: Trace Analysis and the Role of Magnetization". Adv. Funct. Mater. 23: 4888–4896. doi:10.1002/adfm.201300696.
64. Yung C. W.; Fiering J.; Mueller A. J.; Ingber D. E. (2009). "Micromagnetic–microfluidic blood cleansing device". Lab. Chip. 9: 1171–7. doi:10.1039/b816986a. PMID 19370233.
65. Herrmann, I. K., Grass, R. N. & Stark, W. J. High-strength metal nanomagnets for diagnostics and medicine: carbon shells allow long-term stability and reliable linker chemistry. Nanomed. 4, 787–798 (2009).
66. Stacy Shepherd,"Harvard Engineers Invented an Artificial Spleen to Treat Sepsis", Boston Magazine. Retrieved on 20 April 2015.
67. Lalwani Gaurav; Henslee Allan M.; Farshid Behzad; Lin Liangjun; Kasper F. Kurtis, Yi-; Qin Xian; Mikos Antonios G.; Sitharaman Balaji; et al. (2013). "Two-dimensional nanostructure-reinforced biodegradable polymeric nanocomposites for bone tissue engineering". Biomacromolecules. 14 (3): 900–909. doi:10.1021/bm301995s. PMC 3601907Freely accessible. PMID 23405887.

68. Lalwani, Gaurav (September 2013). "Tungsten disulfide nanotubes reinforced biodegradable polymers for bone tissue engineering". Acta Biomaterialia. 9 (9): 8365–8373. doi:10.1016/j.actbio.2013.05.018. PMC 3732565Freely accessible. PMID 23727293.

69. Gobin AM; O'Neal DP; Watkins DM; Halas NJ; Drezek RA; West JL (2005). "Near infrared laser-tissue welding using nanoshells as an exogenous absorber". Lasers Surg Med. 37 (2): 123–9. doi:10.1002/lsm.20206. PMID 16047329.

70. http://www.nanowerk.com/spotlight/spotid=19573.php

71. Nanomedicine, Volume IIA: Biocompatibility, by Robert A. Freitas Jr. 2003, ISBN 1-57059-700-6

72. Freitas, Robert A., Jr. (2005). "Current Status of Nanomedicine and Medical Nanorobotics" (PDF). Journal of Computational and Theoretical Nanoscience. 2 (4): 1–25. doi:10.1166/jctn.2005.001.

73. Nanofactory Collaboration

74. Kurzweil, Ray (2005). The Singularity Is Near. New York City: Viking Press. ISBN 978-0-670-03384-3. OCLC 57201348.

75. Richard P. Feynman (December 1959). "There's Plenty of Room at the Bottom". Retrieved March 2010. Check date values in: |access-date= (help)

76. Ehud Gazit, Plenty of room for biology at the bottom: An introduction to bionanotechnology. Imperial College Press, 2007, ISBN 978-1-86094-677-6

77. "Nanobiology". Nanotech-Now.com.

78. "Nanobiology". Swiss Nanoscience Institute.

79. Ng, CK; Sivakumar K; Liu X; Madhaiyan M; Ji L; Yang L; Tang C; Song H; Kjelleberg S; Cao B. (4 Feb 2013). "Influence of outer membrane c-type cytochromes on particle size and activity of extracellular nanoparticles produced by Shewanella oneidensis.". Biotechnology and Bioengineering. 110 (7): 1831–7. doi:10.1002/bit.24856. PMID 23381725.

80. Bionanotechnology - Definition, wordiQ.com

81. Nolting B, "Biophysical Nanotechnology". In: "Methods in Modern Biophysics", Springer, 2005, ISBN 3-540-27703-X

82. NBTC Homepage | Nanobiotechnology Center

83. Raja muthuramalingam thangavelu et al (2016) Nanobiotechnological approach using plant rooting hormones synthesized silver nanoparticle as a "nanobullets" for the dynamic applications in horticulture -An in vitro and ex vitro study, Arabian Journal of chemistry,http://dx.doi.org/10.1016/j.arabjc.2016.09.022

84. Venkatesan M, Jolad B, editors. Emerging Trends in Robotics and Communication Technologies (INTERACT). 2010 International Conference on . Nanorobots in cancer treatment; 12/3-5; Chennai: IEEE; 2010. doi:10.1109/INTERACT.2010.5706154

85. "The future of nano-biology". ZD Net.

86. "Nanobiology: from physics and engineering to biology". IOP Science.

87. "The Nanobiology Imperative". HistorianoftheFuture.com.

88. Zadegan, Reza M.; Norton, Michael L. (June 2012). "Structural DNA Nanotechnology: From Design to Applications". Int. J. Mol. Sci. 13 (6): 7149–7162. doi:10.3390/ijms13067149. PMC 3397516Freely accessible. PMID 22837684.

89. Nguyen, Peter; Botyanszki, Zsofia; Tay, Pei-Kun; Joshi, Neel (Sep 17, 2014). "Programmable biofilm-based materials from engineered curli nanofibres". Nature Communications. 5: 4945. doi:10.1038/ncomms5945. PMID 25229329.

90. Mashaghi S.; Jadidi T.; Koenderink G.; Mashaghi A. (2013). "Lipid Nanotechnology". Int. J. Mol. Sci. 2013 (14): 4242–4282. doi:10.3390/ijms14024242. PMC 3588097Freely accessible. PMID 23429269.

91. Raja muthuramalingam thangavelu et al (2016) Nanobiotechnological approach using plant rooting hormones synthesized silver nanoparticle as a nanobullets for the dynamic applications in horticulture -An in vitro and ex vitro study, Arabian Journal of chemistry,http://dx.doi.org/10.1016/j.arabjc.2016.09.022

92. Raja muthuramalingam thangavelu et al (2016) Nanobiotechnological approach using plant rooting hormones synthesized silver nanoparticle as a "nanobullets" for the dynamic applications in horticulture -An in vitro and ex vitro study, Arabian Journal of chemistry,http://dx.doi.org/10.1016/j.arabjc.2016.09.022

93. Raja muthuramalingam, T., Chandrasekar, S., Dharanivasan, G., Nallusamy, D., Rajendran, N., Kathiravan, K., 2015. Bioactive bile salt capped silver nanoparticle activity against destructive plant pathogenic fungi through in vitro system. RSC advances. 5, 71174-71182

94. Raqual, B., Eudald, C., Joan, C., Xavier, F., Antoni, S., Victor, P., 2009. Evaluation of the ecotoxicity of model nanoparticles. Chemosphere. 75, 850-857

95. Hediat Salama, M. H., 2012. Effects of silver nanoparticles in some crop plants, common bean (Phaseolus vulgaris L.) and corn (Zea mays L.). International research journal of biotechnology. 3(10), 190-197(

96. Sandeep arora., Priyadarshini sharma., Sumit kumar., Rajeev nayan., Khanna, P. K., Zaidi. M. G. N., 2012. Gold nanoparticles induced enhancement in growth and seed yield of Brassica juncea. Plant Growth Regul. 66, 303-310

CHAPTER 5

Nanomaterials: Cornerstones of Nanoscience and Nanotechnology

Chapter Contents

- **Introduction**
- **Types**
- **Synthesis**
- **Characterization**
- **Uniformity**
- **Fullerene**
- **Carbon Nanotube**
- **Nanoparticle**

Nanomaterials are cornerstones of nanoscience and nanotechnology. Nanostructure science and technology is a broad and interdisciplinary area of research and development activity that has been growing explosively worldwide in the past few years. It has the potential for revolutionizing the ways in which materials and products are created and the range and nature of functionalities that can be accessed. It is already having a significant commercial impact, which will assuredly increase in the future.

INTRODUCTION

Nanomaterials describe, in principle, materials of which a single unit is sized (in at least one dimension) between 1 and 1000 nanometres (10^{-9} meter) but is usually 1—100 nm (the usual definition of nanoscale).

Nanomaterials research takes a materials science-based approach to nanotechnology, leveraging advances in materials metrology and synthesis which have been developed in support of microfabrication research. Materials with structure at the nanoscale often have unique optical, electronic, or mechanical properties.

Nanomaterials are slowly becoming commercialized and beginning to emerge as commodities.

TYPES

Natural Nanomaterials

Biological systems often feature natural, functional nanomaterials. The structure of foraminifera (mainly chalk) and viruses (protein, capsid), the wax crystals covering a lotus or nasturtium leaf, spider and spider-mite silk, the blue hue of tarantulas, the "spatulae" on the bottom of gecko feet, some butterfly wing scales, natural colloids (milk, blood), horny materials (skin, claws, beaks, feathers, horns, hair), paper, cotton, nacre, corals, and even our own bone matrix are all natural *organic* nanomaterials.

Natural *inorganic* nanomaterials occur through crystal growth in the diverse chemical conditions of the Earth's crust. For example, clays display complex nanostructures due to anisotropy of their underlying crystal structure, and volcanic activity can give rise to opals, which are an instance of a naturally occurring photonic crystals due to their nanoscale structure. Fires represent particularly complex reactions and can produce pigments, cement, fumed silica etc.

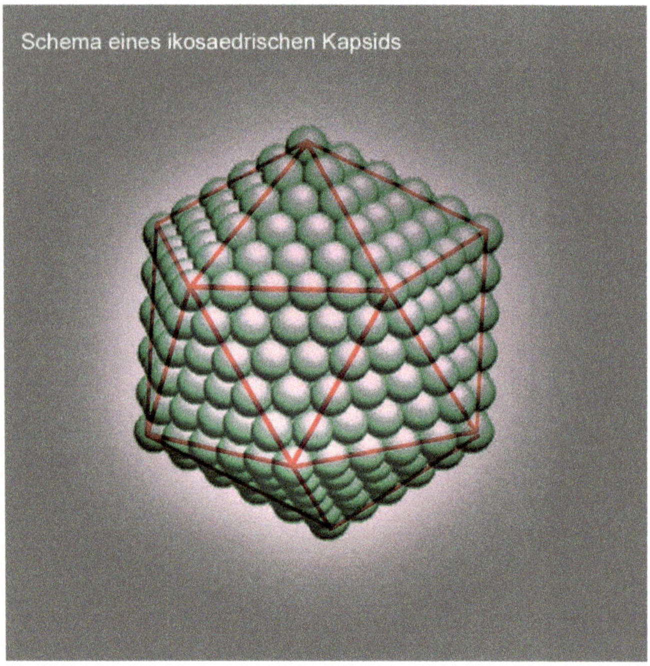

Viral capsid

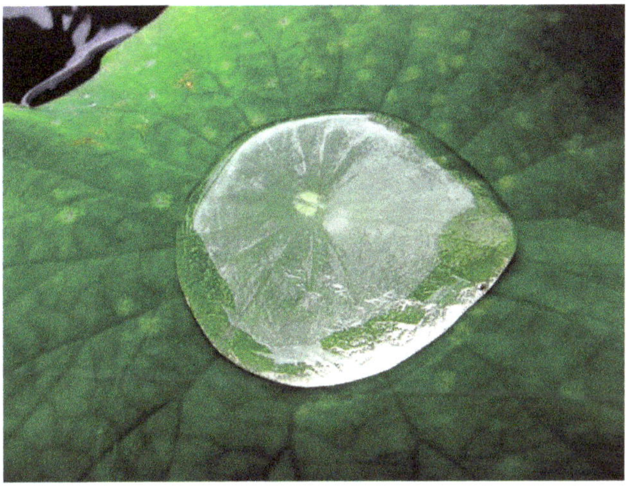

"Lotus effect", hydrophobic effect with self-cleaning ability

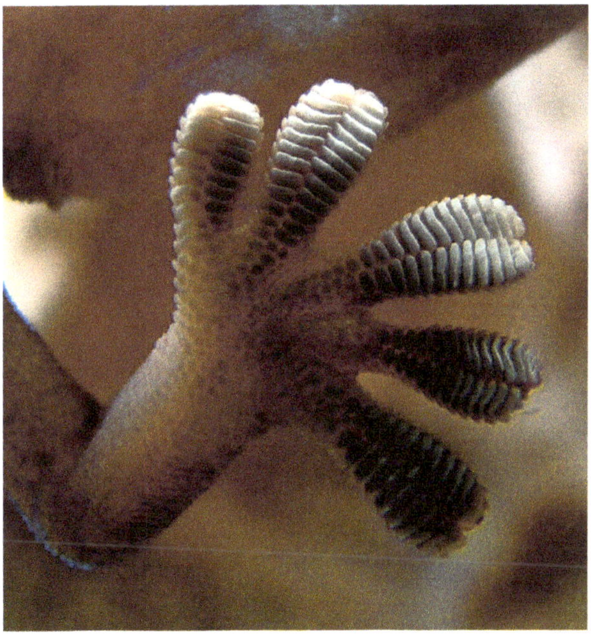

Close-up of the underside of a gecko's foot as it walks on a glass wall. (spatula: 200 × 10-15 nm).

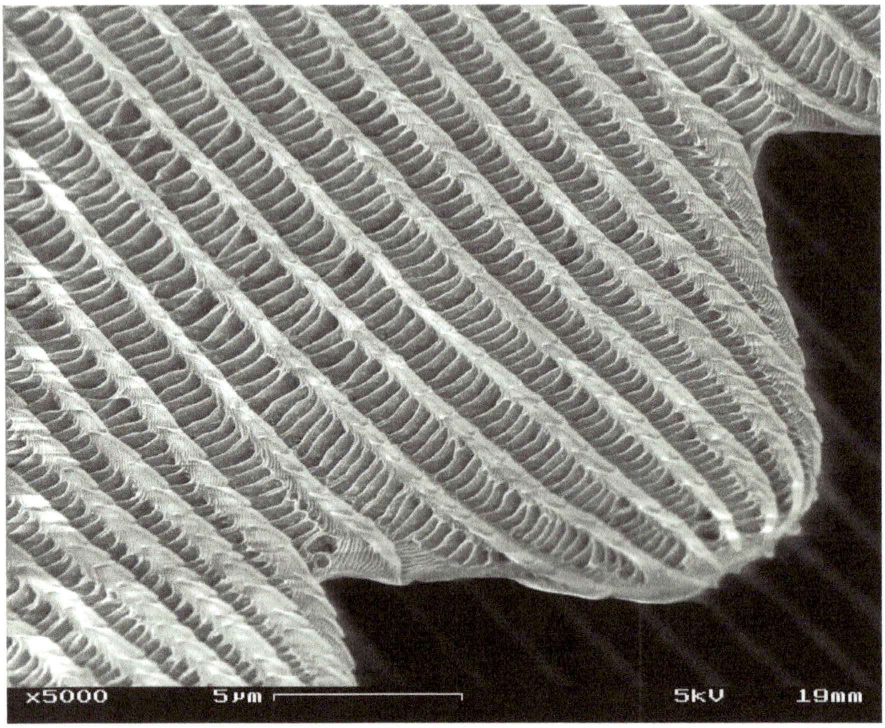

SEM micrograph of a butterfly wing scale (× 5000)

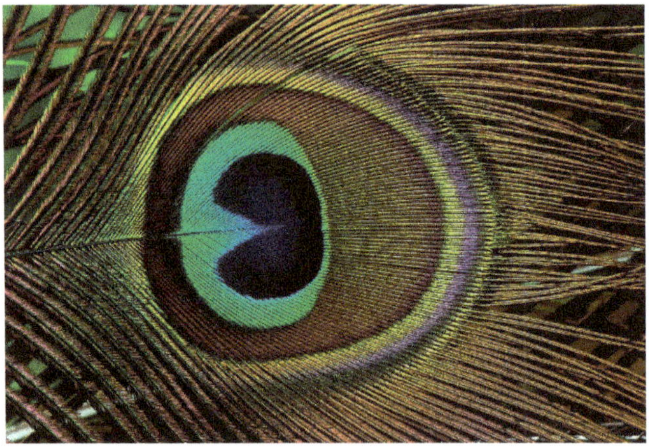

Peacock feather (detail)

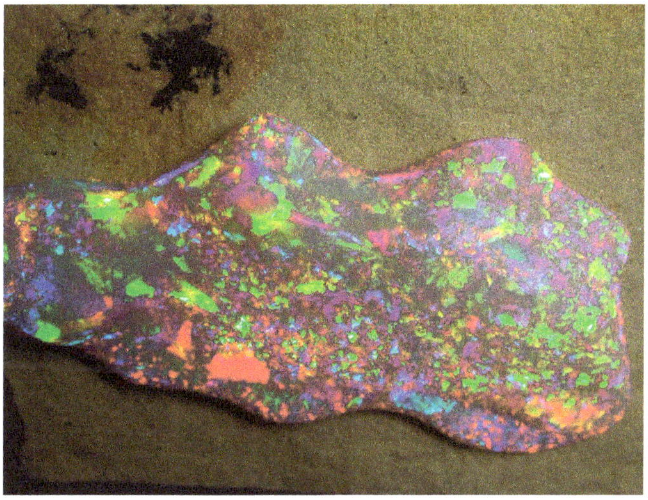

Brazilian Crystal Opal. The play of color is caused by the interference and diffraction of light between silica spheres (150 - 300 nm in diameter).

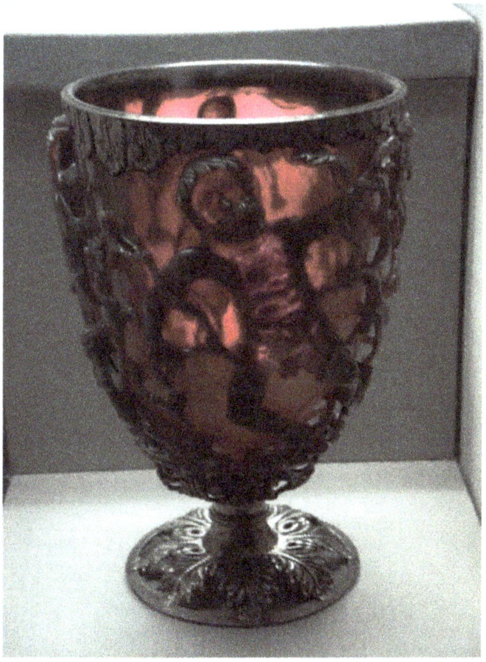

Lycurgus Cup, glass, 4th century, Roman. Nanoparticles (70 nm) of gold and silver, dispersed in colloidal form, are responsible for the dichroic effect (red/green).

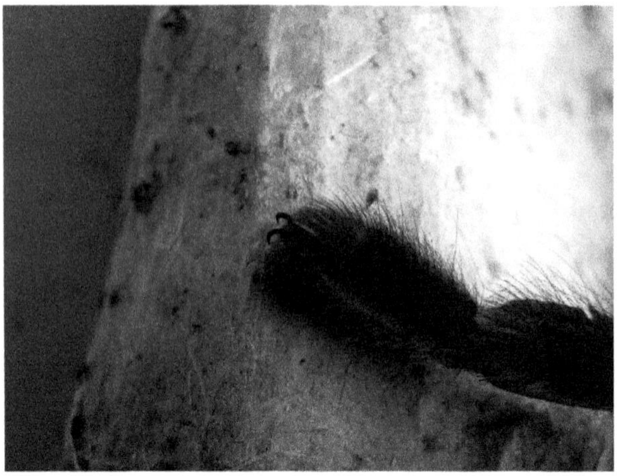

Blue hue of a species of tarantula (450 nm ± 20 nm)

Fullerenes

The fullerenes are a class of allotropes of carbon which conceptually are graphene sheets rolled into tubes or spheres. These include the carbon nanotubes (or silicon nanotubes) which are of interest both because of their mechanical strength and also because of their electrical properties.

The first fullerene molecule to be discovered, and the family's namesake, buckminsterfullerene (C_{60}), was prepared in 1985 by Richard Smalley, Robert Curl, James Heath, Sean O'Brien, and Harold Kroto at Rice University. The name was a homage to Buckminster Fuller, whose geodesic domes it resembles. Fullerenes have since been found to occur in nature. More recently, fullerenes have been detected in outer space.

For the past decade, the chemical and physical properties of fullerenes have been a hot topic in the field of research and development, and are likely to continue to be for a long time. In April 2003, fullerenes were under study for potential medicinal use: binding specific antibiotics to the structure of resistant bacteria and even target certain types of cancer cells such as melanoma. The October 2005 issue of Chemistry and Biology contains an article describing the use of fullerenes as light-activated antimicrobial agents. In the field of nanotechnology, heat resistance and superconductivity are among the properties attracting intense research.

A common method used to produce fullerenes is to send a large current between two nearby graphite electrodes in an inert atmosphere. The resulting carbon plasma arc between the electrodes cools into sooty residue from which many fullerenes can be isolated.

There are many calculations that have been done using ab-initio Quantum Methods applied to fullerenes. By DFT and TDDFT methods one can obtain IR, Raman and UV spectra. Results of such calculations can be compared with experimental results.

Graphene Nanostructures

2D materials are crystalline materials consisting of a two-dimensional single layer of atoms. The most important representative graphene was discovered in 2004. Other 2D materials based on other elements have since been reported.

Box-shaped graphene (BSG) nanostructure is an example of 3D nanomaterial. BSG nanostructure has appeared after mechanical cleavage of pyrolytic graphite. This nanostructure is a multilayer system of parallel hollow nanochannels located along the surface and having quadrangular cross-section. The thickness of the channel walls is approximately equal to 1 nm. The typical width of channel facets makes about 25 nm.

Nanoparticles

Inorganic nanomaterials, (e.g. quantum dots, nanowires and nanorods) because of their interesting optical and electrical properties, could be used in optoelectronics. Furthermore, the optical and electronic properties of nanomaterials which depend on their size and shape can be tuned via synthetic techniques. There are the possibilities to use those materials in organic material based optoelectronic devices such as Organic solar cells, OLEDs etc. The operating principles of such devices are governed by photoinduced processes like electron transfer and energy transfer. The performance of the devices depends on the efficiency of the photoinduced process responsible for their functioning. Therefore, better understanding of those photoinduced processes in organic/inorganic nanomaterial composite systems is necessary in order to use them in organic optoelectronic devices.

Nanoparticles or nanocrystals made of metals, semiconductors, or oxides are of particular interest for their mechanical, electrical, magnetic, optical, chemical and other properties. Nanoparticles have been used as quantum dots and as chemical catalysts such as nanomaterial-based catalysts. Recently, a range of nanoparticles are extensively investigated for biomedical applications including tissue engineering, drug delivery, biosensor.

Nanoparticles are of great scientific interest as they are effectively a bridge between bulk materials and atomic or molecular structures. A bulk material should have constant physical properties regardless of its size, but at the nano-scale this is often not the case. Size-dependent properties are observed such as quantum confinement in semiconductor particles, surface plasmon resonance in some metal particles and superparamagnetism in magnetic materials.

Nanoparticles exhibit a number of special properties relative to bulk material. For example, the bending of bulk copper (wire, ribbon, etc.) occurs with movement of copper atoms/clusters at about the 50 nm scale. Copper nanoparticles smaller than 50 nm are considered super hard materials that do not exhibit the same malleability and ductility as bulk copper. The change in properties is not always desirable. Ferroelectric materials smaller than 10 nm can switch their magnetisation direction using room temperature thermal energy, thus making them useless for memory storage. Suspensions of nanoparticles are possible because the interaction of the particle surface with the solvent is strong enough to overcome differences in density, which usually result in a material either sinking or floating in a liquid. Nanoparticles often have unexpected visual properties because they are small enough to confine their electrons and produce quantum effects. For example, gold nanoparticles appear deep red to black in solution.

The often very high surface area to volume ratio of nanoparticles provides a tremendous driving force for diffusion, especially at elevated temperatures. Sintering is possible at lower temperatures and over shorter durations than for larger particles. This theoretically does not affect the density of the final product, though flow difficulties and the tendency of nanoparticles to agglomerate do complicate matters. The surface effects of nanoparticles also reduces the incipient melting temperature.

Nanozymes

Nanozymes are nanomaterials with enzyme-like characteristics. They are an emerging type of artificial enzyme, which have been used for wide applications in such as biosensing, bioimaging, tumor diagnosis and therapy, antibiofouling, etc.

SYNTHESIS

The goal of any synthetic method for nanomaterials is to yield a material that exhibits properties that are a result of their characteristic length scale being in the nanometer range (~1 – 100 nm). Accordingly, the synthetic method should exhibit control of size in this range so that one property or another can be attained. Often the methods are divided into two main types "Bottom Up" and "Top Down."

Bottom up Methods

Bottom up methods involve the assembly of atoms or molecules into nanostructured arrays. In these methods the raw material sources can be in the form of gases, liquids or solids. The latter requiring some sort of disassembly prior to their incorporation onto a nanostructure. Bottom methods generally fall into two categories: chaotic and controlled.

Chaotic Processes

Chaotic processes involve elevating the constituent atoms or molecules to a chaotic state and then suddenly changing the conditions so as to make that state unstable. Through the clever manipulation of any number of parameters, products form largely as a result of the insuring kinetics. The collapse from the chaotic state can be difficult or impossible to control and so ensemble statistics often govern the resulting size distribution and average size. Accordingly, nanoparticle formation is controlled through manipulation of the end state of the products.

Examples of Chaotic Processes are: Laser ablation, Exploding wire, Arc, Flame pyrolysis, Combustion, Precipitation synthesis techniques.

Controlled Processes

Controlled Processes involve the controlled delivery of the constituent atoms or molecules to the site(s) of nanoparticle formation such that the nanoparticle can grow to a prescribed sizes in a controlled manner. Generally the state of the constituent atoms or molecules are never far from that needed for nanoparticle formation. Accordingly, nanoparticle formation is controlled through the control of the state of the reactants.

Examples of controlled processes are self-limiting growth solution, self-limited chemical vapor deposition, shaped pulse femtosecond laser techniques, and molecular beam epitaxy.

CHARACTERIZATION

Novel effects can occur in materials when structures are formed with sizes comparable to any one of many possible length scales, such as the de Broglie wavelength of electrons, or the optical wavelengths of high energy photons. In these cases quantum mechanical effects can dominate material properties. One example is quantum confinement where the electronic properties of solids are altered with great reductions in particle size. The optical properties of nanoparticles, e.g. fluorescence, also become a function of the particle diameter. This effect does not come into play by going from macrosocopic to micrometer dimensions, but becomes pronounced when the nanometer scale is reached.

In addition to optical and electronic properties, the novel mechanical properties of many nanomaterials is the subject of nanomechanics research. When added to a bulk material, nanoparticles can strongly influence the mechanical properties of the material, such as the stiffness or elasticity. For example, traditional polymers can be reinforced by nanoparticles (such as carbon nanotubes) resulting in novel materials which can be used as lightweight replacements for metals. Such composite materials may enable a weight reduction accompanied by an increase in stability and improved functionality.

Finally, nanostructured materials with small particle size such as zeolites, and asbestos, are used as catalysts in a wide range of critical industrial chemical reactions. The further development of such catalysts can form the basis of more efficient, environmentally friendly chemical processes.

The first observations and size measurements of nano-particles were made during the first decade of the 20th century. Zsigmondy made detailed studies of gold sols and other nanomaterials with sizes down to 10 nm and less. He published a book in 1914. He used an ultramicroscope that employs a *dark field* method for seeing particles with sizes much less than light wavelength.

There are traditional techniques developed during 20th century in Interface and Colloid Science for characterizing nanomaterials. These are widely used for *first generation* passive nanomaterials specified in the next section.

These methods include several different techniques for characterizing particle size distribution. This characterization is imperative because many materials that are expected to be nano-sized are actually aggregated in solutions. Some of methods are based on light scattering. Others apply ultrasound, such as ultrasound attenuation spectroscopy for testing concentrated nano-dispersions and microemulsions.

There is also a group of traditional techniques for characterizing surface charge or zeta potential of nano-particles in solutions. This information is required for proper system stabilzation, preventing its aggregation or flocculation. These methods include microelectrophoresis, electrophoretic light scattering and electroacoustics. The last one, for instance colloid vibration current method is suitable for characterizing concentrated systems.

UNIFORMITY

The chemical processing and synthesis of high performance technological components for the private, industrial and military sectors requires the use of high purity ceramics, polymers, glass-ceramics and material composites. In condensed bodies formed from fine powders, the irregular sizes and shapes of nanoparticles in a typical powder often lead to non-uniform packing morphologies that result in packing density variations in the powder compact.

Uncontrolled agglomeration of powders due to attractive van der Waals forces can also give rise to in microstructural inhomogeneities. Differential stresses that develop as a result of non-uniform drying shrinkage are directly related to the rate at which the solvent can be removed, and thus highly dependent upon the distribution of porosity. Such stresses have been associated with a plastic-to-brittle transition in consolidated bodies, and can yield to crack propagation in the unfired body if not relieved.

In addition, any fluctuations in packing density in the compact as it is prepared for the kiln are often amplified during the sintering process, yielding inhomogeneous densification. Some pores and other structural defects associated with density variations have been shown to play a detrimental role in the sintering process by growing and thus limiting end-point densities. Differential stresses arising from inhomogeneous densification have also been shown to result in the propagation of internal cracks, thus becoming the strength-controlling flaws.

It would therefore appear desirable to process a material in such a way that it is physically uniform with regard to the distribution of components and porosity, rather than using particle size distributions which will maximize the green density. The containment of a uniformly dispersed assembly of strongly interacting particles in suspension requires total control over particle-particle interactions. It should be noted here that a number of dispersants such as ammonium citrate (aqueous) and imidazoline or oleyl alcohol (nonaqueous) are promising solutions as possible additives for enhanced dispersion and deagglomeration. Monodisperse nanoparticles and colloids provide this potential.

Monodisperse powders of colloidal silica, for example, may therefore be stabilized sufficiently to ensure a high degree of order in the colloidal crystal or polycrystalline colloidal solid which results from aggregation. The degree of order appears to be limited by the time and space allowed for longer-range correlations to be established. Such defective polycrystalline colloidal structures would appear to be the basic elements of sub-micrometer colloidal materials science, and, therefore, provide the first step in developing a more rigorous understanding of the mechanisms involved in microstructural evolution in high performance materials and components.

Legal Definition

On 18 October 2011, the European Commission adopted the following definition of a nanomaterial: “A natural, incidental or manufactured material containing particles, in an unbound state or as an aggregate or as an agglomerate and where, for 50% or more of the particles in the number size distribution, one or more external dimensions is in the size range 1 nm – 100 nm. In specific cases and where warranted by concerns for the environment, health, safety or competitiveness the number size distribution threshold of 50% may be replaced by a threshold between 1 and 50%.”

However, this differs from the definition adopted by the International Organization for Standardization (ISO), which is: “Material with any external dimension in the nanoscale or having internal structure in the nanoscale.”

“Nanoscale” is, in turn, defined as: “Size range from approximately 1 nm to 100 nm.”

It is not currently known which of these, if any, will prevail in courts of law.

Safety

Health Impact

While nanomaterials and nanotechnologies are expected to yield numerous health and health care advances, such as more targeted methods of delivering drugs, new cancer therapies, and methods of early detection of diseases, they also may have unwanted effects. Increased rate of absorption is the main concern associated with manufactured nanoparticles.

When materials are made into nanoparticles, their surface area to volume ratio increases. The greater specific surface area (surface area per unit weight) may lead to increased rate of absorption through the skin, lungs, or digestive tract and may cause unwanted effects to the lungs as well as other organs. However, the particles must be absorbed in sufficient quantities in order to pose health risks.

Nanoparticles created adventitiously (e.g., through the rubbing of prostheses) have long been known to be a health hazard, but as the use of nanomaterials increases worldwide, concerns for worker and user safety are mounting. To address such concerns, the Swedish Karolinska Institute conducted a study in which various nanoparticles were introduced to human lung epithelial cells. The results, released in 2008, showed that iron oxide nanoparticles caused little DNA damage and were non-toxic. Zinc oxide nanoparticles were slightly worse. Titanium dioxide caused only DNA damage. Carbon nanotubes caused DNA damage at low levels. Copper oxide was found to be the worst offender, and was the only nanomaterial identified by the researchers as a clear health risk. Though nanomaterials are not confirmed as a health risk to workers who produce them, NIOSH recommends that exposure precautions and personal protective equipment be used to protect workers until the risks of nanomaterial manufacture are better understood.

Occupational Safety

Beyond normal chemical safety practices such as using personal protective equipment, The United States National Institute for Occupational Safety and Health recommends the use of HEPA filtration on local exhaust ventilation such as fume hoods. General laboratory ventilation is often not sufficient to effectively clear nanomaterials released into the general room air over a 30-minute period; therefore, researchers should leave the hood fan on even after synthesis is complete. Nanomaterials in dry powder form have the most risk of airborne dust generation and dermal contact, followed by liquid suspensions and then by nanomaterials embedded in a solid matrix.

Nanoparticles behave differently than other similarly sized particles. It is therefore necessary to develop specialized approaches to testing and monitoring their effects on human health and on the environment. The OECD Chemicals Committee has established the Working Party on Manufactured Nanomaterials to address this issue and to study the practices of OECD member countries in regards to nanomaterial safety.

FULLERENE

A fullerene is a molecule of carbon in the form of a hollow sphere, ellipsoid, tube, and many other shapes. Spherical fullerenes, also referred to as Buckminsterfullerenes (buckyballs), resemble the balls used in football (soccer). Cylindrical fullerenes are also called carbon nanotubes (buckytubes). Fullerenes are similar in structure to graphite, which is composed of stacked graphene sheets of linked hexagonal rings; they may also contain pentagonal (or sometimes heptagonal) rings.

The first fullerene molecule to be discovered, and the family's namesake, buckminsterfullerene (C_{60}), was manufactured in 1985 by Richard Smalley, Robert Curl, James Heath, Sean O'Brien, and Harold Kroto at Rice University. The name was an homage to Buckminster Fuller, whose geodesic domes it resembles. The structure was also identified some five years earlier by Sumio Iijima, from an electron microscope image, where it formed the core of a "bucky onion". Fullerenes have since been found to occur in nature. More recently, fullerenes have been detected in outer space. According to astronomer Letizia Stanghellini, "It's possible that buckyballs from outer space provided seeds for life on Earth."

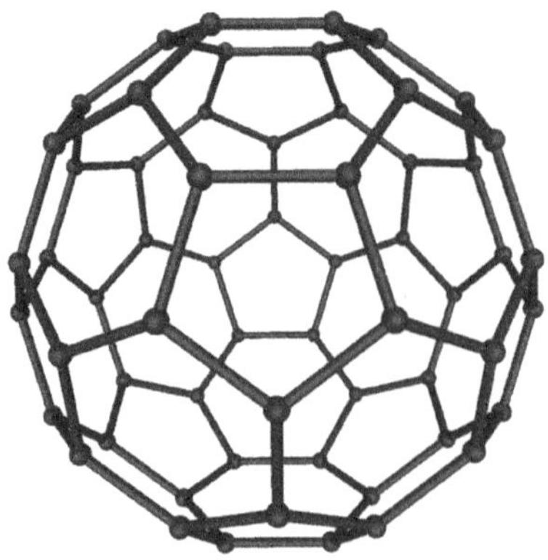

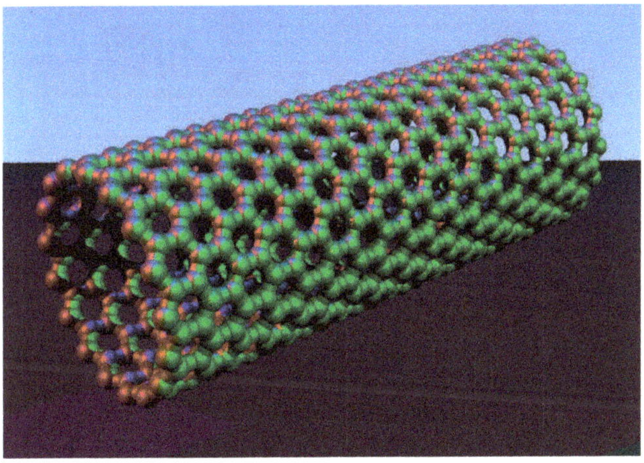

Buckminsterfullerene C_{60} (left) and carbon nanotubes (right) are two examples of structures in the fullerene family.

The discovery of fullerenes greatly expanded the number of known carbon allotropes, which until recently were limited to graphite, graphene, diamond, and amorphous carbon such as soot and charcoal. Buckyballs and buckytubes have been the subject of intense research, both for their unique chemistry and for their technological applications, especially in materials science, electronics, and nanotechnology.

History

The icosahedral $C_{60}H_{60}$ cage was mentioned in 1965 as a possible topological structure. Eiji Osawa of Toyohashi University of Technology predicted the existence of C_{60} in 1970. He noticed that the structure of a corannulene molecule was a subset of an Association football shape, and he hypothesized that a full ball shape could also exist. Japanese scientific journals reported his idea, but neither it nor any translations of it reached Europe or the Americas.

Also in 1970, R. W. Henson (then of the Atomic Energy Research Establishment) proposed the structure and made a model of C_{60}. Unfortunately, the evidence for this new form of carbon was very weak and was not accepted, even by his colleagues. The results were never published but were acknowledged in *Carbon* in 1999.

In 1973 independently from Henson, a group of scientists from the USSR, directed by Prof. Bochvar, made a quantum-chemical analysis of the stability of C_{60} and calculated its electronic structure. As in the previous cases, the scientific community did not accept the theoretical prediction. The paper was published in 1973 in *Proceedings of the USSR Academy of Sciences* (in Russian).

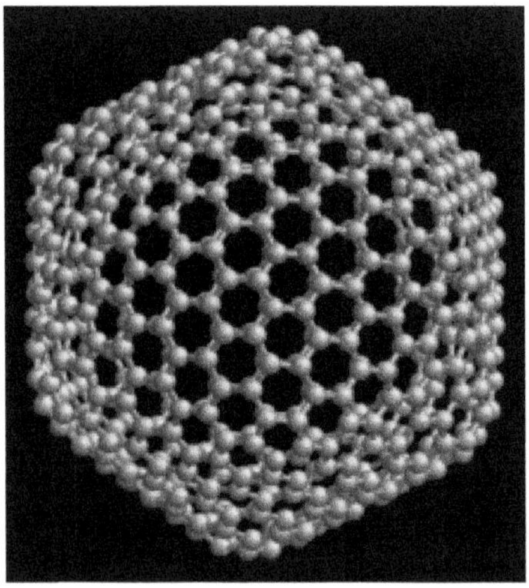

The icosahedral fullerene C_{540}, another member of the family of fullerenes.

In mass spectrometry discrete peaks appeared corresponding to molecules with the exact mass of sixty or seventy or more carbon atoms. In 1985 Harold Kroto of the University of Sussex, James R. Heath, Sean O'Brien, Robert Curl and Richard Smalley from Rice University, discovered C_{60}, and shortly thereafter came to discover the fullerenes. Kroto, Curl, and Smalley were awarded the 1996 Nobel Prize in Chemistry for their roles in the discovery of this class of molecules. C_{60} and other fullerenes were later noticed occurring outside the laboratory (for example, in normal candle-soot). By 1990 it was relatively easy to produce gram-sized samples of fullerene powder using the techniques of Donald Huffman, Wolfgang Krätschmer, Lowell D. Lamb, and Konstantinos Fostiropoulos. Fullerene purification remains a challenge to chemists and to a large extent determines fullerene prices. So-called endohedral fullerenes have ions or small molecules incorporated inside the cage atoms. Fullerene is an unusual reactant in many organic reactions such as the Bingel reaction discovered in 1993. Carbon nanotubes were first discovered and synthesized in 1991. Minute quantities of the fullerenes, in the form of C_{60}, C_{70}, C_{76}, C_{82} and C_{84} molecules, are produced in nature, hidden in soot and formed by lightning discharges in the atmosphere. In 1992, fullerenes were found in a family of minerals known as Shungites in Karelia, Russia.

In 2010, fullerenes (C_{60}) have been discovered in a cloud of cosmic dust surrounding a distant star 6500 light years away. Using NASA's Spitzer infrared telescope the scientists spotted the molecules' unmistakable infrared signature. Sir Harry Kroto, who shared the 1996 Nobel Prize in Chemistry for the discovery of buckyballs commented: "This most exciting breakthrough provides convincing evidence that the buckyball has, as I long suspected, existed since time immemorial in the dark recesses of our galaxy."

Naming

The discoverers of the Buckminsterfullerene (C_{60}) allotrope of carbon named it after Richard Buckminster Fuller, a noted architectural modeler who popularized the geodesic dome. Since buckminsterfullerenes have a similar shape to those of such domes, they thought the name appropriate. As the discovery of the fullerene family came *after* buckminsterfullerene, the shortened name 'fullerene' is used to refer to the family of fullerenes. The suffix "-ene" indicates that each C atom is covalently bonded to three others (instead of the maximum of four), a situation that classically would correspond to the existence of bonds involving two pairs of electrons ("double bonds").

Types of fullerene

Since the discovery of fullerenes in 1985, structural variations on fullerenes have evolved well beyond the individual clusters themselves. Examples include:

- Buckyball clusters: smallest member is C20 (unsaturated version of dodecahedrane) and the most common is C60;
- Nanotubes: hollow tubes of very small dimensions, having single or multiple walls; potential applications in electronics industry;
- Megatubes: larger in diameter than nanotubes and prepared with walls of different thickness; potentially used for the transport of a variety of molecules of different sizes;
- polymers: chain, two-dimensional and three-dimensional polymers are formed under high-pressure high-temperature conditions; single-strand polymers are formed using the Atom Transfer Radical Addition Polymerization (ATRAP) route;
- nano"onions": spherical particles based on multiple carbon layers surrounding a buckyball core; proposed for lubricants;
- linked "ball-and-chain" dimers: two buckyballs linked by a carbon chain;
- fullerene rings.

Buckyballs

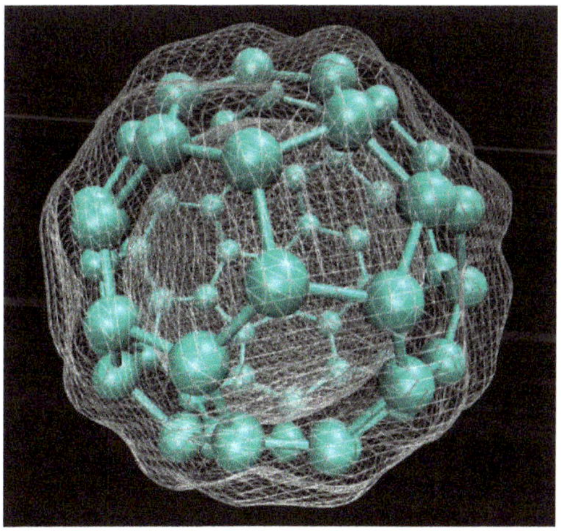

C_{60} with isosurface of ground state electron density as calculated with DFT

Buckminsterfullerene

Buckminsterfullerene is the smallest fullerene molecule containing pentagonal and hexagonal rings in which no two pentagons share an edge (which can be destabilizing, as in pentalene). It is also most common in terms of natural occurrence, as it can often be found in soot.

The structure of C_{60} is a truncated icosahedron, which resembles an association football ball of the type made of twenty hexagons and twelve pentagons, with a carbon atom at the vertices of each polygon and a bond along each polygon edge.

The van der Waals diameter of a C_{60} molecule is about 1.1 nanometers (nm). The nucleus to nucleus diameter of a C_{60} molecule is about 0.71 nm.

The C_{60} molecule has two bond lengths. The 6:6 ring bonds (between two hexagons) can be considered "double bonds" and are shorter than the 6:5 bonds (between a hexagon and a pentagon). Its average bond length is 1.4 angstroms.

Silicon buckyballs have been created around metal ions.

Boron Buckyball

A type of buckyball which uses boron atoms, instead of the usual carbon, was predicted and described in 2007. The B_{80} structure, with each atom forming 5 or 6 bonds, is predicted to be more stable than the C_{60}buckyball. One reason for this given by the researchers is that B_{80} is actually more like the original geodesic dome structure popularized by Buckminster Fuller, which uses triangles rather than hexagons. However, this work has been subject to much criticism by quantum chemists as it was concluded that the predicted I_h symmetric structure was vibrationally unstable and the resulting cage undergoes a spontaneous symmetry break, yielding a puckered cage with rare T_h symmetry (symmetry of a volleyball). The number of six-member rings in this molecule is 20 and number of five-member rings is 12. There is an additional atom in the center of each six-member ring, bonded to each atom surrounding it. By employing a systematic global search algorithm, later it was found that the previously proposed B80 fullerene is not global minimum for 80 atom boron clusters and hence can not be found in nature. In the same paper by Sandip De et al., it was concluded that boron's energy landscape is significantly different from other fullerenes already found in nature hence pure boron fullerenes are unlikely to exist in nature.

Other Buckyballs

Another fairly common fullerene is C_{70}, but fullerenes with 72, 76, 84 and even up to 100 carbon atoms are commonly obtained.

In mathematical terms, the structure of a fullerene is a trivalent convex polyhedron with pentagonal and hexagonal faces. In graph theory, the term fullerene refers to any 3-regular, planar graph with all faces of size 5 or 6 (including the external face). It follows from Euler's polyhedron formula, $V - E + F = 2$ (where V, E, F are the numbers of vertices, edges, and faces), that there are exactly 12 pentagons in a fullerene and $V/2 - 10$ hexagons.

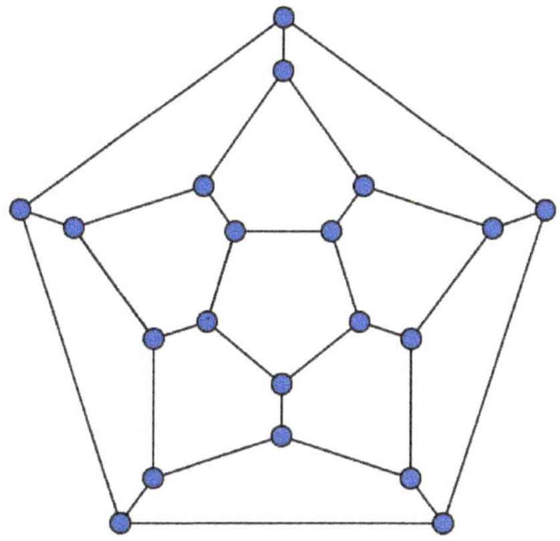

20-fullerene (dodecahedral graph)

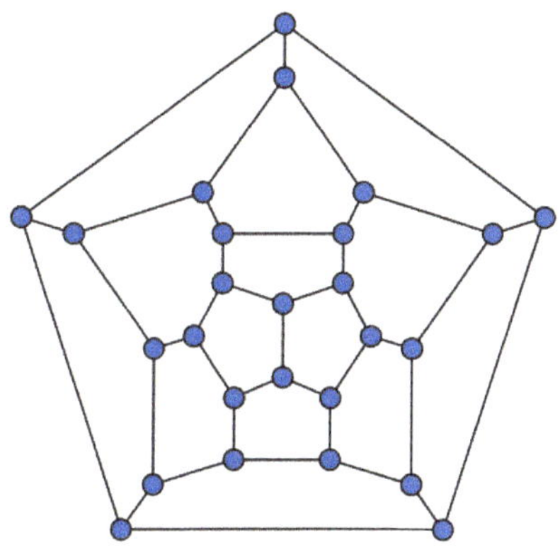

26-fullerene graph

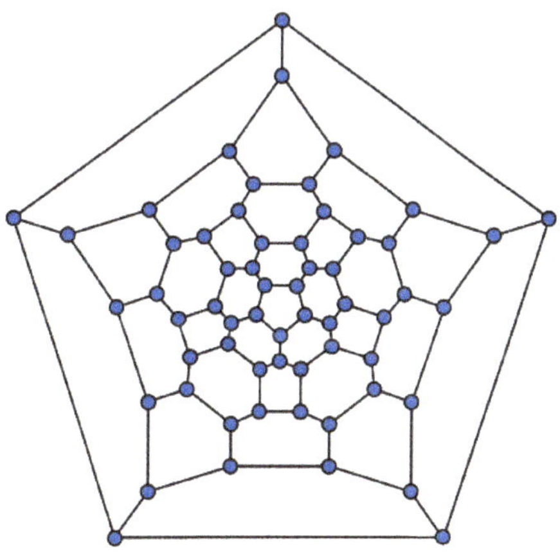

60-fullerene (truncated icosahedral graph)

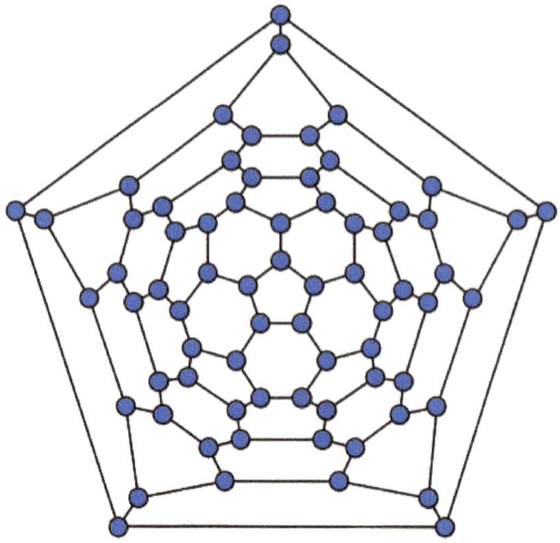

70-fullerene graph

The smallest fullerene is the dodecahedral C_{20}. There are no fullerenes with 22 vertices. The number of fullerenes C_{2n} grows with increasing n = 12, 13, 14, ..., roughly in proportion to n^9 (sequence A007894 in the OEIS). For instance, there are 1812 non-isomorphic fullerenes C_{60}. Note that only one form of C_{60}, the buckminsterfullerene alias truncated icosahedron, has no pair of adjacent pentagons (the smallest such fullerene). To further illustrate the growth, there are 214,127,713 non-isomorphic fullerenes C_{200}, 15,655,672 of which have no adjacent pentagons. Optimized structures of many fullerene isomers are published and listed on the web.

Heterofullerenes have heteroatoms substituting carbons in cage or tube-shaped structures. They were discovered in 1993 and greatly expand the overall fullerene class of compounds. Notable examples include boron, nitrogen (azafullerene), oxygen, and phosphorus derivatives.

Trimetasphere carbon nanomaterials were discovered by researchers at Virginia Tech and licensed exclusively to Luna Innovations. This class of novel molecules comprises 80 carbon atoms (C80) forming a sphere which encloses a complex of three metal atoms and one nitrogen atom. These fullerenes encapsulate metals which puts them in the subset referred to as metallofullerenes. Trimetaspheres have the potential for use in diagnostics (as safe imaging agents), therapeutics and in organic solar cells.

Carbon Nanotubes

Nanotubes are cylindrical fullerenes. These tubes of carbon are usually only a few nanometres wide, but they can range from less than a micrometer to several millimeters in length. They often have closed ends, but can be open-ended as well.

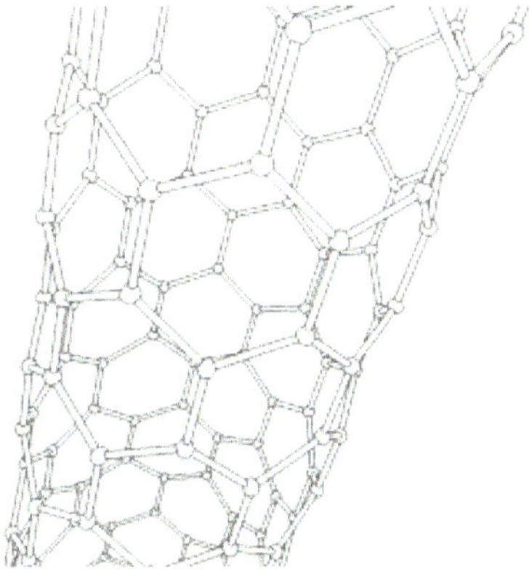

This rotating model of a carbon nanotube shows its 3D structure.

There are also cases in which the tube reduces in diameter before closing off. Their unique molecular structure results in extraordinary macroscopic properties, including high tensile strength, high electrical conductivity, high ductility, high heat conductivity, and relative chemical inactivity (as it is cylindrical and "planar" — that is, it has no "exposed" atoms that can be easily displaced). One proposed use of carbon nanotubes is in paper batteries, developed in 2007 by researchers at Rensselaer Polytechnic Institute. Another highly speculative proposed use in the field of space technologies is to produce high-tensile carbon cables required by a space elevator.

Carbon Nanobuds

Nanobuds have been obtained by adding buckminsterfullerenes to carbon nanotubes.

Fullerite

Fullerites are the solid-state manifestation of fullerenes and related compounds and materials.

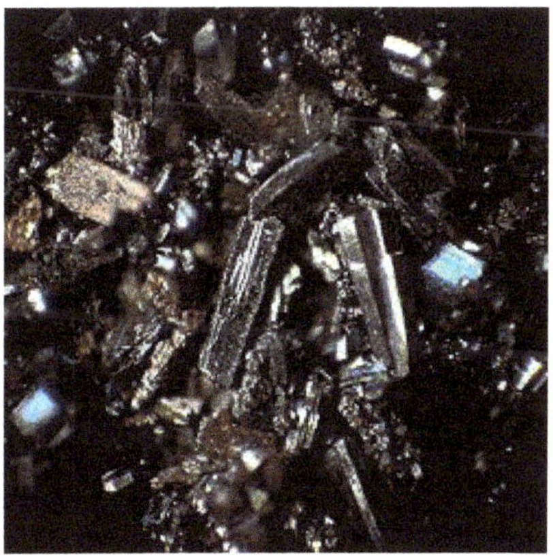

The C_{60} fullerene in crystalline form

"Ultrahard fullerite" is a coined term frequently used to describe material produced by high-pressure high-temperature (HPHT) processing of fullerite. Such treatment converts fullerite into a nanocrystalline form of diamond which has been reported to exhibit remarkable mechanical properties.

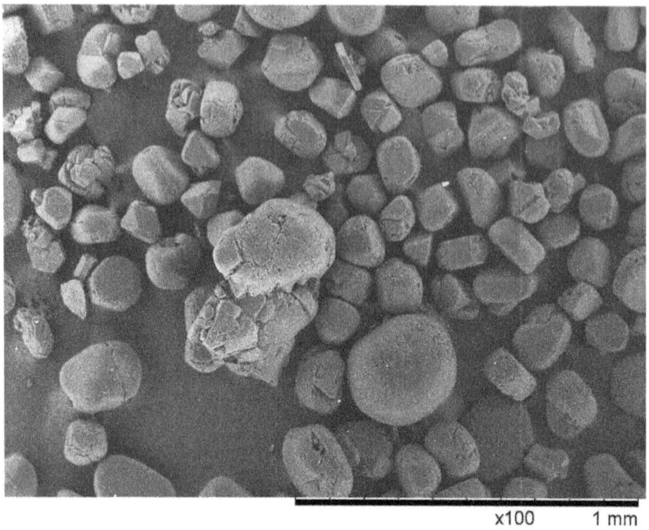

Fullerite (scanning electron microscope image)

Inorganic Fullerenes

Materials with fullerene-like molecular structures but lacking carbon include MoS_2, WS_2, TiS_2 and NbS_2. Prof. J. M. Martin from Ecole Centrale de Lyon in France tested the new material under isostatic pressure and found it to be stable up to at least 350 tons/cm^2.

Properties

For the past decade, the chemical and physical properties of fullerenes have been a hot topic in the field of research and development, and are likely to continue to be for a long time. *Popular Science* has discussed possible uses of fullerenes (graphene) in armor. In April 2003, fullerenes were under study for potential medicinal use: binding specific antibiotics to the structure to target resistant bacteria and even target certain cancer cells such as melanoma. The October 2005 issue of *Chemistry & Biology* contains an article describing the use of fullerenes as light-activated antimicrobial agents.

In the field of nanotechnology, heat resistance and superconductivity are some of the more heavily studied properties.

A common method used to produce fullerenes is to send a large current between two nearby graphite electrodes in an inert atmosphere. The resulting carbon plasma arc between the electrodes cools into sooty residue from which many fullerenes can be isolated.

There are many calculations that have been done using ab-initio quantum methods applied to fullerenes. By DFT and TD-DFT methods one can obtain IR, Raman and UV spectra. Results of such calculations can be compared with experimental results.

Aromaticity

Researchers have been able to increase the reactivity of fullerenes by attaching active groups to their surfaces. Buckminsterfullerene does not exhibit "superaromaticity": that is, the electrons in the hexagonal rings do not delocalize over the whole molecule.

A spherical fullerene of *n* carbon atoms has *n* pi-bonding electrons, free to delocalize. These should try to delocalize over the whole molecule. The quantum mechanics of such an arrangement should be like one shell only of the well-known quantum mechanical structure of a single atom, with a stable filled shell for $n = 2, 8, 18, 32, 50, 72, 98, 128$, etc.; i.e. twice a perfect square number; but this series does not include 60. This $2(N + 1)^2$ rule (with N integer) for spherical aromaticity is the three-dimensional analogue of Hückel's rule. The 10+ cation would satisfy this rule, and should be aromatic. This has been shown to be the case using quantum chemical modelling, which showed the existence of strong diamagnetic sphere currents in the cation.

As a result, C_{60} in water tends to pick up two more electrons and become an anion. The nC_{60} described below may be the result of C_{60} trying to form a loose metallic bond.

Chemistry

Fullerenes are stable, but not totally unreactive. The sp^2-hybridized carbon atoms, which are at their energy minimum in planar graphite, must be bent to form the closed sphere or tube, which produces angle strain. The characteristic reaction of fullerenes is electrophilic addition at 6,6-double bonds, which reduces angle strain by changing sp^2-hybridized carbons into sp^3-hybridized ones. The change in hybridized orbitals causes the bond angles to decrease from about 120° in the sp^2 orbitals to about 109.5° in the sp^3 orbitals. This decrease in bond angles allows for the bonds to bend less when closing the sphere or tube, and thus, the molecule becomes more stable.

Other atoms can be trapped inside fullerenes to form inclusion compounds known as endohedral fullerenes. An unusual example is the egg-shaped fullerene $Tb_3N@C_{84}$, which violates the isolated pentagon rule. Recent evidence for a meteor impact at the end of the Permian period was found by analyzing noble gases so preserved. Metallofullerene-based inoculates using the rhonditic steel process are beginning production as one of the first commercially viable uses of buckyballs.

Solubility

Fullerenes are sparingly soluble in many solvents. Common solvents for the fullerenes include aromatics, such as toluene, and others like carbon disulfide. Solutions of pure buckminsterfullerene have a deep purple color. Solutions of C_{70} are a reddish brown. The higher fullerenes C_{76} to C_{84} have a variety of colors. C_{76} has two optical forms, while other higher fullerenes have several structural isomers. Fullerenes are the only known allotrope of carbon that can be dissolved in common solvents at room temperature.

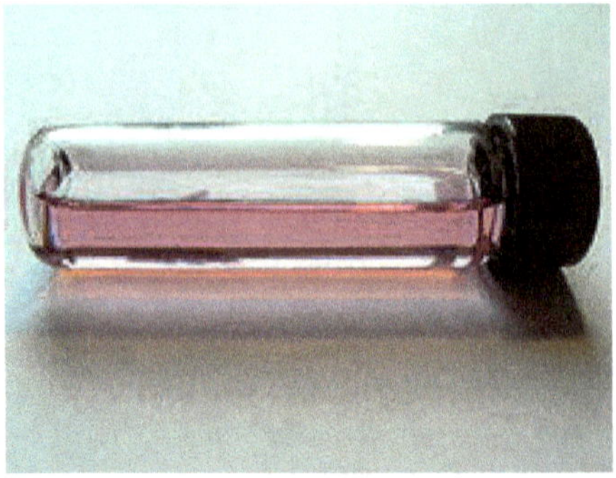

C_{60} in solution

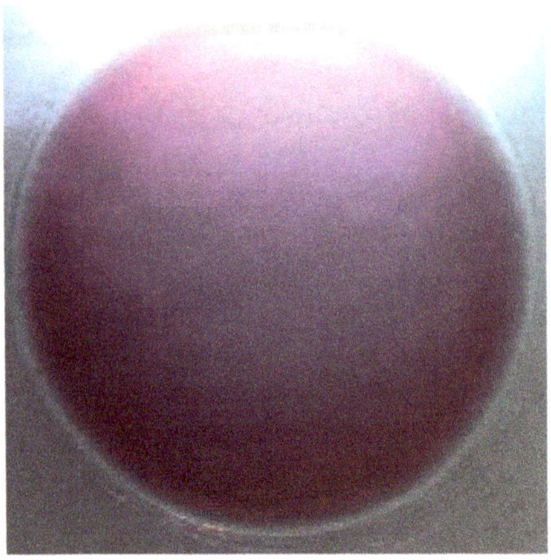

C_{60} in extra virgin olive oil showing the characteristic purple color of pristine C_{60} solutions.

Some fullerene structures are not soluble because they have a small band gap between the ground and excited states. These include the small fullerenes C_{28}, C_{36} and C_{50}. The C_{72} structure is also in this class, but the endohedral version with a trapped lanthanide-group atom is soluble due to the interaction of the metal atom and the electronic states of the fullerene. Researchers had originally been puzzled by C_{72}being absent in fullerene plasma-generated soot extract, but found in endohedral samples. Small band gap fullerenes are highly reactive and bind to other fullerenes or to soot particles.

Solvents that are able to dissolve buckminsterfullerene (C_{60} and C_{70}) are listed at left in order from highest solubility. The solubility value given is the approximate saturated concentration.

Solubility of C_{60} in some solvents shows unusual behaviour due to existence of solvate phases (analogues of crystallohydrates). For example, solubility of C_{60} in benzene solution shows maximum at about 313 K. Crystallization from benzene solution at temperatures below maximum results in formation of triclinic solid solvate with four benzene molecules $C_{60}·4C_6H_6$ which is rather unstable in air. Out of solution, this structure decomposes into usual face-centered cubic (fcc) C_{60} in few minutes' time. At temperatures above solubility maximum the solvate is not stable even when immersed in saturated solution and melts with formation of fcc C_{60}. Crystallization at temperatures above the solubility maximum results in formation of pure fcc C_{60}. Millimeter-sized crystals of C_{60} and C_{70}can be grown from solution both for solvates and for pure fullerenes.

Quantum Mechanics

In 1999, researchers from the University of Vienna demonstrated that wave-particle duality applied to molecules such as fullerene.

Superconductivity

Chirality

Some fullerenes (e.g. C_{76}, C_{78}, C_{80}, and C_{84}) are inherently chiral because they are D_2-symmetric, and have been successfully resolved. Research efforts are ongoing to develop specific sensors for their enantiomers.

Construction

Two theories have been proposed to describe the molecular mechanisms that make fullerenes. The older, "bottom-up" theory proposes that they are built atom-by-atom. The alternative "top-down" approach claims that fullerenes form when much larger structures break into constituent parts.

In 2013 researchers discovered that asymmetrical fullerenes formed from larger structures settle into stable fullerenes. The synthesized substance was a particular metallofullerene consisting of 84 carbon atoms with two additional carbon atoms and two yttrium atoms inside the cage. The process produced approximately 100 micrograms.

However, they found that the asymmetrical molecule could theoretically collapse to form nearly every known fullerene and metallofullerene. Minor perturbations involving the breaking of a few molecular bonds cause the cage to become highly symmetrical and stable. This insight supports the theory that fullerenes can be formed from graphene when the appropriate molecular bonds are severed.

Production Technology

Fullerene production processes comprise the following five subprocesses: (i) synthesis of fullerenes or fullerene-containing soot; (ii) extraction; (iii) separation (purification) for each fullerene molecule, yielding pure fullerenes such as C_{60}; (iv) synthesis of derivatives (mostly using the techniques of organic synthesis); (v) other post-processing such as dispersion into a matrix. The two synthesis methods used in practice are the arc method, and the combustion method. The latter, discovered at the Massachusetts Institute of Technology, is preferred for large scale industrial production.

Solvent	C_{60} mg/mL	C_{70} mg/mL
1-chloronaphthalene	51	ND
1-methylnaphthalene	33	ND
1,2-dichlorobenzene	24	36.2
1,2,4-trimethylbenzene	18	ND
tetrahydronaphthalene	16	ND
carbon disulfide	8	9.875
1,2,3-tribromopropane	8	ND
chlorobenzene	7	ND
p-xylene	5	3.985
bromoform	5	ND
cumene	4	ND
toluene	3	1.406
benzene	1.5	1.3
carbon tetrachloride	0.447	0.121
chloroform	0.25	ND
n-hexane	0.046	0.013
cyclohexane	0.035	0.08
tetrahydrofuran	0.006	ND
acetonitrile	0.004	ND
methanol	4.0×10^{-5}	ND
water	1.3×10^{-11}	ND
pentane	0.004	0.002
heptane	ND	0.047
octane	0.025	0.042
isooctane	0.026	ND
decane	0.070	0.053
dodecane	0.091	0.098
tetradecane	0.126	ND
acetone	ND	0.0019
isopropanol	ND	0.0021
dioxane	0.0041	ND
mesitylene	0.997	1.472
dichloromethane	0.254	0.080
ND, not determined		

Applications

Fullerenes have been extensively used for several biomedical applications including the design of high-performance MRI contrast agents, X-Ray imaging contrast agents, photodynamic therapy and drug and gene delivery, summarized in several comprehensive reviews.

Tumor Research

While past cancer research has involved radiation therapy, photodynamic therapy is important to study because breakthroughs in treatments for tumor cells will give more options to patients with different conditions. More recent experiments using HeLa cells in cancer research involves the development of new photosensitizers with increased ability to be absorbed by cancer cells and still trigger cell death. It is also important that a new photosensitizer does not stay in the body for a long time to prevent unwanted cell damage.

Fullerenes can be made to be absorbed by HeLa cells. The C_{60} derivatives can be delivered to the cells by using the functional groups L-phenylalanine, folic acid, and L-arginine among others. The purpose for functionalizing the fullerenes is to increase the solubility of the molecule by the cancer cells. Cancer cells take up these molecules at an increased rate because of an upregulation of transporters in the cancer cell, in this case amino acid transporters will bring in the L-arginine and L-phenylalanine functional groups of the fullerenes.

Once absorbed by the cells, the C_{60} derivatives would react to light radiation by turning molecular oxygen into reactive oxygen which triggers apoptosis in the HeLa cells and other cancer cells that can absorb the fullerene molecule. This research shows that a reactive substance can target cancer cells and then be triggered by light radiation, minimizing damage to surrounding tissues while undergoing treatment.

When absorbed by cancer cells and exposed to light radiation, the reaction that creates reactive oxygen damages the DNA, proteins, and lipids that make up the cancer cell. This cellular damage forces the cancerous cell to go through apoptosis, which can lead to the reduction in size of a tumor. Once the light radiation treatment is finished the fullerene will reabsorb the free radicals to prevent damage of other tissues. Since this treatment focuses on cancer cells, it is a good option for patients whose cancer cells are within reach of light radiation. As this research continues into the future, it will be able to penetrate deeper into the body and be absorbed by cancer cells more effectively.

Safety and Toxicity

A comprehensive and recent review on fullerene toxicity is given by Lalwani et al. These authors review the works on fullerene toxicity beginning in the early 1990s to present, and conclude that very little evidence gathered since the discovery of fullerenes indicate that C_{60} is toxic. The toxicity of these carbon nanoparticles is not only dose and time-dependent, but also depends on a number of other factors such as: type (e.g., C_{60}, C_{70}, $M@C_{60}$, $M@C_{82}$, functional groups used to water solubilize these nanoparticles (e.g., OH, COOH), and method of administration (e.g., intravenous, intraperitoneal). The authors therefore recommend that pharmacology of every new fullerene- or metallofullerene-based complex must be assessed individually as a different compound.

Popular Culture

Examples of fullerenes in popular culture are numerous. Fullerenes appeared in fiction well before scientists took serious interest in them. In a humorously speculative 1966 column for *New Scientist*, David Jones suggested that it may be possible to create giant hollow carbon molecules by distorting a plane hexagonal net by the addition of impurity atoms.

On 4 September 2010, Google used an interactively rotatable fullerene C_{60} as the second 'o' in their logo to celebrate the 25th anniversary of the discovery of the fullerenes.

CARBON NANOTUBE

Carbon nanotubes (CNTs) are allotropes of carbon with a cylindrical nanostructure. These cylindrical carbon molecules have unusual properties, which are valuable for nanotechnology, electronics, optics and other fields of materials science and technology. Owing to the material's exceptional strength and stiffness, nanotubes have been constructed with length-to-diameter ratio of up to 132,000,000:1, significantly larger than for any other material.

In addition, owing to their extraordinary thermal conductivity, mechanical, and electrical properties, carbon nanotubes find applications as additives to various structural materials. For instance, nanotubes form a tiny portion of the material(s) in some (primarily carbon fiber) baseball bats, golf clubs, car parts or damascus steel.

Nanotubes are members of the fullerene structural family. Their name is derived from their long, hollow structure with the walls formed by one-atom-thick sheets of carbon, called graphene. These sheets are rolled at specific and discrete ("chiral") angles, and the combination of the rolling angle and radius decides the nanotube properties; for example, whether the individual nanotube shell is a metal or semiconductor. Nanotubes are categorized as single-walled nanotubes (SWNTs) and multi-walled nanotubes (MWNTs). Individual nanotubes naturally align themselves into "ropes" held together by van der Waals forces, more specifically, pi-stacking.

Applied quantum chemistry, specifically, orbital hybridization best describes chemical bonding in nanotubes. The chemical bonding of nanotubes is composed entirely of sp^2 bonds, similar to those of graphite. These bonds, which are stronger than the sp^3 bonds found in alkanes and diamond, provide nanotubes with their unique strength.

Types of Carbon Nanotubes and Related Structures

Terminology

There is no consensus on some terms describing carbon nanotubes in scientific literature: both "-wall" and "-walled" are being used in combination with "single", "double", "triple" or "multi", and the letter C is often omitted in the abbreviation; for example, multi-walled carbon nanotube (MWNT).

Single-Walled

Most single-walled nanotubes (SWNTs) have a diameter of close to 1 nanometer, and can be many millions of times longer. The structure of a SWNT can be conceptualized by wrapping a one-atom-thick layer of graphite called graphene into a seamless cylinder.

The way the graphene sheet is wrapped is represented by a pair of indices (*n*,*m*). The integers *n* and *m* denote the number of unit vectors along two directions in the honeycomb crystal lattice of graphene. If $m = 0$, the nanotubes are called **zigzag** nanotubes, and if $n = m$, the nanotubes are called **armchair** nanotubes. Otherwise, they are called **chiral**. The diameter of an ideal nanotube can be calculated from its (n,m) indices as follows

$$d = \frac{a}{\pi}\sqrt{(n^2 + nm + m^2)} = 78.3\sqrt{((n+m)^2 - nm)}\mathrm{pm},$$

where $a = 0.246$ nm.

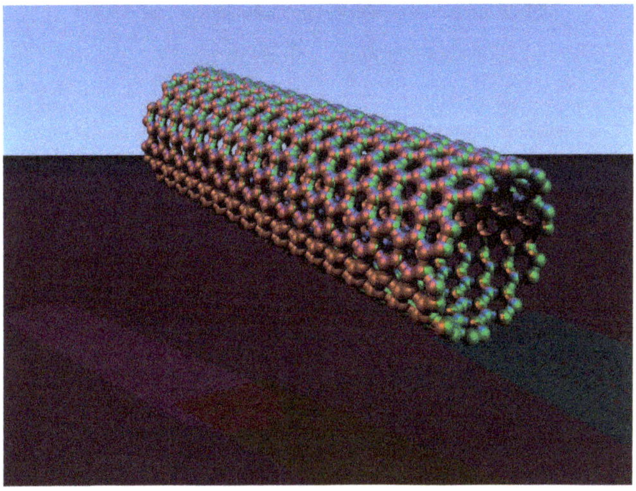

Armchair (*n*,*n*) i.e.: m=n

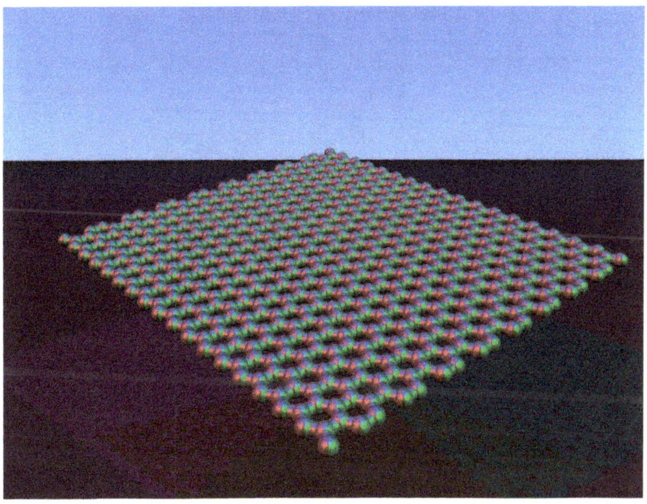

The translation vector is bent, while the chiral vector stays straight

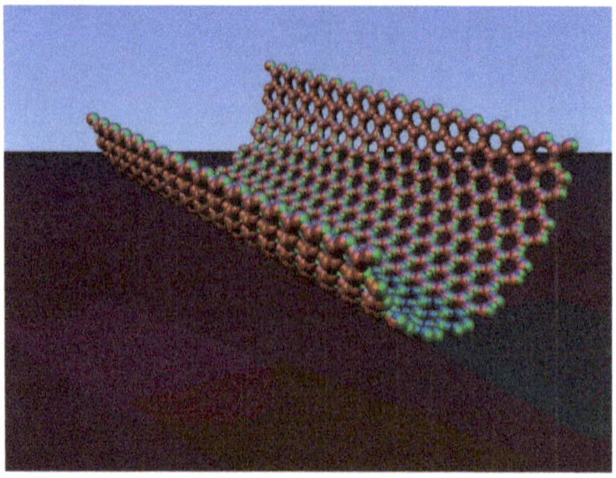

Graphene nanoribbon

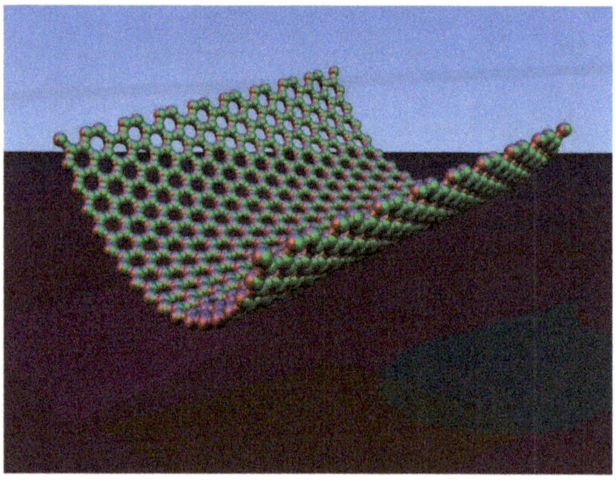

The chiral vector is bent, while the translation vector stays straight

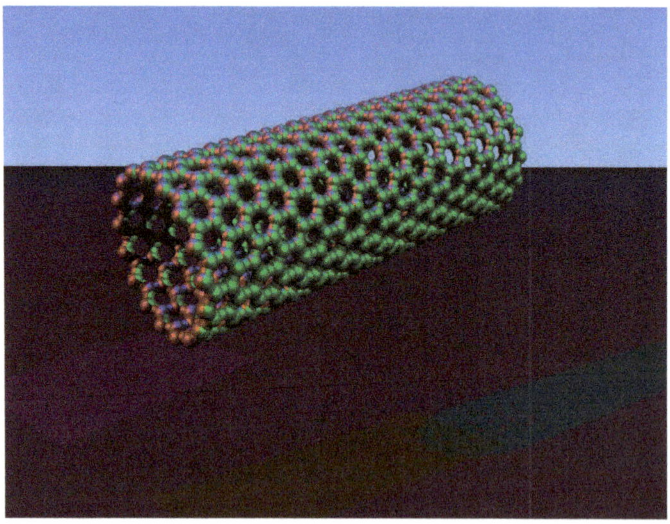

Zigzag $(n,0)$

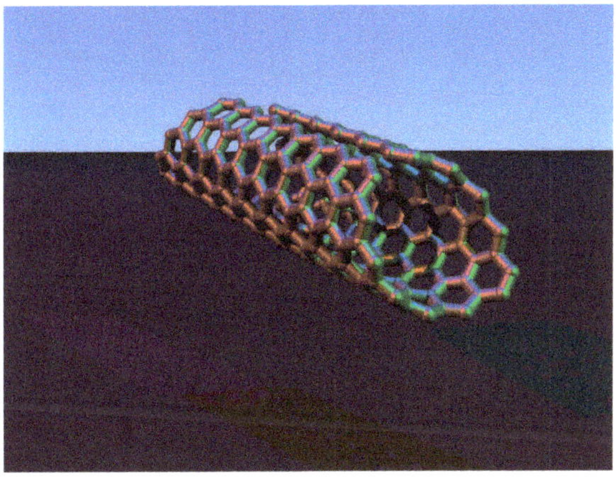

Chiral (n,m)

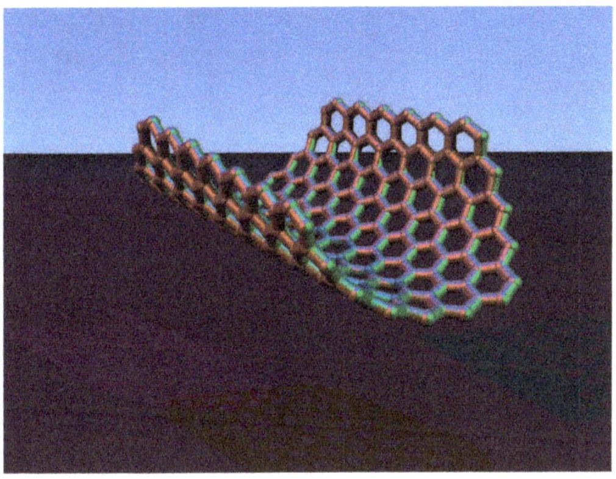

n and m can be counted at the end of the tube

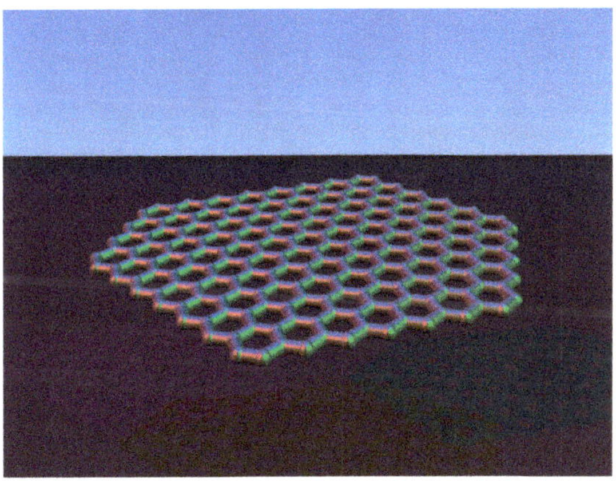

Graphene nanoribbon

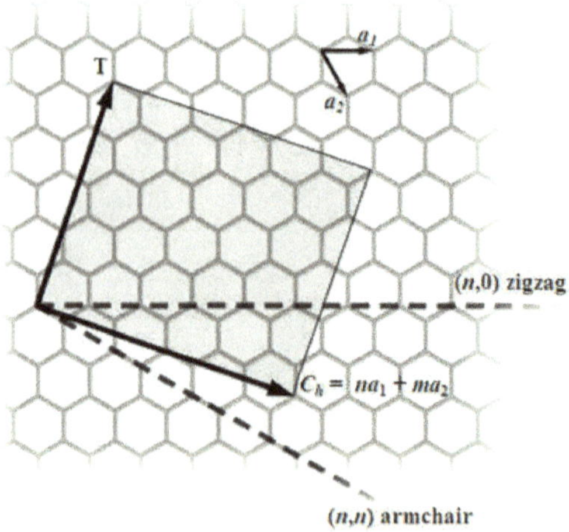

The (n,m) nanotube naming scheme can be thought of as a vector ($\mathbf{C}_h$) in an infinite graphene sheet that describes how to "roll up" the graphene sheet to make the nanotube. **T** denotes the tube axis, and $\mathbf{a}_1$ and $\mathbf{a}_2$ are the unit vectors of graphene in real space.

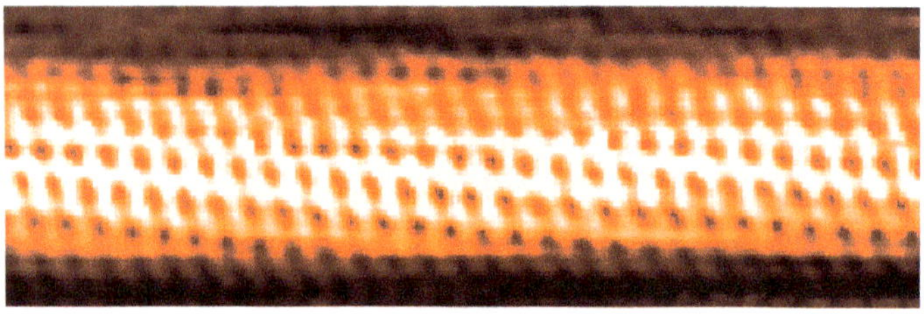

A scanning tunneling microscopy image of single-walled carbon nanotube

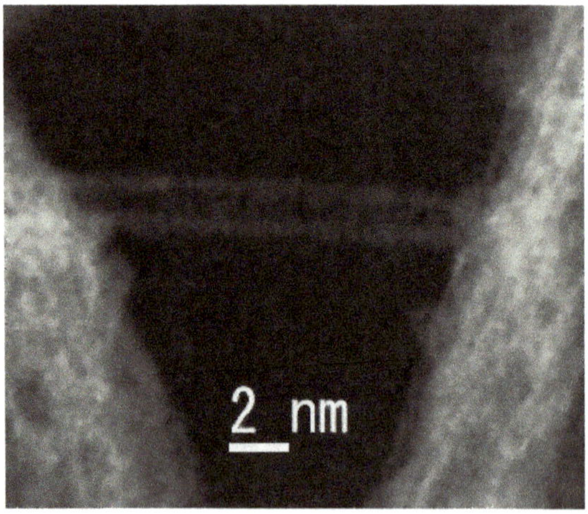

A transmission electron microscopy image of a single-walled carbon nanotube

SWNTs are an important variety of carbon nanotube because most of their properties change significantly with the (n,m) values, and this dependence is non-monotonic. In particular, their band gap can vary from zero to about 2 eV and their electrical conductivity can show metallic or semiconducting behavior. Single-walled nanotubes are likely candidates for miniaturizing electronics. The most basic building block of these systems is the electric wire, and SWNTs with diameters of an order of a nanometer can be excellent conductors. One useful application of SWNTs is in the development of the first intermolecular field-effect transistors (FET). The first intermolecular logic gate using SWCNT FETs was made in 2001. A logic gate requires both a p-FET and an n-FET. Because SWNTs are p-FETs when exposed to oxygen and n-FETs otherwise, it is possible to expose half of an SWNT to oxygen and protect the other half from it. The resulting SWNT acts as a *not* logic gate with both p and n-type FETs in the same molecule.

Prices for single-walled nanotubes declined from around $1500 per gram as of 2000 to retail prices of around $50 per gram of as-produced 40–60% by weight SWNTs as of March 2010. As of 2016 the retail price of as-produced 75% by weight SWNTs were $2 per gram, cheap enough for widespread use.SWNTs are forecast to make a large impact in electronics applications by 2020 according to the *The Global Market for Carbon Nanotubes* report.

Multi-Walled

Multi-walled nanotubes (MWNTs) consist of multiple rolled layers (concentric tubes) of graphene. There are two models that can be used to describe the structures of multi-walled nanotubes. In the *Russian Doll* model, sheets of graphite are arranged in concentric cylinders, e.g., a (0,8) single-walled nanotube (SWNT) within a larger (0,17) single-walled nanotube. In the *Parchment* model, a single sheet of graphite is rolled in around itself, resembling a scroll of parchment or a rolled newspaper. The interlayer distance in multi-walled nanotubes is close to the distance between graphene layers in graphite, approximately 3.4 Å. The Russian Doll structure is observed more commonly. Its individual shells can be described as SWNTs, which can be metallic or semiconducting. Because of statistical probability and restrictions on the relative diameters of the individual tubes, one of the shells, and thus the whole MWNT, is usually a zero-gap metal.

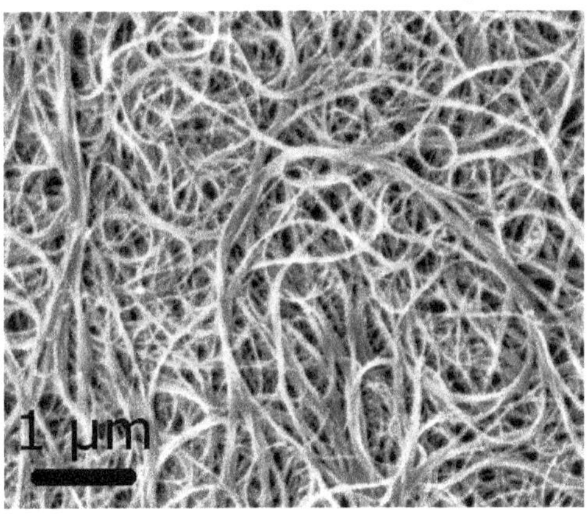

A scanning electron microscopy image of carbon nanotubes bundles

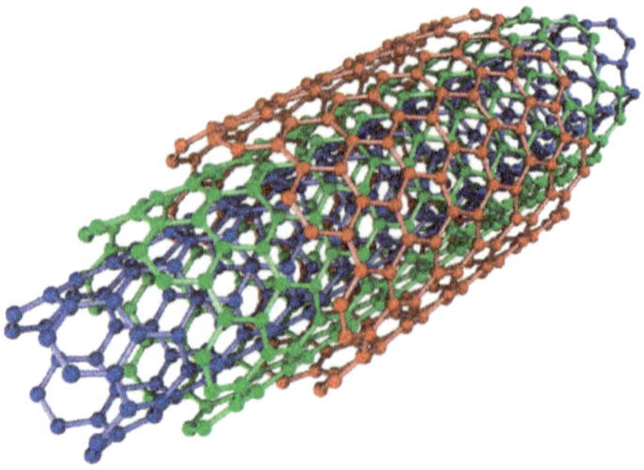

Triple-walled armchair carbon nanotube

Double-walled carbon nanotubes (DWNTs) form a special class of nanotubes because their morphology and properties are similar to those of SWNTs but they are more resistant to chemicals. This is especially important when it is necessary to graft chemical functions to the surface of the nanotubes (functionalization) to add properties to the CNT. Covalent functionalization of SWNTs will break some C=C double bonds, leaving "holes" in the structure on the nanotube, and thus modifying both its mechanical and electrical properties. In the case of DWNTs, only the outer wall is modified. DWNT synthesis on the gram-scale was first proposed in 2003 by the CCVD technique, from the selective reduction of oxide solutions in methane and hydrogen.

The telescopic motion ability of inner shells and their unique mechanical properties will permit the use of multi-walled nanotubes as main movable arms in coming nanomechanical devices. Retraction force that occurs to telescopic motion caused by the Lennard-Jones interaction between shells and its value is about 1.5 nN.

Nanotube Junctions

Junctions between 2 or more nanotubes have been widely discussed theoretically. Such junctions are quite frequently observed in samples prepared by arc discharge as well as by Chemical vapor deposition. The electronic properties of such junctions were first considered theoretically by Lambin et al. , who pointed out that a connection between metallic tube and a semiconducting one would represent a nanoscale heterojunction. Such a junction could therefore form a component of a nanotube-based electronic circuit. The image on the right shows a junction between two multiwalled nanotubes.

Junctions between nanotubes and graphene have been considered theoretically , but not widely studied experimentally. Such junctions form the basis of pillared graphene, in which parallel graphene sheets are separated by short nanotubes. Pillared graphene represents a class of three-dimensional carbon nanotube architectures.

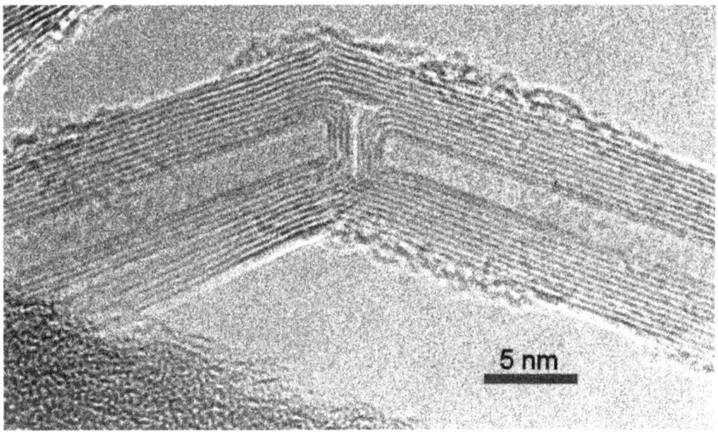

Transmission electron microscope image of carbon nanotube junction

Torus

In theory, a nanotorus is a carbon nanotube bent into a torus (doughnut shape). Nanotori are predicted to have many unique properties, such as magnetic moments 1000 times larger than previously expected for certain specific radii. Properties such as magnetic moment, thermal stability, etc. vary widely depending on radius of the torus and radius of the tube.

Nanobud

Carbon nanobuds are a newly created material combining two previously discovered allotropes of carbon: carbon nanotubes and fullerenes. In this new material, fullerene-like "buds" are covalently bonded to the outer sidewalls of the underlying carbon nanotube.

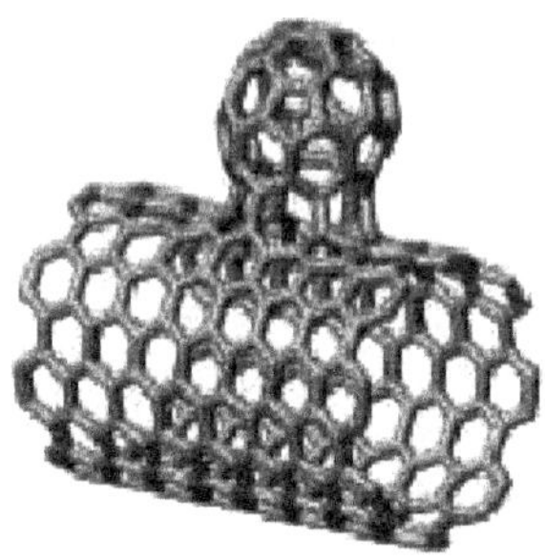

A stable nanobud structure

This hybrid material has useful properties of both fullerenes and carbon nanotubes. In particular, they have been found to be exceptionally good field emitters. In composite materials, the attached fullerene molecules may function as molecular anchors preventing slipping of the nanotubes, thus improving the composite's mechanical properties.

Three-Dimensional Carbon Nanotube Architectures

Recently, several studies have highlighted the prospect of using carbon nanotubes as building blocks to fabricate three-dimensional macroscopic (>100 nm in all three dimensions) all-carbon devices. Lalwani et al. have reported a novel radical initiated thermal crosslinking method to fabricate macroscopic, free-standing, porous, all-carbon scaffolds using single- and multi-walled carbon nanotubes as building blocks. These scaffolds possess macro-, micro-, and nano- structured pores and the porosity can be tailored for specific applications. These 3D all-carbon scaffolds/architectures may be used for the fabrication of the next generation of energy storage, supercapacitors, field emission transistors, high-performance catalysis, photovoltaics, and biomedical devices and implants.

Graphenated Carbon Nanotubes (g-CNTs)

Graphenated CNTs are a relatively new hybrid that combines graphitic foliates grown along the sidewalls of multiwalled or bamboo style CNTs. Yu *et al.* reported on "chemically bonded graphene leaves" growing along the sidewalls of CNTs. Stoner *et al.* described these structures as "graphenated CNTs" and reported in their use for enhanced supercapacitor performance. Hsu *et al.* further reported on similar structures formed on carbon fiber paper, also for use in supercapacitor applications. Pham *et al.* also reported a similar structure, namely "graphene-carbon nanotube hybrids", grown directly onto carbon fiber paper to form an integrated, binder free, high surface area conductive catalyst support for Proton Exchange Membrane Fuel Cells electrode applications with enhanced performance and durability. The foliate density can vary as a function of deposition conditions (e.g. temperature and time) with their structure ranging from few layers of graphene (< 10) to thicker, more graphite-like.

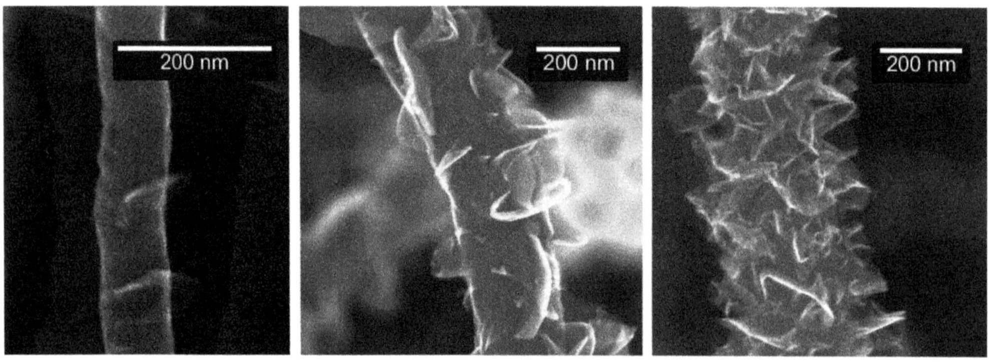

SEM series of graphenated CNTs with varying foliate density

The fundamental advantage of an integrated graphene-CNT structure is the high surface area three-dimensional framework of the CNTs coupled with the high edge density of graphene. Graphene edges provide significantly higher charge density and reactivity than the basal plane, but they are difficult to arrange in a three-dimensional, high volume-density geometry. CNTs are readily aligned in a high density geometry (i.e., a vertically aligned forest) but lack high charge density surfaces—the sidewalls of the CNTs are similar to the basal plane of graphene and exhibit low charge density except where edge defects exist. Depositing a high density of graphene foliates along the length of aligned CNTs can significantly increase the total charge capacity per unit of nominal area as compared to other carbon nanostructures.

Nitrogen-Doped Carbon Nanotubes

Nitrogen doped carbon nanotubes (N-CNTs) can be produced through five main methods, chemical vapor deposition, high-temperature and high-pressure reactions, gas-solid reaction of amorphous carbon with NH_3 at high temperature, solid reaction, and solvothermal synthesis.

N-CNTs can also be prepared by a CVD method of pyrolyzing melamine under Ar at elevated temperatures of 800–980 °C. However synthesis by CVD of melamine results in the formation of bamboo-structured CNTs. XPS spectra of grown N-CNTs reveal nitrogen in five main components, pyridinic nitrogen, pyrrolic nitrogen, quaternary nitrogen, and nitrogen oxides. Furthermore, synthesis temperature affects the type of nitrogen configuration.

Nitrogen doping plays a pivotal role in lithium storage, as it creates defects in the CNT walls allowing for Li ions to diffuse into interwall space. It also increases capacity by providing more favorable bind of N-doped sites. N-CNTs are also much more reactive to metal oxide nanoparticle deposition which can further enhance storage capacity, especially in anode materials for Li-ion batteries. However boron-doped nanotubes have been shown to make batteries with triple capacity.

Peapod

A carbon peapod is a novel hybrid carbon material which traps fullerene inside a carbon nanotube. It can possess interesting magnetic properties with heating and irradiation. It can also be applied as an oscillator during theoretical investigations and predictions.

Cup-Stacked Carbon Nanotubes

Cup-stacked carbon nanotubes (CSCNTs) differ from other quasi-1D carbon structures, which normally behave as quasi-metallic conductors of electrons. CSCNTs exhibit semiconducting behaviors due to the stacking microstructure of graphene layers.

Extreme Carbon Nanotubes

The observation of the *longest* carbon nanotubes grown so far are over 1/2 m (550 mm long) was reported in 2013. These nanotubes were grown on Si substrates using an improved chemical vapor deposition (CVD) method and represent electrically uniform arrays of single-walled carbon nanotubes.

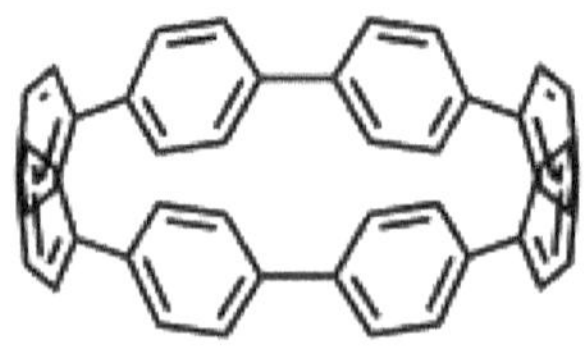

Cycloparaphenylene

The *shortest* carbon nanotube is the organic compound cycloparaphenylene, which was synthesized in 2008.

The *thinnest* carbon nanotube is the armchair (2,2) CNT with a diameter of 0.3 nm. This nanotube was grown inside a multi-walled carbon nanotube. Assigning of carbon nanotube type was done by a combination of high-resolution transmission electron microscopy (HRTEM), Raman spectroscopy and density functional theory (DFT) calculations.

The *thinnest freestanding* single-walled carbon nanotube is about 0.43 nm in diameter. Researchers suggested that it can be either (5,1) or (4,2) SWCNT, but the exact type of carbon nanotube remains questionable. (3,3), (4,3) and (5,1) carbon nanotubes (all about 0.4 nm in diameter) were unambiguously identified using aberration-corrected high-resolution transmission electron microscopy inside double-walled CNTs.

The *highest density* of CNTs was achieved in 2013, grown on a conductive titanium-coated copper surface that was coated with co-catalysts cobalt and molybdenum at lower than typical temperatures of 450 °C. The tubes averaged a height of 380 nm and a mass density of 1.6 g cm^{-3}. The material showed ohmic conductivity (lowest resistance ~22 kΩ).

Properties

Strength

Carbon nanotubes are the strongest and stiffest materials yet discovered in terms of tensile strength and elastic modulus respectively. This strength results from the covalent sp^2 bonds formed between the individual carbon atoms. In 2000, a multi-walled carbon nanotube was tested to have a tensile strength of 63 gigapascals (9,100,000 psi). (For illustration, this translates into the ability to endure tension of a weight equivalent to 6,422 kilograms-force (62,980 N; 14,160 lbf) on a cable with cross-section of 1 square millimetre (0.0016 sq in).) Further studies, such as one conducted in 2008, revealed that individual CNT shells have strengths of up to ≈100 gigapascals (15,000,000 psi), which is in agreement with quantum/atomistic models. Since carbon nanotubes have a low density for a solid of 1.3 to 1.4 g/cm^3, its specific strength of up to 48,000 kN·m·kg^{-1} is the best of known materials, compared to high-carbon steel's 154 kN·m·kg^{-1}.

Under excessive tensile strain, the tubes will undergo plastic deformation, which means the deformation is permanent. This deformation begins at strains of approximately 5% and can increase the maximum strain the tubes undergo before fracture by releasing strain energy.

Although the strength of individual CNT shells is extremely high, weak shear interactions between adjacent shells and tubes lead to significant reduction in the effective strength of multi-walled carbon nanotubes and carbon nanotube bundles down to only a few GPa. This limitation has been recently addressed by applying high-energy electron irradiation, which crosslinks inner shells and tubes, and effectively increases the strength of these materials to ≈60 GPa for multi-walled carbon nanotubes and ≈17 GPa for double-walled carbon nanotube bundles.

CNTs are not nearly as strong under compression. Because of their hollow structure and high aspect ratio, they tend to undergo buckling when placed under compressive, torsional, or bending stress.

Comparison of mechanical properties			
Material	**Young's modulus (TPa)**	**Tensile strength (GPa)**	**Elongation at break (%)**
SWNT^E	≈1 (from 1 to 5)	13–53	16
Armchair SWNT^T	0.94	126.2	23.1
Zigzag SWNT^T	0.94	94.5	15.6–17.5
Chiral SWNT	0.92		
MWNT^E	0.2–0.8–0.95	11–63–150	
Stainless steel^E	0.186–0.214	0.38–1.55	15–50
Kevlar–29&149^E	0.06–0.18	3.6–3.8	≈2

^{E}Experimental observation; ^{T}Theoretical prediction

The above discussion referred to axial properties of the nanotube, whereas simple geometrical considerations suggest that carbon nanotubes should be much softer in the radial direction than along the tube axis. Indeed, TEM observation of radial elasticity suggested that even the van der Waals forces can deform two adjacent nanotubes. Nanoindentation experiments, performed by several groups on multiwalled carbon nanotubes and tapping/contact mode atomic force microscope measurements performed on single-walled carbon nanotubes, indicated a Young's modulus of the order of several GPa, confirming that CNTs are indeed rather soft in the radial direction.

Hardness

Standard single-walled carbon nanotubes can withstand a pressure up to 25 GPa without [plastic/permanent] deformation. They then undergo a transformation to superhard phase nanotubes. Maximum pressures measured using current experimental techniques are around 55 GPa. However, these new superhard phase nanotubes collapse at an even higher, albeit unknown, pressure.

The bulk modulus of superhard phase nanotubes is 462 to 546 GPa, even higher than that of diamond (420 GPa for single diamond crystal).

Wettability

The surface wettability of CNT is of importance for its applications in various settings. Although the intrinsic contact angle of graphite is around 90°, the contact angles of most as-synthesized CNT arrays are over 160°, exhibiting a superhydrophobic property. By applying a voltage as low as 1.3V, the extreme water repellant surface can be switched to a superhydrophilic one.

Kinetic Properties

Multi-walled nanotubes are multiple concentric nanotubes precisely nested within one another. These exhibit a striking telescoping property whereby an inner nanotube core may slide, almost without friction, within its outer nanotube shell, thus creating an atomically perfect linear or rotational bearing. This is one of the first true examples of molecular nanotechnology, the precise positioning of atoms to create useful machines. Already, this property has been utilized to create the world's smallest rotational motor. Future applications such as a gigahertz mechanical oscillator are also envisioned.

Electrical Properties

Unlike graphene, which is a two-dimensional semimetal, carbon nanotubes are either metallic or semiconducting along the tubular axis. For a given (n,m) nanotube, if $n = m$, the nanotube is metallic; if $n - m$ is a multiple of 3, then the nanotube is semiconducting with a very small band gap, otherwise the nanotube is a moderate semiconductor. Thus all armchair $(n = m)$ nanotubes are metallic, and nanotubes (6,4), (9,1), etc. are semiconducting. Carbon nanotubes are not semimetallic because the degenerate point (that point where the π [bonding] band meets the π^* [anti-bonding] band, at which the energy goes to zero) is slightly shifted away from the K point in the Brillouin zone due to the curvature of the tube surface, casing hybridization between the σ^* and π^* anti-bonding bands, modifying the band dispersion.

The rule regarding metallic versus semiconductor behavior has exceptions, because curvature effects in small diameter tubes can strongly influence electrical properties. Thus, a (5,0) SWCNT that should be semiconducting in fact is metallic according to the calculations. Likewise, zigzag and chiral SWCNTs with small diameters that should be metallic have a finite gap (armchair nanotubes remain metallic). In theory, metallic nanotubes can carry an electric current density of 4×10^9 A/cm^2, which is more than 1,000 times greater than those of metals such as copper, where for copper interconnects current densities are limited by electromigration. Carbon nanotubes are thus being explored as conductivity enhancing components in composite materials and many groups are attempting to commercialize highly conducting electrical wire assembled from individual carbon nanotubes. There are significant challenges to be overcome, however, such as the much more resistive nanotube-to-nanotube junctions and impurities, all of which lower the electrical conductivity of the macroscopic nanotube wires by orders of magnitude, as compared to the conductivity of the individual nanotubes.

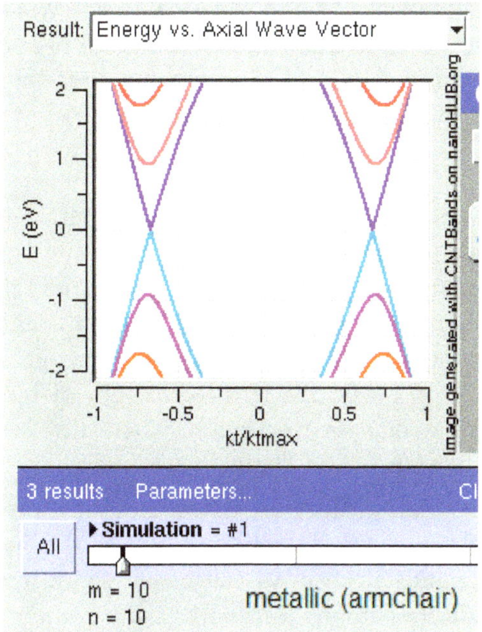

Band structures computed using tight binding approximation for (6,0) CNT (zigzag, metallic), (10,2) CNT (semiconducting) and (10,10) CNT (armchair, metallic).

Because of its nanoscale cross-section, electrons propagate only along the tube's axis. As a result, carbon nanotubes are frequently referred to as one-dimensional conductors. The maximum electrical conductance of a single-walled carbon nanotube is $2G_0$, where $G_0 = 2e^2/h$ is the conductance of a single ballistic quantum channel.

Due to the role of the π-electron system in determining the electronic properties of graphene, doping in carbon nanotubes differs from that of bulk crystalline semiconductors from the same group of the periodic table (e.g. silicon). Graphitic substitution of carbon atoms in the nanotube wall by boron or nitrogen dopants leads to p-type and n-type behavior, respectively, as would be expected in silicon. However, some non-substitutional (intercalated or adsorbed) dopants introduced into a carbon nanotube, such as alkali metals as well as electron-rich metallocenes, result in n-type conduction because they donate electrons to the π-electron system of the nanotube. By contrast, π-electron acceptors such as $FeCl_3$ or electron-deficient metallocenes function as p-type dopants since they draw π-electrons away from the top of the valence band.

Intrinsic superconductivity has been reported, although other experiments found no evidence of this, leaving the claim a subject of debate.

Thermal Properties

All nanotubes are expected to be very good thermal conductors along the tube, exhibiting a property known as "ballistic conduction", but good insulators lateral to the tube axis. Measurements show that a SWNT has a room-temperature thermal conductivity along its axis of about 3500 $W \cdot m^{-1} \cdot K^{-1}$; compare this to copper, a metal well known for its good thermal conductivity, which transmits 385 $W \cdot m^{-1} \cdot K^{-1}$. A SWNT has a room-temperature thermal conductivity across its axis (in the radial direction) of about 1.52 $W \cdot m^{-1} \cdot K^{-1}$, which is about as thermally conductive as soil. The temperature stability of carbon nanotubes is estimated to be up to 2800 °C in vacuum and about 750 °C in air.

Defects

As with any material, the existence of a crystallographic defect affects the material properties. Defects can occur in the form of atomic vacancies. High levels of such defects can lower the tensile strength by up to 85%. An important example is the Stone Wales defect, which creates a pentagon and heptagon pair by rearrangement of the bonds. Because of the very small structure of CNTs, the tensile strength of the tube is dependent on its weakest segment in a similar manner to a chain, where the strength of the weakest link becomes the maximum strength of the chain.

Crystallographic defects also affect the tube's electrical properties. A common result is lowered conductivity through the defective region of the tube. A defect in armchair-type tubes (which can conduct electricity) can cause the surrounding region to become semiconducting, and single monatomic vacancies induce magnetic properties.

Crystallographic defects strongly affect the tube's thermal properties. Such defects lead to phonon scattering, which in turn increases the relaxation rate of the phonons. This reduces the mean free path and reduces the thermal conductivity of nanotube structures. Phonon transport simulations indicate that substitutional defects such as nitrogen or boron will primarily lead to scattering of high-frequency optical phonons. However, larger-scale defects such as Stone Wales defects cause phonon scattering over a wide range of frequencies, leading to a greater reduction in thermal conductivity.

Safety and Health

The toxicity of carbon nanotubes has been an important question in nanotechnology. As of 2007, such research had just begun. The data is still fragmentary and subject to criticism. Preliminary results highlight the difficulties in evaluating the toxicity of this heterogeneous material. Parameters such as structure, size distribution, surface area, surface chemistry, surface charge, and agglomeration state as well as purity of the samples, have considerable impact on the reactivity of carbon nanotubes. However, available data clearly show that, under some conditions, nanotubes can cross membrane barriers, which suggests that, if raw materials reach the organs, they can induce harmful effects such as inflammatory and fibrotic reactions.

As of October 2016, single wall carbon nanotubes have been registered through the European Union's Registration, Evaluation, Authorization and Restriction of Chemicals (REACH) regulations, based on evaluation of the potentially hazardous properties of SWCNT. Based on this registration, SWCNT commercialization is allowed in the EU up to 10 metric tons. Currently, the type of SWCNT registered through REACH is limited to the specific type of single wall carbon nanotubes manufactured by OCSiAl, which submitted the application.

Synthesis

Techniques have been developed to produce nanotubes in sizable quantities, including arc discharge, laser ablation, high-pressure carbon monoxide disproportionation, and chemical vapor deposition (CVD). Most of these processes take place in a vacuum or with process gases. CVD growth of CNTs can occur in vacuum or at atmospheric pressure. Large quantities of nanotubes can be synthesized by these methods; advances in catalysis and continuous growth are making CNTs more commercially viable.

Chemical Modification

Carbon nanotubes can be functionalized to attain desired properties that can be used in a wide variety of applications. The two main methods of carbon nanotube functionalization are covalent and non-covalent modifications. Because of their hydrophobic nature, carbon nanotubes tend to agglomerate hindering their dispersion is solvents or viscous polymer melts. The resulting nanotube bundles or aggregates reduce the mechanical performance of the final composite. The surface of the carbon nanotubes can be modified to reduce the hydrophobicity and improve interfacial adhesion to a bulk polymer through chemical attachment.

Applications

Current

Current use and application of nanotubes has mostly been limited to the use of bulk nanotubes, which is a mass of rather unorganized fragments of nanotubes. Bulk nanotube materials may never achieve a tensile strength similar to that of individual tubes, but such composites may, nevertheless, yield strengths sufficient for many applications. Bulk carbon nanotubes have already been used as composite fibers in polymers to improve the mechanical, thermal and electrical properties of the bulk product.

- Easton-Bell Sports, Inc. have been in partnership with Zyvex Performance Materials, using CNT technology in a number of their bicycle components—including flat and riser handlebars, cranks, forks, seatposts, stems and aero bars.
- Zyvex Technologies has also built a 54’ maritime vessel, the Piranha Unmanned Surface Vessel, as a technology demonstrator for what is possible using CNT technology. CNTs help improve the structural performance of the vessel, resulting in a lightweight 8,000 lb boat that can carry a payload of 15,000 lb over a range of 2,500 miles.
- Amroy Europe Oy manufactures Hybtonite carbon nanoepoxy resins where carbon nanotubes have been chemically activated to bond to epoxy, resulting in a composite material that is 20% to 30% stronger than other composite materials. It has been used for wind turbines, marine paints and variety of sports gear such as skis, ice hockey sticks, baseball bats, hunting arrows, and surfboards.

Other current applications include:

- tips for atomic force microscope probes
- in tissue engineering, carbon nanotubes can act as scaffolding for bone growth

There is also ongoing research in using carbon nanotubes as a scaffold for diverse microfabrication techniques.

Potential

The strength and flexibility of carbon nanotubes makes them of potential use in controlling other nanoscale structures, which suggests they will have an important role in nanotechnology engineering. The highest tensile strength of an individual multi-walled carbon nanotube has been tested to be 63 GPa. Carbon nanotubes were found in Damascus steel from the 17th century, possibly helping to account for the legendary strength of the swords made of it. Recently, several studies have highlighted the prospect of using carbon nanotubes as building blocks to fabricate three-dimensional macroscopic (>1mm in all three dimensions) all-carbon devices. Lalwani et al. have reported a novel radical initiated thermal crosslinking method to fabricated macroscopic, free-standing, porous, all-carbon scaffolds using single- and multi-walled carbon nanotubes as building blocks. These scaffolds possess macro-, micro-, and nano- structured pores and the porosity can be tailored for specific applications. These 3D all-carbon scaffolds/architectures maybe used for the fabrication of the next generation of energy storage, supercapacitors, field emission transistors, high-performance catalysis, photovoltaics, and biomedical devices and implants.

Discovery

The true identity of the discoverers of carbon nanotubes is a subject of some controversy. For years, scientists assumed that Sumio Iijima of NEC had discovered carbon nanotubes in 1991. He published a paper describing his discovery which initiated a flurry of excitement and could be credited by inspiring the many scientists now studying applications of carbon nanotubes. Though Iijima has been given much of the credit for discovering carbon nanotubes, it turns out that the timeline of carbon nanotubes goes back much further than 1991. In 1952 L. V. Radushkevich and V. M. Lukyanovich published clear images of 50 nanometer diameter tubes made of carbon in the Soviet *Journal of Physical Chemistry*. This discovery was largely unnoticed, as the article was published in Russian, and Western scientists' access to Soviet press was limited during the Cold War. Before they came to be known as carbon nanotubes, in 1976, Morinobu Endo of CNRS observed hollow tubes of rolled up graphite sheets synthesised by a chemical vapour-growth technique. The first specimens observed would later come to be known as single-walled carbon nanotubes (SWNTs). The three scientists have been the first ones to show images of a nanotube with a solitary graphene wall.

Endo, in his early review of vapor-phase-grown carbon fibers (VPCF), also reminded us that he had observed a hollow tube, linearly extended with parallel carbon layer faces near the fiber core. This appears to be the observation of multi-walled carbon nanotubes at the center of the fiber.The mass-produced MWCNTs today are strongly related to the VPGCF developed by Endo. In fact, they call it the "Endo-process", out of respect for his early work and patents.

In 1979, John Abrahamson presented evidence of carbon nanotubes at the 14th Biennial Conference of Carbon at Pennsylvania State University. The conference paper described carbon nanotubes as carbon fibers that were produced on carbon anodes during arc discharge. A characterization of these fibers was given as well as hypotheses for their growth in a nitrogen atmosphere at low pressures.

In 1981, a group of Soviet scientists published the results of chemical and structural characterization of carbon nanoparticles produced by a thermocatalytical disproportionation of carbon monoxide. Using TEM images and XRD patterns, the authors suggested that their "carbon multi-layer tubular crystals" were formed by rolling graphene layers into cylinders. They speculated that by rolling graphene layers into a cylinder, many different arrangements of graphene hexagonal nets are possible. They suggested two possibilities of such arrangements: circular arrangement (armchair nanotube) and a spiral, helical arrangement (chiral tube).

In 1987, Howard G. Tennent of Hyperion Catalysis was issued a U.S. patent for the production of "cylindrical discrete carbon fibrils" with a "constant diameter between about 3.5 and about 70 nanometers..., length 10^2 times the diameter, and an outer region of multiple essentially continuous layers of ordered carbon atoms and a distinct inner core...."

Iijima's discovery of multi-walled carbon nanotubes in the insoluble material of arc-burned graphite rods in 1991 and Mintmire, Dunlap, and White's independent prediction that if single-walled carbon nanotubes could be made, then they would exhibit remarkable conducting properties helped create the initial buzz that is now associated with carbon nanotubes. Nanotube research accelerated greatly following the independent discoveries by Bethune at IBM and Iijima at NEC of *single-walled* carbon nanotubes and methods to specifically produce them by adding transition-metal catalysts to the carbon in an arc discharge. The arc discharge technique was well-known to produce the famed Buckminster fullerene on a preparative scale, and these results appeared to extend the run of accidental discoveries relating to fullerenes. The discovery of nanotubes remains a contentious issue. Many believe that Iijima's report in 1991 is of particular importance because it brought carbon nanotubes into the awareness of the scientific community as a whole.

NANOPARTICLE

Nanoparticles are particles between 1 and 100 nanometers in size. In nanotechnology, a particle is defined as a small object that behaves as a whole unit with respect to its transport and properties. Particles are further classified according to diameter. Ultrafine particles are the same as nanoparticles and between 1 and 100 nanometers in size, fine particles are sized between 100 and 2,500 nanometers, and coarse particles cover a range between 2,500 and 10,000 nanometers. Scientific research on nanoparticles is intense as they have many potential applications in medicine, optics, and electronics. The U.S. National Nanotechnology Initiative offers government funding focused on nanoparticle research.

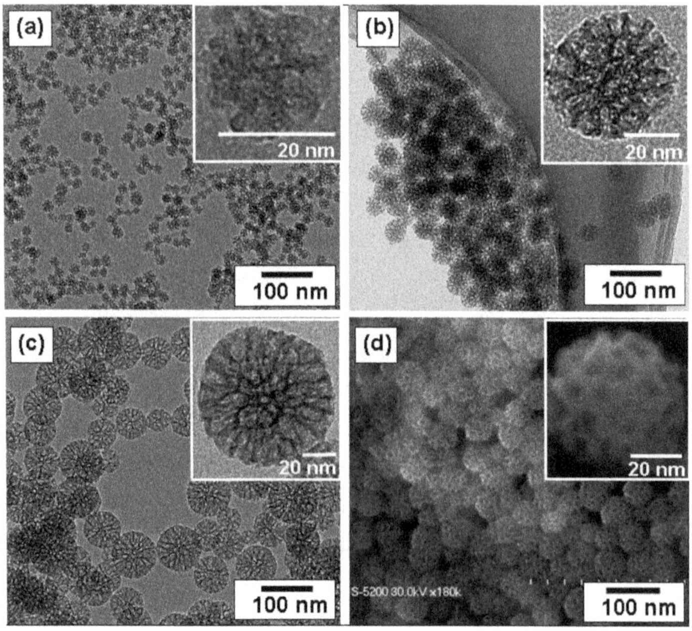

TEM (a, b, and c) images of prepared mesoporous silica nanoparticles with mean outer diameter: (a) 20nm, (b) 45nm, and (c) 80nm. SEM (d) image corresponding to (b). The insets are a high magnification of mesoporous silica particle.

Definition

The term "nanoparticle" is not usually applied to individual molecules; it usually refers to inorganic materials.

The reason for the synonymous definition of nanoparticles and ultrafine particles is that, during the 1970s and 80s, when the first thorough fundamental studies with "nanoparticles" were underway in the USA (by Granqvist and Buhrman)and Japan, (within an ERATO Project) they were called "ultrafine particles" (UFP). However, during the 1990s before the National Nanotechnology Initiative was launched in the USA, the new name, "nanoparticle," had become more common (for example, see the same senior author's paper 20 years later addressing the same issue, lognormal distribution of sizes). Nanoparticles can exhibit size-related properties significantly different from those of either fine particles or bulk materials.

Nanoclusters have at least one dimension between 1 and 10 nanometers and a narrow size distribution. Nanopowders are agglomerates of ultrafine particles, nanoparticles, or nanoclusters. Nanometer-sized single crystals, or single-domain ultrafine particles, are often referred to as nanocrystals.

Background

Although nanoparticles are associated with modern science, they have a long history. Nanoparticles were used by artisans as far back as Rome in the fourth century in the famous Lycurgus cup made of dichroic glass as well as the ninth century in Mesopotamia for creating a glittering effect on the surface of pots.

In modern times, pottery from the Middle Ages and Renaissance often retains a distinct gold- or copper-colored metallic glitter. This luster is caused by a metallic film that was applied to the transparent surface of a glazing. The luster can still be visible if the film has resisted atmospheric oxidation and other weathering.

The luster originates within the film itself, which contains silver and copper nanoparticles dispersed homogeneously in the glassy matrix of the ceramic glaze. These nanoparticles are created by the artisans by adding copper and silver salts and oxides together with vinegar, ochre, and clay on the surface of previously-glazed pottery. The object is then placed into a kiln and heated to about 600 °C in a reducing atmosphere.

In the heat the glaze softens, causing the copper and silver ions to migrate into the outer layers of the glaze. There the reducing atmosphere reduced the ions back to metals, which then came together forming the nanoparticles that give the color and optical effects.

Luster technique showed that ancient craftsmen had a sophisticated empirical knowledge of materials. The technique originated in the Muslim world. As Muslims were not allowed to use gold in artistic representations, they sought a way to create a similar effect without using real gold. The solution they found was using luster.

Michael Faraday provided the first description, in scientific terms, of the optical properties of nanometer-scale metals in his classic 1857 paper. In a subsequent paper, the author (Turner) points out that: «It is well known that when thin leaves of gold or silver are mounted upon glass and heated to a temperature that is well below a red heat (~500 °C), a remarkable change of properties takes place, whereby the continuity of the metallic film is destroyed. The result is that white light is now freely transmitted, reflection is correspondingly diminished, while the electrical resistivity is enormously increased.»

Uniformity

The chemical processing and synthesis of high-performance technological components for the private, industrial, and military sectors requires the use of high-purity ceramics, polymers, glass-ceramics, and composite materials. In condensed bodies formed from fine powders, the irregular particle sizes and shapes in a typical powder often lead to non-uniform packing morphologies that result in packing density variations in the powder compact.

Uncontrolled agglomeration of powders due to attractive van der Waals forces can also give rise to microstructural heterogeneity. Differential stresses that develop as a result of non-uniform drying shrinkage are directly related to the rate at which the solvent can be removed, and thus highly dependent upon the distribution of porosity. Such stresses have been associated with a plastic-to-brittle transition in consolidated bodies, and can yield to crack propagation in the unfired body if not relieved.

In addition, any fluctuations in packing density in the compact as it is prepared for the kiln are often amplified during the sintering process, yielding inhomogeneous densification. Some pores and other structural defects associated with density variations have been shown to play a detrimental role in the sintering process by growing and thus limiting end-point densities. Differential stresses arising from inhomogeneous densification have also been shown to result in the propagation of internal cracks, thus becoming the strength-controlling flaws.

Inert gas evaporation and inert gas deposition are free many of these defects due to the distillation (cf. purification) nature of the process and having enough time to form single crystal particles, however even their non-aggreated deposits have lognormal size distribution, which is typical with nanoparticles. The reason why modern gas evaporation techniques can produce a relatively narrow size distribution is that aggregation can be avoided. However, even in this case, random residence times in the growth zone, due to the combination of drift and diffusion, result in a size distribution appearing lognormal.

It would, therefore, appear desirable to process a material in such a way that it is physically uniform with regard to the distribution of components and porosity, rather than using particle size distributions that will maximize the green density. The containment of a uniformly dispersed assembly of strongly interacting particles in suspension requires total control over interparticle forces. Monodisperse nanoparticles and colloids provide this potential.

Monodisperse powders of colloidal silica, for example, may therefore be stabilized sufficiently to ensure a high degree of order in the colloidal crystal or polycrystalline colloidal solid that results from aggregation. The degree of order appears to be limited by the time and space allowed for longer-range correlations to be established. Such defective polycrystalline colloidal structures would appear to be the basic elements of submicrometer colloidal materials science and, therefore, provide the first step in developing a more rigorous understanding of the mechanisms involved in microstructural evolution in high performance materials and components.

Properties

Nanoparticles are of great scientific interest as they are, in effect, a bridge between bulk materials and atomic or molecular structures. A bulk material should have constant physical properties regardless of its size, but at the nano-scale size-dependent properties are often observed. Thus, the properties of materials change as their size approaches the nanoscale and as the percentage of the surface in relation to the percentage of the volume of a material becomes significant. For bulk materials larger than one micrometer (or micron), the percentage of the surface is insignificant in relation to the volume in the bulk of the material. *The interesting and sometimes unexpected properties of nanoparticles are therefore largely due to the large surface area of the material, which dominates the contributions made by the small bulk of the material.*

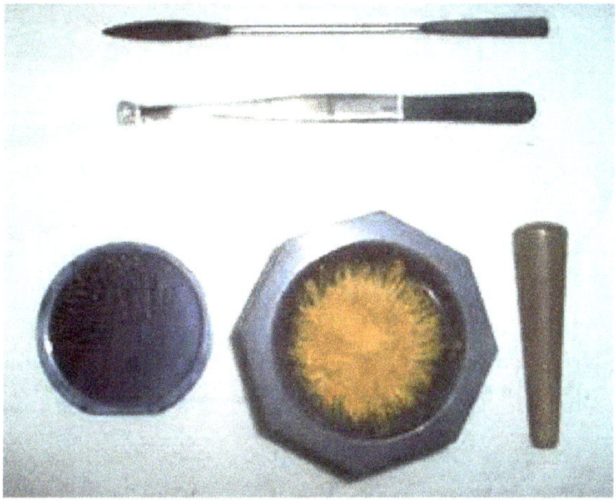

Silicon nanopowder

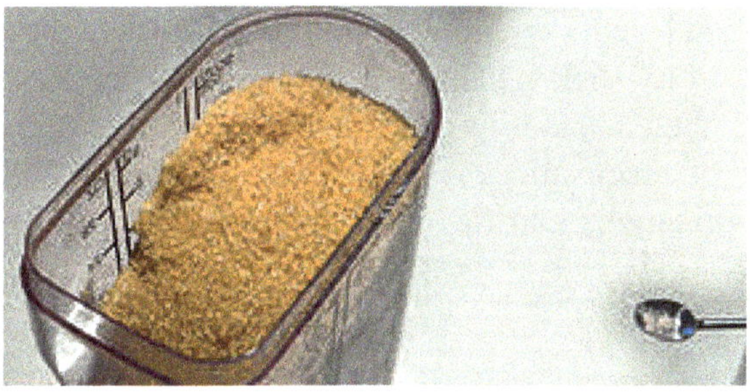

1 kg of particles of 1 mm^3 has the same surface area as 1 mg of particles of 1 nm^3

Nanoparticles often possess unexpected optical properties as they are small enough to confine their electrons and produce quantum effects. For example, gold nanoparticles appear deep-red to black in solution. Nanoparticles of yellow gold and grey silicon are red in color. Gold nanoparticles melt at much lower temperatures (~300 °C for 2.5 nm size) than the gold slabs (1064 °C);. Absorption of solar radiation is much higher in materials composed of nanoparticles than it is in thin films of continuous sheets of material. In both solar PV and solar thermal applications, controlling the size, shape, and material of the particles, it is possible to control solar absorption.

Other size-dependent property changes include quantum confinement in semiconductor particles, surface plasmon resonance in some metal particles and superparamagnetism in magnetic materials. What would appear ironic is that the changes in physical properties are not always desirable. Ferromagnetic materials smaller than 10 nm can switch their magnetisation direction using room temperature thermal energy, thus making them unsuitable for memory storage.

Suspensions of nanoparticles are possible since the interaction of the particle surface with the solvent is strong enough to overcome density differences, which otherwise usually result in a material either sinking or floating in a liquid.

The high surface area to volume ratio of nanoparticles provides a tremendous driving force for diffusion, especially at elevated temperatures. Sintering can take place at lower temperatures, over shorter time scales than for larger particles. In theory, this does not affect the density of the final product, though flow difficulties and the tendency of nanoparticles to agglomerate complicates matters. Moreover, nanoparticles have been found to impart some extra properties to various day to day products. For example, the presence of titanium dioxide nanoparticles imparts what we call the self-cleaning effect, and, the size being nano-range, the particles cannot be observed. Zinc oxide particles have been found to have superior UV blocking properties compared to its bulk substitute. This is one of the reasons why it is often used in the preparation of sunscreen lotions, is completely photostable and toxic.

Clay nanoparticles when incorporated into polymer matrices increase reinforcement, leading to stronger plastics, verifiable by a higher glass transition temperature and other mechanical property tests. These nanoparticles are hard, and impart their properties to the polymer (plastic). Nanoparticles have also been attached to textile fibers in order to create smart and functional clothing.

Metal, dielectric, and semiconductor nanoparticles have been formed, as well as hybrid structures (e.g., core–shell nanoparticles). Nanoparticles made of semiconducting material may also be labeled quantum dots if they are small enough (typically sub 10 nm) that quantization of electronic energy levels occurs. Such nanoscale particles are used in biomedical applications as drug carriers or imaging agents.

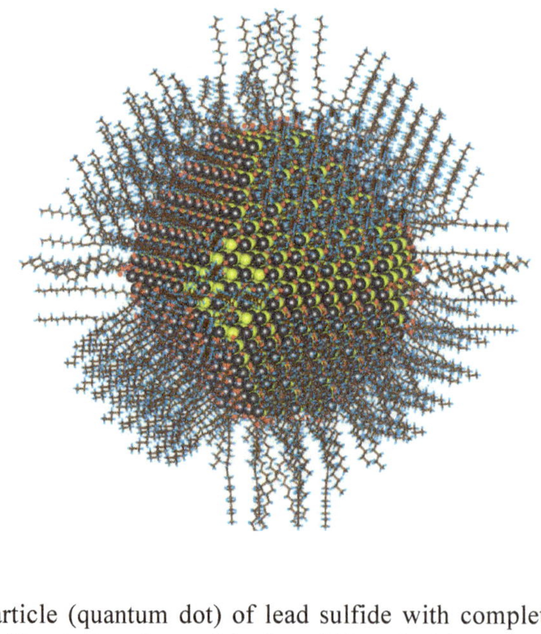

Semiconductor nanoparticle (quantum dot) of lead sulfide with complete passivation by oleic acid, oleyl amine and hydroxyl ligands (size ~5nm)

Semi-solid and soft nanoparticles have been manufactured. A prototype nanoparticle of semi-solid nature is the liposome. Various types of liposome nanoparticles are currently used clinically as delivery systems for anticancer drugs and vaccines.

Nanoparticles with one half hydrophilic and the other half hydrophobic are termed Janus particles and are particularly effective for stabilizing emulsions. They can self-assemble at water/oil interfaces and act as solid surfactants.

Synthesis

There are several methods for creating nanoparticles, including attrition, pyrolysis and hydrothermal synthesis. In attrition, macro- or micro-scale particles are ground in a ball mill, a planetary ball mill, or other size-reducing mechanism. The resulting particles are air classified to recover nanoparticles. In pyrolysis, a vaporous precursor (liquid or gas) is forced through an orifice at high pressure and burned. The resulting solid (a version of soot) is air classified to recover oxide particles from by-product gases. Traditional pyrolysis often results in aggregates and agglomerates rather than single primary particles. Ultrasonic nozzle spray pyrolysis (USP) on the other hand aids in preventing agglomerates from forming.

A thermal plasma can deliver the energy to vaporize small micrometer-size particles. The thermal plasma temperatures are in the order of 10,000 K, so that solid powder easily evaporates. Nanoparticles are formed upon cooling while exiting the plasma region. The main types of the thermal plasma torches used to produce nanoparticles are dc plasma jet, dc arc plasma, and radio frequency (RF) induction plasmas. In the arc plasma reactors, the energy necessary for evaporation and reaction is provided by an electric arc formed between the anode and the cathode. For example, silica sand can be vaporized with an arc plasma at atmospheric pressure, or thin aluminum wires can be vaporized by exploding wire method. The resulting mixture of plasma gas and silica vapour can be rapidly cooled by quenching with oxygen, thus ensuring the quality of the fumed silica produced.

In RF induction plasma torches, energy coupling to the plasma is accomplished through the electromagnetic field generated by the induction coil. The plasma gas does not come in contact with electrodes, thus eliminating possible sources of contamination and allowing the operation of such plasma torches with a wide range of gases including inert, reducing, oxidizing, and other corrosive atmospheres. The working frequency is typically between 200 kHz and 40 MHz. Laboratory units run at power levels in the order of 30–50 kW, whereas the large-scale industrial units have been tested at power levels up to 1 MW. As the residence time of the injected feed droplets in the plasma is very short, it is important that the droplet sizes are small enough in order to obtain complete evaporation. The RF plasma method has been used to synthesize different nanoparticle materials, for example synthesis of various ceramic nanoparticles such as oxides, carbours/carbides, and nitrides of Ti and Si.

Inert-gas condensation is frequently used to make nanoparticles from metals with low melting points. The metal is vaporized in a vacuum chamber and then supercooled with an inert gas stream. The supercooled metal vapor condenses into nanometer-size particles, which can be entrained in the inert gas stream and deposited on a substrate or studied in situ.

Nanoparticles can also be formed using radiation chemistry. Radiolysis from gamma rays can create strongly active free radicals in solution. This relatively simple technique uses a minimum number of chemicals. These including water, a soluble metallic salt, a radical scavenger (often a secondary alcohol), and a surfactant (organic capping agent). High gamma doses on the order of 10^4 Gray are required. In this process, reducing radicals will drop metallic ions down to the zero-valence state. A scavenger chemical will preferentially interact with oxidizing radicals to prevent the re-oxidation of the metal. Once in the zero-valence state, metal atoms begin to coalesce into particles. A chemical surfactant surrounds the particle during formation and regulates its growth. In sufficient concentrations, the surfactant molecules stay attached to the particle. This prevents it from dissociating or forming clusters with other particles. Formation of nanoparticles using the radiolysis method allows for tailoring of particle size and shape by adjusting precursor concentrations and gamma dose.

Sol-gel

The sol-gel process is a wet-chemical technique (also known as chemical solution deposition) widely used recently in the fields of materials science and ceramic engineering. Such methods are used primarily for the fabrication of materials (typically a metal oxide) starting from a chemical solution (*sol*, short for solution), which acts as the precursor for an integrated network (or *gel*) of either discrete particles or network polymers.

Typical precursors are metal alkoxides and metal chlorides, which undergo hydrolysis and polycondensation reactions to form either a network "elastic solid" or a colloidal suspension (or dispersion) – a system composed of discrete (often amorphous) submicrometer particles dispersed to various degrees in a host fluid. Formation of a metal oxide involves connecting the metal centers with oxo (M-O-M) or hydroxo (M-OH-M) bridges, therefore generating metal-oxo or metal-hydroxo polymers in solution. Thus, the sol evolves toward the formation of a gel-like diphasic system containing both a liquid phase and solid phase whose morphologies range from discrete particles to continuous polymer networks.

In the case of the colloid, the volume fraction of particles (or particle density) may be so low that a significant amount of fluid may need to be removed initially for the gel-like properties to be recognized. This can be accomplished in a number of ways. The most simple method is to allow time for sedimentation to occur, and then pour off the remaining liquid. Centrifugation can also be used to accelerate the process of phase separation.

Removal of the remaining liquid (solvent) phase requires a drying process, which is typically causes shrinkage and densification. The rate at which the solvent can be removed is ultimately determined by the distribution of porosity in the gel. The ultimate microstructure of the final component will clearly be strongly influenced by changes implemented during this phase of processing. Afterward, a thermal treatment, or firing process, is often necessary in order to favor further polycondensation and enhance mechanical properties and structural stability via final sintering, densification, and grain growth. One of the distinct advantages of using this methodology as opposed to the more traditional processing techniques is that densification is often achieved at a much lower temperature.

The precursor sol can be either deposited on a substrate to form a film (e.g., by dip-coating or spin-coating), cast into a suitable container with the desired shape (e.g., to obtain a monolithic ceramics, glasses, fibers, membranes, aerogels), or used to synthesize powders (e.g., microspheres, nanospheres). The sol-gel approach is a cheap and low-temperature technique that allows for the fine control of the product's chemical composition. Even small quantities of dopants, such as organic dyes and rare earth metals, can be introduced in the sol and end up uniformly dispersed in the final product. It can be used in ceramics processing and manufacturing as an investment casting material, or as a means of producing very thin films of metal oxides for various purposes. Sol-gel derived materials have diverse applications in optics, electronics, energy, space, (bio) sensors, medicine (e.g., controlled drug release) and separation (e.g., chromatography) technology.

Colloids

The term colloid is used primarily to describe a range of mixtures which have solid particles dispersed in a liquid medium. The term applies only if the particles are larger than atomic dimensions but small enough to exhibit Brownian motion. If the particles are large enough, their dynamic behavior in any given period of time in suspension would be governed by forces of gravity and sedimentation. If the particles are small enough, their irregular motion in suspension can be attributed to the collective bombardment of a myriad of thermally agitated molecules in the liquid suspending medium, as described originally by Albert Einstein in his dissertation. Einstein showed evidence that water was made up of discrete molecules by characterizing the observed erratic particle behavior using the theory of Brownian motion, with sedimentation being a possible result. The critical size range (or particle diameter) typically ranges from nanometers (10^{-9} m) to micrometers (10^{-6} m).

Morphology

Scientists have taken to naming their particles after the real-world shapes that they might represent. Nanospheres, nanochains, nanoreefs, nanoboxes and more have appeared in the literature. These morphologies sometimes arise spontaneously as an effect of a templating or directing agent present in the synthesis such as miscellar emulsions or anodized alumina pores, or from the innate crystallographic growth patterns of the materials themselves. Some of these morphologies may serve a purpose, such as long carbon nanotubes used to bridge an electrical junction, or just a scientific curiosity like the stars shown at right.

Amorphous particles usually adopt a spherical shape (due to their microstructural isotropy), whereas the shape of anisotropic microcrystalline whiskers corresponds to their particular crystal habit. At the small end of the size range, nanoparticles are often referred to as clusters. Spheres, rods, fibers, and cups are just a few of the shapes that have been grown. The study of fine particles is called micromeritics.

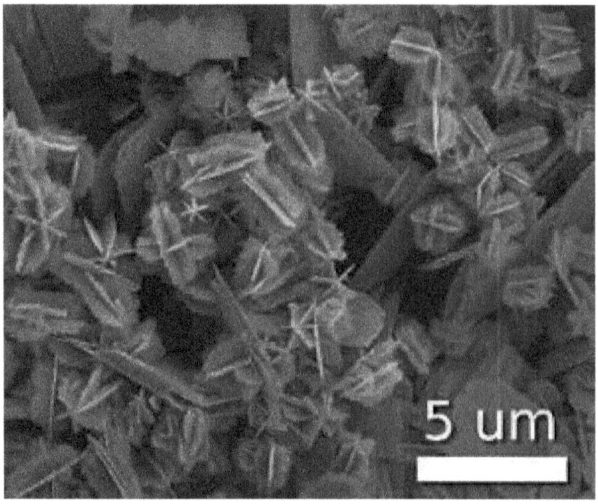

Nanostars of vanadium(IV) oxide

Characterization

The majority of nanoparticle characterization techniques are light-based, but a non-optical nanoparticle characterization technique called Tunable Resistive Pulse Sensing (TRPS) has been developed that enables the simultaneous measurement of size, concentration and surface charge for a wide variety of nanoparticles. This technique, which applies the Coulter Principle, allows for particle-by-particle quantification of these three nanoparticle characteristics with high resolution.

Functionalization

The surface coating of nanoparticles determines many of their properties, notably stability, solubility, and targeting. A coating that is multivalent or polymeric confers high stability. Functionalized nanomaterial-based catalysts can be used for catalysis of many known organic reactions.

Surface Coating for Biological Applications

For biological applications, the surface coating should be polar to give high aqueous solubility and prevent nanoparticle aggregation. In serum or on the cell surface, highly charged coatings promote non-specific binding, whereas polyethylene glycol linked to terminal hydroxyl or methoxy groups repel non-specific interactions. Nanoparticles can be linked to biological molecules that can act as address tags, to direct the nanoparticles to specific sites within the body, specific organelles within the cell, or to follow specifically the movement of individual protein or RNA molecules in living cells. Common address tags are monoclonal antibodies, aptamers, streptavidin or peptides. These targeting agents should ideally be covalently linked to the nanoparticle and should be present in a controlled number per nanoparticle. Multivalent nanoparticles, bearing multiple targeting groups, can cluster receptors, which can activate cellular signaling pathways, and give stronger anchoring. Monovalent nanoparticles, bearing a single binding site, avoid clustering and so are preferable for tracking the behavior of individual proteins.

Red blood cell coatings can help nanoparticles evade the immune system.

Safety

Nanoparticles present possible dangers, both medically and environmentally. Most of these are due to the high surface to volume ratio, which can make the particles very reactive or catalytic. They are also able to pass through cell membranes in organisms, and their interactions with biological systems are relatively unknown. However, it is unlikely the particles would enter the cell nucleus, Golgi complex, endoplasmic reticulum or other internal cellular components due to the particle size and intercellular agglomeration. A recent study looking at the effects of ZnO nanoparticles on human immune cells has found varying levels of susceptibility to cytotoxicity. There are concerns that pharmaceutical companies, seeking regulatory approval for nano-reformulations of existing medicines, are relying on safety data produced during clinical studies of the earlier, pre-reformulation version of the medicine. This could result in regulatory bodies, such as the FDA, missing new side effects that are specific to the nano-reformulation.

Whether cosmetics and sunscreens containing nanomaterials pose health risks remains largely unknown at this stage. However considerable research has demonstrated that zinc nanoparticles are not absorbed into the bloodstream in vivo.

Concern has also been raised over the health effects of respirable nanoparticles from certain combustion processes. As of 2013 the U.S. Environmental Protection Agency was investigating the safety of the following nanoparticles:

- Carbon Nanotubes: Carbon materials have a wide range of uses, ranging from composites for use in vehicles and sports equipment to integrated circuits for electronic components. The interactions between nanomaterials such as carbon nanotubes and natural organic matter strongly influence both their aggregation and deposition, which strongly affects their transport, transformation, and exposure in aquatic environments. In past research, carbon nanotubes exhibited some toxicological impacts that will be evaluated in various environmental settings in current EPA chemical safety research. EPA research will provide data, models, test methods, and best practices to discover the acute health effects of carbon nanotubes and identify methods to predict them.
- Cerium oxide: Nanoscale cerium oxide is used in electronics, biomedical supplies, energy, and fuel additives. Many applications of engineered cerium oxide nanoparticles naturally disperse themselves into the environment, which increases the risk of exposure. There is ongoing exposure to new diesel emissions using fuel additives containing CeO_2 nanoparticles, and the environmental and public health impacts of this new technology are unknown. EPA's chemical safety research is assessing the environmental, ecological, and health implications of nanotechnology-enabled diesel fuel additives.

- Titanium dioxide: Nano titanium dioxide is currently used in many products. Depending on the type of particle, it may be found in sunscreens, cosmetics, and paints and coatings. It is also being investigated for use in removing contaminants from drinking water.
- Nano Silver: Nano silver is being incorporated into textiles, clothing, food packaging, and other materials to eliminate bacteria. EPA and the U.S. Consumer Product Safety Commission are studying certain products to see whether they transfer nano-size silver particles in real-world scenarios. EPA is researching this topic to better understand how much nano-silver children come in contact with in their environments.
- Iron: While nano-scale iron is being investigated for many uses, including "smart fluids" for uses such as optics polishing and as a better-absorbed iron nutrient supplement, one of its more prominent current uses is to remove contamination from groundwater. This use, supported by EPA research, is being piloted at a number of sites across the country.

Laser Applications

The use of nanoparticles in laser dye-doped poly(methyl methacrylate) (PMMA) laser gain media was demonstrated in 2003 and it has been shown to improve conversion efficiencies and to decrease laser beam divergence. Researchers attribute the reduction in beam divergence to improved dn/dT characteristics of the organic-inorganic dye-doped nanocomposite. The optimum composition reported by these researchers is 30% w/w of SiO_2 (~ 12 nm) in dye-doped PMMA.

REFERENCES

1. Buzea, Cristina; Pacheco, Ivan; Robbie, Kevin (2007). "Nanomaterials and Nanoparticles: Sources and Toxicity". Biointerphases. 2 (4): MR17–MR71. doi:10.1116/1.2815690. PMID 20419892.
2. Eldridge, T. (8 January 2014). "Achieving industry integration with nanomaterials through financial markets". Nanotechnology_Now.
3. McGovern, C. (2010). "Commoditization of nanomaterials". Nanotechnol. Perceptions. 6 (3): 155–178. doi:10.4024/N15GO10A.ntp.06.03.
4. Novel natural nanomaterial spins off from spider-mite genome sequencing. Phys. Org (May 23, 2013)
5. Why Are Tarantulas Blue?
6. "Fullerenes". Encyclopaedia Britannica.
7. Buseck, P.R.; Tsipursky, S.J.; Hettich, R. (1992). "Fullerenes from the Geological Environment". Science. 257 (5067): 215–7. Bibcode:1992Sci...257..215B. doi:10.1126/science.257.5067.215. PMID 17794751.
8. Cami, J; Bernard-Salas, J.; Peeters, E.; Malek, S. E. (2 September 2010). "Detection of C60 and C70 in a Young Planetary Nebula". Science. 329 (5996):

1180–2. Bibcode:2010Sci...329.1180C. doi:10.1126/science.1192035. PMID 20651118.

9. R. V. Lapshin (2016). "STM observation of a box-shaped graphene nanostructure appeared after mechanical cleavage of pyrolytic graphite" (PDF). Applied Surface Science. Netherlands: Elsevier B. V. 360: 451–460. doi:10.1016/j.apsusc.2015.09.222. ISSN 0169-4332.
10. Zeng, S.; Baillargeat, Dominique; Ho, Ho-Pui; Yong, Ken-Tye (2014). "Nanomaterials enhanced surface plasmon resonance for biological and chemical sensing applications". Chemical Society Reviews. 43 (10): 3426–3452. doi:10.1039/C3CS60479A. PMID 24549396.
11. Kerativitayanan, P; Carrow, JK; Gaharwar, AK (26 May 2015). "Nanomaterials for Engineering Stem Cell Responses.". Advanced healthcare materials. 4: 1600–27. doi:10.1002/adhm.201500272. PMID 26010739.
12. Wei, Hui; Wang, Erkang (2013-06-21). "Nanomaterials with enzyme-like characteristics (nanozymes): next-generation artificial enzymes". Chemical Society Reviews. 42 (14). doi:10.1039/C3CS35486E. ISSN 1460-4744.
13. Ramsden, J.J. (2011) Nanotechnology: An Introduction, Elsevier, Amsterdam
14. Zsigmondy, R. (1914) "Colloids and the Ultramicroscope", J. Wiley and Sons, NY
15. Dukhin, A.S. & Goetz, P.J. (2002). Ultrasound for characterizing colloids. Elsevier.
16. Onoda, G.Y. Jr.; Hench, L.L., eds. (1979). Ceramic Processing Before Firing. New York: Wiley & Sons. ISBN 0-471-65410-8.
17. Aksay, I.A.; Lange, F.F.; Davis, B.I. (1983). "Uniformity of Al2O3-ZrO2 Composites by Colloidal Filtration". J. Am. Ceram. Soc. 66 (10): C–190. doi:10.1111/j.1151-2916.1983.tb10550.x.
18. Franks, G.V. & Lange, F.F. (1996). "Plastic-to-Brittle Transition of Saturated, Alumina Powder Compacts". J. Am. Ceram. Soc. 79 (12): 3161–3168. doi:10.1111/j.1151-2916.1996.tb08091.x.
19. Evans, A.G.; Davidge, R.W. (1969). "The strength and fracture of fully dense polycrystalline magnesium oxide". Phil. Mag. 20 (164): 373–388. Bibcode:1969PMag...20..373E. doi:10.1080/14786436908228708.
20. Lange, F.F. & Metcalf, M. (1983). "Processing-Related Fracture Origins: II, Agglomerate Motion and Cracklike Internal Surfaces Caused by Differential Sintering". J. Am. Ceram. Soc. 66 (6): 398–406. doi:10.1111/j.1151-2916.1983.tb10069.x.
21. Evans, A.G. (1987). "Considerations of Inhomogeneity Effects in Sintering". J. Am. Ceram. Soc. 65 (10): 497–501. doi:10.1111/j.1151-2916.1982.tb10340.x.
22. Whitesides, George M.; et al. (1991). "Molecular Self-Assembly and Nanochemistry: A Chemical Strategy for the Synthesis of Nanostructures". Science. 254 (5036): 1312–9. Bibcode:1991Sci...254.1312W. doi:10.1126/science.1962191. PMID 1962191.
23. Dubbs D. M; Aksay I.A. (2000). "Self-Assembled Ceramics Produced by Complex-Fluid Templation". Annu. Rev. Phys. Chem. 51: 601–22.

Bibcode:2000ARPC...51..601D. doi:10.1146/annurev.physchem.51.1.601. PMID 11031294.

24. Nanomaterials. European Commission. Last updated 18 October 2011
25. ISO/TS 800004-1 Nanotechnologies—Vocabulary—Part 1: Core terms. Geneva: 2011.
26. Kerativitayanan, Punyavee; Carrow, James K.; Gaharwar, Akhilesh K. (May 2015). "Nanomaterials for Engineering Stem Cell Responses". Advanced Healthcare Materials. 4: n/a–n/a. doi:10.1002/adhm.201500272. PMID 26010739.
27. Lauterwasser, C. (18 July 2007). "Opportunities and risks of Nanotechnologies" (PDF). OECD.org.
28. Revell, P.A. (2006). "The biological effects of nanoparticles". Nanotechnology Perceptions. 2 (3): 283–298. ISSN 1660-6795.
29. "Study Sizes up Nanomaterial Toxicity". Chemical & Engineering News. 86 (35): 44. 2008.
30. Topmiller, Jennifer L.; Dunn, Kevin H. (9 December 2013). "Controlling Exposures to Workers Who Make or Use Nanomaterials". National Institute of Occupational Safety and Health. Retrieved 6 January 2015.
31. "Current Strategies for Engineering Controls in Nanomaterial Production and Downstream Handling Processes" (PDF). National Institute of Occupational Safety and Health. November 2013. Retrieved 6 January 2015.
32. "General Safe Practices for Working with Engineered Nanomaterials in Research Laboratories". National Institute of Occupational Safety and Health. May 2012. pp. 6–8. Retrieved 2016-07-15.
33. "Safety of Manufactured Nanomaterials: About, OECD Environment Directorate". OECD.org. 18 July 2007.
34. Module 3: Characteristics of Particles – Particle Size Categories. epa.gov
35. Taylor, Robert; Coulombe, Sylvain; Otanicar, Todd; Phelan, Patrick; Gunawan, Andrey; Lv, Wei; Rosengarten, Gary; Prasher, Ravi; Tyagi, Himanshu (2013). "Small particles, big impacts: A review of the diverse applications of nanofluids". Journal of Applied Physics. 113: 011301. Bibcode:2013JAP...113a1301T. doi:10.1063/1.4754271.
36. Taylor, Robert A; Otanicar, Todd; Rosengarten, Gary (2012). "Nanofluid-based optical filter optimization for PV/T systems". Light: Science & Applications. 1 (10): e34. doi:10.1038/lsa.2012.34.
37. Hewakuruppu, Y. L.; Dombrovsky, L. A.; Chen, C.; Timchenko, V.; Jiang, X.; Baek, S.; Taylor, R. A. (2013). "Plasmonic "pump–probe" method to study semi-transparent nanofluids". Applied Optics. 52 (24): 6041–6050. Bibcode:2013ApOpt..52.6041H. doi:10.1364/AO.52.006041. PMID 24085009.
38. Taylor, Robert A.; Otanicar, Todd P.; Herukerrupu, Yasitha; Bremond, Fabienne; Rosengarten, Gary; Hawkes, Evatt R.; Jiang, Xuchuan; Coulombe, Sylvain (2013). "Feasibility of nanofluid-based optical filters". Applied Optics. 52 (7): 1413–22. Bibcode:2013ApOpt..52.1413T. doi:10.1364/AO.52.001413. PMID 23458793.

39. Vert, M.; Doi, Y.; Hellwich, K. H.; Hess, M.; Hodge, P.; Kubisa, P.; Rinaudo, M.; Schué, F. O. (2012). "Terminology for biorelated polymers and applications (IUPAC Recommendations 2012)". Pure and Applied Chemistry. 84 (2). doi:10.1351/PAC-REC-10-12-04.
40. MacNaught, Alan D.; Wilkinson, Andrew R., eds. (1997). Compendium of Chemical Terminology: IUPAC Recommendations (2nd ed.). Blackwell Science. ISBN 0865426848.
41. Alemán, J.; Chadwick, A. V.; He, J.; Hess, M.; Horie, K.; Jones, R. G.; Kratochvíl, P.; Meisel, I.; Mita, I.; Moad, G.; Penczek, S.; Stepto, R. F. T. (2007). "Definitions of terms relating to the structure and processing of sols, gels, networks, and inorganic-organic hybrid materials (IUPAC Recommendations 2007)". Pure and Applied Chemistry. 79 (10): 1801. doi:10.1351/pac200779101801.
42. Vert, Michel; Doi, Yoshiharu; Hellwich, Karl-Heinz; Hess, Michael; Hodge, Philip; Kubisa, Przemyslaw; Rinaudo, Marguerite; Schué, François (2012). "Terminology for biorelated polymers and applications (IUPAC Recommendations 2012)" (PDF). Pure and Applied Chemistry. 84 (2): 377–410. doi:10.1351/PAC-REC-10-12-04.
43. Granqvist, C.; Buhrman, R.; Wyns, J.; Sievers, A. (1976). "Far-Infrared Absorption in Ultrafine Al Particles". Physical Review Letters. 37 (10): 625–629. Bibcode:1976PhRvL..37..625G. doi:10.1103/PhysRevLett.37.625.
44. Hayashi, C.; Uyeda, R & Tasaki, A. (1997). Ultra-fine particles: exploratory science and technology (1997 Translation of the Japan report of the related ERATO Project 1981–86). Noyes Publications.
45. Kiss, L. B.; Söderlund, J.; Niklasson, G. A.; Granqvist, C. G. (1999). "New approach to the origin of lognormal size distributions of nanoparticles". Nanotechnology. 10: 25–28. Bibcode:1999Nanot..10...25K. doi:10.1088/0957-4484/10/1/006.
46. Buzea, C.; Pacheco, I. I.; Robbie, K. (2007). "Nanomaterials and nanoparticles: Sources and toxicity". Biointerphases. 2 (4): MR17–MR71. doi:10.1116/1.2815690. PMID 20419892.
47. ASTM E 2456 – 06 Standard Terminology Relating to Nanotechnology
48. Fahlman, B. D. (2007). Materials Chemistry. Springer. pp. 282–283. ISBN 1-4020-6119-6. Retrieved 2016-12-06.
49. "Nanotechnology Timeline | Nano". www.nano.gov. Retrieved 2016-12-12.
50. Reiss, Gunter; Hutten, Andreas (2010). "Magnetic Nanoparticles". In Sattler, Klaus D. Handbook of Nanophysics: Nanoparticles and Quantum Dots. CRC Press. pp. 2–1. ISBN 9781420075458. Retrieved 2016-12-06.
51. Khan, Firdos Alam (2012). Biotechnology Fundamentals. CRC Press. p. 328. ISBN 9781439820094. Retrieved 2016-12-06.
52. Rawson, Philip S. (1984). Ceramics. University of Pennsylvania Press. ISBN 0-8122-1156-1. Retrieved 2016-12-06.
53. Faraday, Michael (1857). "Experimental relations of gold (and other metals) to

light". Phil. Trans. Roy. Soc. London. 147: 145–181. doi:10.1098/rstl.1857.0011.

54. Beilby, G.T. (1903). "The Effects of Heat and of Solvents on Thin Films of Metal". Proceedings of the Royal Society A. 72 (477–486): 226–235. doi:10.1098/rspl.1903.0046. JSTOR 116470.
55. Turner, T. (1908). "Transparent Silver and Other Metallic Films". Proceedings of the Royal Society A (Transparent silver and other metallic films). 81 (548): 301–310. Bibcode:1908RSPSA..81..301T. doi:10.1098/rspa.1908.0084. JSTOR 93060.
56. Onoda, G.Y. Jr.; Hench, L.L., eds. (1979). Ceramic Processing Before Firing. New York: Wiley & Sons. ISBN 0-471-65410-8.
57. Aksay, I.A., Lange, F.F., Davis, B.I. (1983). "Uniformity of Al2O3-ZrO2 Composites by Colloidal Filtration". J. Am. Ceram. Soc. 66 (10): C–190. doi:10.1111/j.1151-2916.1983.tb10550.x.
58. Franks, G.V. & Lange, F.F. (1996). "Plastic-to-Brittle Transition of Saturated, Alumina Powder Compacts". J. Am. Ceram. Soc. 79 (12): 3161–3168. doi:10.1111/j.1151-2916.1996.tb08091.x.
59. Evans, A.G. & Davidge, R.W. (1969). "The strength and fracture of fully dense polycrystalline magnesium oxide". Phil. Mag. 20 (164): 373–388. Bibcode:1969PMag...20..373E. doi:10.1080/14786436908228708.
60. Evans, A. G.; Davidge, R. W. (1970). "The strength and oxidation of reaction-sintered silicon nitride". J Mat. Sci. 5 (4): 314–325. Bibcode:1970JMatS...5..314E. doi:10.1007/BF02397783.
61. Lange, F.F. & Metcalf, M. (1983). "Processing-Related Fracture Origins: II, Agglomerate Motion and Cracklike Internal Surfaces Caused by Differential Sintering". J. Am. Ceram. Soc. 66 (6): 398–406. doi:10.1111/j.1151-2916.1983.tb10069.x.
62. Evans, A.G. (1987). "Considerations of Inhomogeneity Effects in Sintering". J. Am. Ceram. Soc. 65 (10): 497–501. doi:10.1111/j.1151-2916.1982.tb10340.x.
63. Whitesides, G.M.; et al. (1991). "Molecular Self-Assembly and Nanochemistry: A Chemical Strategy for the Synthesis of Nanostructures". Science. 254 (5036): 1312–9. Bibcode:1991Sci...254.1312W. doi:10.1126/science.1962191. PMID 1962191.
64. Dabbs D. M, Aksay I.A.; Aksay (2000). "Self-Assembled Ceramics". Annu. Rev. Phys. Chem. 51: 601–22. Bibcode:2000ARPC...51..601D. doi:10.1146/annurev.physchem.51.1.601. PMID 11031294.
65. Buffat, Ph.; Borel, J.-P. (1976). "Size effect on the melting temperature of gold particles". Physical Review A. 13 (6): 2287–2298. Bibcode:1976PhRvA..13.2287B. doi:10.1103/PhysRevA.13.2287.
66. Taylor, Robert A; Phelan, Patrick E; Otanicar, Todd P; Adrian, Ronald; Prasher, Ravi (2011). "Nanofluid optical property characterization: Towards efficient direct absorption solar collectors". Nanoscale Research Letters. 6 (1): 225. Bibcode:2011NRL.....6..225T. doi:10.1186/1556-276X-6-225. PMC 3211283Freely

accessible. PMID 21711750.

67. Gubin, Sergey P. (2009). Magnetic nanoparticles. Wiley-VCH. ISBN 3-527-40790-1.
68. "Sunscreen". U.S. Food and Drug Administration. Retrieved 2016-12-06.
69. Mitchnick, MA; Fairhurst, D; Pinnell, SR (1999). "Microfine zinc oxide (Z-cote) as a photostable UVA/UVB sunblock agent". Journal of the American Academy of Dermatology. 40 (1): 85–90. doi:10.1016/S0190-9622(99)70532-3. PMID 9922017.
70. Heim, J; Felder, E; Tahir, MN; Kaltbeitzel, A; Heinrich, UR; Brochhausen, C; Mailänder, V; Tremel, W; Brieger, J (21 May 2015). "Genotoxic effects of zinc oxide nanoparticles.". Nanoscale. 7 (19): 8931–8. Bibcode:2015Nanos...7.8931H. doi:10.1039/c5nr01167a. PMID 25916659.
71. Wang, B; Zhang, Y; Mao, Z; Yu, D; Gao, C (August 2014). "Toxicity of ZnO nanoparticles to macrophages due to cell uptake and intracellular release of zinc ions.". Journal of Nanoscience and Nanotechnology. 14 (8): 5688–96. doi:10.1166/jnn.2014.8876. PMID 25935990.
72. Gosens, I; Kermanizadeh, A; Jacobsen, NR; Lenz, AG; Bokkers, B; de Jong, WH; Krystek, P; Tran, L; Stone, V; Wallin, H; Stoeger, T; Cassee, FR (2015). "Comparative hazard identification by a single dose lung exposure of zinc oxide and silver nanomaterials in mice.". PLOS ONE. 10 (5): e0126934. doi:10.1371/journal.pone.0126934. PMC 4429007Freely accessible. PMID 25966284.
73. Hanagata, N; Morita, H (2015). "Calcium ions rescue human lung epithelial cells from the toxicity of zinc oxide nanoparticles.". The Journal of toxicological sciences. 40 (5): 625–35. doi:10.2131/jts.40.625. PMID 26354379.
74. Kim, YH; Kwak, KA; Kim, TS; Seok, JH; Roh, HS; Lee, JK; Jeong, J; Meang, EH; Hong, JS; Lee, YS; Kang, JS (June 2015). "Retinopathy Induced by Zinc Oxide Nanoparticles in Rats Assessed by Micro-computed Tomography and Histopathology.". Toxicological research. 31 (2): 157–63. doi:10.5487/tr.2015.31.2.157. PMID 26191382.
75. Moridian, M; Khorsandi, L; Talebi, AR (2015). "Morphometric and stereological assessment of the effects of zinc oxide nanoparticles on the mouse testicular tissue.". Bratislavske lekarske listy. 116 (5): 321–5. doi:10.4149/bll_2015_060. PMID 25924642.
76. "The Textiles Nanotechnology Laboratory". nanotextiles.human.cornell.edu. Retrieved 2016-12-06.
77. Belloni, J.; Mostafavi, M.; Remita, H.; Marignier, J. L.; Delcourt, A. M. O. (1998). "Radiation-induced synthesis of mono- and multi-metallic clusters and nanocolloids". New Journal of Chemistry. 22 (11): 1239–1255. doi:10.1039/A801445K.
78. Brinker, C.J. & Scherer, G.W. (1990). Sol-Gel Science: The Physics and Chemistry of Sol-Gel Processing. Academic Press. ISBN 0-12-134970-5.
79. Hench, L. L.; West, J. K. (1990). "The sol-gel process". Chemical Reviews.

90: 33–72. doi:10.1021/cr00099a003.

80. Klein, L. (1994). Sol-Gel Optics: Processing and Applications. Springer Verlag. ISBN 0-7923-9424-0. Retrieved 2016-12-06.
81. Corriu, Robert & Anh, Nguyên Trong (2009). Molecular Chemistry of Sol-Gel Derived Nanomaterials. John Wiley and Sons. ISBN 0-470-72117-0. Retrieved 2016-12-06.
82. Pais, A. (2005). Subtle is the Lord: The Science and the Life of Albert Einstein. Oxford University Press. ISBN 0-19-280672-6. Retrieved 2016-12-06.
83. Agam, M. A.; Guo, Q (2007). "Electron Beam Modification of Polymer Nanospheres". Journal of Nanoscience and Nanotechnology. 7 (10): 3615–9. doi:10.1166/jnn.2007.814. PMID 18330181.
84. Kralj, Slavko; Makovec, Darko (27 October 2015). "Magnetic Assembly of Superparamagnetic Iron Oxide Nanoparticle Clusters into Nanochains and Nanobundles". ACS Nano. 9 (10): 9700–9707. doi:10.1021/acsnano.5b02328.
85. Choy J.H.; Jang E.S.; Won J.H.; Chung J.H.; Jang D.J. & Kim Y.W. (2004). "Hydrothermal route to ZnO nanocoral reefs and nanofibers". Appl. Phys. Lett. 84 (2): 287. Bibcode:2004ApPhL..84..287C. doi:10.1063/1.1639514.
86. Sun, Y; Xia, Y; Xia (2002). "Shape-controlled synthesis of gold and silver nanoparticles". Science. 298 (5601): 2176–9. Bibcode:2002Sci...298.2176S. doi:10.1126/science.1077229. PMID 12481134.
87. Murphy, C.J. (2002). "Materials science. Nanocubes and nanoboxes". Science. 298 (5601): 2139–41. doi:10.1126/science.1080007. PMID 12481122.
88. Anderson, Will; Kozak, Darby; Coleman, Victoria; Jamting, Asa; Trau, Matt (1 September 2013), "A comparative study of submicron particle sizing platforms: Accuracy, precision and resolution analysis of polydisperse particle size distributions", Journal of Colloid and Interface Science, UK, 405: 322–330, doi:10.1016/j.jcis.2013.02.030
89. Prime, KL; Whitesides, GM (1991). "Self-assembled organic monolayers: model systems for studying adsorption of proteins at surfaces". Science. 252 (5009): 1164–7. Bibcode:1991Sci...252.1164P. doi:10.1126/science.252.5009.1164. PMID 2031186.
90. Liu, W; Greytak, AB; Lee, J; Wong, CR; Park, J; Marshall, LF; Jiang, W; Curtin, PN; Ting, AY; Nocera, Daniel G.; Fukumura, Dai; Jain, Rakesh K.; Bawendi, Moungi G. (2010). "Compact biocompatible quantum dots via RAFT-mediated synthesis of imidazole-based random copolymer ligand". Journal of the American Chemical Society. 132 (2): 472–83. doi:10.1021/ja908137d. PMC 2871316Freely accessible. PMID 20025223.
91. Akerman ME, Chan WC, Laakkonen P, Bhatia SN, Ruoslahti E.; Chan; Laakkonen; Bhatia; Ruoslahti (2002). "Nanocrystal targeting in vivo". Proceedings of the National Academy of Sciences of the United States of America. 99 (20): 12617–21. Bibcode:2002PNAS...9912617A. doi:10.1073/pnas.152463399. PMC 130509Freely accessible. PMID 12235356.

92. Hoshino, A; Fujioka, K; Oku, T; Nakamura, S; Suga, M; Yamaguchi, Y; Suzuki, K; Yasuhara, M; Yamamoto, K (2004). "Quantum dots targeted to the assigned organelle in living cells". Microbiology and immunology. 48 (12): 985–94. doi:10.1111/j.1348-0421.2004.tb03621.x. PMID 15611617.

93. Suzuki, KG; Fujiwara, TK; Edidin, M; Kusumi, A (2007). "Dynamic recruitment of phospholipase Cγ at transiently immobilized GPI-anchored receptor clusters induces IP3–Ca2+ signaling: single-molecule tracking study 2". The Journal of Cell Biology. 177 (4): 731–42. doi:10.1083/jcb.200609175. PMC 2064217Freely accessible. PMID 17517965.

94. Sung, KM; Mosley, DW; Peelle, BR; Zhang, S; Jacobson, JM (2004). "Synthesis of monofunctionalized gold nanoparticles by fmoc solid-phase reactions". Journal of the American Chemical Society. 126 (16): 5064–5. doi:10.1021/ja049578p. PMID 15099078.

95. Fu, A; Micheel, CM; Cha, J; Chang, H; Yang, H; Alivisatos, AP (2004). "Discrete nanostructures of quantum dots/Au with DNA". Journal of the American Chemical Society. 126 (35): 10832–3. doi:10.1021/ja046747x. PMID 15339154.

96. Howarth, M; Liu, W; Puthenveetil, S; Zheng, Y; Marshall, LF; Schmidt, MM; Wittrup, KD; Bawendi, MG; Ting, AY (2008). "Monovalent, reduced-size quantum dots for imaging receptors on living cells". Nature Methods. 5 (5): 397–9. doi:10.1038/nmeth.1206. PMC 2637151Freely accessible. PMID 18425138.

97. Nanoparticles play at being red blood cells

98. Mnyusiwalla, Anisa; Daar, Abdallah S; Singer, Peter A (2003). "Mind the gap : science and ethics in nanotechnology". Nanotechnology. 14 (3): R9. Bibcode:2003Nanot..14R...9M. doi:10.1088/0957-4484/14/3/201.

99. "Toxic Nanoparticles Might be Entering Human Food Supply, MU Study Finds". University of Missouri. 22 August 2013. Retrieved 23 August 2013.

100. Ying, Jackie (2001). Nanostructured Materials. New York: Academic Press. ISBN 0-12-744451-3. Retrieved 2016-12-06.

101. Nanotechnologies: 6. What are potential harmful effects of nanoparticles? europa.eu

102. Greulich, C.; Diendorf, J.; Simon, T.; Eggeler, G.; Epple, M.; Köller, M. (2011). "Uptake and intracellular distribution of silver nanoparticles in human mesenchymal stem cells". Acta Biomaterialia. 7 (1): 347–354. doi:10.1016/j.actbio.2010.08.003. ISSN 1742-7061.

103. Hanley, C; Thurber, A; Hanna, C; Punnoose, A; Zhang, J; Wingett, DG; Thurber; Hanna; Punnoose; Zhang; Wingett (2009). "The Influences of Cell Type and ZnO Nanoparticle Size on Immune Cell Cytotoxicity and Cytokine Induction". Nanoscale Res Lett. 4 (12): 1409–20. Bibcode:2009NRL.....4.1409H. doi:10.1007/s11671-009-9413-8. PMC 2894345Freely accessible. PMID 20652105.

104. Vines T, Faunce T (2009). "Assessing the safety and cost-effectiveness of early nanodrugs". Journal of law and medicine. 16 (5): 822–45. PMID 19554862.

105. Davidson, Keay (2006-05-17). "FDA urged to limit nanoparticle use in cosmetics

and sunscreens". San Francisco Chronicle. Retrieved 2007-04-20.

106. Benson, H., Sarveiya, V., Risk, S. and Roberts, M. S. (2005) . "Influence of anatomical site and topical formulation on skin penetration of sunscreens. Therapeutics and Clinical Risk Management, 1 3: 209–218." [dead link] Retrieved 2012-04-01.

107. Howard, V. (2009). "Statement of Evidence: Particulate Emissions and Health (An Bord Plenala, on Proposed Ringaskiddy Waste-to-Energy Facility)." Retrieved 2011-04-26.

108. "Nanomaterials EPA is Assessing". Environmental Protection Agency. Retrieved February 6, 2013.

109. Duarte, F. J. and James, R. O. (2003). "Tunable solid-state lasers incorporating dye-doped polymer-nanoparticle gain media". Opt. Lett. 28 (21): 2088–2090. Bibcode:2003OptL...28.2088D. doi:10.1364/OL.28.002088. PMID 14587824.

CHAPTER 6

Molecular Self-Assembly

Chapter Contents

- **Introduction**
- **Supramolecular Systems**
- **Self-Assembled Monolayer**
- **Supramolecular Assembly**
- **DNA Nanotechnology**

Molecular self-assembly is the assembly of molecules without guidance or management from an outside source. Self-assembly can occur spontaneously in nature, for example, in cells such as the self-assembly of the lipid bilayer membrane. It usually results in an increase in internal organization of the system. Many biological systems use self-assembly to assemble various molecules and structures. Imitating these strategies and creating novel molecules with the ability to self-assemble into supramolecular assemblies is an important technique in nanotechnology.

INTRODUCTION

Molecular self-assembly is the process by which molecules adopt a defined arrangement without guidance or management from an outside source. There are two types of self-assembly. These are intramolecular self-assembly and intermolecular self-assembly. Commonly, the term molecular self-assembly refers to intermolecular self-assembly, while the intramolecular analog is more commonly called folding.

SUPRAMOLECULAR SYSTEMS

Molecular self-assembly is a key concept in supramolecular chemistry. This is because assembly of molecules in such systems is directed through noncovalent interactions (e.g., hydrogen bonding, metal coordination, hydrophobic forces, van der Waals forces, π-π interactions, and/or electrostatic) as well as electromagnetic interactions. Common examples include the formation of micelles, vesicles, liquid crystal phases, and Langmuir monolayers by surfactant molecules. Further examples of supramolecular assemblies demonstrate that a variety of different shapes and sizes can be obtained using molecular self-assembly.

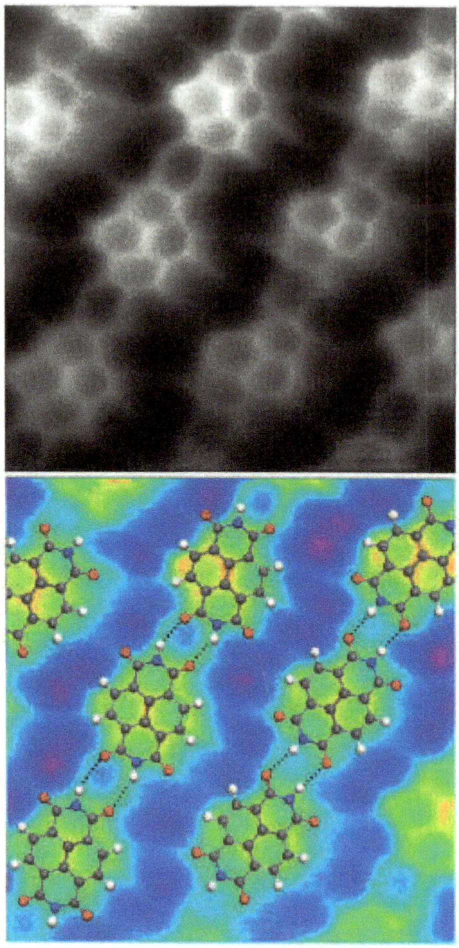

AFM image of napthalenetetracarboxylic diimide molecules on silver interacting via hydrogen bonding at 77 K.("Hydrogen bonds" in the top image are exaggerated by artifacts of the imaging technique.)

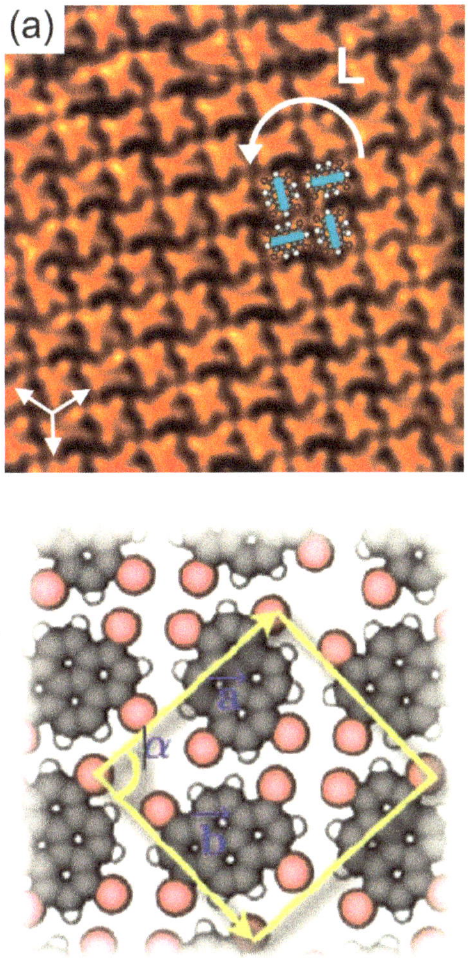

STM image of self-assembled Br_4-pyrene molecules on Au(111) surface (top) and its model (bottom; pink spheres are Br atoms).

Molecular self-assembly allows the construction of challenging molecular topologies. One example is Borromean rings, interlocking rings wherein removal of one ring unlocks each of the other rings. DNA has been used to prepare a molecular analog of Borromean rings. More recently, a similar structure has been prepared using non-biological building blocks. While a mechanistic understanding of how supramolecular self-assembly occurs remains largely unknown, both experimental and theoretic work has been pursued on this topic.

Biological Systems

Molecular self-assembly underlies the construction of biologic macromolecular assemblies in living organisms, and so is crucial to the function of cells. It is exhibited in the self-assembly of lipids to form the membrane, the formation of double helical DNA through hydrogen bonding of the individual strands, and the assembly of proteins to form quaternary structures. Molecular self-assembly of incorrectly folded proteins into insoluble amyloid fibers is responsible for infectious prion-related neurodegenerative diseases. Molecular self-assembly of nanoscale structures plays a role in the growth of the remarkable β-keratin lamellae/setae/spatulae structures used to give geckos the ability to climb walls and adhere to ceilings and rock overhangs.

Nanotechnology

Molecular self-assembly is an important aspect of bottom-up approaches to nanotechnology. Using molecular self-assembly the final (desired) structure is programmed in the shape and functional groups of the molecules. Self-assembly is referred to as a 'bottom-up' manufacturing technique in contrast to a 'top-down' technique such as lithography where the desired final structure is carved from a larger block of matter. In the speculative vision of molecular nanotechnology, microchips of the future might be made by molecular self-assembly. An advantage to constructing nanostructure using molecular self-assembly for biological materials is that they will degrade back into individual molecules that can be broken down by the body.

DNA Nanotechnology

DNA nanotechnology is an area of current research that uses the bottom-up, self-assembly approach for nanotechnological goals. DNA nanotechnology uses the unique molecular recognition properties of DNA and other nucleic acids to create self-assembling branched DNA complexes with useful properties. DNA is thus used as a structural material rather than as a carrier of biological information, to make structures such as two-dimensional periodic lattices (both tile-based as well as using the "DNA origami" method) and three-dimensional structures in the shapes of polyhedra. These DNA structures have also been used as templates in the assembly of other molecules such as gold nanoparticles and streptavidin proteins.

Two-Dimensional Monolayers

The spontaneous assembly of a single layer of molecules at interfaces is usually referred to as two-dimensional self-assembly. Early direct proofs showing that molecules can assembly into higher-order architectures at solid interfaces came with the development of scanning tunneling microscopy and shortly thereafter. Eventually two strategies became popular for the self-assembly of 2D architectures, namely self-assembly following ultra-high-vacuum deposition and annealing and self-assembly at the solid-liquid interface. The design of molecules and conditions leading to the formation of highly-crystalline architectures is considered today a form of 2D crystal engineering at the nanoscopic scale.

SELF-ASSEMBLED MONOLAYER

Self-assembled monolayers (SAM) of organic molecules are molecular assemblies formed spontaneously on surfaces by adsorption and are organized into more or less large ordered domains. In some cases molecules that form the monolayer do not interact strongly with the substrate. This is the case for instance of the two-dimensional supramolecular networks of e.g. Perylene-tetracarboxylicacid-dianhydride (PTCDA) on gold or of e.g. porphyrins on highly oriented pyrolitic graphite (HOPG). In other cases the molecules possess a head group that has a strong affinity to the substrate and anchors the molecule to it. Such a SAM consisting of a head group, tail and functional end group is depicted in Figure 1. Common head groups include thiols, silanes, phosphonates, etc.

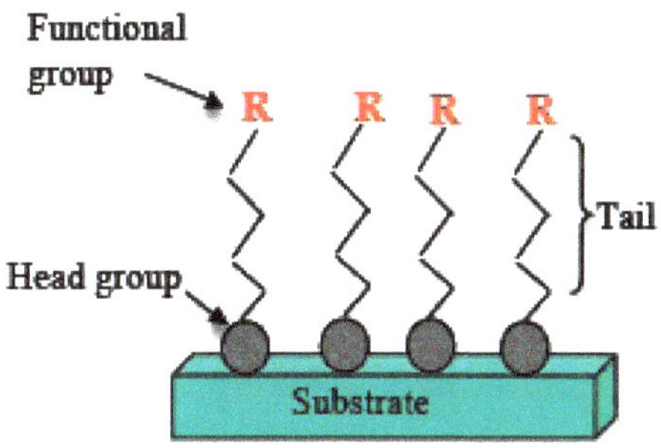

Representation of a SAM structure

SAMs are created by the chemisorption of “head groups” onto a substrate from either the vapor or liquid phase followed by a slow organization of “tail groups”. Initially, at small molecular density on the surface, adsorbate molecules form either a disordered mass of molecules or form an ordered two-dimensional “lying down phase”, and at higher molecular coverage, over a period of minutes to hours, begin to form three-dimensional crystalline or semicrystalline structures on the substrate surface. The “head groups” assemble together on the substrate, while the tail groups assemble far from the substrate. Areas of close-packed molecules nucleate and grow until the surface of the substrate is covered in a single monolayer.

Adsorbate molecules adsorb readily because they lower the surface free-energy of the substrate and are stable due to the strong chemisorption of the “head groups.” These bonds create monolayers that are more stable than the physisorbed bonds of Langmuir–Blodgett films. A Trichlorosilane based “head group”, for example in a FDTS molecule, reacts with an hydroxyl group on a substrate, and forms very stable, covalent bond [R-Si-O-substrate] with an energy of 452 kJ/mol. Thiol-metal bonds are on the order of 100 kJ/mol, making them fairly stable in a variety of temperatures, solvents, and potentials. The monolayer packs tightly due to van der Waals interactions, thereby reducing its own free energy. The adsorption can be described by the Langmuir adsorption isotherm if lateral interactions are neglected. If they cannot be neglected, the adsorption is better described by the Frumkin isotherm.

Types

Selecting the type of head group depends on the application of the SAM. Typically, head groups are connected to a molecular chain in which the terminal end can be functionalized (i.e. adding –OH, –NH2, –COOH, or –SH groups) to vary the wetting and interfacial properties. An appropriate substrate is chosen to react with the head group. Substrates can be planar surfaces, such as silicon and metals, or curved surfaces, such as nanoparticles. Alkanethiols are the most commonly used molecules for SAMs. Alkanethiols are molecules with an alkyl chain, $(C\text{-}C)^n$ chain, as the back bone, a tail group, and a S-H head group. Other types of interesting molecules include aromatic thiols, of interest in molecular electronics, in which the alkane chain is (partly) replaced by aromatic rings. An example is the dithiol 1,4-Benzenedimethanethiol ($SHCH_2C_6H_4CH_2SH$)). Interest in such dithiols stems from the possibility of linking the two sulfur ends to metallic contacts, which was first used in molecular conduction measurements. Thiols are frequently used on noble metal substrates because of the strong affinity of sulfur for these metals. The sulfur gold interaction is semi-covalent and has a strength of approximately 45kcal/mol. In addition, gold is an inert and biocompatible material that is easy to acquire. It is also easy to pattern via lithography, a useful feature for applications in nanoelectromechanical systems (NEMS). Additionally, it can withstand harsh chemical cleaning treatments. Recently other chalcogenide SAMs: selenides and tellurides have attracted attention in a search for different bonding characteristics to substrates affecting the SAM characteristics and which could be of interest in some applications such as molecular electronics. Silanes are generally used on nonmetallic oxide surfaces; however monolayers formed from covalent bonds between silicon and carbon or oxygen cannot be considered self assembled because they do not form reversibly. Self-assembled monolayers of thiolates on noble metals are a special case because the metal-metal bonds become reversible after the formation of the thiolate-metal complex. This reversibility is what gives rise to vacancy islands and it is why SAMs of alkanethiolates can be thermally desorbed and undergo exchange with free thiols.

Preparation

Metal substrates for use in SAMs can be produced through physical vapor deposition techniques, electrodeposition or electroless deposition.Thiol or selenium SAMs produced by adsorption from solution are typically made by immersing a substrate into a dilute solution of alkane thiol in ethanol, though many different solvents can be used besides use of pure liquids. While SAMs are often allowed to form over 12 to 72 hours at room temperature, SAMs of alkanethiolates form within minutes. Special attention is essential in some cases, such as that of dithiol SAMs to avoid problems due to oxidation or photoinduced processes, which can affect terminal groups and lead to disorder and multilayer formation. In this case appropriate choice of solvents, their degassing by inert gasses and preparation in the absence of light is crucialand allows formation of "standing up" SAMs with free –SH groups. Self-assembled monolayers can also be adsorbed from the vapor phase. In some cases when obtaining an ordered assembly is difficult or when different density phases need to be obtained substitutional self-assembly is used. Here one first forms the SAM of a given type of molecules, which give rise to ordered assembly and then a second assembly phase is performed (e.g. by immersion into a different solution). This method has also been used to give information on relative binding strengths of SAMs with different head groups and more generally on self-assembly characteristics.

Characterization

The thicknesses of SAMs can be measured using ellipsometry and X-ray photoelectron spectroscopy (XPS), which also give information on interfacial properties. The order in the SAM and orientation of molecules can be probed by Near Edge Xray Absorption Fine Structure (NEXAFS) and Fourier Transform Infrared Spectroscopy in Reflection Absorption Infrared Spectroscopy (RAIRS) studies. Numerous other spectroscopic techniques are used such as Second-harmonic generation (SHG), Sum-frequency generation (SFG), Surface-enhanced Raman scattering (SERS), as well as High-resolution electron energy loss spectroscopy (HREELS). The structures of SAMs are commonly determined using scanning probe microscopy techniques such as atomic force microscopy (AFM) and scanning tunneling microscopy (STM). STM has been able to help understand the mechanisms of SAM formation as well as determine the important structural features that lend SAMs their integrity as surface-stable entities. In particular STM can image the shape, spatial distribution, terminal groups and their packing structure. AFM offers an equally powerful tool without the requirement of the SAM being conducting or semi-conducting. AFM has been used to determine chemical functionality, conductance, magnetic properties, surface charge, and frictional forces of SAMs. More recently, however, diffractive methods have also been used. The structure can be used to characterize the kinetics and defects found on the monolayer surface. These techniques have also shown physical differences between SAMs with planar substrates and nanoparticle substrates. An alternative characterization instrument for measuring the self-assembly in real time is dual polarisation interferometry where the refractive index, thickness, mass and birefringence of the self assembled layer are quantified at high resolution. Contact angle measurements can be used to determine the surface free-energy which reflects the average composition of the surface of the SAM and can be used to probe the kinetics and thermodynamics of the formation of SAMs. The kinetics of adsorption and temperature induced desorption as well as information on structure can also be obtained in real time by ion scattering techniques such as low energy ion scattering (LEIS) and time of flight direct recoil spectroscopy (TOFDRS).

Defects

Defects due to both external and intrinsic factors may appear. External factors include the cleanliness of the substrate, method of preparation, and purity of the adsorbates. SAMs intrinsically form defects due to the thermodynamics of formation, e.g. thiol SAMs on gold typically exhibit etch pits (monatomic vacancy islands) likely due to extraction of adatoms from the substrate and formation of adatom-adsorbate moieties. Recently, a new type of fluorosurfactants have found that can form nearly perfect monolayer on gold substrate due to the increase of mobility of gold surface atoms.

Nanoparticle Properties

The structure of SAMs is also dependent on the curvature of the substrate. SAMs on nanoparticles, including colloids and nanocrystals, "stabilize the reactive surface of the particle and present organic functional groups at the particle-solvent interface". These organic functional groups are useful for applications, such as immunoassays, that are dependent on chemical composition of the surface.

Kinetics

There is evidence that SAM formation occurs in two steps: an initial fast step of adsorption and a second slower step of monolayer organization. Adsorption occurs at the liquid–liquid, liquid–vapor, and liquid-solid interfaces. The transport of molecules to the surface occurs due to a combination of diffusion and convective transport. According to the Langmuir or Avrami kinetic model the rate of deposition onto the surface is proportional to the free space of the surface.

$$\mathbf{k}(1-\theta) = \frac{d\theta}{dt}.$$

Where θ is the proportional amount of area deposited and **k** is the rate constant. Although this model is robust it is only used for approximations because it fails to take into account intermediate processes. Dual polarisation interferometry being a real time technique with ~10 Hz resolution can measure the kinetics of monolayer self-assembly directly.

Once the molecules are at the surface the self-organization occurs in three phases:

1. A low-density phase with random dispersion of molecules on the surface.
2. An intermediate-density phase with conformational disordered molecules or molecules lying flat on the surface.
3. A high-density phase with close-packed order and molecules standing normal to the substrate's surface.

The phase transitions in which a SAM forms depends on the temperature of the environment relative to the triple point temperature, the temperature in which the tip of the low-density phase intersects with the intermediate-phase region. At temperatures below the triple point the growth goes from phase 1 to phase 2 where many islands form with the final SAM structure, but are surrounded by random molecules. Similar to nucleation in metals, as these islands grow larger they intersect forming boundaries until they end up in phase 3, as seen below.

At temperatures above the triple point the growth is more complex and can take two paths. In the first path the heads of the SAM organize to their near final locations with the tail groups loosely formed on top. Then as they transit to phase 3, the tail groups become ordered and straighten out. In the second path the molecules start in a lying down position along the surface. These then form into islands of ordered SAMs, where they grow into phase 3, as seen below.

The nature in which the tail groups organize themselves into a straight ordered monolayer is dependent on the inter-molecular attraction, or Van der Waals forces, between the tail groups. To minimize the free energy of the organic layer the molecules adopt conformations that allow high degree of Van der Waals forces with some hydrogen bonding. The small size of the SAM molecules are important here because Van der Waals forces arise from the dipoles of molecules and are thus much weaker than the surrounding surface forces at larger scales. The assembly process begins with a small group of molecules, usually two, getting close enough that the Van der Waals forces overcome the surrounding force. The forces between the molecules orient them so they are in their straight, optimal, configuration. Then as other molecules come close by they interact with these already organized molecules in the same fashion and become a part of the conformed group. When this occurs across a large area the molecules support each other into forming their SAM shape. The orientation of the molecules can be described with two parameters: α and β. α is the angle of tilt of the backbone from the surface normal. In typical applications α varies from 0 to 60 degrees depending on the substrate and type of SAM molecule. β is the angle of rotation along the long axis of tee molecule. β is usually between 30 and 40 degrees. In some cases existence of kinetic traps hindering the final ordered orientation has been pointed out. Thus in case of dithiols formation of a lying down phase was considered an impediment to formation of standing up phase, however various recent studies indicate this is not the case.

Many of the SAM properties, such as thickness, are determined in the first few minutes. However, it may take hours for defects to be eliminated via annealing and for final SAM properties to be determined. The exact kinetics of SAM formation depends on the adsorbate, solvent and substrate properties. In general, however, the kinetics are dependent on both preparations conditions and material properties of the solvent, adsorbate and substrate. Specifically, kinetics for adsorption from a liquid solution are dependent on:

- Temperature – room-temperature preparation improves kinetics and reduces defects.
- Concentration of adsorbate in the solution – low concentrations require longer immersion times and often create highly crystalline domains.
- Purity of the adsorbate – impurities can affect the final physical properties of the SAM
- Dirt or contamination on the substrate – imperfections can cause defects in the SAM

The final structure of the SAM is also dependent on the chain length and the structure of both the adsorbate and the substrate. Steric hindrance and metal substrate properties, for example, can affect the packing density of the film, while chain length affects SAM thickness. Longer chain length also increases the thermodynamic stability.

Patterning

1. Locally Attract

This first strategy involves locally depositing self-assembled monolayers on the surface only where the nanostructure will later be located. This strategy is advantageous because it involves high throughput methods that generally involve fewer steps than the other two strategies. The major techniques that use this strategy are:

- Micro-contact printing

Micro-contact printing or soft lithography is analogous to printing ink with a rubber stamp. The SAM molecules are inked onto a pre-shaped elastomeric stamp with a solvent and transferred to the substrate surface by stamping. The SAM solution is applied to the entire stamp but only areas that make contact with the surface allow transfer of the SAMs. The transfer of the SAMs is a complex diffusion process that depends on the type of molecule, concentration, duration of contact, and pressure applied. Typical stamps use PDMS because its elastomeric properties, $E = 1.8$ MPa, allow it to fit the countour of micro surfaces and its low surface energy, $\gamma = 21.6$ dyn/cm^2. This is a parallel process and can thus place nanoscale objects over a large area in a short time.

- Dip-pen nanolithography

Dip-pen nanolithography is a process that uses an atomic force microscope to transfer molecules on the tip to a substrate. Initially the tip is dipped into a reservoir with an ink. The ink on the tip evaporates and leaves the desired molecules attached to the tip. When the tip is brought into contact with the surface a water meniscus forms between the tip and the surface resulting in the diffusion of molecules from the tip to the surface. These tips can have radii in the tens of nanometers, and thus SAM molecules can be very precisely deposited onto a specific location of the surface. This process was discovered by Chad Mirkin and co-workers at Northwestern University.

2. Locally Remove

The locally remove strategy begins with covering the entire surface with a SAM. Then individual SAM molecules are removed from locations where the deposition of nanostructures is not desired. The end result is the same as in the locally attract strategy, the difference being in the way this is achieved. The major techniques that use this strategy are:

- Scanning tunneling microscope

The scanning tunneling microscope can remove SAM molecules in many different ways. The first is to remove them mechanically by dragging the tip across the substrate surface. This is not the most desired technique as these tips are expensive and dragging them causes a lot of wear and reduction of the tip quality. The second way is to degrade or desorb the SAM molecules by shooting them with an electron beam. The scanning tunneling microscope can also remove SAMs by field desorption and field enhanced surface diffusion.

- Atomic force microscope

The most common use of this technique is to remove the SAM molecules in a process called shaving, where the atomic force microscope tip is dragged along the surface mechanically removing the molecules. An atomic force microscope can also remove SAM molecules by local oxidation nanolithography.

- Ultraviolet irradiation

In this process, UV light is projected onto the surface with a SAM through a pattern of apperatures in a chromium film. This leads to photo oxidation of the SAM molecules. These can then be washed away in a polar solvent. This process has 100 nm resolutions and requires exposure time of 15–20 minutes.

3. Modify Tail Groups

The final strategy focuses not on the deposition or removal of SAMS, but the modification of terminal groups. In the first case the terminal group can be modified to remove functionality so that SAM molecule will be inert. In the same regards the terminal group can be modified to add functionality so it can accept different materials or have different properties than the original SAM terminal group. The major techniques that use this strategy are:

- Focused electron beam and ultraviolet irradiation

Exposure to electron beams and UV light changes the terminal group chemistry. Some of the changes that can occur include the cleavage of bonds, the forming of double carbon bonds, cross-linking of adjacent molecules, fragmentation of molecules, and confromational disorder.

- Atomic force microscope

A conductive AFM tip can create an electrochemical reaction that can change the terminal group.

Applications

Thin-film SAMs

SAMs are an inexpensive and versatile surface coating for applications including control of wetting and adhesion, chemical resistance, bio compatibility, sensitization, and molecular recognition for sensors and nano fabrication. Areas of application for SAMs include biology, electrochemistry and electronics, nanoelectromechanical systems (NEMS) and microelectromechanical systems (MEMS), and everyday household goods. SAMs can serve as models for studying membrane properties of cells and organelles and cell attachment on surfaces. SAMs can also be used to modify the surface properties of electrodes for electrochemistry, general electronics, and various NEMS and MEMS. For example, the properties of SAMs can be used to control electron transfer in electrochemistry. They can serve to protect metals from harsh chemicals and etchants. SAMs can also reduce sticking of NEMS and MEMS components in humid environments. In the same way, SAMs can alter the properties of glass. A common household product, Rain-X, utilizes SAMs to create a hydrophobic monolayer on car windshields to keep them clear of rain. Another application is an anti-adhesion coating on nanoimprint lithography (NIL) tools and stamps. One can also coat injection molding tools for polymer replication with a Perfluordecyltrichlorosilane SAM.

Thin film SAMs can also be placed on nanostructures. In this way they functionalize the nanostructure. This is advantageous because the nanostructure can now selectively attach itself to other molecules or SAMs. This technique is useful in biosensors or other MEMS devices that need to separate one type of molecule from its environment. One example is the use of magnetic nanoparticles to remove a fungus from a blood stream. The nanoparticle is coated with a SAM that binds to the fungus. As the contaminated blood is filtered through a MEMS device the magnetic nanoparticles are inserted into the blood where they bind to the fungus and are then magnetically driven out of the blood stream into a nearby laminar waste stream.

Patterned SAMs

SAMs are also useful in depositing nanostructures, because each adsorbate molecule can be tailored to attract two different materials. Current techniques utilize the head to attract to a surface, like a plate of gold. The terminal group is then modified to attract a specific material like a particular nanoparticle, wire, ribbon, or other nanostructure. In this way, wherever the a SAM is patterned to a surface there will be nanostructures attached to the tail groups. One example is the use of two types of SAMs to align single wall carbon nanotubes, SWNTs. Dip pen nanolithography was used to pattern a 16-mercaptohexadecanoic acid (MHA)SAM and the rest of the surface was passivated with 1-octadecanethiol (ODT) SAM. The polar solvent that is carrying the SWNTs is attracted to the hydrophilic MHA; as the solvent evaporates, the SWNTs are close enough to the MHA SAM to attach to it due to Van der Waals forces. The nanotubes thus line up with the MHA-ODT boundary. Using this technique Chad Mirkin, Schatz and their co-workers were able to make complex two-dimensional shapes, a representation of a shape created is shown to the right.Another application of patterned SAMs is the functionalization of biosensors. The tail groups can be modified so they have an affinity for cells, proteins, or molecules. The SAM can then be placed onto a biosensor so that binding of these molecules can be detected. The ability to pattern these SAMs allows them to be placed in configurations that increase sensitivity and do not damage or interfere with other components of the biosensor.

Metal Organic Superlattices

There has been considerable interest in use of SAMs for new materials e.g. via formation of two- or three-dimensional metal organic superlattices by assembly of SAM capped nanoparticles or layer by layer SAM-nanoparticle arrays using dithiols.

SUPRAMOLECULAR ASSEMBLY

A supramolecular assembly or "supermolecule" is a well defined complex of molecules held together by noncovalent bonds. While a supramolecular assembly can be simply composed of two molecules (e.g., a DNA double helix or an inclusion compound), it is more often used to denote larger complexes of molecules that form sphere-, rod-, or sheet-like species. Micelles, liposomes and biological membranes are examples of supramolecular assemblies. The dimensions of supramolecular assemblies can range from nanometers to micrometers. Thus they allow access to nanoscale objects using a bottom-up approach in far fewer steps than a single molecule of similar dimensions.

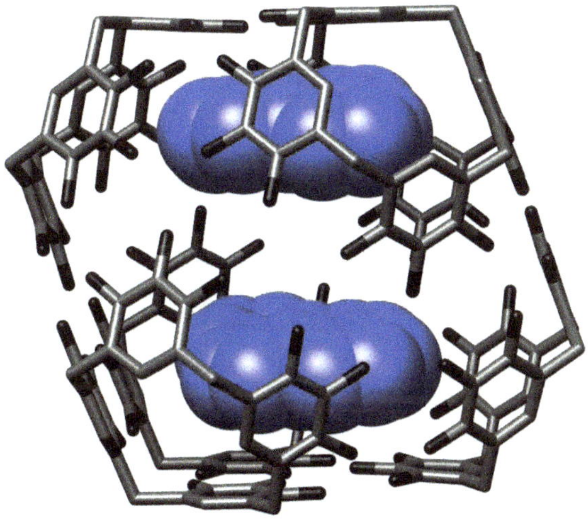

In this example two pyrene butyric acids are bound within a hexameric nanocapsule composed of six C-hexylpyrogallolarenes held together by hydrogen bonds. The side chains of the pyrene butyric acids are omitted.

The process by which a supramolecular assembly forms is called molecular self-assembly. Some try to distinguish self-assembly as the process by which individual molecules form the defined aggregate. Self-organization, then, is the process by which those aggregates create higher-order structures. This can become useful when talking about liquid crystals and block copolymers.

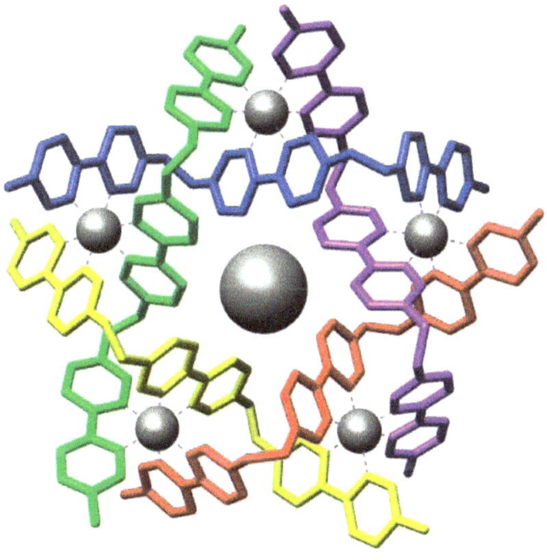

Circular hellcate $[(Fe_5L_5)Cl]^{9+}$, where L stands for s tris-bpy ligand strand; the central gray atom is Cl, while the smaller gray spheres are Fe.

Templating Reactions

As studied in coordination chemistry, metals (usually transition metals) exist in solution bound to ligands, In many cases, the coordination sphere defines geometries conducive to reactions either between ligands or involving ligands and other external reagents.

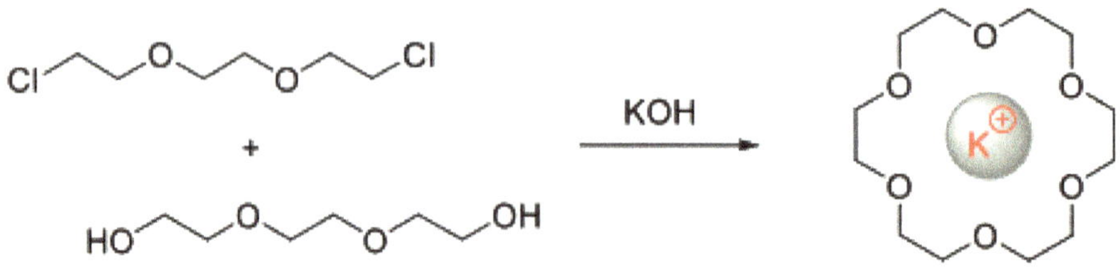

18-crown-6 can be synthesized from using potassium ion as the template cation

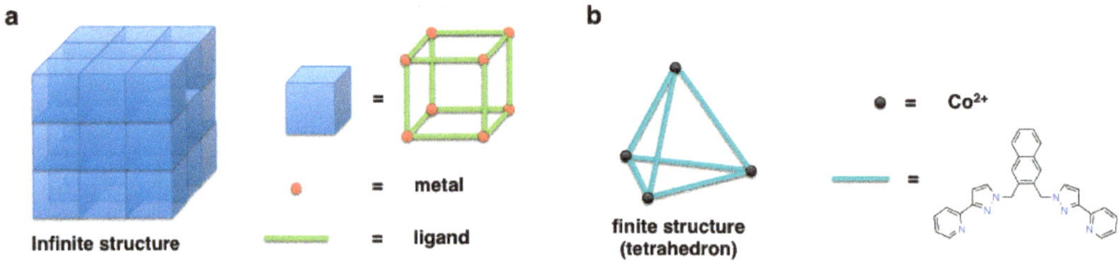

Illustrations of a. metal-organic frameworks and b. supramolecular coordination complexes

A well known metal-templating was described by Charles Pederson in his synthesis of various crown ethers using metal cations as template. For example, 18-crown-6 strongly coordinates potassium ion thus can be prepared through the Williamson ether synthesis using potassium ion as the template metal.

Metals are frequently used for assembly of large supramolecular structures. Metal organic frameworks (MOFs) are one example. MOFs are infinite structures where metal serve as nodes to connect organic ligands together. SCCs are discrete systems where selected metals and ligands undergo self-assembly to form finite supramolecular complexes, usually the size and structure of the complex formed can be determined by the angularity of chosen metal-ligand bonds.

Hydrogen Bond Assisted Supramolecular Assembly

Hydrogen bond-assisted supramolecular assembly is the process of assembling small organic molecules to form large supramolecular structures by non-covalent hydrogen bonding interactions. The directionality, reversibility, and strong bonding nature of hydrogen bond make it an attractive and useful approach in supramolecular assembly. Functional groups such as carboxylic acids, ureas, amines, and amides are commonly used to assemble higher order structures upon hydrogen bonding.

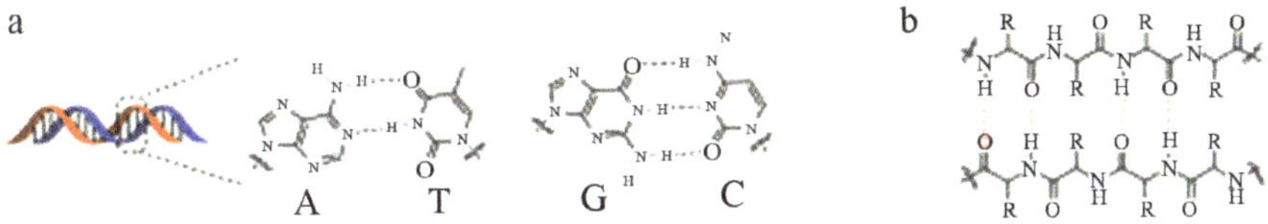

Hydrogen bonds in (a) DNA duplex formation and (b) protein β-sheet structure

(a) Representative hydrogen bond patterns in supramolecular assembly. (b) Hydrogen bond network in cyanuric acid-melamine crystals.

Hydrogen bond play an essential role in the assembly of secondary and tertiary structures of large biomolecules. DNA double helix is formed by hydrogen bonding between nucleobases: adenine and thymine forms two hydrogen bonds, while guanine and cytosine forms three hydrogen bonds (Figure Hydrogen bonds in (a) DNA duplex formation). Another prominent example of hydrogen bond-assisted assembly in nature is the formation of protein secondary structures. Both the α-helix and β-sheet are formed through hydrogen bonding between the amide hydrogen and the amide carbonyl oxygen (Figure Hydrogen bonds in (b) protein β-sheet structure).

In supramolecular chemistry, hydrogen bonds have been broadly applied to crystal engineering, molecular recognition, and catalysis. Hydrogen bonds are among the mostly used synthons in bottom-up approach to engineering molecular interactions in crystals. Representative hydrogen bond patterns for supramolecular assembly is shown in Figure Representative hydrogen bond patterns in supramolecular assembly. A 1: 1 mixture of cyanuric acid and melamine forms crystal with a highly dense hydrogen-bonding network. This supramolecular aggregates has been used as templates to engineering other crystal structures.

Applications

Supramolecular assemblies have no specific applications but are the subject of many intriguing reactions. A supramolecular assembly of peptide amphiphiles in the form of nanofibers has been shown to promote the growth of neurons. An advantage to this supramolecular approach is that the nanofibers will degrade back into the individual peptide molecules that can be broken down by the body. By self-assembling of dendritic dipeptides, hollow cylinders can be produced. The cylindrical assemblies possess internal helical order and self-organize into columnar liquid crystalline lattices. When inserted into vesicular membranes, the porous cylindrical assemblies mediate transport of protons across the membrane. Self-assembly of dendrons generates arrays of nanowires. Electron donor-acceptor complexes comprise the core of the cylindrical supramolecular assemblies, which further self-organize into two-dimensional columnar liquid crystaline lattices. Each cylindrical supramolecular assembly functions as an individual wire. High charge carrier mobilities for holes and electrons were obtained.

DNA NANOTECHNOLOGY

DNA nanotechnology is the design and manufacture of artificial nucleic acid structures for technological uses. In this field, nucleic acids are used as non-biological engineering materials for nanotechnology rather than as the carriers of genetic information in living cells. Researchers in the field have created static structures such as two- and three-dimensional crystal lattices, nanotubes, polyhedra, and arbitrary shapes, and functional devices such as molecular machines and DNA computers. The field is beginning to be used as a tool to solve basic science problems in structural biology and biophysics, including applications in X-ray crystallography and nuclear magnetic resonance spectroscopy of proteins to determine structures. Potential applications in molecular scale electronics and nanomedicine are also being investigated.

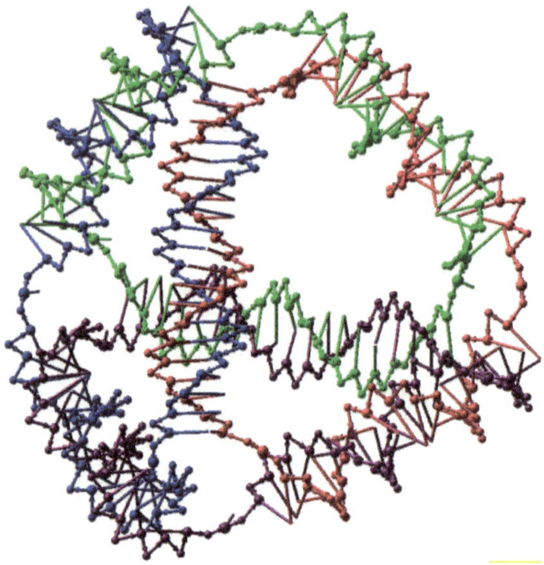

DNA nanotechnology involves forming artificial, designed nanostructures out of nucleic acids, such as this DNA tetrahedron.Each edge of the tetrahedron is a 20 base pair DNA double helix, and each vertex is a three-arm junction. The 4 DNA strands that form the 4 tetrahedral faces are color-coded.

The conceptual foundation for DNA nanotechnology was first laid out by Nadrian Seeman in the early 1980s, and the field began to attract widespread interest in the mid-2000s. This use of nucleic acids is enabled by their strict base pairing rules, which cause only portions of strands with complementary base sequences to bind together to form strong, rigid double helix structures. This allows for the rational design of base sequences that will selectively assemble to form complex target structures with precisely controlled nanoscale features. Several assembly methods are used to make these structures, including tile-based structures that assemble from smaller structures, folding structures using the DNA origami method, and dynamically reconfigurable structures using strand displacement methods. While the field's name specifically references DNA, the same principles have been used with other types of nucleic acids as well, leading to the occasional use of the alternative name *nucleic acid nanotechnology*.

Fundamental Concepts

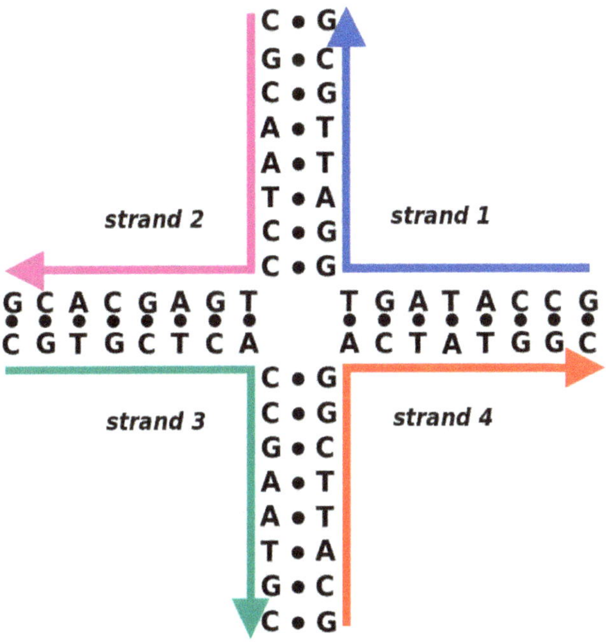

These four strands associate into a DNA four-arm junction because this structure maximizes the number of correct base pairs, with A matched to T and C matched to G. See this image for a more realistic model of the four-arm junction showing its tertiary structure.

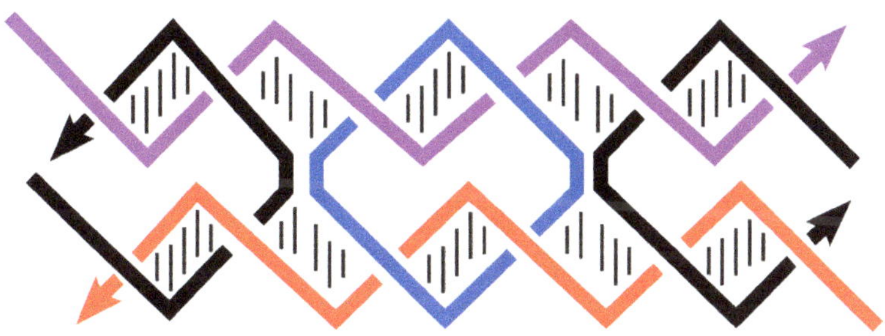

This double-crossover (DX) supramolecular complex consists of five DNA single strands that form two double-helical domains, on the top and the bottom in this image. There are two crossover points where the strands cross from one domain into the other.

Properties of Nucleic Acids

Nanotechnology is often defined as the study of materials and devices with features on a scale below 100 nanometers. DNA nanotechnology, specifically, is an example of bottom-up molecular self-assembly, in which molecular components spontaneously organize into stable structures; the particular form of these structures is induced by the physical and chemical properties of the components selected by the designers. In DNA nanotechnology, the component materials are strands of nucleic acids such as DNA; these strands are often synthetic and are almost always used outside the context of a living cell. DNA is well-suited to nanoscale construction because the binding between two nucleic acid strands depends on simple base pairing rules which are well understood, and form the specific nanoscale structure of the nucleic acid double helix. These qualities make the assembly of nucleic acid structures easy to control through nucleic acid design. This property is absent in other materials used in nanotechnology, including proteins, for which protein design is very difficult, and nanoparticles, which lack the capability for specific assembly on their own.

The structure of a nucleic acid molecule consists of a sequence of nucleotides distinguished by which nucleobase they contain. In DNA, the four bases present are adenine (A), cytosine (C), guanine (G), and thymine (T). Nucleic acids have the property that two molecules will only bind to each other to form a double helix if the two sequences are complementary, meaning that they form matching sequences of base pairs, with A only binding to T, and C only to G. Because the formation of correctly matched base pairs is energetically favorable, nucleic acid strands are expected in most cases to bind to each other in the conformation that maximizes the number of correctly paired bases. The sequences of bases in a system of strands thus determine the pattern of binding and the overall structure in an easily controllable way. In DNA nanotechnology, the base sequences of strands are rationally designed by researchers so that the base pairing interactions cause the strands to assemble in the desired conformation. While DNA is the dominant material used, structures incorporating other nucleic acids such as RNA and peptide nucleic acid (PNA) have also been constructed.

Subfields

DNA nanotechnology is sometimes divided into two overlapping subfields: structural DNA nanotechnology and dynamic DNA nanotechnology. Structural DNA nanotechnology, sometimes abbreviated as SDN, focuses on synthesizing and characterizing nucleic acid complexes and materials that assemble into a static, equilibrium end state. On the other hand, dynamic DNA nanotechnology focuses on complexes with useful non-equilibrium behavior such as the ability to reconfigure based on a chemical or physical stimulus. Some complexes, such as nucleic acid nanomechanical devices, combine features of both the structural and dynamic subfields.

The complexes constructed in structural DNA nanotechnology use topologically branched nucleic acid structures containing junctions. (In contrast, most biological DNA exists as an unbranched double helix.) One of the simplest branched structures is a four-arm junction that consists of four individual DNA strands, portions of which are complementary in a specific pattern. Unlike in natural Holliday junctions, each arm in the artificial immobile four-arm junction has a different base sequence, causing the junction point to be fixed at a certain position. Multiple junctions can be combined in the same complex, such as in the widely used double-crossover (DX) structural motif, which contains two parallel double helical domains with individual strands crossing between the domains at two crossover points. Each crossover point is, topologically, a four-arm junction, but is constrained to one orientation, in contrast to the flexible single four-arm junction, providing a rigidity that makes the DX motif suitable as a structural building block for larger DNA complexes.

Dynamic DNA nanotechnology uses a mechanism called toehold-mediated strand displacement to allow the nucleic acid complexes to reconfigure in response to the addition of a new nucleic acid strand. In this reaction, the incoming strand binds to a single-stranded toehold region of a double-stranded complex, and then displaces one of the strands bound in the original complex through a branch migration process. The overall effect is that one of the strands in the complex is replaced with another one. In addition, reconfigurable structures and devices can be made using functional nucleic acids such as deoxyribozymes and ribozymes, which can perform chemical reactions, and aptamers, which can bind to specific proteins or small molecules.

Structural DNA Nanotechnology

Structural DNA nanotechnology, sometimes abbreviated as SDN, focuses on synthesizing and characterizing nucleic acid complexes and materials where the assembly has a static, equilibrium endpoint. The nucleic acid double helix has a robust, defined three-dimensional geometry that makes it possible to predict and design the structures of more complicated nucleic acid complexes. Many such structures have been created, including two- and three-dimensional structures, and periodic, aperiodic, and discrete structures.

Extended Lattices

Small nucleic acid complexes can be equipped with sticky ends and combined into larger two-dimensional periodic lattices containing a specific tessellated pattern of the individual molecular tiles. The earliest example of this used double-crossover (DX) complexes as the basic tiles, each containing four sticky ends designed with sequences that caused the DX units to combine into periodic two-dimensional flat sheets that are essentially rigid two-dimensional crystals of DNA. Two-dimensional arrays have been made from other motifs as well, including the Holliday junction rhombus lattice, and various DX-based arrays making use of a double-cohesion scheme. The top two images at right show examples of tile-based periodic lattices.

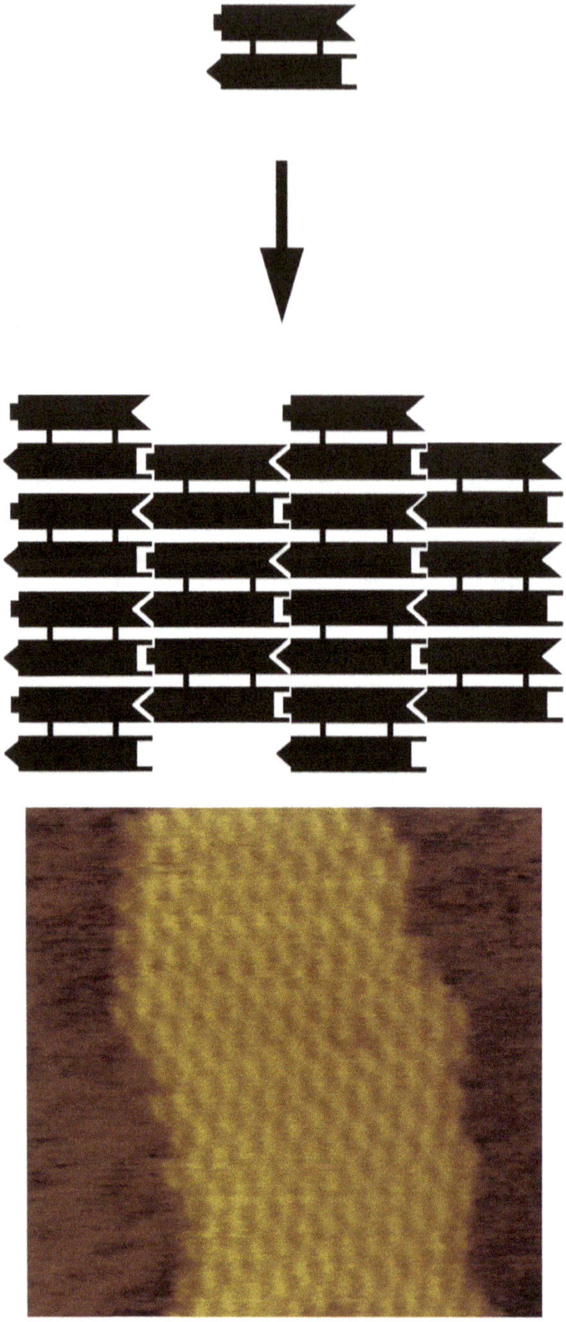

The assembly of a DX array. *Left*, schematic diagram. Each bar represents a double-helical domain of DNA, with the shapes representing complementary sticky ends. The DX complex at top will combine with other DX complexes into the two-dimensional array shown at bottom. *Right*, an atomic force microscopy image of the assembled array. The individual DX tiles are clearly visible within the assembled structure. The field is 150 nm across.

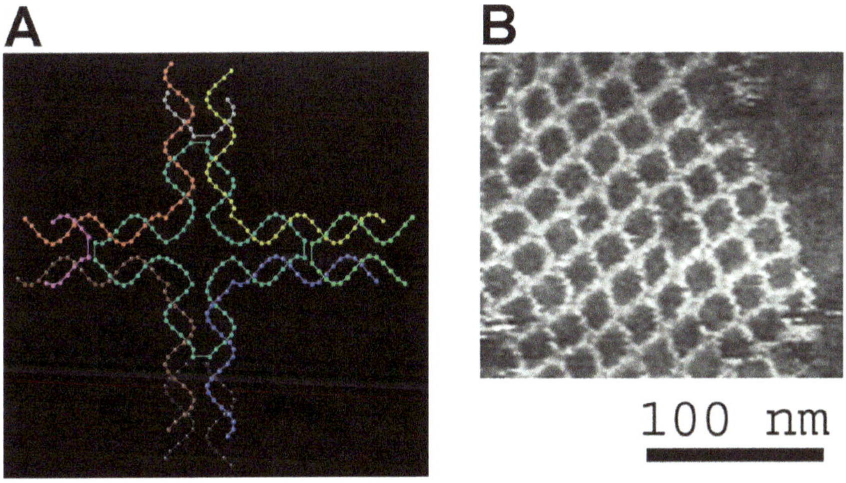

Left, a model of a DNA tile used to make another two-dimensional periodic lattice. *Right*, an atomic force micrograph of the assembled lattice.

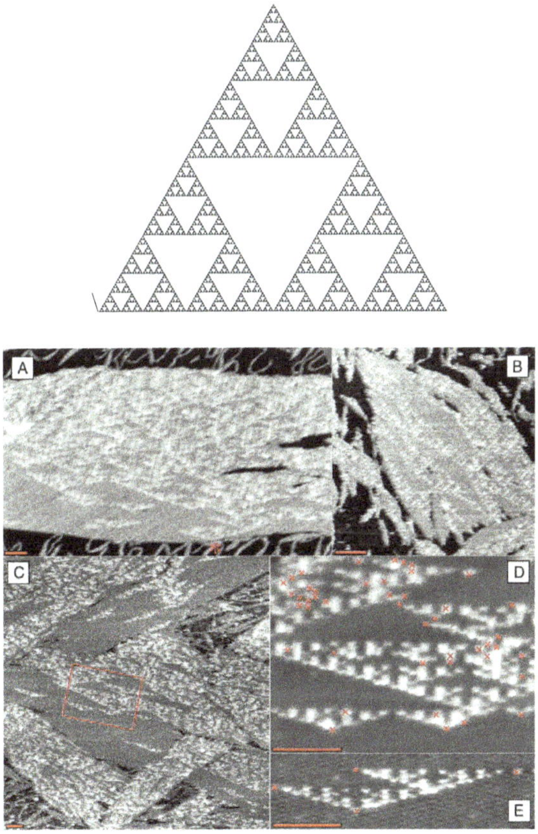

An example of an aperiodic two-dimensional lattice that assembles into a fractal pattern. *Left*, the Sierpinski gasket fractal. *Right*, DNA arrays that display a representation of the Sierpinski gasket on their surfaces

Two-dimensional arrays can be made to exhibit aperiodic structures whose assembly implements a specific algorithm, exhibiting one form of DNA computing. The DX tiles can have their sticky end sequences chosen so that they act as Wang tiles, allowing them to perform computation. A DX array whose assembly encodes an XOR operation has been demonstrated; this allows the DNA array to implement a cellular automaton that generates a fractal known as the Sierpinski gasket. The third image at right shows this type of array. Another system has the function of a binary counter, displaying a representation of increasing binary numbers as it grows. These results show that computation can be incorporated into the assembly of DNA arrays.

DX arrays have been made to form hollow nanotubes 4–20 nm in diameter, essentially two-dimensional lattices which curve back upon themselves. These DNA nanotubes are somewhat similar in size and shape to carbon nanotubes, and while they lack the electrical conductance of carbon nanotubes, DNA nanotubes are more easily modified and connected to other structures. One of many schemes for constructing DNA nanotubes uses a lattice of curved DX tiles that curls around itself and closes into a tube. In an alternative method that allows the circumference to be specified in a simple, modular fashion using single-stranded tiles, the rigidity of the tube is an emergent property.

Forming three-dimensional lattices of DNA was the earliest goal of DNA nanotechnology, but this proved to be one of the most difficult to realize. Success using a motif based on the concept of tensegrity, a balance between tension and compression forces, was finally reported in 2009.

Discrete Structures

Researchers have synthesized many three-dimensional DNA complexes that each have the connectivity of a polyhedron, such as a cube or octahedron, meaning that the DNA duplexes trace the edges of a polyhedron with a DNA junction at each vertex. The earliest demonstrations of DNA polyhedra were very work-intensive, requiring multiple ligations and solid-phase synthesis steps to create catenated polyhedra. Subsequent work yielded polyhedra whose synthesis was much easier. These include a DNA octahedron made from a long single strand designed to fold into the correct conformation, and a tetrahedron that can be produced from four DNA strands in one step, pictured at the top of this article.

Nanostructures of arbitrary, non-regular shapes are usually made using the DNA origami method. These structures consist of a long, natural virus strand as a "scaffold", which is made to fold into the desired shape by computationally designed short "staple" strands. This method has the advantages of being easy to design, as the base sequence is predetermined by the scaffold strand sequence, and not requiring high strand purity and accurate stoichiometry, as most other DNA nanotechnology methods do. DNA origami was first demonstrated for two-dimensional shapes, such as a smiley face and a coarse map of the Western Hemisphere. Solid three-dimensional structures can be made by using parallel DNA helices arranged in a honeycomb pattern, and structures with two-dimensional faces can be made to fold into a hollow overall three-dimensional shape, akin to a cardboard box. These can be programmed to open and reveal or release a molecular cargo in response to a stimulus, making them potentially useful as programmable molecular cages.

Templated Assembly

Nucleic acid structures can be made to incorporate molecules other than nucleic acids, sometimes called heteroelements, including proteins, metallic nanoparticles, quantum dots, and fullerenes. This allows the construction of materials and devices with a range of functionalities much greater than is possible with nucleic acids alone. The goal is to use the self-assembly of the nucleic acid structures to template the assembly of the nanoparticles hosted on them, controlling their position and in some cases orientation. Many of these schemes use a covalent attachment scheme, using oligonucleotides with amide or thiol functional groups as a chemical handle to bind the heteroelements. This covalent binding scheme has been used to arrange gold nanoparticles on a DX-based array, and to arrange streptavidin protein molecules into specific patterns on a DX array. A non-covalent hosting scheme using Dervan polyamides on a DX array was used to arrange streptavidin proteins in a specific pattern on a DX array. Carbon nanotubes have been hosted on DNA arrays in a pattern allowing the assembly to act as a molecular electronic device, a carbon nanotube field-effect transistor. In addition, there are nucleic acid metallization methods, in which the nucleic acid is replaced by a metal which assumes the general shape of the original nucleic acid structure, and schemes for using nucleic acid nanostructures as lithography masks, transferring their pattern into a solid surface.

Dynamic DNA Nanotechnology

Dynamic DNA nanotechnology focuses on forming nucleic acid systems with designed dynamic functionalities related to their overall structures, such as computation and mechanical motion.

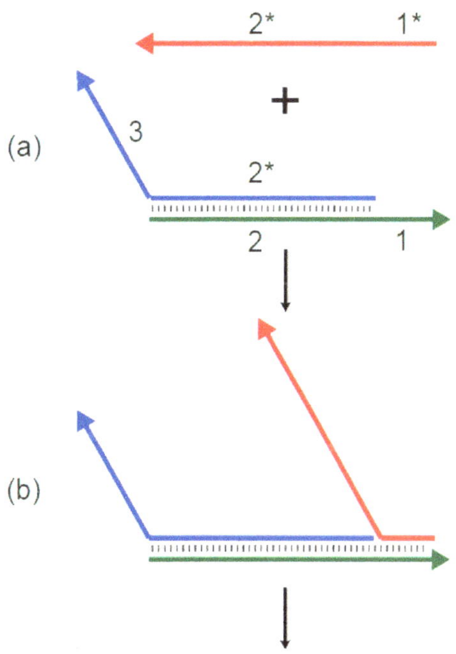

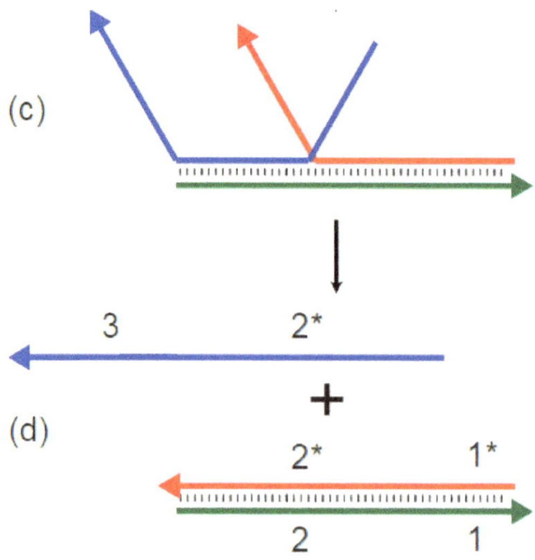

Dynamic DNA nanotechnology often makes use of toehold-mediated strand displacement reactions. In this example, the red strand binds to the single stranded toehold region on the green strand (region 1), and then in a branch migration process across region 2, the blue strand is displaced and freed from the complex. Reactions like these are used to dynamically reconfigure or assemble nucleic acid nanostructures. In addition, the red and blue strands can be used as signals in a molecular logic gate.

There is some overlap between structural and dynamic DNA nanotechnology, as structures can be formed through annealing and then reconfigured dynamically, or can be made to form dynamically in the first place.

Nanomechanical Devices

DNA complexes have been made that change their conformation upon some stimulus, making them one form of nanorobotics. These structures are initially formed in the same way as the static structures made in structural DNA nanotechnology, but are designed so that dynamic reconfiguration is possible after the initial assembly. The earliest such device made use of the transition between the B-DNA and Z-DNA forms to respond to a change in buffer conditions by undergoing a twisting motion. This reliance on buffer conditions, however, caused all devices to change state at the same time. Subsequent systems could change states based upon the presence of control strands, allowing multiple devices to be independently operated in solution. Some examples of such systems are a "molecular tweezers" design that has an open and a closed state, a device that could switch from a paranemic-crossover (PX) conformation to a double-junction (JX2) conformation, undergoing rotational motion in the process, and a two-dimensional array that could dynamically expand and contract in response to control strands. Structures have also been made that dynamically open or close, potentially acting as a molecular cage to release or reveal a functional cargo upon opening.

DNA walkers are a class of nucleic acid nanomachines that exhibit directional motion along a linear track. A large number of schemes have been demonstrated. One strategy is to control the motion of the walker along the track using control strands that need to be manually added in sequence. Another approach is to make use of restriction enzymes or deoxyribozymes to cleave the strands and cause the walker to move forward, which has the advantage of running autonomously. A later system could walk upon a two-dimensional surface rather than a linear track, and demonstrated the ability to selectively pick up and move molecular cargo. Additionally, a linear walker has been demonstrated that performs DNA-templated synthesis as the walker advances along the track, allowing autonomous multistep chemical synthesis directed by the walker. The synthetic DNA walkers' function is similar to that of the proteins dynein and kinesin.

Strand Displacement Cascades

Cascades of strand displacement reactions can be used for either computational or structural purposes. An individual strand displacement reaction involves revealing a new sequence in response to the presence of some initiator strand. Many such reactions can be linked into a cascade where the newly revealed output sequence of one reaction can initiate another strand displacement reaction elsewhere. This in turn allows for the construction of chemical reaction networks with many components, exhibiting complex computational and information processing abilities. These cascades are made energetically favorable through the formation of new base pairs, and the entropy gain from disassembly reactions. Strand displacement cascades allow isothermal operation of the assembly or computational process, in contrast to traditional nucleic acid assembly's requirement for a thermal annealing step, where the temperature is raised and then slowly lowered to ensure proper formation of the desired structure. They can also support catalytic function of the initiator species, where less than one equivalent of the initiator can cause the reaction to go to completion.

Strand displacement complexes can be used to make molecular logic gates capable of complex computation. Unlike traditional electronic computers, which use electric current as inputs and outputs, molecular computers use the concentrations of specific chemical species as signals. In the case of nucleic acid strand displacement circuits, the signal is the presence of nucleic acid strands that are released or consumed by binding and unbinding events to other strands in displacement complexes. This approach has been used to make logic gates such as AND, OR, and NOT gates. More recently, a four-bit circuit was demonstrated that can compute the square root of the integers 0–15, using a system of gates containing 130 DNA strands.

Another use of strand displacement cascades is to make dynamically assembled structures. These use a hairpin structure for the reactants, so that when the input strand binds, the newly revealed sequence is on the same molecule rather than disassembling. This allows new opened hairpins to be added to a growing complex. This approach has been used to make simple structures such as three- and four-arm junctions and dendrimers.

Applications

DNA nanotechnology provides one of the few ways to form designed, complex structures with precise control over nanoscale features. The field is beginning to see application to solve basic science problems in structural biology and biophysics. The earliest such application envisaged for the field, and one still in development, is in crystallography, where molecules that are difficult to crystallize in isolation could be arranged within a three-dimensional nucleic acid lattice, allowing determination of their structure. Another application is the use of DNA origami rods to replace liquid crystals in residual dipolar coupling experiments in protein NMR spectroscopy; using DNA origami is advantageous because, unlike liquid crystals, they are tolerant of the detergents needed to suspend membrane proteins in solution. DNA walkers have been used as nanoscale assembly lines to move nanoparticles and direct chemical synthesis. Further, DNA origami structures have aided in the biophysical studies of enzyme function and protein folding.

DNA nanotechnology is moving toward potential real-world applications. The ability of nucleic acid arrays to arrange other molecules indicates its potential applications in molecular scale electronics. The assembly of a nucleic acid structure could be used to template the assembly of a molecular electronic elements such as molecular wires, providing a method for nanometer-scale control of the placement and overall architecture of the device analogous to a molecular breadboard. DNA nanotechnology has been compared to the concept of programmable matter because of the coupling of computation to its material properties.

In a study conducted by a group of scientists from iNANO center and CDNA Center in Aarhus university (Aarhus), researchers were able to construct a small multi-switchable 3D DNA Box Origami. The proposed nanoparticle was characterized by atomic force microscopy (AFM), transmission electron microscopy (TEM) and Förster resonance energy transfer (FRET). The constructed box was shown to have a unique reclosing mechanism, which enabled it to repeatedly open and close in response to a unique set of DNA or RNA keys. The authors proposed that this "DNA device can potentially be used for a broad range of applications such as controlling the function of single molecules, controlled drug delivery, and molecular computing.".

There are potential applications for DNA nanotechnology in nanomedicine, making use of its ability to perform computation in a biocompatible format to make "smart drugs" for targeted drug delivery. One such system being investigated uses a hollow DNA box containing proteins that induce apoptosis, or cell death, that will only open when in proximity to a cancer cell. There has additionally been interest in expressing these artificial structures in engineered living bacterial cells, most likely using the transcribed RNA for the assembly, although it is unknown whether these complex structures are able to efficiently fold or assemble in the cell's cytoplasm. If successful, this could enable directed evolution of nucleic acid nanostructures. Scientists at Oxford University reported the self-assembly of four short strands of synthetic DNA into a cage which can enter cells and survive for at least 48 hours. The fluorescently labeled DNA tetrahedra were found to remain intact in the laboratory cultured human kidney cells despite the attack by cellular enzymes after two days. This experiment showed the potential of drug delivery inside the living cells using the DNA 'cage'. A DNA tetrahedron was used to deliver RNA Interference (RNAi) in a mouse model, reported a team of researchers in MIT. Delivery of the interfering RNA for treatment has showed some success using polymer or lipid, but there are limits of safety and imprecise targeting, in addition to short shelf life in the blood stream. The DNA nanostructure created by the team consists of six strands of

DNA to form a tetrahedron, with one strand of RNA affixed to each of the six edges. The tetrahedron is further equipped with targeting protein, three folate molecules, which lead the DNA nanoparticles to the abundant folate receptors found on some tumors. The result showed that the gene expression targeted by the RNAi, luciferase, dropped by more than half. This study shows promise in using DNA nanotechnology as an effective tool to deliver treatment using the emerging RNA Interference technology.

Design

DNA nanostructures must be rationally designed so that individual nucleic acid strands will assemble into the desired structures. This process usually begins with specification of a desired target structure or function. Then, the overall secondary structure of the target complex is determined, specifying the arrangement of nucleic acid strands within the structure, and which portions of those strands should be bound to each other. The last step is the primary structure design, which is the specification of the actual base sequences of each nucleic acid strand.

Structural Design

The first step in designing a nucleic acid nanostructure is to decide how a given structure should be represented by a specific arrangement of nucleic acid strands. This design step determines the secondary structure, or the positions of the base pairs that hold the individual strands together in the desired shape. Several approaches have been demonstrated:

- Tile-based structures. This approach breaks the target structure into smaller units with strong binding between the strands contained in each unit, and weaker interactions between the units. It is often used to make periodic lattices, but can also be used to implement algorithmic self-assembly, making them a platform for DNA computing. This was the dominant design strategy used from the mid-1990s until the mid-2000s, when the DNA origami methodology was developed.
- Folding structures. An alternative to the tile-based approach, folding approaches make the nanostructure from one long strand, which can either have a designed sequence that folds due to its interactions with itself, or it can be folded into the desired shape by using shorter, “staple” strands. This latter method is called DNA origami, which allows forming nanoscale two- and three-dimensional shapes.
- Dynamic assembly. This approach directly controls the kinetics of DNA self-assembly, specifying all of the intermediate steps in the reaction mechanism in addition to the final product. This is done using starting materials which adopt a hairpin structure; these then assemble into the final conformation in a cascade reaction, in a specific order. This approach has the advantage of proceeding isothermally, at a constant temperature. This is in contrast to the thermodynamic approaches, which require a thermal annealing step where a temperature change is required to trigger the assembly and favor proper formation of the desired structure.

Sequence Design

After any of the above approaches are used to design the secondary structure of a target complex, an actual sequence of nucleotides that will form into the desired structure must be devised. Nucleic acid design is the process of assigning a specific nucleic acid base sequence to each of a structure's constituent strands so that they will associate into a desired conformation. Most methods have the goal of designing sequences so that the target structure has the lowest energy, and is thus the most thermodynamically favorable, while incorrectly assembled structures have higher energies and are thus disfavored. This is done either through simple, faster heuristic methods such as sequence symmetry minimization, or by using a full nearest-neighbor thermodynamic model, which is more accurate but slower and more computationally intensive. Geometric models are used to examine tertiary structure of the nanostructures and to ensure that the complexes are not overly strained.

Nucleic acid design has similar goals to protein design. In both, the sequence of monomers is designed to favor the desired target structure and to disfavor other structures. Nucleic acid design has the advantage of being much computationally easier than protein design, because the simple base pairing rules are sufficient to predict a structure's energetic favorability, and detailed information about the overall three-dimensional folding of the structure is not required. This allows the use of simple heuristic methods that yield experimentally robust designs. However, nucleic acid structures are less versatile than proteins in their function because of proteins' increased ability to fold into complex structures, and the limited chemical diversity of the four nucleotides as compared to the twenty proteinogenic amino acids.

Materials and Methods

The sequences of the DNA strands making up a target structure are designed computationally, using molecular modeling and thermodynamic modeling software. The nucleic acids themselves are then synthesized using standard oligonucleotide synthesis methods, usually automated in an oligonucleotide synthesizer, and strands of custom sequences are commercially available. Strands can be purified by denaturing gel electrophoresis if needed, and precise concentrations determined via any of several nucleic acid quantitation methods using ultraviolet absorbance spectroscopy.

The fully formed target structures can be verified using native gel electrophoresis, which gives size and shape information for the nucleic acid complexes. An electrophoretic mobility shift assay can assess whether a structure incorporates all desired strands. Fluorescent labeling and Förster resonance energy transfer (FRET) are sometimes used to characterize the structure of the complexes.

Nucleic acid structures can be directly imaged by atomic force microscopy, which is well suited to extended two-dimensional structures, but less useful for discrete three-dimensional structures because of the microscope tip's interaction with the fragile nucleic acid structure; transmission electron microscopy and cryo-electron microscopy are often used in this case. Extended three-dimensional lattices are analyzed by X-ray crystallography.

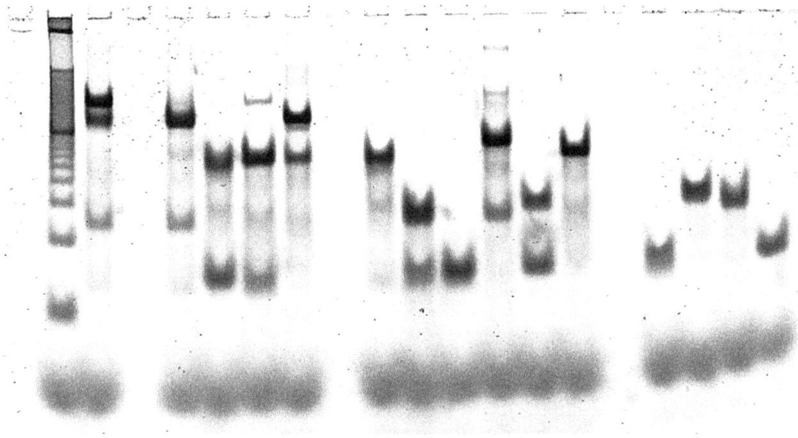

Gel electrophoresis methods, such as this formation assay on a DX complex, are used to ascertain whether the desired structures are forming properly. Each vertical lane contains a series of bands, where each band is characteristic of a particular reaction intermediate.

History

The conceptual foundation for DNA nanotechnology was first laid out by Nadrian Seeman in the early 1980s. Seeman's original motivation was to create a three-dimensional DNA lattice for orienting other large molecules, which would simplify their crystallographic study by eliminating the difficult process of obtaining pure crystals. This idea had reportedly come to him in late 1980, after realizing the similarity between the woodcut *Depth* by M. C. Escher and an array of DNA six-arm junctions. Several natural branched DNA structures were known at the time, including the DNA replication fork and the mobile Holliday junction, but Seeman's insight was that immobile nucleic acid junctions could be created by properly designing the strand sequences to remove symmetry in the assembled molecule, and that these immobile junctions could in principle be combined into rigid crystalline lattices. The first theoretical paper proposing this scheme was published in 1982, and the first experimental demonstration of an immobile DNA junction was published the following year.

In 1991, Seeman's laboratory published a report on the synthesis of a cube made of DNA, the first synthetic three-dimensional nucleic acid nanostructure, for which he received the 1995 Feynman Prize in Nanotechnology. This was followed by a DNA truncated octahedron. However, it soon became clear that these structures, polygonal shapes with flexible junctions as their vertices, were not rigid enough to form extended three-dimensional lattices. Seeman developed the more rigid double-crossover (DX) structural motif, and in 1998, in collaboration with Erik Winfree, published the creation of two-dimensional lattices of DX tiles. These tile-based structures had the advantage that they provided the ability to implement DNA computing, which was demonstrated by Winfree and Paul Rothemund in their 2004 paper on the algorithmic self-assembly of a Sierpinski gasket structure, and for which they shared the 2006 Feynman Prize in Nanotechnology. Winfree's key insight was that the DX tiles could be used as Wang tiles, meaning that their assembly could perform computation. The synthesis of a three-dimensional lattice was finally published by Seeman in 2009, nearly thirty years after he had set out to achieve it.

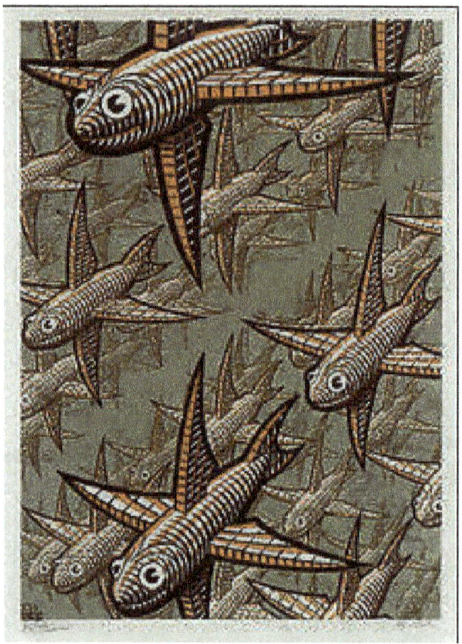

The woodcut *Depth* (pictured) by M. C. Escher reportedly inspired Nadrian Seeman to consider using three-dimensional lattices of DNA to orient hard-to-crystallize molecules. This led to the beginning of the field of DNA nanotechnology.

New abilities continued to be discovered for designed DNA structures throughout the 2000s. The first DNA nanomachine—a motif that changes its structure in response to an input—was demonstrated in 1999 by Seeman. An improved system, which was the first nucleic acid device to make use of toehold-mediated strand displacement, was demonstrated by Bernard Yurke the following year. The next advance was to translate this into mechanical motion, and in 2004 and 2005, several DNA walker systems were demonstrated by the groups of Seeman, Niles Pierce, Andrew Turberfield, and Chengde Mao. The idea of using DNA arrays to template the assembly of other molecules such as nanoparticles and proteins, first suggested by Bruche Robinson and Seeman in 1987, was demonstrated in 2002 by Seeman, Kiehl et al. and subsequently by many other groups.

In 2006, Rothemund first demonstrated the DNA origami method for easily and robustly forming folded DNA structures of arbitrary shape. Rothemund had conceived of this method as being conceptually intermediate between Seeman's DX lattices, which used many short strands, and William Shih's DNA octahedron, which consisted mostly of one very long strand. Rothemund's DNA origami contains a long strand which folding is assisted by several short strands. This method allowed forming much larger structures than formerly possible, and which are less technically demanding to design and synthesize. DNA origami was the cover story of *Nature* on March 15, 2006. Rothemund's research demonstrating two-dimensional DNA origami structures was followed by the demonstration of solid three-dimensional DNA origami by Douglas *et al.* in 2009, while the labs of Jørgen Kjems and Yan demonstrated hollow three-dimensional structures made out of two-dimensional faces.

DNA nanotechnology was initially met with some skepticism due to the unusual non-biological use of nucleic acids as materials for building structures and doing computation, and the preponderance of proof of principle experiments that extended the abilities of the field but were far from actual applications. Seeman's 1991 paper on the synthesis of the DNA cube was rejected by the journal *Science* after one reviewer praised its originality while another criticized it for its lack of biological relevance. By the early 2010s, however, the field was considered to have increased its abilities to the point that applications for basic science research were beginning to be realized, and practical applications in medicine and other fields were beginning to be considered feasible. The field had grown from very few active laboratories in 2001 to at least 60 in 2010, which increased the talent pool and thus the number of scientific advances in the field during that decade.

REFERENCES

1. Sweetman, A. M.; Jarvis, S. P.; Sang, Hongqian; Lekkas, I.; Rahe, P.; Wang, Yu; Wang, Jianbo; Champness, N.R.; Kantorovich, L.; Moriarty, P. (2014). "Mapping the force field of a hydrogen-bonded assembly". Nature Communications. 5. doi:10.1038/ncomms4931.
2. Hapala, Prokop; Kichin, Georgy; Wagner, Christian; Tautz, F. Stefan; Temirov, Ruslan; Jelínek, Pavel (2014-08-19). "Mechanism of high-resolution STM/AFM imaging with functionalized tips". Physical Review B. 90 (8): 085421. doi:10.1103/PhysRevB.90.085421.
3. Hämäläinen, Sampsa K.; van der Heijden, Nadine; van der Lit, Joost; den Hartog, Stephan; Liljeroth, Peter; Swart, Ingmar (2014-10-31). "Intermolecular Contrast in Atomic Force Microscopy Images without Intermolecular Bonds". Physical Review Letters. 113 (18): 186102. doi:10.1103/PhysRevLett.113.186102. PMID 25396382.
4. Pham, Tuan Anh; Song, Fei; Nguyen, Manh-Thuong; Stöhr, Meike (2014). "Self-assembly of pyrene derivatives on Au(111): Substituent effects on intermolecular interactions". Chem. Commun. 50 (91): 14089. doi:10.1039/C4CC02753A.
5. Lehn, J.-M. (1988). "Perspectives in Supramolecular Chemistry-From Molecular Recognition towards Molecular Information Processing and Self-Organization". Angew. Chem. Int. Ed. Engl. 27 (11): 89–121. doi:10.1002/anie.198800891.
6. Lehn, J.-M. (1990). "Supramolecular Chemistry-Scope and Perspectives: Molecules, Supermolecules, and Molecular Devices (Nobel Lecture)". Angew. Chem. Int. Ed. Engl. 29 (11): 1304–1319. doi:10.1002/anie.199013041.
7. Lehn, J.-M. Supramolecular Chemistry: Concepts and Perspectives. Wiley-VCH. ISBN 978-3-527-29311-7.
8. Rosen, Milton J. (2004). Surfactants and interfacial phenomena. Hoboken, NJ: Wiley-Interscience. ISBN 978-0-471-47818-8.

9. Ariga, Katsuhiko; Hill, Jonathan P; Lee, Michael V; Vinu, Ajayan; Charvet, Richard; Acharya, Somobrata (2008). "Challenges and breakthroughs in recent research on self-assembly". Science and Technology of Advanced Materials. 9 (1): 014109. Bibcode:2008STAdM...9a4109A. doi:10.1088/1468-6996/9/1/014109. PMC 5099804Freely accessible. PMID 27877935.

10. Mao, C; Sun, W; Seeman, N. C. (1997). "Assembly of Borromean rings from DNA". Nature. 386 (6621): 137–138. Bibcode:1997Natur.386..137M. doi:10.1038/386137b0. PMID 9062186.

11. Chichak, K. S.; Cantrill, S. J.; Pease, A. R.; Chiu, S. H.; Cave, G. W.; Atwood, J. L.; Stoddart, J. F. (2004). "Molecular Borromean Rings". Science. 304 (5675): 1308–1312. Bibcode:2004Sci...304.1308C. doi:10.1126/science.1096914. PMID 15166376.

12. Larsen, Randy (2008). "How fast do metal organic polyhedra form in solution? Kinetics of [Cu2(5-OH-bdc)2L2]12 formation in methanol". Journal of the American Chemical Society. 130 (34): 11246–11247. doi:10.1021/ja802605v.

13. Alkordi, Mohamed; Belof, Jonathan; Rivera, Edwin; Wojtas, Lukasz; Eddaoudi, Mohamed (2011). "Insight into the construction of metal–organic polyhedra: metal–organic cubes as a case study". Chemical Science. 2 (9): 1695–1705. doi:10.1039/C1SC00269D.

14. Min, Younjin; et al. (2008). "The role of interparticle and external forces in nanoparticle assembly". Nature Materials. 7 (7): 527–38. Bibcode:2008NatMa...7..527M. doi:10.1038/nmat2206. PMID 18574482.

15. Santos, Daniel; Spenko, Matthew; Parness, Aaron; Kim, Sangbae; Cutkosky, Mark (2007). "Directional adhesion for climbing: theoretical and practical considerations". Journal of Adhesion Science and Technology. 21 (12–13): 1317–1341. doi:10.1163/156856107782328399. Gecko "feet and toes are a hierarchical system of complex structures consisting of lamellae, setae,and spatulae. The distinguishing characteristics of the gecko adhesion system have been described [as] (1) anisotropic attachment, (2) high pulloff force to preload ratio, (3) low detachment force, (4) material independence, (5) self-cleaning, (6) anti-self sticking and (7) non-sticky default state. ... The gecko's adhesive structures are made from ß-keratin (modulus of elasticity [approx.] 2 GPa). Such a stiff material is not inherently sticky; however, because of the gecko adhesive's hierarchical nature and extremely small distal features (spatulae are [approx.] 200 nm in size), the gecko's foot is able to intimately conform to the surface and generate significant attraction using van der Waals forces.

16. Seeman, N. C. (2003). DNA in a material world. Nature. 421 (6921): 427–431. Bibcode:2003Natur.421..427S. doi:10.1038/nature01406. PMID 12540916.

17. Chen, J. & Seeman, N. C. (1991). Synthesis from DNA of a molecule with the connectivity of a cube. Nature. 350 (6319): 631–633. Bibcode:1991Natur.350..631C. doi:10.1038/350631a0. PMID 2017259.

18. Mirkin, C. A.; Letsinger, R. L.; Mucic, R. C.; Storhoff, J. J. (1996). A DNA-based method for rationally assembling nanoparticles into macroscopic materials. Nature.

382 (6592): 607–609. Bibcode:1996Natur.382..607M. doi:10.1038/382607a0. PMID 8757129.

19. Yan, H; Park, S. H.; Finkelstein, G; Reif, J. H.; Labean, T. H. (2003). DNA-Templated Self-Assembly of Protein Arrays and Highly Conductive Nanowires. Science. 301 (5641): 1882–1884. Bibcode:2003Sci...301.1882Y. doi:10.1126/science.1089389. PMID 14512621.
20. Foster, J. S. & Frommer, J. E. (1988). Imaging of liquid crystals using a tunnelling microscope. Nature. 333 (6173): 542–545. Bibcode:1988Natur.333..542F. doi:10.1038/333542a0.
21. Rabe, J.P. & Buchholz, S. (1991). Commensurability and Mobility in Two-Dimensional Molecular Patterns on Graphite. Science. 353 (5018): 424–427. Bibcode:1991Sci...253..424R. doi:10.1126/science.253.5018.424. JSTOR 2878886.
22. Love; et al. (2005). Self-Assembled Monolayers of Thiolates on Metals as a Form of Nanotechnology. Chem. Rev. 105 (4): 1103–1170. doi:10.1021/cr0300789. PMID 15826011.
23. Barlow, S.M.; Raval R.. (2003). Complex organic molecules at metal surfaces: bonding, organisation and chirality. Surface Science reports. 50 (6–8): 201–341. Bibcode:2003SurSR..50..201B. doi:10.1016/S0167-5729(03)00015-3.
24. Elemans, J.A.A.W.; Lei S., De Feyter S. (2009). Molecular and Supramolecular Networks on Surfaces: From Two-Dimensional Crystal Engineering to Reactivity. Angew. Chem. Int. Ed. 48 (40): 7298–7332. doi:10.1002/anie.200806339.
25. Witte, G.; Wöll Ch. (2004). Growth of aromatic molecules on solid substrates for applications in organic electronics. Journal of Material Research. 19 (7): 1889–1916. Bibcode:2004JMatR..19.1889W. doi:10.1557/JMR.2004.0251.
26. De Feyter, S.; De Schreyer F.C. (2003). Two-dimensional supramolecular self-assembly probed by scanning tunneling microscopy. Chemical Society Reviews. 32 (3): 139–150. doi:10.1039/b206566p. PMID 12792937.
27. Schwartz, D.K., Mechanisms and Kinetics of Self-Assembled Monolayer Formation (2001). Mechanisms and kinetics of self-assembled monolayer formation. Annu. Rev. Phys. Chem. 52: 107–37. Bibcode:2001ARPC...52..107S. doi:10.1146/annurev.physchem.52.1.107. PMID 11326061.
28. Schreiber, F (30 November 2000). Structure and growth of self-assembling monolayers. Progress in Surface Science. 65 (5–8): 151–257. Bibcode:2000PrSS...65..151S. doi:10.1016/S0079-6816(00)00024-1.
29. Wnek, Gary, Gary L. Bowlin (2004). Encyclopedia of Biomaterials and Biomedical Engineering. Informa Healthcare. pp. 1331–1333.
30. Vos, Johannes G., Robert J. Forster, Tia E. Keyes (2003). Interfacial Supramolecular Assemblies. Wiley. pp. 88–94.
31. Madou, Marc (2002). Fundamentals of Microfabrication: The Science of Miniaturization. CRC. pp. 62–63.
32. Kaifer, Angel (2001). Supramolecular Electrochemistry. Coral Gables. Wiley VCH. pp. 191–193.

33. Saliterman, Steven (2006). Self-assembled monolayers (SAMs). Fundamentals of BioMEMS and Medical Microdevices. SPIE Press. pp. 94–96.

34. Andres, R.P.; Bein T.; Dorogi M.; Feng S.; Henderson J.I.; Kubiak C.P.; Mahoney W.; Osifchin R.G.; Reifenberger R. (1996). Coulomb Staircase at Room Temperature in a Self-Assembled Molecular Nanostructure. Science. 272 (5266): 1323–1325. Bibcode:1996Sci...272.1323A. doi:10.1126/science.272.5266.1323. PMID 8662464.

35. Shaporenko, A.; Muller J.; Weidner T.; Terfort A.; Zharnikov M. (2007). Balance of Structure-Building Forces in Selenium-Based Self-Assembled Monolayers. Journal of the American Chemical Society. 129 (8): 2232–2233. doi:10.1021/ja068916e.

36. Subramanian, S.; Sampath S. (2007). Enhanced stability of short- and long-chain diselenide self-assembled monolayers on gold probed by electrochemistry, spectroscopy, and microscopy. Journal of Colloid and Interface Science. 312 (2): 413–424. doi:10.1016/j.jcis.2007.03.021. PMID 17451727.

37. Bucher, Jean-Pierre; Santesson, Lars, Kern, Klaus (31 March 1994). Thermal Healing of Self-Assembled Organic Monolayers: Hexane- and Octadecanethiol on Au(111) and Ag(111). Langmuir. 10 (4): 979–983. doi:10.1021/la00016a001.

38. Schlenoff, Joseph B.; Li, Ming, Ly, Hiep (30 November 1995). Stability and Self-Exchange in Alkanethiol Monolayers. Journal of the American Chemical Society. 117 (50): 12528–12536. doi:10.1021/ja00155a016.

39. Wysocki. Self-Assembled Monolayers (SAMs) as Collision Surfaces for Ion Activation (PDF).

40. Nuzzo, Ralph G.; Allara, David L. (31 May 1983). Adsorption of bifunctional organic disulfides on gold surfaces. Journal of the American Chemical Society. 105 (13): 4481–4483. doi:10.1021/ja00351a063.

41. Bain, Colin D.; Troughton, E. Barry; Tao, Yu Tai; Evall, Joseph; Whitesides, George M.; Nuzzo, Ralph G. (31 December 1988). Formation of monolayer films by the spontaneous assembly of organic thiols from solution onto gold. Journal of the American Chemical Society. 111 (1): 321–335. doi:10.1021/ja00183a049.

42. Hamoudi, H.; Prato M., Dablemont C., Cavalleri O., Canepa M., Esaulov, V. A. (2010). Self-Assembly of 1,4-Benzenedimethanethiol Self-Assembled Monolayers on Gold. Langmuir. 26 (10): 7242–7247. doi:10.1021/la904317b. PMID 20199099.

43. Hamoudi, H.; Guo Z.,Prato M., Dablemont C., Zheng W.Q., Bourguignon B., Canepa M., Esaulov, V. A.; Prato, Mirko; Dablemont, Céline; Zheng, Wan Quan; Bourguignon, Bernard; Canepa, Maurizio; Esaulov, Vladimir A. (2008). On the self assembly of short chain alkanedithiols. Physical Chemistry Chemical Physics. 10 (45): 6836–6841. Bibcode:2008PCCP...10.6836H. doi:10.1039/B809760G. PMID 19015788.

44. Alarcon, L.S.; Chen L., Esaulov, V. A., Gayone J.E., Sanchez E., Grizzi O. (2010). Thiol Terminated 1,4-Benzenedimethanethiol Self-Assembled Monolayers on Au(111) and InP(110) from Vapor Phase. Journal of Physical Chemistry C. 114 (47): 19993–19999. doi:10.1021/jp1044157.

45. Chaudhari, V.; Harish N.M.K.; Sampath S.; Esaulov V.A. (2011). Substitutional Self-Assembly of Alkanethiol and Selenol SAMs from a Lying-Down Doubly Tethered Butanedithiol SAM on Gold. Journal of Physical Chemistry C. 115 (33): 16518–16523. doi:10.1021/jp2042922.

46. Prato, M.; Moroni R.; Bisio F.; Rolandi R.; Mattera L.; Cavalleri O.; Canepa M. (2008). Optical Characterization of Thiolate Self-Assembled Monolayers on Au(111). Journal of Physical Chemistry C. 112 (10): 3899–3906. doi:10.1021/jp711194s.

47. Kato, H.; Noh J.; Hara M.; Kawai M. (2002). An HREELS Study of Alkanethiol Self-Assembled Monolayers on Au(111). Journal of Physical Chemistry C. 106 (37): 9655–9658. doi:10.1021/jp020968c.

48. Smith; et al. (2004). Patterning Self-Assembled Monolayers. Progress in Surface Science. 75: 1–68. Bibcode:2004PrSS...75....1S. doi:10.1016/j.progsurf.2003.12.001.

49. Yongan Tang, Jiawei Yan, Xiaoshun Zhou, Yongchun Fu, Bingwei Mao. An STM study on nonionic fluorosurfactant zonyl FSN self-assembly on Au(111): large domains, few defects, and good stability. Langmuir 2008, 24, 13245-13249.

50. Jiawei Yan, Yongan Tang, Chunfeng Sun, Yuzhuan Su, Bingwei Mao. STM Study on Nonionic Fluorosurfactant Zonyl FSN Self-Assembly on Au(100): (3/1/-1/1) Molecular Lattice, Corrugations, and Adsorbate-Enhanced Mobility. Langmuir 2010, 26, 3829-3834

51. Yongan Tang, Jiawei Yan, Feng Zhu, Chunfeng Sun, Bingwei Mao. Comparative electrochemical scanning tunneling microscopy study of nonionic fluorosurfactant zonyl FSN self-assembled monolayers on Au(111) and Au(100): a potential-induced structural transition. Langmuir 2011, 27, 943-947

52. Seong, Jin Koh (2007). Strategies for Controlled Placement of Nanoscale Building Blocks. Nanoscale Res Lett. 2 (11): 519–545. Bibcode:2007NRL.....2..519K. doi:10.1007/s11671-007-9091-3. PMC 3246612Freely accessible. PMID 21794185.

53. Piner, R.D; Zhu, J; Xu, F; Hong, S; Mirkin, C.A (1999). Dip-Pen Nanolithography. Science. 283 (5402): 661–663. doi:10.1126/science.283.5402.661. PMID 9924019.

54. Lud, S.Q; Neppl, S; Xu, F; Feulner, P; Stutzmann, M; Jordan, Rainer; Feulner, Peter; Stutzmann, Martin; Garrido, Jose A. (2010). Controlling Surface Functionality through Generation of Thiol Groups in a Self-Assembled Monolayer. Langmuir. 26 (20): 15895–900. doi:10.1021/la102225r.

55. Laibinis, Paul E.; Whitesides, George M.; Allara, David L.; Tao, Yu Tai; Parikh, Atul N.; Nuzzo, Ralph G. (1991-09-01). Comparison of the structures and wetting properties of self-assembled monolayers of n-alkanethiols on the coinage metal surfaces, copper, silver, and gold. Journal of the American Chemical Society. 113 (19): 7152–7167. doi:10.1021/ja00019a011. ISSN 0002-7863.

56. Noyhouzer, Tomer; Mandler, Daniel (2011-01-17). Determination of low levels of cadmium ions by the under potential deposition on a self-assembled monolayer

on gold electrode. Analytica Chimica Acta. 684 (1–2): 1–7. doi:10.1016/j.aca.2010.10.021.

57. Lud, S.Q; Steenackers, M; Bruno, P; Gruen, D.M; Feulner, P; Garrido, J.A; Stutzmann, M; Stutzmann, M (2006). Chemical Grafting of Biphenyl Self-Assembled Monolayers on Ultrananocrystalline Diamond. Journal of the American Chemical Society. 128 (51): 16884–16891. doi:10.1021/ja0657049. PMID 17177439.
58. Cech J; Taboryski R (2012). Stability of FDTS monolayer coating on aluminum injection molding tools. Applied Surface Science. 259: 538–541. Bibcode:2012ApSS..259..538C. doi:10.1016/j.apsusc.2012.07.078.
59. Yung et all; Fiering, J; Mueller, AJ; Ingber, DE (2009). Micromagnetic–microfluidic blood cleansing device. Lab on a Chip. 9 (9): 1171–1177. doi:10.1039/b816986a. PMID 19370233.
60. Garcia, R.; Martinez, R.V; Martinez, J (2005). Nano Chemistry and Scanning Probe Nanolithographies. Chemical Society Reviews. 35 (1): 29–38. doi:10.1039/b501599p. PMID 16365640.
61. Kiely, C.J.; Fink J., Brust M., Bethell D? Schiffrin D.J. (1999). Spontaneous ordering of bimodal ensembles of nanoscopic gold clusters. Nature. 396 (3): 444–446. doi:10.1038/24808.
62. Vijaya Sarathy, K.; John Thomas P.,Kulkarni G.U., Rao C.N.R. (1999). Superlattices of Metal and Metal–Semiconductor Quantum Dots Obtained by Layer-by-Layer Deposition of Nanoparticle Arrays. Journal of Physical Chemistry. 103 (3): 399–401. doi:10.1021/jp983836l.

CHAPTER 7

NANOELECTRONICS

Chapter Contents

- **Introduction**
- **Fundamental Concepts**
- **Approaches To Nanoelectronics**
- **Nanoelectronic Devices**
- **Molecular Scale Electronics**
- **Nanolithography**

Nanoelectronics refer to the field of study which is concerned with understanding, exploring and exploiting the characteristics of devices and instruments, which have directional dimensions at the nano scale. Its one of the most powerful and useful study which has helped engineers to implement new properties. It is used for building the nano electronics components just like transistors. Devices and machines are developed at the rate of 100 nanometers which is extremely small and efficient rate for processing. Nano electronics is also known as the disruptive technology because of its various properties.

INTRODUCTION

Nanoelectronics refer to the use of nanotechnology in electronic components. The term covers a diverse set of devices and materials, with the common characteristic that they are so small that inter-atomic interactions and quantum mechanical properties need to be studied extensively. Some of these candidates include: hybrid molecular/semiconductor electronics, one-dimensional nanotubes/nanowires, or advanced molecular electronics. Recent silicon CMOS technology generations, such as the 22 nanometer node, are already within this regime. Nanoelectronics are sometimes considered as disruptive technology because present candidates are significantly different from traditional transistors.

FUNDAMENTAL CONCEPTS

In 1965 Gordon Moore observed that silicon transistors were undergoing a continual process of scaling downward, an observation which was later codified as Moore's law. Since his observation transistor minimum feature sizes have decreased from 10 micrometers to the 28-22 nm range in 2011. The field of nanoelectronics aims to enable the continued realization of this law by using new methods and materials to build electronic devices with feature sizes on the nanoscale.

The volume of an object decreases as the third power of its linear dimensions, but the surface area only decreases as its second power. This somewhat subtle and unavoidable principle has huge ramifications. For example, the power of a drill (or any other machine) is proportional to the volume, while the friction of the drill's bearings and gears is proportional to their surface area. For a normal-sized drill, the power of the device is enough to handily overcome any friction. However, scaling its length down by a factor of 1000, for example, decreases its power by 1000^3 (a factor of a billion) while reducing the friction by only 1000^2 (a factor of only a million). Proportionally it has 1000 times less power per unit friction than the original drill. If the original friction-to-power ratio was, say, 1%, that implies the smaller drill will have 10 times as much friction as power; the drill is useless.

For this reason, while super-miniature electronic integrated circuits are fully functional, the same technology cannot be used to make working mechanical devices beyond the scales where frictional forces start to exceed the available power. So even though you may see microphotographs of delicately etched silicon gears, such devices are currently little more than curiosities with limited real world applications, for example, in moving mirrors and shutters. Surface tension increases in much the same way, thus magnifying the tendency for very small objects to stick together. This could possibly make any kind of "micro factory" impractical: even if robotic arms and hands could be scaled down, anything they pick up will tend to be impossible to put down. The above being said, molecular evolution has resulted in working cilia, flagella, muscle fibers and rotary motors in aqueous environments, all on the nanoscale. These machines exploit the increased frictional forces found at the micro or nanoscale. Unlike a paddle or a propeller which depends on normal frictional forces (the frictional forces perpendicular to the surface) to achieve propulsion, cilia develop motion from the exaggerated drag or laminar forces (frictional forces parallel to the surface) present at micro and nano dimensions. To build meaningful "machines" at the nanoscale, the relevant forces need to be considered. We are faced with the development and design of intrinsically pertinent machines rather than the simple reproductions of macroscopic ones.

All scaling issues therefore need to be assessed thoroughly when evaluating nanotechnology for practical applications.

APPROACHES TO NANOELECTRONICS

Nanofabrication

For example, single electron transistors, which involve transistor operation based on a single electron. Nanoelectromechanical systems also fall under this category. Nanofabrication can be used to construct ultradense parallel arrays of nanowires, as an alternative to synthesizing nanowires individually.

Nanomaterials Electronics

Besides being small and allowing more transistors to be packed into a single chip, the uniform and symmetrical structure of nanotubes allows a higher electron mobility (faster electron movement in the material), a higher dielectric constant (faster frequency), and a symmetrical electron/hole characteristic.

Also, nanoparticles can be used as quantum dots.

Molecular Electronics

Single molecule devices are another possibility. These schemes would make heavy use of molecular self-assembly, designing the device components to construct a larger structure or even a complete system on their own. This can be very useful for reconfigurable computing, and may even completely replace present FPGA technology.

Molecular electronics is a new technology which is still in its infancy, but also brings hope for truly atomic scale electronic systems in the future. One of the more promising applications of molecular electronics was proposed by the IBM researcher Ari Aviram and the theoretical chemist Mark Ratner in their 1974 and 1988 papers *Molecules for Memory, Logic and Amplification*.

This is one of many possible ways in which a molecular level diode / transistor might be synthesized by organic chemistry. A model system was proposed with a spiro carbon structure giving a molecular diode about half a nanometre across which could be connected by polythiophene molecular wires. Theoretical calculations showed the design to be sound in principle and there is still hope that such a system can be made to work.

Other Approaches

Nanoionics studies the transport of ions rather than electrons in nanoscale systems.

Nanophotonics studies the behavior of light on the nanoscale, and has the goal of developing devices that take advantage of this behavior.

NANOELECTRONIC DEVICES

Current high-technology production processes are based on traditional top down strategies, where nanotechnology has already been introduced silently. The critical length scale of integrated circuits is already at the nanoscale (50 nm and below) regarding the gate length of transistors in CPUs or DRAM devices.

Computers

Nanoelectronics holds the promise of making computer processors more powerful than are possible with conventional semiconductor fabrication techniques. A number of approaches are currently being researched, including new forms of nanolithography, as well as the use of nanomaterials such as nanowires or small molecules in place of traditional CMOS components. Field effect transistors have been made using both semiconducting carbon nanotubes and with heterostructured semiconductor nanowires.

In 1999, the CMOS transistor developed at the Laboratory for Electronics and Information Technology in Grenoble, France, tested the limits of the principles of the MOSFET transistor with a diameter of 18 nm (approximately 70 atoms placed side by side). This was almost one tenth the size of the smallest industrial transistor in 2003 (130 nm in 2003, 90 nm in 2004, 65 nm in 2005 and 45 nm in 2007). It enabled the theoretical integration of seven billion junctions on a €1 coin. However, the CMOS transistor, which was created in 1999, was not a simple research experiment to study how CMOS technology functions, but rather a demonstration of how this technology functions now that we ourselves are getting ever closer to working on a molecular scale. Today it would be impossible to master the coordinated assembly of a large number of these transistors on a circuit and it would also be impossible to create this on an industrial level.

Memory Storage

Electronic memory designs in the past have largely relied on the formation of transistors. However, research into crossbar switch based electronics have offered an alternative using reconfigurable interconnections between vertical and horizontal wiring arrays to create ultra high density memories. Two leaders in this area are Nantero which has developed a carbon nanotube based crossbar memory called Nano-RAM and Hewlett-Packard which has proposed the use of memristor material as a future replacement of Flash memory.

An example of such novel devices is based on spintronics.The dependence of the resistance of a material (due to the spin of the electrons) on an external field is called magnetoresistance. This effect can be significantly amplified (GMR - Giant Magneto-Resistance) for nanosized objects, for example when two ferromagnetic layers are separated by a nonmagnetic layer, which is several nanometers thick (e.g. Co-Cu-Co). The GMR effect has led to a strong increase in the data storage density of hard disks and made the gigabyte range possible. The so-called tunneling magnetoresistance (TMR) is very similar to GMR and based on the spin dependent tunneling of electrons through adjacent ferromagnetic layers. Both GMR and TMR effects can be used to create a non-volatile main memory for computers, such as the so-called magnetic random access memory or MRAM.

Novel Optoelectronic Devices

In the modern communication technology traditional analog electrical devices are increasingly replaced by optical or optoelectronic devices due to their enormous bandwidth and capacity, respectively. Two promising examples are photonic crystals and quantum dots. Photonic crystals are materials with a periodic variation in the refractive index with a lattice constant that is half the wavelength of the light used. They offer a selectable band gap for the propagation of a certain wavelength, thus they resemble a semiconductor, but for light or photons instead of electrons. Quantum dots are nanoscaled objects, which can be used, among many other things, for the construction of lasers. The advantage of a quantum dot laser over the traditional semiconductor laser is that their emitted wavelength depends on the diameter of the dot. Quantum dot lasers are cheaper and offer a higher beam quality than conventional laser diodes.

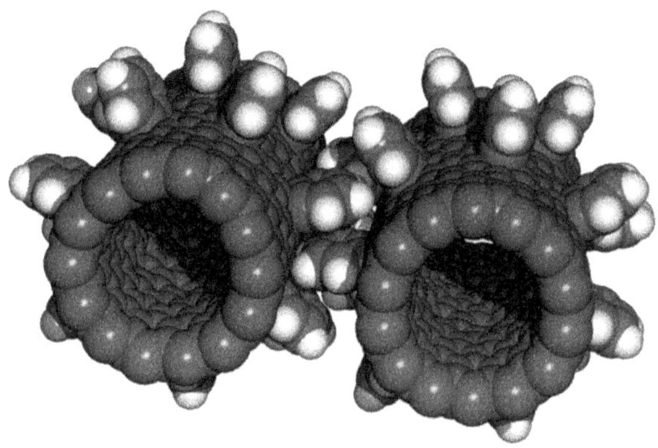

Displays

The production of displays with low energy consumption might be accomplished using carbon nanotubes (CNT). Carbon nanotubes are electrically conductive and due to their small diameter of several nanometers, they can be used as field emitters with extremely high efficiency for field emission displays (FED). The principle of operation resembles that of the cathode ray tube, but on a much smaller length scale.

Quantum Computers

Entirely new approaches for computing exploit the laws of quantum mechanics for novel quantum computers, which enable the use of fast quantum algorithms. The Quantum computer has quantum bit memory space termed "Qubit" for several computations at the same time. This facility may improve the performance of the older systems.

Radios

Nanoradios have been developed structured around carbon nanotubes.

Energy Production

Research is ongoing to use nanowires and other nanostructured materials with the hope to create cheaper and more efficient solar cells than are possible with conventional planar silicon solar cells. It is believed that the invention of more efficient solar energy would have a great effect on satisfying global energy needs.

There is also research into energy production for devices that would operate *in vivo*, called bio-nano generators. A bio-nano generator is a nanoscale electrochemical device, like a fuel cell or galvanic cell, but drawing power from blood glucose in a living body, much the same as how the body generates energy from food. To achieve the effect, an enzyme is used that is capable of stripping glucose of its electrons, freeing them for use in electrical devices. The average person's body could, theoretically, generate 100 watts of electricity (about 2000 food calories per day) using a bio-nano generator. However, this estimate is only true if all food was converted to electricity, and the human body needs some energy consistently, so possible power generated is likely much lower. The electricity generated by such a device could power devices embedded in the body (such as pacemakers), or sugar-fed nanorobots. Much of the research done on bio-nano generators is still experimental, with Panasonic's Nanotechnology Research Laboratory among those at the forefront.

Medical Diagnostics

There is great interest in constructing nanoelectronic devices that could detect the concentrations of biomolecules in real time for use as medical diagnostics, thus falling into the category of nanomedicine. A parallel line of research seeks to create nanoelectronic devices which could interact with single cells for use in basic biological research. These devices are called nanosensors. Such miniaturization on nanoelectronics towards in vivo proteomic sensing should enable new approaches for health monitoring, surveillance, and defense technology.

MOLECULAR SCALE ELECTRONICS

Molecular scale electronics, also called single-molecule electronics, is a branch of nanotechnology that uses single molecules, or nanoscale collections of single molecules, as electronic components. Because single molecules constitute the smallest stable structures imaginable, this miniaturization is the ultimate goal for shrinking electrical circuits.

The field is often termed simply as "molecular electronics", but this term is also used to refer to the distantly related field of conductive polymers and organic electronics, which uses the properties of molecules to affect the bulk properties of a material. A nomenclature distinction has been suggested so that *molecular materials for electronics* refers to this latter field of bulk applications, while *molecular scale electronics* refers to the nanoscale single-molecule applications treated here.

Fundamental Concepts

Conventional electronics have traditionally been made from bulk materials. Ever since their invention in 1958, the performance and complexity of integrated circuits has undergone exponential growth, a trend named Moore's law, as feature sizes of the embedded components have shrunk accordingly. As the structures shrink, the sensitivity to deviations increases. In a few technology generations, when the minimum feature sizes reaches 13 nm, the composition of the devices must be controlled to a precision of a few atoms for the devices to work. With bulk methods growing increasingly demanding and costly as they near inherent limits, the idea was born that the components could instead be built up atom by atom in a chemistry lab (bottom up) versus carving them out of bulk material (top down). This is the idea behind molecular electronics, with the ultimate miniaturization being components contained in single molecules.

In single-molecule electronics, the bulk material is replaced by single molecules. Instead of forming structures by removing or applying material after a pattern scaffold, the atoms are put together in a chemistry lab. In this way, billions of billions of copies are made simultaneously (typically more than 10^{20} molecules are made at once) while the composition of molecules are controlled down to the last atom. The molecules used have properties that resemble traditional electronic components such as a wire, transistor or rectifier.

Single-molecule electronics is an emerging field, and entire electronic circuits consisting exclusively of molecular sized compounds are still very far from being realized. However, the unceasing demand for more computing power, along with the inherent limits of lithographic methods as of 2016, make the transition seem unavoidable. Currently, the focus is on discovering molecules with interesting properties and on finding ways to obtain reliable and reproducible contacts between the molecular components and the bulk material of the electrodes.

Theoretical Basis

Molecular electronics operates in the quantum realm of distances less than 100 nanometers. The miniaturization down to single molecules brings the scale down to a regime where quantum mechanics effects are important. In conventional electronic components, electrons can be filled in or drawn out more or less like a continuous flow of electric charge. In contrast, in molecular electronics the transfer of one electron alters the system significantly. For example, when an electron has been transferred from a source electrode to a molecule, the molecule gets charged up, which makes it far harder for the next electron to transfer . The significant amount of energy due to charging must be accounted for when making calculations about the electronic properties of the setup, and is highly sensitive to distances to conducting surfaces nearby.

The theory of single-molecule devices is especially interesting since the system under consideration is an open quantum system in nonequilibrium (driven by voltage).

In the low bias voltage regime, the nonequilibrium nature of the molecular junction can be ignored, and the current-voltage traits of the device can be calculated using the equilibrium electronic structure of the system. However, in stronger bias regimes a more sophisticated treatment is required, as there is no longer a variational principle. In the elastic tunneling case (where the passing electron does not exchange energy with the system), the formalism of Rolf Landauer can be used to calculate the transmission through the system as a function of bias voltage, and hence the current. In inelastic tunneling, an elegant formalism based on the non-equilibrium Green's functions of Leo Kadanoff and Gordon Baym, and independently by Leonid Keldysh was advanced by Ned Wingreen and Yigal Meir. This Meir-Wingreen formulation has been used to great success in the molecular electronics community to examine the more difficult and interesting cases where the transient electron exchanges energy with the molecular system (for example through electron-phonon coupling or electronic excitations).

Further, connecting single molecules reliably to a larger scale circuit has proven a great challenge, and constitutes a significant hindrance to commercialization.

Examples

Common for molecules used in molecular electronics is that the structures contain many alternating double and single bonds. This is done because such patterns delocalize the molecular orbitals, making it possible for electrons to move freely over the conjugated area.

Wires

The sole purpose of molecular wires is to electrically connect different parts of a molecular electrical circuit. As the assembly of these and their connection to a macroscopic circuit is still not mastered, the focus of research in single-molecule electronics is primarily on the functionalized molecules: molecular wires are characterized by containing no functional groups and are hence composed of plain repetitions of a conjugated building block. Among these are the carbon nanotubes that are quite large compared to the other suggestions but have shown very promising electrical properties.

The main problem with the molecular wires is to obtain good electrical contact with the electrodes so that electrons can move freely in and out of the wire.

Transistors

Single-molecule transistors are fundamentally different from the ones known from bulk electronics. The gate in a conventional (field-effect) transistor determines the conductance between the source and drain electrode by controlling the density of charge carriers between them, whereas the gate in a single-molecule transistor controls the possibility of a single electron to jump on and off the molecule by modifying the energy of the molecular orbitals. One of the effects of this difference is that the single-molecule transistor is almost binary: it is either *on* or *off*. This opposes its bulk counterparts, which have quadratic responses to gate voltage.

It is the quantization of charge into electrons that is responsible for the markedly different behavior compared to bulk electronics. Because of the size of a single molecule, the charging due to a single electron is significant and provides means to turn a transistor *on* or *off*. For this to work, the electronic orbitals on the transistor molecule cannot be too well integrated with the orbitals on the electrodes. If they are, an electron cannot be said to be located on the molecule or the electrodes and the molecule will function as a wire.

A popular group of molecules, that can work as the semiconducting channel material in a molecular transistor, is the oligopolyphenylenevinylenes (OPVs) that works by the Coulomb blockade mechanism when placed between the source and drain electrode in an appropriate way. Fullerenes work by the same mechanism and have also been commonly used.

Semiconducting carbon nanotubes have also been demonstrated to work as channel material but although molecular, these molecules are sufficiently large to behave almost as bulk semiconductors.

The size of the molecules, and the low temperature of the measurements being conducted, makes the quantum mechanical states well defined. Thus, it is being researched if the quantum mechanical properties can be used for more advanced purposes than simple transistors (e.g. spintronics).

Physicists at the University of Arizona, in collaboration with chemists from the University of Madrid , have designed a single-molecule transistor using a ring-shaped molecule similar to benzene. Physicists at Canada's National Institute for Nanotechnology have designed a single-molecule transistor using styrene. Both groups expect (the designs were experimentally unverified as of June 2005) their respective devices to function at room temperature, and to be controlled by a single electron.

Rectifiers (diodes)

Molecular rectifiers are mimics of their bulk counterparts and have an asymmetric construction so that the molecule can accept electrons in one end but not the other. The molecules have an electron donor (D) in one end and an electron acceptor (A) in the other. This way, the unstable state $D^+ - A^-$ will be more readily made than $D^- - A^+$. The result is that an electric current can be drawn through the molecule if the electrons are added through the acceptor end, but less easily if the reverse is attempted.

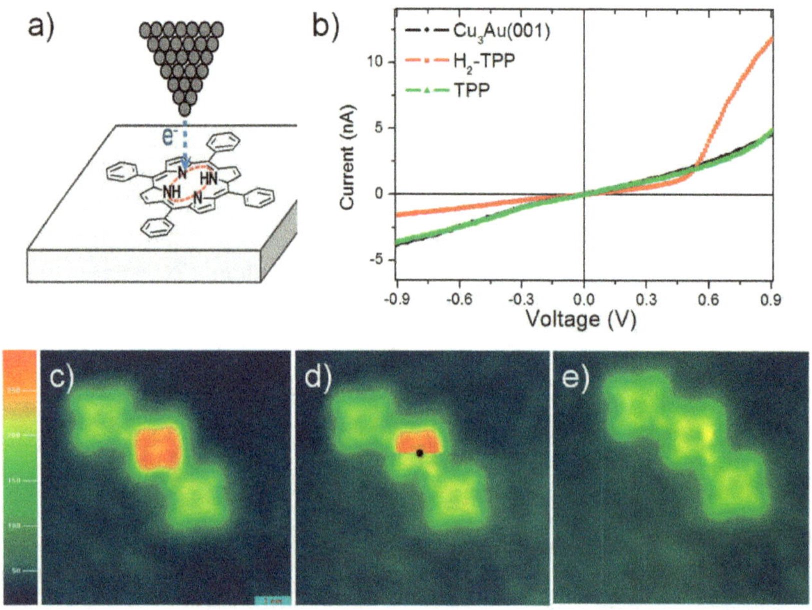

Hydrogen can be removed from individual tetraphenylporphyrin (H_2TPP) molecules by applying excess voltage to the tip of a scanning tunneling microscope (STAM, a); this removal alters the current-voltage (I-V) curves of TPP molecules, measured using the same STM tip, from diode-like (red curve in b) to resistor-like (green curve). Image (c) shows a row of TPP, H_2TPP and TPP molecules. While scanning image (d), excess voltage was applied to H_2TPP at the black dot, which instantly removed hydrogen, as shown in the bottom part of (d) and in the re-scan image (e). Such manipulations can be used in single-molecule electronics.

Methods

One of the biggest problems with measuring on single molecules is to establish reproducible electrical contact with only one molecule and doing so without shortcutting the electrodes. Because the current photolithographic technology is unable to produce electrode gaps small enough to contact both ends of the molecules tested (on the order of nanometers), alternative strategies are applied.

Molecular Gaps

One way to produce electrodes with a molecular sized gap between them is break junctions, in which a thin electrode is stretched until it breaks. Another is electromigration. Here a current is led through a thin wire until it melts and the atoms migrate to produce the gap. Further, the reach of conventional photolithography can be enhanced by chemically etching or depositing metal on the electrodes.

Probably the easiest way to conduct measurements on several molecules is to use the tip of a scanning tunneling microscope (STM) to contact molecules adhered at the other end to a metal substrate.

Anchoring

A popular way to anchor molecules to the electrodes is to make use of sulfur's high chemical affinity to gold. In these setups, the molecules are synthesized so that sulfur atoms are placed strategically to function as crocodile clips connecting the molecules to the gold electrodes. Though useful, the anchoring is non-specific and thus anchors the molecules randomly to all gold surfaces. Further, the contact resistance is highly dependent on the precise atomic geometry around the site of anchoring and thereby inherently compromises the reproducibility of the connection.

To circumvent the latter issue, experiments has shown that fullerenes could be a good candidate for use instead of sulfur because of the large conjugated π-system that can electrically contact many more atoms at once than one atom of sulfur.

Fullerene Nanoelectronics

In polymers, classical organic molecules are composed of both carbon and hydrogen (and sometimes additional compounds such as nitrogen, chlorine or sulphur). They are obtained from petrol and can often be synthesized in large amounts. Most of these molecules are insulating when their length exceeds a few nanometers. However, naturally occurring carbon is conducting, especially graphite recovered from coal or encountered otherwise. From a theoretical viewpoint, graphite is a semi-metal, a category in between metals and semi-conductors. It has a layered structure, each sheet being one atom thick. Between each sheet, the interactions are weak enough to allow an easy manual cleavage.

Tailoring the graphite sheet to obtain well defined nanometer-sized objects remains a challenge. However, by the close of the twentieth century, chemists were exploring methods to fabricate extremely small graphitic objects that could be considered single molecules. After studying the interstellar conditions under which carbon is known to form clusters, Richard Smalley's group (Rice University, Texas) set up an experiment in which graphite was vaporized via laser irradiation. Mass spectrometry revealed that clusters containing specific *magic numbers* of atoms were stable, especially those clusters of 60 atoms. Harry Kroto, an English chemist who assisted in the experiment, suggested a possible geometry for these clusters – atoms covalently bound with the exact symmetry of a soccer ball. Coined buckminsterfullerenes, buckyballs, or C_{60}, the clusters retained some properties of graphite, such as conductivity. These objects were rapidly envisioned as possible building blocks for molecular electronics.

Problems

Artifacts

When trying to measure electronic traits of molecules, artificial phenomena can occur that can be hard to distinguish from truly molecular behavior. Before they were discovered, these artifacts have mistakenly been published as being features pertaining to the molecules in question.

Applying a voltage drop on the order of volts across a nanometer sized junction results in a very strong electrical field. The field can cause metal atoms to migrate and eventually close the gap by a thin filament, which can be broken again when carrying a current. The two levels of conductance imitate molecular switching between a conductive and an isolating state of a molecule.

Another encountered artifact is when the electrodes undergo chemical reactions due to the high field strength in the gap. When the voltage bias is reversed, the reaction will cause hysteresis in the measurements that can be interpreted as being of molecular origin.

A metallic grain between the electrodes can act as a single electron transistor by the mechanism described above, thus resembling the traits of a molecular transistor. This artifact is especially common with nanogaps produced by the electromigration method.

Commercialization

One of the biggest hindrances for single-molecule electronics to be commercially exploited is the lack of methods to connect a molecular sized circuit to bulk electrodes in a way that gives reproducible results. At the current state, the difficulty of connecting single molecules vastly outweighs any possible performance increase that could be gained from such shrinkage. The difficulties grow worse if the molecules are to have a certain spatial orientation and/or have multiple poles to connect.

Also problematic is that some measurements on single molecules are carried out in cryogenic temperatures (near absolute zero), which is very energy consuming. This is done to reduce signal noise enough to measure the faint currents of single molecules.

History and Recent Progress

In their treatment of so-called *donor-acceptor* complexes in the 1940s, Robert Mulliken and Albert Szent-Györgyi advanced the concept of charge transfer in molecules. They subsequently further refined the study of both charge transfer and energy transfer in molecules. Likewise, a 1974 paper from Mark Ratner and Ari Aviram illustrated a theoretical molecular rectifier. In 1988, Aviram described in detail a theoretical single-molecule field-effect transistor. Further concepts were proposed by Forrest Carter of the Naval Research Laboratory, including single-molecule logic gates. A wide range of ideas were presented, under his aegis, at a conference entitled *Molecular Electronic Devices* in 1988. These were all theoretical constructs and not concrete devices. The *direct* measurement of the electronic traits of individual molecules awaited the development of methods for making molecular-scale electrical contacts. This was no easy task. Thus, the first experiment directly-measuring the conductance of a single molecule was only reported in 1995 on a single C_{60} molecule by C. Joachim and J. K. Gimzewsky in their seminal Physical Revie Letter paper and later in 1997 by Mark Reed and co-workers on a few hundred molecules. Since then, this branch of the field has advanced rapidly. Likewise, as it has grown possible to measure such properties directly, the theoretical predictions of the early workers have been confirmed substantially.

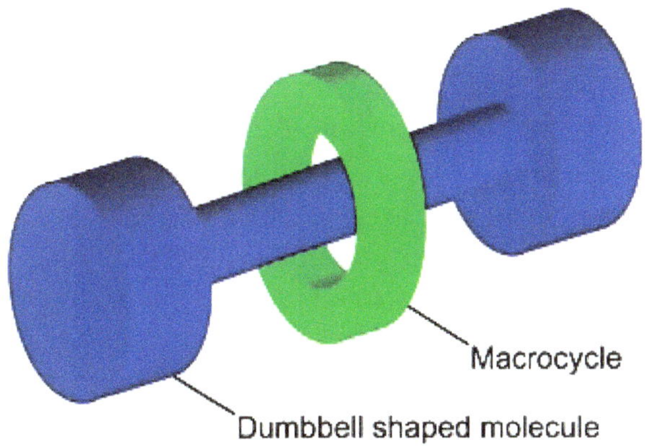

Graphical representation of a rotaxane, useful as a molecular switch.

Recent progress in nanotechnology and nanoscience has facilitated both experimental and theoretical study of molecular electronics. Development of the scanning tunneling microscope (STM) and later the atomic force microscope (AFM) have greatly facilitated manipulating single-molecule electronics. Also, theoretical advances in molecular electronics have facilitated further understanding of non-adiabatic charge transfer events at electrode-electrolyte interfaces.

The concept of molecular electronics was first published in 1974 when Aviram and Ratner suggested an organic molecule that could work as a rectifier. Having both huge commercial and fundamental interest, much effort was put into proving its feasibility, and 16 years later in 1990, the first demonstration of an intrinsic molecular rectifier was realized by Ashwell and coworkers for a thin film of molecules.

The first measurement of the conductance of a single molecule was realised in 1994 by C. Joachim and J. K. Gimzewski and published in 1995. This was the conclusion of 10 years of research started at IBM TJ Watson, using the scanning tunnelling microscope tip apex to switch a single molecule as already explored by A. Aviram, C. Joachim and M. Pomerantz at the end of the 80's. The trick was to use an UHV Scanning Tunneling microscope to allow the tip apex to gently touch the top of a single C60 molecule adsorbed on an Au(110) surface. A resistance of 55 MOhms was recorded along with a low voltage linear I-V. The contact was certified by recording the I-z current distance property, which allows measurement of the deformation of the C60 cage under contact. This first experiment was followed by the reported result using a mechanical break junction method to connect two gold electrodes to a sulfur-terminated molecular wire by Mark Reed and James Tour in 1997.

A single-molecule amplifier was implemented by C. Joachim and J.K. Gimzewski in IBM Zurich. This experiment, involving one C60 molecule, demonstrated that one such molecule can provide gain in a circuit via intramolecular quantum interference effects alone.

A collaboration of researchers at Hewlett-Packard (HP) and University of California, Los Angeles (UCLA), led by James Heath, Fraser Stoddart, R. Stanley Williams, and Philip Kuekes, has developed molecular electronics based on rotaxanes and catenanes.

Work is also occurring on the use of single-wall carbon nanotubes as field-effect transistors. Most of this work is being done by International Business Machines (IBM).

Some specific reports of a field-effect transistor based on molecular self-assembled monolayers were shown to be fraudulent in 2002 as part of the Schön scandal.

Until recently entirely theoretical, the Aviram-Ratner model for a unimolecular rectifier has been confirmed unambiguously in experiments by a group led by Geoffrey J. Ashwell at Bangor University, UK. Many rectifying molecules have so far been identified, and the number and efficiency of these systems is growing rapidly.

Supramolecular electronics is a new field involving electronics at a supramolecular level.

An important issue in molecular electronics is the determination of the resistance of a single molecule (both theoretical and experimental). For example, Bumm, et al. used STM to analyze a single molecular switch in a self-assembled monolayer to determine how conductive such a molecule can be. Another problem faced by this field is the difficulty of performing direct characterization since imaging at the molecular scale is often difficult in many experimental devices.

NANOLITHOGRAPHY

Nanolithography is the branch of nanotechnology concerned with the study and application of fabricating nanometer-scale structures, meaning patterns with at least one lateral dimension between 1 and 100 nm. Different approaches can be categorized in serial or parallel, mask or maskless/direct-write, top-down or bottom-up, beam or tip-based, resist-based or resist-less methods. As of 2015, nanolithography is a very active area of research in academia and in industry. Applications of nanolithography include among others: Multigate devices such as Field effect transistors (FET), Quantum dots, Nanowires, Gratings, Zone plates and Photomasks, nanoelectromechanical systems (NEMS), or semiconductor integrated circuits (nanocircuitry).

Optical Lithography

Optical lithography, which has been the predominant patterning technique since the advent of the semiconductor age, is capable of producing sub-100-nm patterns with the use of very short optical wavelengths. Several optical lithography techniques require the use of liquid immersion and a host of resolution enhancement technologies like phase-shift masks (PSM) and optical proximity correction (OPC). Multiple patterning is a method of increasing the resolution by printing features in between pre-printed features on the same layer by etching or creating sidewall spacers, and has been used in commercial production of microprocessors since the 32 nm process node e.g. by directed self-assembly (DSA). Extreme ultraviolet lithography (EUVL) uses ultrashort wavelengths (13.5 nm) and as of 2015, is the most popularly considered Next-generation lithography (NGL) technique for mass-fabrication.

Electron-Beam Lithography

Electron beam lithography or *Electron-Beam Direct-Write Lithography* (EBDW) scans a focused beam of electrons on a surface covered with an electron-sensitive film or resist (e.g. PMMA or HSQ) to draw custom shapes. By changing the solubility of the resist and subsequent selective removal of material by immersion in a solvent, sub-10 nm resolutions have been achieved. This form of direct-write, maskless lithography has high resolution and low throughput, limiting single-column e-beams to photomask fabrication, low-volume production of semiconductor devices, and research&development. Multiple-electron beam approaches have as a goal an increase of throughput for semiconductor mass-production.

Nanoimprint Lithography

Nanoimprint lithography (NIL), and its variants, such as Step-and-Flash Imprint Lithography, LISA and LADI are promising nanopattern replication technologies where patterns are created by mechanical deformation of imprint resist, typically a monomer or polymer formulation that is cured by heat or UV light during imprinting. This technique can be combined with contact printing and cold welding.

Multiphoton Lithography

Multiphoton lithography (also known as *direct laser lithography* or *direct laser writing*) patterns surfaces without the use of a photomask, whereby two-photon absorption is utilized to induce a change in the solubility of the resist.

Scanning Probe Lithography

Scanning probe lithography (SPL) is a tool for patterning at the nanometer-scale down to individual atoms using scanning probes. Dip-pen nanolithography is an additive, diffusive method, thermochemical nanolithography triggers chemical reactions, thermal scanning probe lithography creates 3D surfaces from polymers, and local oxidation nanolithography employs a local oxidation reaction for patterning purposes.

Other Techniques

- Molecular self-assembly (as bottom-up approach) of dense lines less than 20 nm wide in large pre-patterned trenches has been demonstrated. The degree of dimension and orientation control as well as prevention of lamella merging still need to be addressed for this to be an effective patterning technique. The important issue of line edge roughness is also highlighted by this technique. Self-assembled ripple patterns and dot arrays formed by low-energy ion-beam sputtering are another emerging form of bottom-up lithography. Aligned arrays of plasmonic and magnetic wires and nanoparticles are deposited on these templates via oblique evaporation. The templates are easily produced over large areas with periods down to 25 nm.

- Stencil lithography is a resist-less and parallel method of fabricating nanometer scale patterns using nanometer-size apertures as shadow-masks.
- X-ray lithography can be extended to a resolution of 15 nm by using the X-ray wavelengths of 1 nm as illumination. This is implemented by the proximity printing approach. The technique is developed to the extent of batch processing. The extension of the method relies on Near Field X-rays in Fresnel diffraction: A clear mask feature is "demagnified" by proximity to a wafer that is set near to a "Critical Condition". This Condition determines the mask-to-wafer gap and depends on both the size of the clear mask feature and on the wavelength. The method is simple because it requires no lenses.
- Laser printing of single nanoparticles In this method, the optical forces induced via scattering and absorption of photons on nanoparticles are used to direct single nanoparticles to specific locations on substrates and attach them via van-der Waals forces. This technique has been demonstrated on metallic nanoparticles, which are easier to print due to their large plasmonically-induced scattering and absorption cross sections, in both serial and parallel printing methods.
- Magnetolithography (ML) based on applying a magnetic field on the substrate using paramagnetic metal masks call "magnetic mask". Magnetic mask which is analog to photomask define the spatial distribution and shape of the applied magnetic field. The second component is ferromagnetic nanoparticles (analog to the Photoresist) that are assembled onto the substrate according to the field induced by the magnetic mask.
- Nanosphere lithography uses self-assembled monolayers of spheres (typically made of Polystyrene) as evaporation masks. This method has been used to fabricate arrays of gold nanodots with precisely controlled spacings.
- Proton beam writing uses a focused beam of high energy (MeV) protons to pattern resist material at nanodimensions.
- Charged-particle lithography, such as ion- or electron-projection lithographies (PREVAIL, SCALPEL, LEEPL), are also capable of high-resolution patterning. Ion beam lithography uses a focused or broad beam of energetic lightweight ions (like He^+) for transferring pattern to a surface. Using Ion Beam Proximity Lithography (IBL) nano-scale features can be transferred on non-planar surfaces.
- Neutral particle lithography (NPL) uses a broad beam of energetic neutral particle for pattern transfer on a surface.

REFERENCES

1. "MEMS Overview". Retrieved 2009-06-06.
2. Melosh, N.; Boukai, Abram; Diana, Frederic; Gerardot, Brian; Badolato, Antonio; Petroff, Pierre & Heath, James R. (2003). "Ultrahigh density nanowire lattices and circuits". Science. 300 (5616): 112–5. Bibcode:2003Sci...300..112M. doi:10.1126/science.1081940. PMID 12637672. Cite uses deprecated parameter |coauthors= (help)

3. Das, S.; Gates, A.J.; Abdu, H.A.; Rose, G.S.; Picconatto, C.A.; Ellenbogen, J.C. (2007). "Designs for Ultra-Tiny, Special-Purpose Nanoelectronic Circuits". IEEE Trans. on Circuits and Systems I. 54 (11): 11. doi:10.1109/TCSI.2007.907864.
4. Goicoechea, J.; Zamarreñoa, C.R.; Matiasa, I.R.; Arregui, F.J. (2007). "Minimizing the photobleaching of self-assembled multilayers for sensor applications". Sensors and Actuators B: Chemical. 126 (1): 41–47. doi:10.1016/j.snb.2006.10.037.
5. Petty, M.C.; Bryce, M.R.; Bloor, D. (1995). An Introduction to Molecular Electronics. London: Edward Arnold. ISBN 0-19-521156-1.
6. Aviram, A.; Ratner, M. A. (1974). "Molecular Rectifier". Chemical Physics Letters. 29 (2): 277–283. Bibcode:1974CPL....29..277A. doi:10.1016/0009-2614(74)85031-1.
7. Aviram, A. (1988). "Molecules for memory, logic, and amplification". Journal of the American Chemical Society. 110 (17): 5687–5692. doi:10.1021/ja00225a017.
8. Postma, Henk W. Ch.; Teepen, Tijs; Yao, Zhen; Grifoni, Milena; Dekker, Cees (2001). "Carbon nanotube single-electron transistors at room temperature". Science. 293 (5527): 76–79. Bibcode:2001Sci...293...76P. doi:10.1126/science.1061797. PMID 11441175.
9. Xiang, Jie; Lu, Wei; Hu, Yongjie; Wu, Yue; Yan; Hao & Lieber, Charles M. (2006). "Ge/Si nanowire heterostructures as highperformance field-effect transistors". Nature. 441 (7092): 489–493. Bibcode:2006Natur.441..489X. doi:10.1038/nature04796. PMID 16724062. Cite uses deprecated parameter |coauthors= (help)
10. Waldner, Jean-Baptiste (2007). Nanocomputers and Swarm Intelligence. London: ISTE. p. 26. ISBN 1-84704-002-0.
11. Jensen, K.; Jensen, K.; Weldon, J.; Garcia, H. & Zettl A. (2007). "Nanotube Radio". Nano Lett. 7 (11): 3508–3511. Bibcode:2007NanoL...7.3508J. doi:10.1021/nl0721113. PMID 17973438. Cite uses deprecated parameter |coauthors= (help)
12. Tian, Bozhi; Zheng, Xiaolin; Kempa, Thomas J.; Fang, Ying;Yu, Nanfang; Yu, Guihua; Huang, Jinlin & Lieber, Charles M. (2007). "Coaxial silicon nanowires as solar cells and nanoelectronic power sources". Nature. 449 (7164): 885–889. Bibcode:2007Natur.449..885T. doi:10.1038/nature06181. PMID 17943126. Cite uses deprecated parameter |coauthors= (help)
13. "Power from blood could lead to 'human batteries'". Sydney Morning Herald. August 4, 2003. Retrieved 2008-10-08.
14. LaVan, D.A.; McGuire, Terry & Langer, Robert (2003). "Small-scale systems for in vivo drug delivery". Nat. Biotechnol. 21 (10): 1184–1191. doi:10.1038/nbt876. PMID 14520404.
15. Grace, D. (2008). "Special Feature: Emerging Technologies". Medical Product Manufacturing News. 12: 22–23.
16. Saito, S. (1997). "Carbon Nanotubes for Next-Generation Electronics Devices". Science. 278 (5335): 77–78. doi:10.1126/science.278.5335.77.
17. Cavalcanti, A.; Shirinzadeh, B.; Freitas Jr, Robert A. & Hogg, Tad (2008). "Nanorobot architecture for medical target identification". Nanotechnology.

19 (1): 015103(15pp). Bibcode:2008Nanot..19a5103C. doi:10.1088/0957-4484/19/01/015103.

18. Cheng, Mark Ming-Cheng; Cuda, Giovanni; Bunimovich, Yuri L; Gaspari, Marco; Heath, James R; Hill, Haley D; Mirkin,Chad A; Nijdam, A Jasper; Terracciano, Rosa; Thundat, Thomas & Ferrari, Mauro (2006). "Nanotechnologies for biomolecular detection and medical diagnostics". Current Opinion in Chemical Biology. 10 (1): 11–19. doi:10.1016/j.cbpa.2006.01.006. PMID 16418011. Cite uses deprecated parameter |coauthors= (help)
19. Patolsky, F.; Timko, B.P.; Yu, G.; Fang, Y.; Greytak, A.B.; Zheng, G.; Lieber, C.M. (2006). "Detection, stimulation, and inhibition of neuronal signals with high-density nanowire transistor arrays". Science. 313 (5790): 1100–1104. Bibcode:2006Sci...313.1100P. doi:10.1126/science.1128640. PMID 16931757.
20. Frist, W.H. (2005). "Health care in the 21st century". N. Engl. J. Med. 352 (3): 267–272. doi:10.1056/NEJMsa045011. PMID 15659726.
21. Cavalcanti, A.; Shirinzadeh, B.; Zhang, M. & Kretly, L.C. (2008). "Nanorobot Hardware Architecture for Medical Defense" (PDF). Sensors. 8 (5): 2932–2958. doi:10.3390/s8052932.
22. Couvreur, P. & Vauthier, C. (2006). "Nanotechnology: intelligent design to treat complex disease". Pharm. Res. 23 (7): 1417–1450. doi:10.1007/s11095-006-0284-8. PMID 16779701.
23. Petty, M.C.; Bryce, M.R. & Bloor, D. (1995). Introduction to Molecular Electronics. New York: Oxford University Press. pp. 1–25. ISBN 0-19-521156-1.
24. Tour, James M.; et al. (1998). "Recent advances in molecular scale electronics". Annals of the New York Academy of Sciences. 852: 197–204. Bibcode:1998NYASA.852..197T. doi:10.1111/j.1749-6632.1998.tb09873.x.
25. Waser, Rainer; Lüssem, B. & Bjørnholm, T. (2008). "Chapter 8: Concepts in Single-Molecule Electronics". Nanotechnology. Volume 4: Information Technology II. Weinheim: Wiley-VCH Verlag GmbH & Co. KGaA. pp. 175–212. ISBN 978-3-527-31737-0.
26. Kubatkin, S.; et al. (2003). "Single-electron transistor of a single organic molecule with access to several redox states". Nature. 425 (6959): 698–701. Bibcode:2003Natur.425..698K. doi:10.1038/nature02010. PMID 14562098.
27. Anderson, Mark (2005-06-09) "Honey, I Shrunk the PC". Wired.com
28. Zoldan, Vinícius Claudio; Faccio, Ricardo & Pasa, André Avelino (2015). "N and p type character of single molecule diodes". Scientific Reports. 5: 8350. Bibcode:2015NatSR...5E8350Z. doi:10.1038/srep08350. PMC 4322354Freely accessible. PMID 25666850.
29. Gimzewski, J.K.; Joachim, C. (1999). "Nanoscale science of single molecules using local probes". Science. 283 (5408): 1683–1688. Bibcode:1999Sci...283.1683G. doi:10.1126/science.283.5408.1683. PMID 10073926.
30. Sørensen, J.K.. (2006). "Synthesis of new components, functionalized with (60)fullerene, for molecular electronics". 4th Annual meeting – CONT 2006, University of Copenhagen.

31. Service, R.F. (2003). "Molecular electronics – Next-generation technology hits an early midlife crisis". Science. 302 (5645): 556–+. doi:10.1126/science.302.5645.556. PMID 14576398.

32. Aviram, Arieh; Ratner, Mark A. (1974). "Molecular rectifiers". Chemical Physics Letters. 29 (2): 277–283. Bibcode:1974CPL....29..277A. doi:10.1016/0009-2614(74)85031-1.

33. Carter, F. L.; Siatkowski, R. E. and Wohltjen, H. (eds.) (1988) Molecular Electronic Devices, pp. 229–244, North Holland, Amsterdam.

34. Gupta, Chaitanya; Shannon, Mark A.; Kenis, Paul J. A. (2009). "Mechanisms of Charge Transport through Monolayer-Modified Polycrystalline Gold Electrodes in the Absence of Redox-Active Moieties". The Journal of Physical Chemistry C. 113 (11): 4687–4705. doi:10.1021/jp8090045.

35. Gupta, Chaitanya; Shannon, Mark A.; Kenis, Paul J. A. (2009). "Electronic Properties of a Monolayer–Electrolyte Interface Obtained from Mechanistic Impedance Analysis". The Journal of Physical Chemistry C. 113 (21): 9375–9391. doi:10.1021/jp900918u.

36. Aviram, Arieh; Ratner, M.A. (1974). "Molecular rectifiers". Chemical Physics Letters. 29 (2): 277–283. Bibcode:1974CPL....29..277A. doi:10.1016/0009-2614(74)85031-1.

37. Reed, M.A.; et al. (1997). "Conductance of a Molecular Junction". Science. 287 (5336): 252–254. doi:10.1126/science.278.5336.252.

38. Jacoby, Mitch (27 January 2003). "Molecule-based circuitry revisited". Chemical and Engineering News. Retrieved 24 February 2011.

39. Ashwell, Geoffrey J.; Hamilton, Richard; High, L. R. Hermann (2003). "Molecular rectification: asymmetric current-voltage curves from self-assembled monolayers of a donor-(n-bridge)-acceptor dye". Journal of Materials Chemistry. 13 (7): 1501. doi:10.1039/B304465N.

40. Ashwell, Geoffrey J.; Chwialkowska, Anna; High, L. R. Hermann (2004). "Au-S-CnH2n-Q3CNQ: self-assembled monolayers for molecular rectification". Journal of Materials Chemistry. 14 (15): 2389. doi:10.1039/B403942D.

41. Ashwell, Geoffrey J.; Chwialkowska, Anna; Hermann High, L. R. (2004). "Rectifying Au-S-CnH2n-P3CNQ derivatives". Journal of Materials Chemistry. 14 (19): 2848. doi:10.1039/B411343H.

42. Bumm, L. A.; Arnold, J. J.; Cygan, M. T.; Dunbar, T. D.; Burgin, T. P.; Jones, L.; Allara, D. L.; Tour, J. M.; Weiss, P. S. (1996). "Are Single Molecular Wires Conducting?". Science. 271 (5256): 1705–1707. Bibcode:1996Sci...271.1705B. doi:10.1126/science.271.5256.1705.

43. "ASML: Press - Press Releases - ASML reaches agreement for delivery of minimum of 15 EUV lithography systems". www.asml.com. Retrieved 2015-05-11.

44. Sundrani D, Darling SB, Sibener SJ (June 2004). "Hierarchical assembly and compliance of aligned nanoscale polymer cylinders in confinement" (PDF). Langmuir. 20 (12): 5091–9. doi:10.1021/la036123p. PMID 15984272.

45. T.W.H. Oates; A. Keller; S. Facsko; A. Muecklich (2007). "Aligned silver nanoparticles on rippled silicon templates exhibiting anisotropic plasmon absorption". Plasmonics. 2 (2): 47–50. doi:10.1007/s11468-007-9025-z.

46. Alexander S. Urban, Andrey A. Lutich, Fenando D. Stefani, and Jochen Feldmann, "Laser Printing Single Gold Nanoparticles", Nano Letters, VOL. 10, NO. 12, OCTOBER 2010

47. Spas Nedev, Alexander S. Urban, Andrey A. Lutich, and Jochen Feldmann, "Optical Force Stamping Lithography", Nano Letters, VOL. 11, NO. 11, OCTOBER 2011

48. A. Hatzor-de Picciotto, A. D. Wissner-Gross, G. Lavallee, P. S. Weiss (2007). "Arrays of Cu(2+)-complexed organic clusters grown on gold nano dots" (PDF). Journal of Experimental Nanoscience. 2: 3–11. Bibcode:2007JENan...2....3P. doi:10.1080/17458080600925807.

49. Dhara Parikh, Barry Craver, Hatem N. Nounu, Fu-On Fong, and John C. Wolfe, "Nanoscale Pattern Definition on Nonplanar Surfaces Using Ion Beam Proximity Lithography and Conformal Plasma-Deposited Resist", Journal of Microelectromechanical Systems, VOL. 17, NO. 3, JUNE 2008

50. J C Wolfe and B P Craver, "Neutral particle lithography: a simple solution to charge-related artefacts in ion beam proximity printing", J. Phys. D: Appl. Phys. 41 (2008) 024007 (12pp)

CHAPTER 8

Nanometrology Concepts

Chapter Contents

- **Introduction**
- **Atomic-Force Microscopy**
- **Super-Resolution Microscopy**
- **Nanotribology**

Metrology is the science of measurements, and nanometrology is that part of metrology that relates to measurements at the nanoscale. Much has been said about the predicted spectacular growth in nanotechnological production in the coming years: what is less well-known is that nanometrology has a key role in this promised growth.

INTRODUCTION

Nanometrology is a subfield of metrology, concerned with the science of measurement at the nanoscale level. Nanometrology has a crucial role in order to produce nanomaterials and devices with a high degree of accuracy and reliability in nanomanufacturing.

A challenge in this field is to develop or create new measurement techniques and standards to meet the needs of next-generation advanced manufacturing, which will rely on nanometer scale materials and technologies. The needs for measurement and characterization of new sample structures and characteristics far exceed the capabilities of current measurement science. Anticipated advances in emerging U.S. nanotechnology industries will require revolutionary metrology with higher resolution and accuracy than has previously been envisioned.

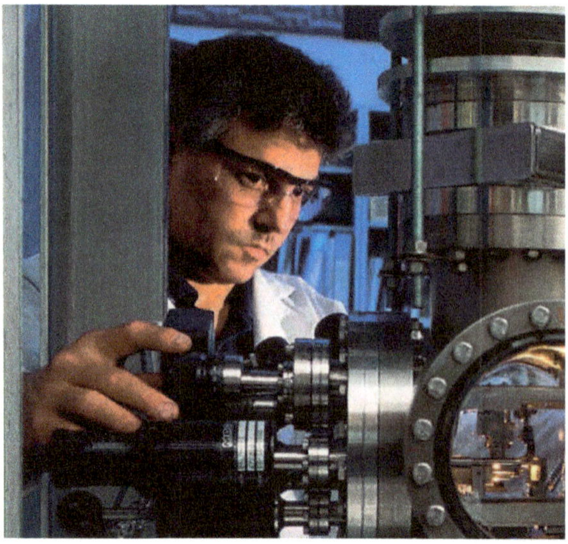

NIST Next-Generation Nanometrology research.

Control of the critical dimensions are the most important factors in nanotechnology. Nanometrology today, is to a large extent based on the development in semiconductor technology. Nanometrology is the science of measurement at the nanoscale level. Nanometre or nm is equivalent to 10-9 m. In Nanotechnology accurate control of dimensions of objects is important. Typical dimensions of nanosystems vary from 10 nm to a few hundred nm and while fabricating such systems measurement up to 0.1 nm is required.

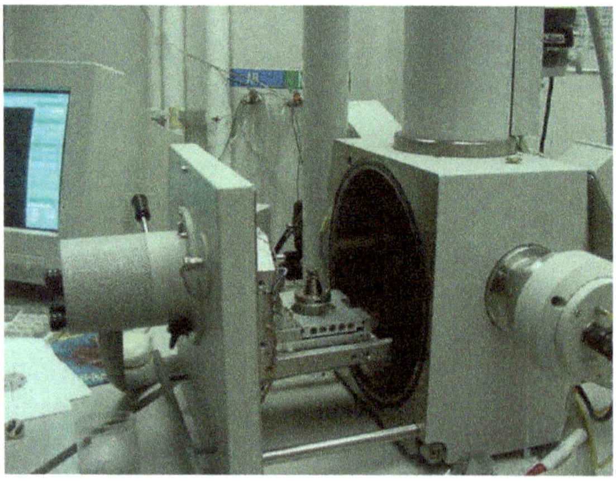

"Scanning Electron Microscope"

At nanoscale due to the small dimensions various new physical phenomena can be observed. For example, when the crystal size is smaller than the electron mean free path the conductivity of the crystal changes. Another example is the discretization of stresses in the system. It becomes important to measure the physical parameters so as to apply these phenomena into engineering of nanosystems and manufacturing them. The measurement of length or size, force, mass, electrical and other properties is included in Nanometrology. The problem is how to measure these with reliability and accuracy. The measurement techniques used for macro systems cannot be directly used for measurement of parameters in nanosystems. Various techniques based on physical phenomena have been developed which can be used for measure or determine the parameters for nanostructures and nanomaterials. Some of the popular ones are X-Ray Diffraction, Transmission Electron Microscopy, High Resolution Transmission Electron Microscopy, Atomic Force Microscopy, Scanning Electron Microscopy, Field Emission Scanning Electron Microscopy and Brunauer, Emmett, Teller method to determine specific surface.

Nanotechnology is an important field because of the large number of applications it has and it has become necessary to develop more precise techniques of measurement and globally accepted standards. Hence progress is required in the field of Nanometrology.

Development Needs

Nanotechnology can be divided into two branches. The first being Molecular Nanotechnology which involves bottom up manufacturing and the second is Engineering Nanotechnology which involve the development and processing of materials and systems at nanoscale. The measurement and manufacturing tools and techniques required for the two branches are slightly different.

Furthermore, Nanometrology requirements are different for the industry and research institutions. Nanometrology of research has progressed faster than that for industry mainly because implementing nanometrology for industry is difficult. In research oriented nanometrology resolution is important whereas in industrial nanometrology accuracy is given precedence over resolution. Further due to economic reasons it is important to have low time costs in industrial nanometrology it is not important for research nanometrology. The various measurement techniques available today require a controlled environment like in vacuum, vibration and noise free environment. Also, in industrial nanometrology requires that the measurements be more quantitative with minimum number of parameters.

Standards

International Standards

Metrology standards are objects or ideas that are designated as being authoritative for some accepted reason. Whatever value they possess is useful for comparison to unknowns for the purpose of establishing or confirming an assigned value based on the standard. The execution of measurement comparisons for the purpose of establishing the relationship between a standard and some other measuring device is calibration. The ideal standard is independently reproducible without uncertainty. The world-wide market for products with nanotechnology applications is projected to be at least a couple of hundred billion dollars in the near future. Until recently, there almost no established internationally accepted standards for nanotechnology related field. The International Organisation for

Standardization TC-229 Technical Committee on Nanotechnology recently published few standards for terminology, characterization of nanomaterials and nanoparticles using measurement tools like AFM, SEM, Interferometers, optoacoustic tools, gas adsorption methods etc. Certain standards for standardization of measurements for electrical properties have been published by the International Electrotechnical Commission. Some important standards which are yet to be established are standards for measuring thickness of thin films or layers, characterization of surface features, standards for force measurement at nanoscale, standards for characterization of critical dimensions of nanoparticles and nanostructures and also Standards for measurement for physical properties like conductivity, elasticity etc.

National Standards

Because of the importance of nanotechnology in the future, countries around the world have programmes to establish national standards for nanometrology and nanotechnology. These programmes are run by the national standard agencies of the respective countries. In the United States, National Institute of Standards and Technology has been working on developing new techniques for measurement at nanoscale and has also established some national standards for nanotechnology. These standards are for nanoparticle characterization, Roughness Characterization, magnification standard, calibration standards etc.

Calibration

It is difficult to provide samples using which precision instruments can be calibrated at nanoscale. Reference or Calibration standards are important for repeatability to be ensured. But there are no international standards for calibration and the calibration artefacts provided by the company along with their equipment is only good for calibrating that particular equipment. Hence it is difficult to select a universal calibration artefact using which we can achieve repeatability at nanoscale. At nanoscale while calibrating care needs to be taken for influence of external factors like vibration, noise, motions caused by thermal drift and creep and internal factors like the interaction between the artefact and the equipment which can cause significant deviations.

Measurement Techniques

In the last 70 years various techniques for measuring at nanoscale have been developed. Most of them based on some physical phenomena observed on particle interactions or forces at nanoscale. Some of the most commonly used techniques are Atomic Force Microscopy, X-Ray Diffraction, Scanning Electron Microscopy, Transmission Electron Microscopy, High Resolution Transmission Electron Microscopy, and Field Emission Scanning Electron Microscopy.

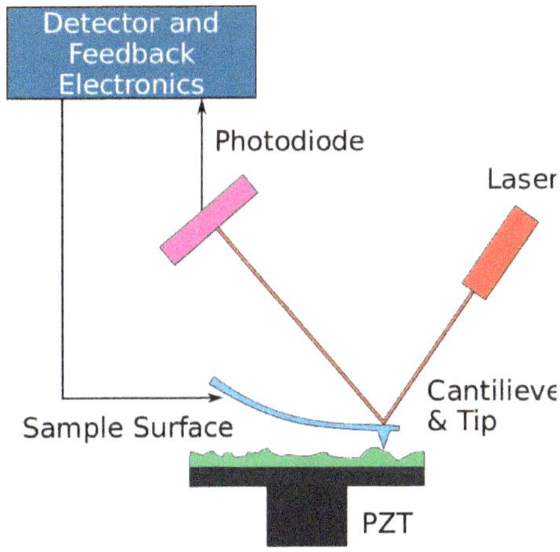

Block Diagram of *Atomic Force Microscope.*

Atomic Force Microscopy (AFM) is one of the most common measurement techniques. It can be used to measure Topology, grain size, frictional characteristics and different forces. It consists of a silicon cantilever with a sharp tip with a radius of curvature of a few nanometers. The tip is used as a probe on the specimen to be measured. The forces acting at the atomic level between the tip and the surface of the specimen cause the tip to deflect and this deflection is detected using a laser spot which is reflected to an array of photodiodes.

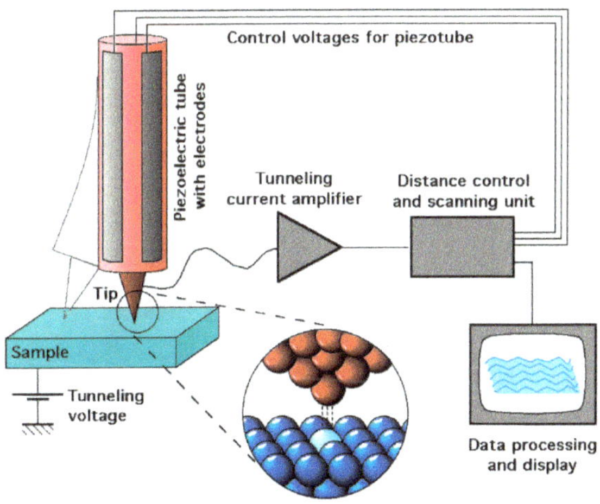

Diagram of *Scanning Tunneling Microscope.*

Scanning Tunneling Microscopy (STM) is another instrument commonly used. It is used to measure 3-D topology of the specimen. The STM is based on the concept of quantum tunneling. When a conducting tip is brought very near to the surface to be examined, a bias (voltage difference) applied between the two can allow electrons to tunnel through the vacuum between them. Measurements are made by monitoring the current as the tip's position scans across the surface, which can then be used to display an image.

Another commonly used instrument is the Scanning Electron Microscopy (SEM) which apart from measuring the shape and size of the particles and topography of the surface can be used to determine the composition of elements and compounds the sample is composed of. In SEM the specimen surface is scanned with a high energy electron beam. The electrons in the beam interact with atoms in the specimen and interactions are detected using detectors. The interactions produced are back scattering of electrons, transmission of electrons, secondary electrons etc. To remove high angle electrons magnetics lenses are used.

The instruments mentioned above produce realistic pictures of the surface are excellent measuring tools for research. Industrial applications of nanotechnology require the measurements to be produced need to be more quantitative. The requirement in industrial nanometrology is for higher accuracy than resolution as compared to research nanometrology.

Nano Coordinate Measuring Machine

A Coordinate Measuring Machine (CMM) that works at the nanoscale would have a smaller frame than the CMM used for macroscale objects. This is so because it may provide the necessary stiffness and stability to achieve nanoscale uncertainties in x,y and z directions. The probes for such a machine need to be small to enable a 3-D measurement of nanometre features from the sides and from inside like nanoholes. Also for accuracy laser interferometers need to be used. NIST has developed a surface measuring instrument, called the Molecular Measuring Machine. This instrument is basically an STM. The x- and y-axes are read out by laser interferometers. The molecules on the surface area can be identified individually and at the same time the distance between any two molecules can be determined. For measuring with molecular resolution, the measuring times become very large for even a very small surface area. Ilmenau Machine is another nanomeasuring machine developed by researchers at the Ilmenau University of Technology.

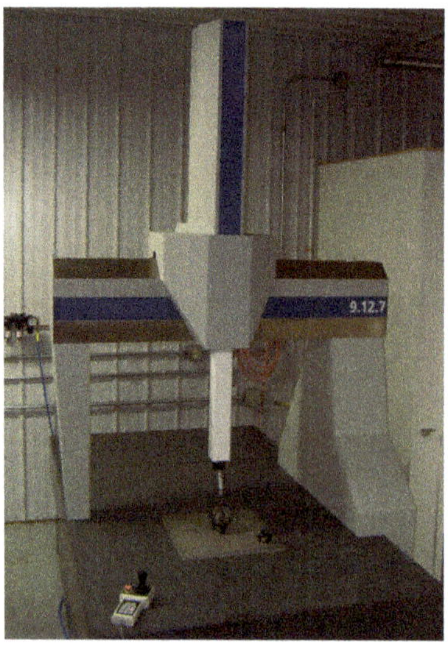

Dimensional Metrology using *CMM*.

Components of a Nano CMM

- Nanoprobes
- Control Hardware
- 3D-nanopositioning platform
- Instruments with high resolution and accuracy for linear measurement
- Instruments with high resolution and accuracy for angular measurement

List of some of the measurement techniques

- Atomic Force Microscopy
- X-ray absorption Spectroscopy
- X- Ray Diffraction
- Small Angle X-Ray Scattering
- Scanning Tunneling Microscopy
- Transmission Electron Microscopy
- Capacitance Spectroscopy
- Polarization Spectroscopy
- Auger Electron Spectroscopy
- Raman Spectroscopy
- Small Angle Neutron Scattering
- Scanning Electron Microscopy
- Cyclic Voltammetry
- Linear Sweep Voltammetry
- Nuclear Magnetic Resonance
- Mössbauer Spectroscopy
- Fourier Transform Infrared Spectroscopy
- Photoluminescence Spectroscopy
- Electroluminescence Spectroscopy
- Differential Scanning Calorimetry
- Secondary Ion Mass Spectrometry
- Cathodoluminescence Spectroscopy
- Electron Energy Loss Spectroscopy
- Energy Dispersive X-Ray Spectroscopy
- Four point probe and I-V technique
- X-Ray Photoelectron Spectroscopy
- Scanning Near-field Optical Microscopy
- Single-molecule Spectroscopy
- Neutron Diffraction

- Interference Microscopy
- Laser Interferometry

Traceability

In metrology at macro scale achieving traceability is quite easy and artefacts like scales, laser interferometers, step gauges, and straight edges are used. At nanoscale a crystalline highly oriented pyrolytic graphite (HOPG), mica or silicon surface is considered suitable used as calibration artefact for achieving traceability. But it is not always possible to ensure traceability. Like what is a straight edge at nanoscale and even if take the same standard as that for macroscale there is no way to calibrate it accurately at nanoscale. This so because the requisite internationally or nationally accepted reference standards are not always there. Also the measurement equipment required to ensure traceability has not been developed. The generally used for traceability are miniaturisation of traditional metrology standards hence there is a need for establishing nanoscale standards. Also there is a need to establish some kind of uncertainty estimation model. Traceability is one of the fundamental requirements for manufacturing and assembly of products when multiple producers are there.

Tolerance

Tolerance is the permissible limit or limits of variation in dimensions, properties, or conditions without significantly affecting functioning of equipment or a process.

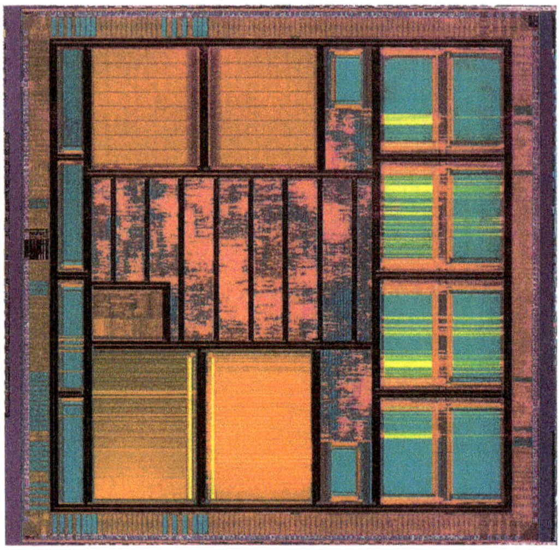

"Integrated Circuit" made using Monolithic Integration Technique.

Tolerances are specified to allow reasonable leeway for imperfections and inherent variability without compromising performance. In nanotechnology the systems have dimensions in the range of nanometers. Defining tolerances at nanoscale with suitable calibration standards for traceability is difficult for different nanomanufacturing methods. There are various integration techniques developed in the semiconductor industry that are used in nanomanufacturing.

Integration Techniques

- In Hetero integration direct fabrication of nanosystems from compound substrates is done. Geometric tolerances are required to achieve the functionality of the assembly.
- In Hybrid integration nanocomponents are placed or assembled on a substrate fabricating functioning nanosystems. In this technique, the most important control parameter is the positional accuracy of the components on the substrate.
- In Monolithic integration all the fabrication process steps are integrated on a single substrate and hence no mating of components or assembly is required. The advantage of this technique is that the geometric measurements are no longer of primary importance for achieving functionality of nanosystem or control of the fabrication process.

Classification of Nanostructures

There are a variety of Nanostructures like nanocomposites, nanowires, nanopowders, nanotubes, fullerenes nanofibers, nanocages, nanocrystallites, nanoneedles, nanofoams, nanomeshes, nanoparticles, nanopillars, thin films, nanorods, nanofabrics, quantumdots etc. The most common way to classify nano structures is by their dimensions.

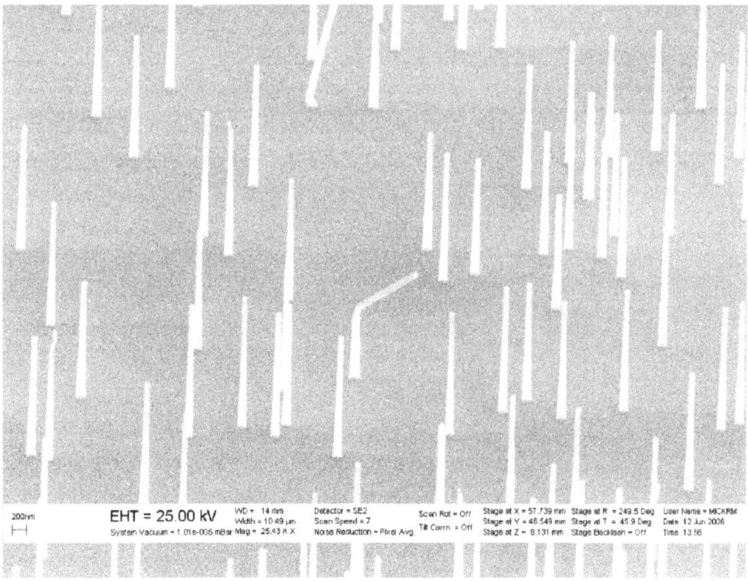

SEM of *Nanowire.*

Dimensional Classification

Dimensions	Criteria	Examples
Zero-dimensional (0-D)	The nanostructure has all dimensions in the nanometer range.	Nanoparticles, quantum dots, nanodots
One-dimensional (1-D)	One dimension of the nanostructure is outside the nanometer range.	Nanowires, nanorods, nanotubes
Two-dimensional (2-D)	Two dimensions of the nanostructure are outside the nanometer range.	Coatings, thin-film-multilayers
Three-dimensional (3-D)	Three dimensions of the nanostructure are outside the nanometer range.	Bulk

Classification of Grain Structure

Nanostructures can be classified on the basis of the grain structure and size there are made up of. This is applicable in the cas of 2-dimensional and 3-Dimensional Nanostructurs.

Surface Area Measurement

For nanopowder to determine the specific surface area the B.E.T. method is commonly used. The drop of pressure of nitrogen in a closed container due to adsorption of the nitrogen molecules to the surface of the material inserted in the container is measured. Also, the shape of the nanopowder particles is assumed to be spherical.

$$D = 6/(\rho * A)$$

Where «D» is the effective diameter, «ρ» is the density and «A» is the surface area fond from the B.E.T. method.

ATOMIC-FORCE MICROSCOPY

Atomic-force microscopy (AFM) or scanning-force Microscopy (SFM) is a very-high-resolution type of scanning probe microscopy (SPM), with demonstrated resolution on the order of fractions of a nanometer, more than 1000 times better than the optical diffraction limit.

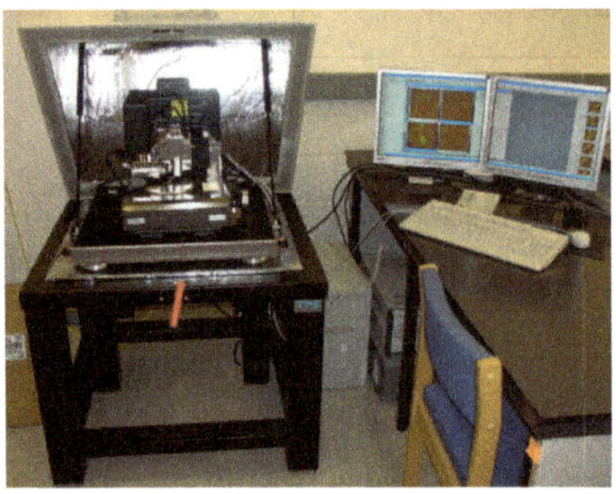

An atomic-force microscope on the left with controlling computer on the right.

Overview

Atomic-force microscopy (AFM) or scanning-force microscopy (SFM) is a type of scanning probe microscopy (SPM), with demonstrated resolution on the order of fractions of a nanometer, more than 1000 times better than the optical diffraction limit. The information is gathered by "feeling" or "touching" the surface with a mechanical probe. Piezoelectric elements that facilitate tiny but accurate and precise movements on (electronic) command enable very precise scanning.

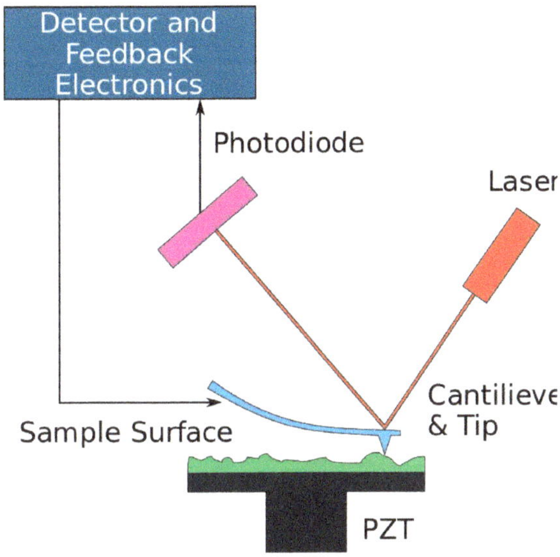

Block diagram of atomic-force microscope using beam deflection detection. As the cantilever is displaced via its interaction with the surface, so too will the reflection of the laser beam be displaced on the surface of the photodiode.

Abilities

The AFM has three major abilities: force measurement, imaging, and manipulation.

In force measurement, AFMs can be used to measure the forces between the probe and the sample as a function of their mutual separation. This can be applied to perform force spectroscopy.

For imaging, the reaction of the probe to the forces that the sample imposes on it can be used to form an image of the three-dimensional shape (topography) of a sample surface at a high resolution. This is achieved by raster scanning the position of the sample with respect to the tip and recording the height of the probe that corresponds to a constant probe-sample interaction. The surface topography is commonly displayed as a pseudocolor plot.

In manipulation, the forces between tip and sample can also be used to change the properties of the sample in a controlled way. Examples of this include atomic manipulation, scanning probe lithography and local stimulation of cells.

Simultaneous with the acquisition of topographical images, other properties of the sample can be measured locally and displayed as an image, often with similarly high resolution. Examples of such properties are mechanical properties like stiffness or adhesion strength and electrical properties such as conductivity or surface potential. In fact, the majority of SPM techniques are extensions of AFM that use this modality.

Other Microscopy Technologies

Compared to competitive technologies such as optical microscopy and electron microscopy, the major difference between these and the atomic-force microscope is that the latter does not use lenses or beam irradiation. Therefore, it does not suffer from a limitation of space resolution due to diffraction limit and aberration, and it is not necessary to prepare a space for guiding the beam (by creating a vacuum) or to stain the sample.

There are several types of scanning microscopy including scanning probe microscopy (which includes AFM, STM and near-field scanning optical microscope (SNOM/NSOM), STED microscopy (STED), and scanning electron microscopy). Although SNOM and STED use visible light to illuminate the sample, their resolution is not constrained by the diffraction limit.

Configuration

Figure shows an AFM typically consisting of the following features:

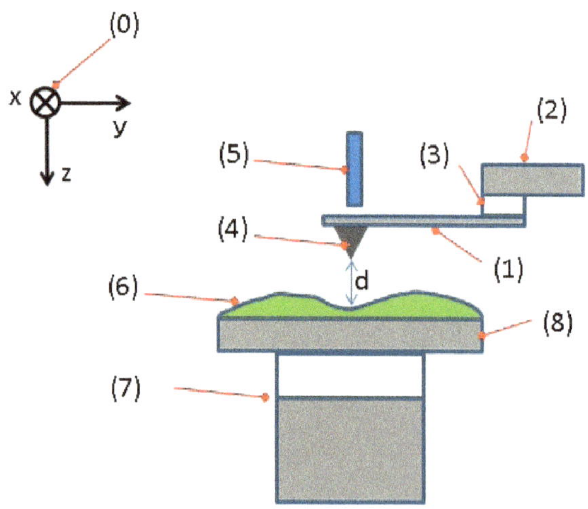

Typical configuration of an AFM.

(1):: Cantilever, **(2)**: Support for cantilever, **(3)**: Piezoelectric element(to oscillate cantilever at its eigen frequency.), **(4)**: Tip (Fixed to open end of a cantilever, acts as the probe), **(5)**: Detector of deflection and motion of the cantilever, **(6)**: Sample to be measured by AFM, **(7)**: xyz drive, (moves sample (6) and stage (8) in x, y, and z directions with respect to a tip apex (4)), and **(8)**: Stage.

The small spring-like cantilever (1) is carried by the support (2). Optionally, a piezoelectric element (3) oscillates the cantilever (1). The sharp tip (4) is fixed to the free end of the cantilever (1). The detector (5) records the deflection and motion of the cantilever (1). The sample (6) is mounted on the sample stage (8). An xyz drive (7) permits to displace the sample (6) and the sample stage (8) in x, y, and z directions with respect to the tip apex (4). Although Figure shows the drive attached to the sample, the drive can also be attached to the tip, or independent drives can be attached to both, since it is the relative displacement of the sample and tip that needs to be controlled. Controllers and plotter are not shown in Figure. Numbers in parentheses correspond to numbered features in Figure above. Coordinate directions are defined by the coordinate system (0).

According to the configuration described above, the interaction between tip and sample, which can be an atomic scale phenomenon, is transduced into changes of the motion of cantilever which is a macro scale phenomenon. Several different aspects of the cantilever motion can be used to quantify the interaction between the tip and sample, most commonly the value of the deflection, the amplitude of an imposed oscillation of the cantilever, or the shift in resonance frequency of the cantilever.

Detector

The detector (5) of AFM measures the deflection (displacement with respect to the equilibrium position) of the cantilever and converts it into an electrical signal. The intensity of this signal will be proportional to the displacement of the cantilever.

Various methods of detection can be used, e.g. interferometry, optical levers, the piezoresistive method, the piezoelectric method, and STM-based detectors.

Image Formation

When using the AFM to image a sample, the tip is brought into contact with the sample, and the sample is raster scanned along an x-y grid. Most commonly, an electronic feedback loop is employed to keep the probe-sample force constant during scanning. This feedback loop has the cantilever deflection as input, and its output controls the distance along the z axis between the probe support and the sample support. As long as the tip remains in contact with the sample, and the sample is scanned in the x-y plane, height variations in the sample will change the deflection of the cantilever. The feedback then adjusts the height of the probe support so that the deflection is restored to a user-defined value (the setpoint). A properly adjusted feedback loop adjusts the support-sample separation continuously during the scanning motion, such that the deflection remains approximately constant. In this situation, the feedback output equals the sample surface topography to within a small error.

Historically, a different operation method has been used, in which the sample-probe support distance is kept constant and not controlled by a feedback (servo mechanism). In this mode, usually referred to as 'constant height mode', the deflection of the cantilever is recorded as a function of the sample x-y position. As long as the tip is in contact with the sample, the deflection then corresponds to surface topography. The main reason this method is not very popular anymore, is that the forces between tip and sample are not controlled, which can lead to forces high enough to damage the tip or the sample. It is however common practice to record the deflection even when scanning in 'constant force mode', with feedback. This reveals the small tracking error of the feedback, and can sometimes reveal features that the feedback was not able to adjust for.

The AFM signals, such as sample height or cantilever deflection, are recorded on a computer during the x-y scan. They are plotted in a pseudocolor image, in which each pixel represents an x-y position on the sample, and the color represents the recorded signal.

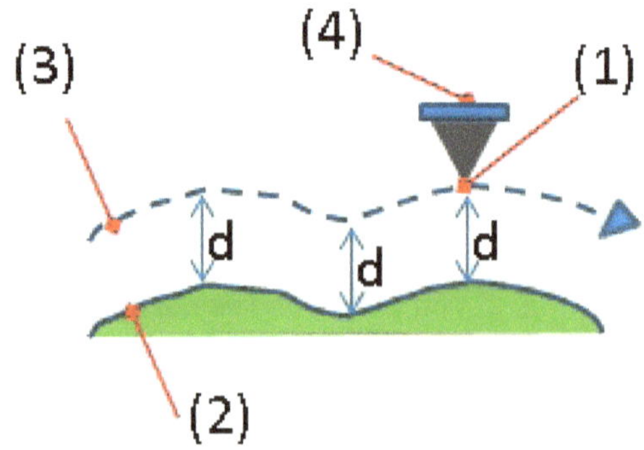

Topographic image forming by AFM. **(1)**: Tip apex, **(2)**: Sample surface, **(3)**: Z-orbit of Tip apex, **(4)**: Cantilever.

History

AFM was invented by IBM Scientists in 1982.The precursor to the AFM, the scanning tunneling microscope (STM), was developed by Gerd Binnig and Heinrich Rohrer in the early 1980s at IBM Research - Zurich, a development that earned them the Nobel Prize for Physics in 1986. Binnig invented the atomic-force microscope and the first experimental implementation was made by Binnig, Quate and Gerber in 1986.

The first commercially available atomic-force microscope was introduced in 1989. The AFM is one of the foremost tools for imaging, measuring, and manipulating matter at the nanoscale.

Applications

The AFM has been applied to problems in a wide range of disciplines of the natural sciences, including solid state physics, semiconductor science and technology, molecular engineering, polymer chemistry and physics, surface chemistry, molecular biology, cell biology and medicine.

Applications in the field of solid state physics include (a) the identification of atoms at a surface, (b) the evaluation of interactions between a specific atom and its neighboring atoms, and (c) the study of changes in physical properties arising from changes in an atomic arrangement through atomic manipulation.

In cellular biology, AFM can be used to (a) attempt to distinguish cancer cells and normal cells based on a hardness of cells, and (b) to evaluate interactions between a specific cell and its neighboring cells in a competitive culture system.

In some variations, electric potentials can also be scanned using conducting cantilevers. In more advanced versions, currents can be passed through the tip to probe the electrical conductivity or transport of the underlying surface, but this is a challenging task with few research groups reporting consistent data (as of 2004).

Principles

The AFM consists of a cantilever with a sharp tip (probe) at its end that is used to scan the specimen surface. The cantilever is typically silicon or silicon nitride with a tip radius of curvature on the order of nanometers. When the tip is brought into proximity of a sample surface, forces between the tip and the sample lead to a deflection of the cantilever according to Hooke's law.

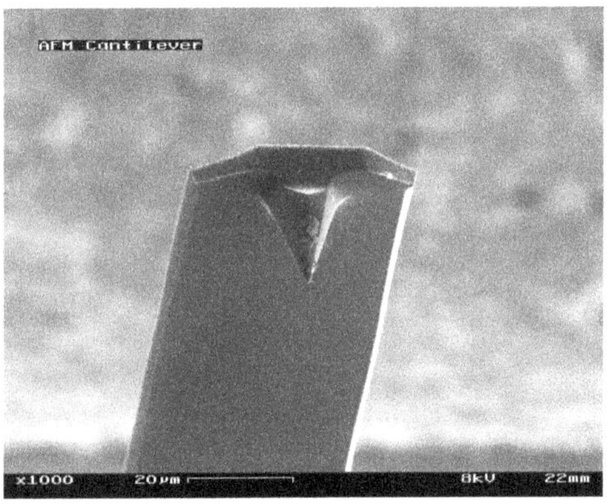

Electron micrograph of a used AFM cantilever. Image width ~100 micrometers

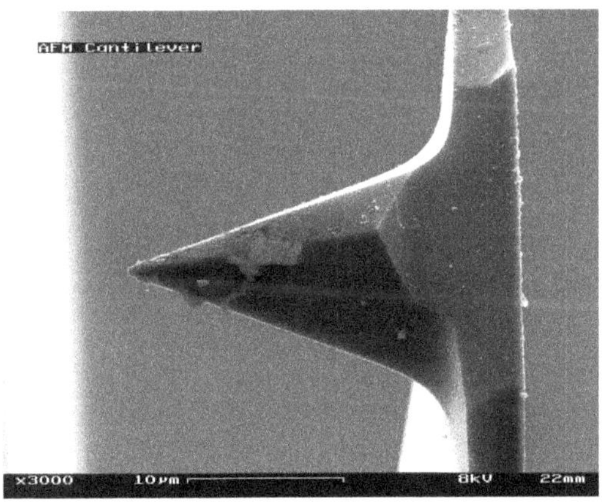

Electron micrograph of a used AFM cantilever. Image width ~30 micrometers

Depending on the situation, forces that are measured in AFM include mechanical contact force, van der Waals forces, capillary forces, chemical bonding, electrostatic forces, magnetic forces, Casimir forces, solvation forces, etc. Along with force, additional quantities may simultaneously be measured through the use of specialized types of probes.

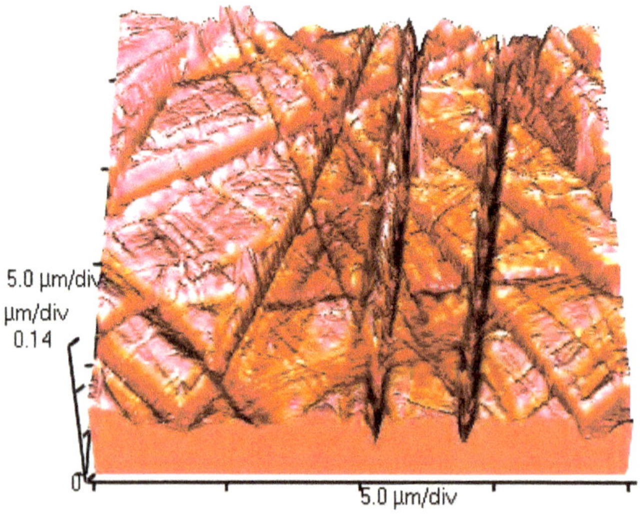

Atomic-force microscope topographical scan of a glass surface. The micro and nano-scale features of the glass can be observed, portraying the roughness of the material. The image space is (x,y,z) = (20 µm × 20 µm × 420 nm).

The AFM can be operated in a number of modes, depending on the application. In general, possible imaging modes are divided into static (also called *contact*) modes and a variety of dynamic (non-contact or "tapping") modes where the cantilever is vibrated or oscillated at a given frequency.

Imaging Modes

AFM operation is usually described as one of three modes, according to the nature of the tip motion: contact mode, also called static mode (as opposed to the other two modes, which are called dynamic modes); tapping mode, also called intermittent contact, AC mode, or vibrating mode, or, after the detection mechanism, amplitude modulation AFM; non-contact mode, or, again after the detection mechanism, frequency modulation AFM.

It should be noted that despite the nomenclature, repulsive contact can occur or be avoided both in amplitude modulation AFM and frequency modulation AFM, depending on the settings.

Contact Mode

In contact mode, the tip is "dragged" across the surface of the sample and the contours of the surface are measured either using the deflection of the cantilever directly or, more commonly, using the feedback signal required to keep the cantilever at a constant position. Because the measurement of a static signal is prone to noise and drift, low stiffness cantilevers (i.e. cantilevers with a low spring constant, k) are used to achieve a large enough deflection signal while keeping the interaction force low. Close to the surface of the sample, attractive forces can be quite strong, causing the tip to "snap-in" to the surface. Thus, contact mode AFM is almost always done at a depth where the overall force is repulsive, that is, in firm "contact" with the solid surface.

Tapping Mode

In ambient conditions, most samples develop a liquid meniscus layer. Because of this, keeping the probe tip close enough to the sample for short-range forces to become detectable while preventing the tip from sticking to the surface presents a major problem for non-contact dynamic mode in ambient conditions. Dynamic contact mode (also called intermittent contact, AC mode or tapping mode) was developed to bypass this problem. Nowadays, tapping mode is the most frequently used AFM mode when operating in ambient conditions or in liquids.

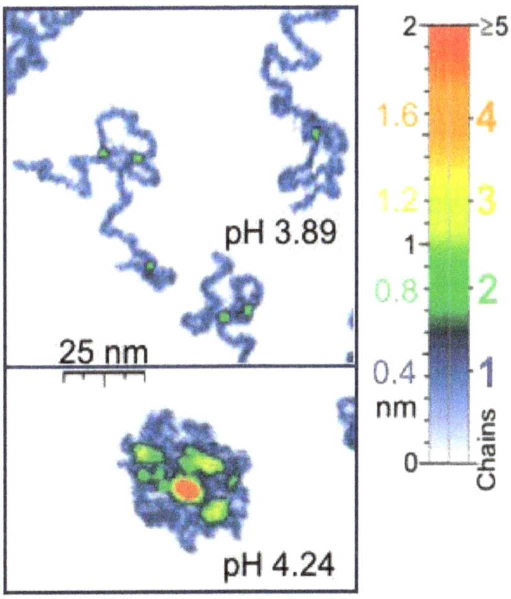

Single polymer chains (0.4 nm thick) recorded in a tapping mode under aqueous media with different pH.

In *tapping mode*, the cantilever is driven to oscillate up and down at or near its resonance frequency. This oscillation is commonly achieved with a small piezo element in the cantilever holder, but other possibilities include an AC magnetic field (with magnetic cantilevers), piezoelectric cantilevers, or periodic heating with a modulated laser beam. The amplitude of this oscillation usually varies from several nm to 200 nm. In tapping mode, the frequency and amplitude of the driving signal are kept constant, leading to a constant amplitude of the cantilever oscillation as long as there is no drift or interaction with the surface. The interaction of forces acting on the cantilever when the tip comes close to the surface, Van der Waals forces, dipole-dipole interactions, electrostatic forces, etc. cause the amplitude of the cantilever's oscillation to change (usually decrease) as the tip gets closer to the sample. This amplitude is used as the parameter that goes into the electronic servo that controls the height of the cantilever above the sample. The servo adjusts the height to maintain a set cantilever oscillation amplitude as the cantilever is scanned over the sample. A *tapping AFM* image is therefore produced by imaging the force of the intermittent contacts of the tip with the sample surface.

Although the peak forces applied during the contacting part of the oscillation can be much higher than typically used in contact mode, tapping mode generally lessens the damage done to the surface and the tip compared to the amount done in contact mode. This can be explained by the short duration of the applied force, and because the lateral forces between tip and sample are significantly lower in tapping mode over contact mode. Tapping mode imaging is gentle enough even for the visualization of supported lipid bilayers or adsorbed single polymer molecules (for instance, 0.4 nm thick chains of synthetic polyelectrolytes) under liquid medium. With proper scanning parameters, the conformation of single molecules can remain unchanged for hours, and even single molecular motors can be imaged while moving.

When operating in tapping mode, the phase of the cantilever's oscillation with respect to the driving signal can be recorded as well. This signal channel contains information about the energy dissipated by the cantilever in each oscillation cycle. Samples that contain regions of varying stiffness or with different adhesion properties can give a contrast in this channel that is not visible in the topographic image. Extracting the sample's material properties in a quantitative manner from phase images, however, is often not feasible.

Non-Contact Mode

In non-contact atomic force microscopy mode, the tip of the cantilever does not contact the sample surface. The cantilever is instead oscillated at either its resonant frequency (frequency modulation) or just above (amplitude modulation) where the amplitude of oscillation is typically a few nanometers (<10 nm) down to a few picometers. The van der Waals forces, which are strongest from 1 nm to 10 nm above the surface, or any other long-range force that extends above the surface acts to decrease the resonance frequency of the cantilever. This decrease in resonant frequency combined with the feedback loop system maintains a constant oscillation amplitude or frequency by adjusting the average tip-to-sample distance. Measuring the tip-to-sample distance at each (x,y) data point allows the scanning software to construct a topographic image of the sample surface.

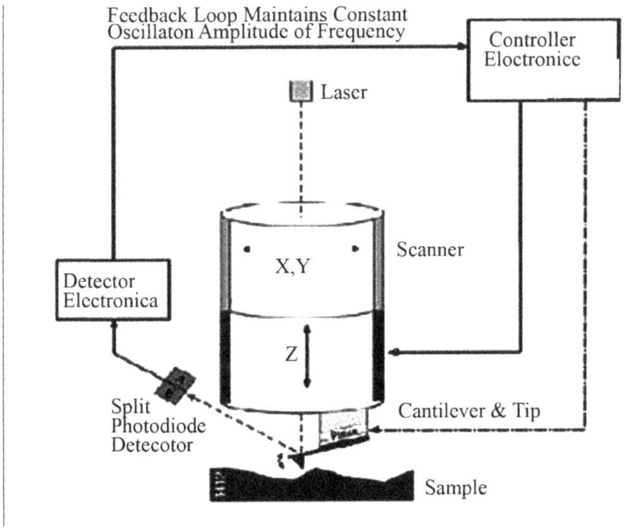

AFM – non-contact mode

Non-contact mode AFM does not suffer from tip or sample degradation effects that are sometimes observed after taking numerous scans with contact AFM. This makes non-contact AFM preferable to contact AFM for measuring soft samples, e.g. biological samples and organic thin film. In the case of rigid samples, contact and non-contact images may look the same. However, if a few monolayers of adsorbed fluid are lying on the surface of a rigid sample, the images may look quite different. An AFM operating in contact mode will penetrate the liquid layer to image the underlying surface, whereas in non-contact mode an AFM will oscillate above the adsorbed fluid layer to image both the liquid and surface.

Schemes for dynamic mode operation include frequency modulation where a phase-locked loop is used to track the cantilever's resonance frequency and the more common amplitude modulation with a servo loop in place to keep the cantilever excitation to a defined amplitude. In frequency modulation, changes in the oscillation frequency provide information about tip-sample interactions. Frequency can be measured with very high sensitivity and thus the frequency modulation mode allows for the use of very stiff cantilevers. Stiff cantilevers provide stability very close to the surface and, as a result, this technique was the first AFM technique to provide true atomic resolution in ultra-high vacuum conditions.

In amplitude modulation, changes in the oscillation amplitude or phase provide the feedback signal for imaging. In amplitude modulation, changes in the phase of oscillation can be used to discriminate between different types of materials on the surface. Amplitude modulation can be operated either in the non-contact or in the intermittent contact regime. In dynamic contact mode, the cantilever is oscillated such that the separation distance between the cantilever tip and the sample surface is modulated.

Amplitude modulation has also been used in the non-contact regime to image with atomic resolution by using very stiff cantilevers and small amplitudes in an ultra-high vacuum environment.

Topographic Image

Image formation is a plotting method that produces a color mapping through changing the x-y position of the tip while scanning and recording the measured variable, i.e. the intensity of control signal, to each x-y coordinate. The color mapping shows the measured value corresponding to each coordinate. The image expresses the intensity of a value as a hue. Usually, the correspondence between the intensity of a value and a hue is shown as a color scale in the explanatory notes accompanying the image.

What is the topographic image of atomic-force microscope?

Operation mode of Image forming of the AFM are generally classified into two groups from the viewpoint whether it uses z-Feedback loop (not shown) to maintain the tip-sample distance to keep signal intensity exported by the detector. The first one (using z-Feedback loop), said to be "constant **XX** mode" (**XX** is something which kept by z-Feedback loop).

Topographic Image Formation Mode is based on abovementioned "constant **XX** mode", z-Feedback loop controls the relative distance between the probe and the sample through outputting control signals to keep constant one of frequency, vibration and phase which typically corresponds to the motion of cantilever (for instance, voltage is applied to the Z-piezoelectric element and it moves the sample up and down towards the Z direction.

Details will be explained in the case that especially "constant df mode"(FM-AFM) among AFM as an instance in next section.

Topographic image of FM-AFM

When the distance between the probe and the sample is brought to the range where atomic force may be detected, while a cantilever is excited in its natural eigen frequency (f_0), a phenomenon that the resonance frequency (f) of the cantilever shifts from the original resonance frequency (natural eigen frequency) of the cantilever. In other words, in the range where atomic force may be detected, the frequency shift ($df=f-f_0$) will be observed. So, when the distance between the probe and the sample is in the **non-contact** region, the frequency shift increases in negative direction as the distance between the probe and the sample gets smaller.

When the sample has concavity and convexity, the distance between the tip-apex and the sample varies in accordance with the concavity and convexity accompanied with a scan of the sample along x-y direction (without height regulation in z-direction) . As a result, the frequency shift arises. The image in which the values of the frequency obtained by a raster scan along the x-y direction of the sample surface are plotted against the x-y coordination of each measurement point is called a constant-height image.

On the other hand, the df may be kept constant by moving the probe upward and downward in z-direction using a negative feedback (by using z-feedback loop) while the raster scan of the sample surface along the x-y direction . The image in which the amounts of the negative feedback (the moving distance of the probe upward and downward in z-direction) are plotted against the x-y coordination of each measurement point is a topographic image. In other words, the topographic image is a trace of the tip of the probe regulated so that the df is constant and it may also be considered to be a plot of a constant-height surface of the df.

Therefore, the topographic image of the AFM is not the exact surface morphology itself, but actually the image influenced by the bond-order between the probe and the sample, however, the topographic image of the AFM is considered to reflect the geographical shape of the surface more than the topographic image of a scanning tunnel microscope.

Force Spectroscopy

Another major application of AFM (besides imaging) is force spectroscopy, the direct measurement of tip-sample interaction forces as a function of the gap between the tip and sample (the result of this measurement is called a force-distance curve). For this method, the AFM tip is extended towards and retracted from the surface as the deflection of the cantilever is monitored as a function of piezoelectric displacement. These measurements have been used to measure nanoscale contacts, atomic bonding, Van der Waals forces, and Casimir forces, dissolution forces in liquids and single molecule stretching and rupture forces. Furthermore, AFM was used to measure, in an aqueous environment, the dispersion force due to polymer adsorbed on the substrate. Forces of the order of a few piconewtons can now be routinely measured with a vertical distance resolution of better than 0.1 nanometers. Force spectroscopy can be performed with either static or dynamic modes. In dynamic modes, information about the cantilever vibration is monitored in addition to the static deflection.

Problems with the technique include no direct measurement of the tip-sample separation and the common need for low-stiffness cantilevers, which tend to 'snap' to the surface. These problems are not insurmountable. An AFM that directly measures the tip-sample separation has been developed. The snap-in can be reduced by measuring in liquids or by using stiffer cantilevers, but in the latter case a more sensitive deflection sensor is needed. By applying a small dither to the tip, the stiffness (force gradient) of the bond can be measured as well.

Biological Applications and Other

Force spectroscopy is used in biophysics to measure the mechanical properties. of living material (such as tissue or cells). Another application was to measure the interaction forces between from one hand a material stuck on the tip of the cantilever, and from another hand the surface of particles either free or occupied by the same material. From the adhesion force distribution curve, a mean value of the forces has been derived. It allowed to make a cartography of the surface of the particles, covered or not by the material.

Identification of Individual Surface Atoms

The AFM can be used to image and manipulate atoms and structures on a variety of surfaces. The atom at the apex of the tip "senses" individual atoms on the underlying surface when it forms incipient chemical bonds with each atom. Because these chemical interactions subtly alter the tip's vibration frequency, they can be detected and mapped.

This principle was used to distinguish between atoms of silicon, tin and lead on an alloy surface, by comparing these 'atomic fingerprints' to values obtained from large-scale density functional theory (DFT) simulations.

The trick is to first measure these forces precisely for each type of atom expected in the sample, and then to compare with forces given by DFT simulations. The team found that the tip interacted most strongly with silicon atoms, and interacted 24% and 41% less strongly with tin and lead atoms, respectively. Thus, each different type of atom can be identified in the matrix as the tip is moved across the surface.

Probe

An AFM probe has a sharp tip on the free-swinging end of a cantilever that is protruding from a holder. The dimensions of the cantilever are in the scale of micrometers. The radius of the tip is usually on the scale of a few nanometers to a few tens of nanometers. (Specialized probes exist with much larger end radii, for example probes for indentation of soft materials.) The cantilever holder, also called holder chip – often 1.6 mm by 3.4 mm in size – allows the operator to hold the AFM cantilever/probe assembly with tweezers and fit it into the corresponding holder clips on the scanning head of the atomic-force microscope.

This device is most commonly called an "AFM probe", but other names include "AFM tip" and "cantilever" (employing the name of a single part as the name of the whole device). An AFM probe is a particular type of SPM (scanning probe microscopy) probe.

AFM probes are manufactured with MEMS technology. Most AFM probes used are made from silicon (Si), but borosilicate glass and silicon nitride are also in use. AFM probes are considered consumables as they are often replaced when the tip apex becomes dull or contaminated or when the cantilever is broken. They can cost from a couple of tens of dollars up to hundreds of dollars per cantilever for the most specialized cantilever/probe combinations.

Just the tip is brought very close to the surface of the object under investigation, the cantilever is deflected by the interaction between the tip and the surface, which is what the AFM is designed to measure. A spatial map of the interaction can be made by measuring the deflection at many points on a 2D surface.

Several types of interaction can be detected. Depending on the interaction under investigation, the surface of the tip of the AFM probe needs to be modified with a coating. Among the coatings used are gold – for covalent bonding of biological molecules and the detection of their interaction with a surface, diamond for increased wear resistance and magnetic coatings for detecting the magnetic properties of the investigated surface. Another solution exists to achieve high resolution magnetic imaging : having the probe equip with a microSQUID. The AFM tips is fabricated using silicon micro machining and the precise positioning of the microSQUID loop is done by electron beam lithography.

The surface of the cantilevers can also be modified. These coatings are mostly applied in order to increase the reflectance of the cantilever and to improve the deflection signal.

AFM Cantilever-Deflection Measurement

Beam-Deflection Measurement

(PSD) consisting of two closely spaced photodiodes whose output signal is collected by a differential amplifier. Angular displacement of the cantilever results in one photodiode collecting more light than the other photodiode, producing an output signal (the difference between the photodiode signals normalized by their sum), which is proportional to the deflection of the cantilever. The sensitivity of the beam-deflection method is very high, a noise floor on the order of 10 fm $Hz^{-1/2}$ can be obtained routinely in a well-designed system. Although this method is sometimes called the 'optical lever' method, the signal is not amplified if the beam path is made longer. A longer beam path increases the motion of the reflected spot on the photodiodes, but also widens the spot by the same amount due to diffraction, so that the same amount of optical power is moved from one photodiode to the other. The 'optical leverage' (output signal of the detector divided by deflection of the cantilever) is inversely proportional to the numerical aperture of the beam focusing optics, as long as the focused laser spot is small enough to fall completely on the cantilever. It is also inversely proportional to the length of the cantilever. The most common method for cantilever-deflection measurements is the beam-deflection method. In this method, laser light from a solid-state diode is reflected off the back of the cantilever and collected by a position-sensitive detector.

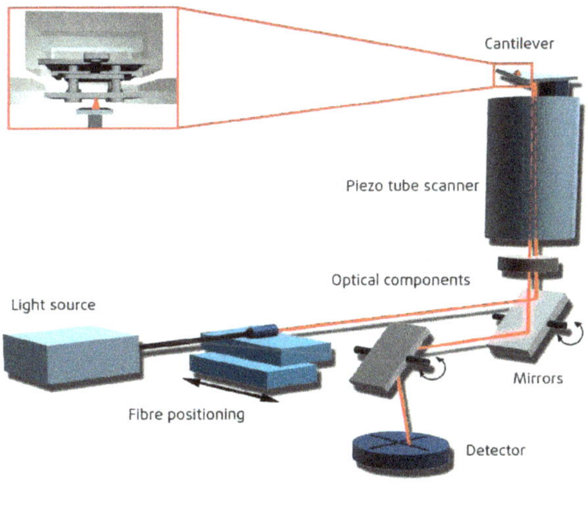

AFM beam-deflection detection

The relative popularity of the beam-deflection method can be explained by its high sensitivity and simple operation, and by the fact that cantilevers do not require electrical contacts or other special treatments, and can therefore be fabricated relatively cheaply with sharp integrated tips.

Other Deflection-Measurement Methods

Many other methods for beam-deflection measurements exist.

- *Piezoelectric detection* – Cantilevers made from quartz (such as the qPlus configuration), or other piezoelectric materials can directly detect deflection as an electrical signal. Cantilever oscillations down to 10pm have been detected with this method.
- *Laser Doppler vibrometry* – A laser Doppler vibrometer can be used to produce very accurate deflection measurements for an oscillating cantilever (thus is only used in non-contact mode). This method is expensive and is only used by relatively few groups.
- *STM* — The first atomic microscope used an STM complete with its own feedback mechanism to measure deflection. This method is very difficult to implement, and is slow to react to deflection changes compared to modern methods.
- *Optical interferometry* – Optical interferometry can be used to measure cantilever deflection. Due to the nanometre scale deflections measured in AFM, the interferometer is running in the sub-fringe regime, thus, any drift in laser power or wavelength has strong effects on the measurement. For these reasons optical interferometer measurements must be done with great care (for example using index matching fluids between optical fibre junctions), with very stable lasers. For these reasons optical interferometry is rarely used.
- *Capacitive detection* – Metal coated cantilevers can form a capacitor with another contact located behind the cantilever. Deflection changes the distance between the contacts and can be measured as a change in capacitance.
- *Piezoresistive detection* – Cantilevers can be fabricated with piezoresistive elements that act as a strain gauge. Using a Wheatstone bridge, strain in the AFM cantilever due to deflection can be measured. This is not commonly used in vacuum applications, as the piezoresistive detection dissipates energy from the system affecting Q of the resonance.

Piezoelectric Scanners

AFM scanners are made from piezoelectric material, which expands and contracts proportionally to an applied voltage. Whether they elongate or contract depends upon the polarity of the voltage applied. Traditionally the tip or sample is mounted on a 'tripod' of three piezo crystals, with each responsible for scanning in the x,y and z directions. In 1986, the same year as the AFM was invented, a new piezoelectric scanner, the tube scanner, was developed for use in STM. Later tube scanners were incorporated into AFMs. The tube scanner can move the sample in the x, y, and z directions using a single tube piezo with a single interior contact and four external contacts. An advantage of the tube scanner compared to the original tripod design, is better vibrational isolation, resulting from the higher resonant frequency of the single element construction, in combination with a low resonant frequency isolation stage. A disadvantage is that the x-y motion can cause unwanted z motion resulting in distortion. Another popular design for AFM scanners is the flexure stage, which uses separate piezos for each axis, and couples them through a flexure mechanism.

Scanners are characterized by their sensitivity, which is the ratio of piezo movement to piezo voltage, i.e., by how much the piezo material extends or contracts per applied volt. Because of differences in material or size, the sensitivity varies from scanner to scanner. Sensitivity varies non-linearly with respect to scan size. Piezo scanners exhibit more sensitivity at the end than at the beginning of a scan. This causes the forward and reverse scans to behave differently and display hysteresis between the two scan directions. This can be corrected by applying a non-linear voltage to the piezo electrodes to cause linear scanner movement and calibrating the scanner accordingly. One disadvantage of this approach is that it requires re-calibration because the precise non-linear voltage needed to correct non-linear movement will change as the piezo ages (see below). This problem can be circumvented by adding a linear sensor to the sample stage or piezo stage to detect the true movement of the piezo. Deviations from ideal movement can be detected by the sensor and corrections applied to the piezo drive signal to correct for non-linear piezo movement. This design is known as a 'closed loop' AFM. Non-sensored piezo AFMs are referred to as 'open loop' AFMs.

The sensitivity of piezoelectric materials decreases exponentially with time. This causes most of the change in sensitivity to occur in the initial stages of the scanner's life. Piezoelectric scanners are run for approximately 48 hours before they are shipped from the factory so that they are past the point where they may have large changes in sensitivity. As the scanner ages, the sensitivity will change less with time and the scanner would seldom require recalibration, though various manufacturer manuals recommend monthly to semi-monthly calibration of open loop AFMs.

Advantages and Disadvantages

Just like any other tool, an AFM's usefulness has limitations. When determining whether or not analyzing a sample with an AFM is appropriate, there are various advantages and disadvantages that must be considered.

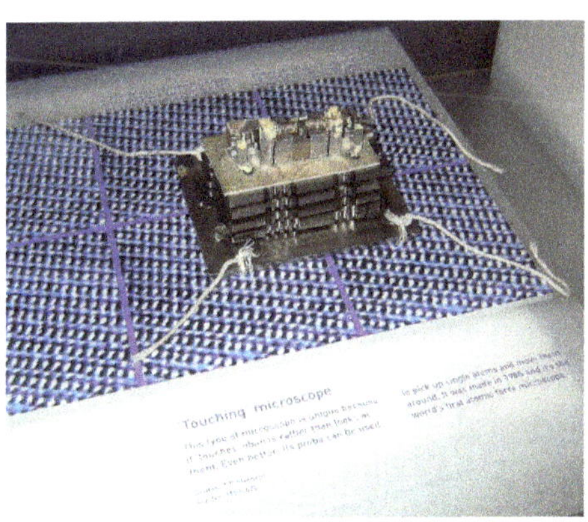

The first atomic-force microscope

Advantages

AFM has several advantages over the scanning electron microscope (SEM). Unlike the electron microscope, which provides a two-dimensional projection or a two-dimensional image of a sample, the AFM provides a three-dimensional surface profile. In addition, samples viewed by AFM do not require any special treatments (such as metal/carbon coatings) that would irreversibly change or damage the sample, and does not typically suffer from charging artifacts in the final image. While an electron microscope needs an expensive vacuum environment for proper operation, most AFM modes can work perfectly well in ambient air or even a liquid environment. This makes it possible to study biological macromolecules and even living organisms. In principle, AFM can provide higher resolution than SEM. It has been shown to give true atomic resolution in ultra-high vacuum (UHV) and, more recently, in liquid environments. High resolution AFM is comparable in resolution to scanning tunneling microscopy and transmission electron microscopy. AFM can also be combined with a variety of optical microscopy techniques such as fluorescent microscopy, further expanding its applicability. Combined AFM-optical instruments have been applied primarily in the biological sciences but have also found a niche in some materials applications, especially those involving photovoltaics research.

Disadvantages

A disadvantage of AFM compared with the scanning electron microscope (SEM) is the single scan image size. In one pass, the SEM can image an area on the order of square millimeters with a depth of field on the order of millimeters, whereas the AFM can only image a maximum scanning area of about 150×150 micrometers and a maximum height on the order of 10-20 micrometers. One method of improving the scanned area size for AFM is by using parallel probes in a fashion similar to that of millipede data storage.

The scanning speed of an AFM is also a limitation. Traditionally, an AFM cannot scan images as fast as an SEM, requiring several minutes for a typical scan, while an SEM is capable of scanning at near real-time, although at relatively low quality. The relatively slow rate of scanning during AFM imaging often leads to thermal drift in the image making the AFM less suited for measuring accurate distances between topographical features on the image. However, several fast-acting designs were suggested to increase microscope scanning productivity including what is being termed videoAFM (reasonable quality images are being obtained with videoAFM at video rate: faster than the average SEM). To eliminate image distortions induced by thermal drift, several methods have been introduced.

AFM images can also be affected by nonlinearity, hysteresis, and creep of the piezoelectric material and cross-talk between the x, y, z axes that may require software enhancement and filtering. Such filtering could "flatten" out real topographical features. However, newer AFMs utilize real-time correction software (for example, feature-oriented scanning) or closed-loop scanners, which practically eliminate these problems. Some AFMs also use separated orthogonal scanners (as opposed to a single tube), which also serve to eliminate part of the cross-talk problems.

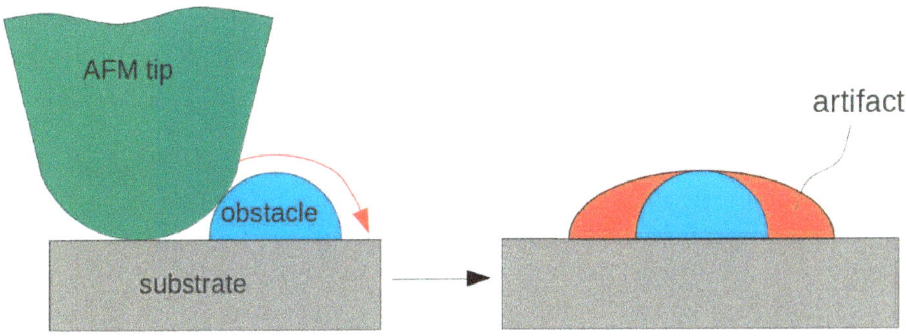

Showing an AFM artifact arising from a tip with a high radius of curvature with respect to the feature that is to be visualized.

As with any other imaging technique, there is the possibility of image artifacts, which could be induced by an unsuitable tip, a poor operating environment, or even by the sample itself, as depicted on the right. These image artifacts are unavoidable; however, their occurrence and effect on results can be reduced through various methods. Artifacts resulting from a too-coarse tip can be caused for example by inappropriate handling or de facto collisions with the sample by either scanning too fast or having an unreasonably rough surface, causing actual wearing of the tip.

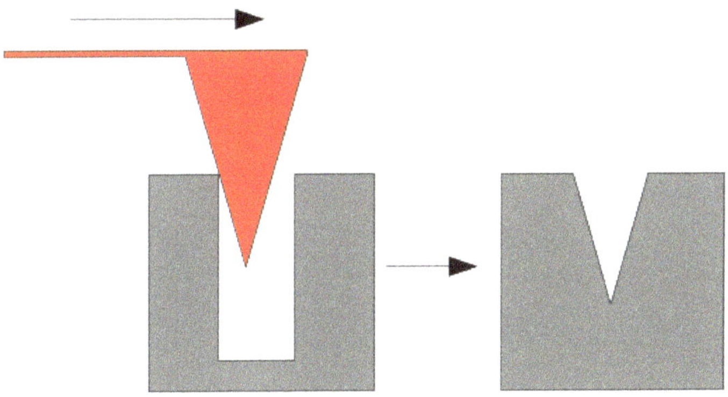

AFM artifact, steep sample topography

Due to the nature of AFM probes, they cannot normally measure steep walls or overhangs. Specially made cantilevers and AFMs can be used to modulate the probe sideways as well as up and down (as with dynamic contact and non-contact modes) to measure sidewalls, at the cost of more expensive cantilevers, lower lateral resolution and additional artifacts.

Other Applications in Various Fields of Study

The latest efforts in integrating nanotechnology and biological research have been successful and show much promise for the future. Since nanoparticles are a potential vehicle of drug delivery, the biological responses of cells to these nanoparticles are continuously being explored to optimize their efficacy and how their design could be improved. Pyrgiotakis et al. were able to study the interaction between CeO2 and Fe2O3 engineered nanoparticles and cells by attaching the engineered nanoparticles to the AFM tip. Beyond the interactions with external synthetic materials, cells have been imaged with X-ray crystallography and there has been much curiosity about their behavior *in vivo*. Studies have taken advantage of AFM to obtain further information on the behavior of live cells in biological media. Real-time atomic force spectroscopy (or nanoscopy) and dynamic atomic force spectroscopy have been used to study live cells and membrane proteins and their dynamic behavior at high resolution, on the nanoscale. Imaging and obtaining information on the topography and the properties of the cells has also given insight into chemical processes and mechanisms that occur through cell-cell interaction and interactions with other signaling molecules (ex. ligands). Evans and Calderwood used single cell force microscopy to study cell adhesion forces, bond kinetics/dynamic bond strength and its role in chemical processes such as cell signaling. Scheuring, Lévy, and Rigaud reviewed studies in which AFM to explore the crystal structure of membrane proteins of photosynthetic bacteria. Alsteen et al. have used AFM-based nanoscopy to perform a real-time analysis of the interaction between live mycobacteria and antimycobacterial drugs (specifically isoniazid, ethionamide, ethambutol, and streptomycine), which serves as an example of the more in-depth analysis of pathogen-drug interactions that can be done through AFM.

SUPER-RESOLUTION MICROSCOPY

Super-resolution microscopy is a form of light microscopy. Due to the diffraction of light, the resolution of conventional light microscopy is limited, as stated by Ernst Abbe in 1873. A good approximation of the resolution attainable is the full width at half maximum (FWHM) of the point spread function, and a precise widefield microscope with high numerical aperture and visible light usually reaches a resolution of ~250 nm.

Super-resolution techniques allow images to be taken with a higher resolution than the diffraction limit.

True subwavelength imaging techniques include those that utilize the Pendry Superlens and near field scanning optical microscopy, the 4Pi Microscope and structured illumination microscopy technologies like SIM and SMI. However, the majority of techniques of importance in biological imaging fall into the functional category.

There are two major groups of methods for functional super-resolution microscopy:

- Deterministic super-resolution: The most commonly used emitters in biological microscopy, fluorophores, show a nonlinear response to excitation, and this nonlinear response can be exploited to enhance resolution. These methods include STED, GSD, RESOLFT and SSIM.
- Stochastic super-resolution: The chemical complexity of many molecular light sources gives them a complex temporal behavior, which can be used to make several close-by fluorophores emit light at separate times and thereby become resolvable in time. These methods include Super-resolution optical fluctuation

imaging (SOFI) and all single-molecule localization methods (SMLM) such as SPDM, SPDMphymod, PALM, FPALM, STORM and dSTORM.

On October 8, 2014, the Nobel Prize in Chemistry was awarded to Eric Betzig, W.E. Moerner and Stefan Hell for "the development of super-resolved fluorescence microscopy," which brings "optical microscopy into the nanodimension".

NANOTRIBOLOGY

Nanotribology is the branch of tribology that studies friction, wear, adhesion and lubrication phenomena at the nanoscale, where atomic interactions and quantum effects are not negligible. The aim of this discipline is characterizing and modifying surfaces for both scientific and technological purposes.

Historically, nanotribological research includes direct investigation with microscopy techniques, such as Scanning Tunneling Microscope (STM), Atomic-Force Microscope (AFM) and Surface Forces Apparatus, (SFA) used to analyze surfaces with extremely high resolution, and thanks to the development of computational methods and power surfaces, we can study these phenomena indirectly as well.

Changing the topology of surfaces at the nanoscale, friction can be either reduced or enhanced more intensively than macroscopic lubrication and adhesion; in this way, superlubrication and superadhesion can be achieved. In micro- and nano-mechanical devices problems of friction and wear, that are critical due to the extremely high surface volume ratio, can be solved covering moving parts with super lubricant coatings. On the other hand, where adhesion is an issue, nanotribological techniques offer a possibility to overcome such difficulties.

REFERENCES

1. This article incorporates public domain material from the National Institute of Standards and Technology website http://www.nist.gov.
2. NIST Manufacturing Engineering (2008).NIST Programs of the Manufacturing Engineering Laboratory. March 2008.
3. NIST 2008, p.31
4. R. V. Lapshin (2015). "Drift-insensitive distributed calibration of probe microscope scanner in nanometer range: Approach description" (PDF). Applied Surface Science. Netherlands: Elsevier B. V. 359: 629–636. arXiv:1501.05545Freely accessible. Bibcode:2015ApSS..359..629L. doi:10.1016/j.apsusc.2015.10.108. ISSN 0169-4332.
5. R. V. Lapshin (2016). "Drift-insensitive distributed calibration of probe microscope scanner in nanometer range: Virtual mode" (PDF). Applied Surface Science. Netherlands: Elsevier B. V. 378: 530–539. doi:10.1016/j.apsusc.2016.03.201. ISSN 0169-4332.
6. http://www.co-nanomet.eu/

7. R. V. Lapshin (1998). "Automatic lateral calibration of tunneling microscope scanners" (PDF). Review of Scientific Instruments. USA: AIP. 69 (9): 3268–3276. Bibcode:1998RScI...69.3268L. doi:10.1063/1.1149091. ISSN 0034-6748.
8. D.J. Whitehouse "Surface and Nanometrlogy"
9. Nanotechnology Global Strategies, Industry Trends and Applications
10. http://www.co-nanomet.eu/.../Eighth%20Nanoforum%20Report_%20 Nanometrology.pdf
11. http://www.wiley-vch.de/books/sample/3527326758_c01.pdf
12. Patent US4724318 - Atomic-force microscope and method for imaging surfaces with atomic resolution
13. Binnig, G.; Quate, C. F.; Gerber, C. (1986). "Atomic-Force Microscope". Physical Review Letters. 56: 930–933. Bibcode:1986PhRvL..56..930B. doi:10.1103/physrevlett.56.930.
14. Lang, K.M.; D. A. Hite; R. W. Simmonds; R. McDermott; D. P. Pappas; John M. Martinis (2004). "Conducting atomic-force microscopy for nanoscale tunnel barrier characterization". Review of Scientific Instruments. 75 (8): 2726–2731. Bibcode:2004RScI...75.2726L. doi:10.1063/1.1777388.
15. Cappella, B; Dietler, G (1999). "Force-distance curves by atomic-force microscopy" (PDF). Surface Science Reports. 34 (1–3): 1–104. Bibcode:1999SurSR..34....1C. doi:10.1016/S0167-5729(99)00003-5. Archived from the original (PDF) on 2012-12-03.
16. Binnig, G.; Quate, C. F.; Gerber, Ch. (1986). "Atomic-Force Microscope". Physical Review Letters. 56 (9): 930–933. Bibcode:1986PhRvL..56..930B. doi:10.1103/PhysRevLett.56.930. ISSN 0031-9007. PMID 10033323.
17. Roiter, Y; Minko, S (Nov 2005). "AFM single molecule experiments at the solid-liquid interface: in situ conformation of adsorbed flexible polyelectrolyte chains". Journal of the American Chemical Society. 127 (45): 15688–9. doi:10.1021/ja0558239. ISSN 0002-7863. PMID 16277495.
18. Zhong, Q; Inniss, D; Kjoller, K; Elings, V (1993). "Fractured polymer/silica fiber surface studied by tapping mode atomic-force microscopy". Surface Science Letters. 290: L688. Bibcode:1993SurSL.290L.688Z. doi:10.1016/0167-2584(93)90906-Y.
19. Geisse, Nicholas A. (July–August 2009). "AFM and Combined Optical Techniques". Materials Today. 12 (7–8): 40–45. doi:10.1016/S1369-7021(09)70201-9. Retrieved 4 November 2011.
20. Gross, L.; Mohn, F.; Moll, N.; Liljeroth, P.; Meyer, G. (27 August 2009). "The Chemical Structure of a Molecule Resolved by Atomic-Force Microscopy". Science. 325 (5944): 1110–1114. Bibcode:2009Sci...325.1110G. doi:10.1126/science.1176210. PMID 19713523.
21. Giessibl, Franz J. (2003). "Advances in atomic-force microscopy". Reviews of Modern Physics. 75 (3): 949–983. arXiv:cond-mat/0305119Freely accessible. Bibcode:2003RvMP...75..949G. doi:10.1103/RevModPhys.75.949.

22. Hinterdorfer, P; Dufrêne, Yf (May 2006). "Detection and localization of single molecular recognition events using atomic-force microscopy". Nature Methods. 3 (5): 347–55. doi:10.1038/nmeth871. ISSN 1548-7091. PMID 16628204.

23. Ferrari, L.; Kaufmann, J.; Winnefeld, F.; Plank, J. (Jul 2010). "Interaction of cement model systems with superplasticizers investigated by atomic-force microscopy, zeta potential, and adsorption measurements". J Colloid Interface Sci. 347 (1): 15–24. doi:10.1016/j.jcis.2010.03.005. PMID 20356605.

24. Butt, H; Cappella, B; Kappl, M (2005). "Force measurements with the atomic-force microscope: Technique, interpretation and applications". Surface Science Reports. 59: 1–152. Bibcode:2005SurSR..59....1B. doi:10.1016/j.surfrep.2005.08.003.

25. Gavin M. King; Ashley R. Carter; Allison B. Churnside; Louisa S. Eberle & Thomas T. Perkins (2009). "Ultrastable Atomic-Force Microscopy: Atomic-Scale Stability and Registration in Ambient Conditions". Nano Letters. 9 (4): 1451–1456. Bibcode:2009NanoL...9.1451K. doi:10.1021/nl803298q. PMC 2953871Freely accessible. PMID 19351191.

26. M. Hoffmann, Ahmet Oral; Ralph A. G, Peter (2001). "Direct measurement of interatomic-force gradients using an ultra-low-amplitude atomic-force microscope". Proceedings of the Royal Society A. 457 (2009): 1161–1174. Bibcode:2001RSPSA.457.1161M. doi:10.1098/rspa.2000.0713.

27. D. Murugesapillai et al, DNA bridging and looping by HMO1 provides a mechanism for stabilizing nucleosome-free chromatin, Nucl Acids Res (2014) 42 (14): 8996-9004

28. D. Murugesapillai et al, Single-molecule studies of high-mobility group B architectural DNA bending proteins, Biophys Rev (2016) doi:10.1007/s12551-016-0236-4

29. Takenaka, Musashi; Miyachi, Yusuke; Ishii, Jun; Ogino, Chiaki; Kondo, Akihiko (2015-03-04). "The mapping of yeast's G-protein coupled receptor with an atomic force microscope". Nanoscale. 7 (11): 4956–4963. doi:10.1039/c4nr05940a. ISSN 2040-3372.

30. Radmacher, M. (1997). "Measuring the elastic properties of biological samples with the AFM". IEEE Eng Med Biol Mag. 16 (2): 47–57. doi:10.1109/51.582176. PMID 9086372.

31. Perkins, Thomas. "Atomic force microscopy measures properties of proteins and protein folding". SPIE Newsroom. Retrieved 4 March 2016.

32. Thomas, G.; Y. Ouabbas; P. Grosseau; M. Baron; A. Chamayou; L. Galet (2009). "Modeling the mean interaction forces between power particles. Application to silice gel-magnesium stearate mixtures". Applied Surface Science. 255: 7500–7507. Bibcode:2009ApSS..255.7500T. doi:10.1016/j.apsusc.2009.03.099.

33. Sugimoto, Y; Pou, P; Abe, M; Jelinek, P; Pérez, R; Morita, S; Custance, O (Mar 2007). "Chemical identification of individual surface atoms by atomic-force microscopy". Nature. 446 (7131): 64–7. Bibcode:2007Natur.446...64S. doi:10.1038/nature05530. ISSN 0028-0836. PMID 17330040.

34. Bryant, P. J.; Miller, R. G.; Yang, R.; "Scanning tunneling and atomic-force microscopy combined". Applied Physics Letters, Jun 1988, Vol: 52 Issue:26, p. 2233–2235, ISSN 0003-6951.
35. Oscar H. Willemsen, Margot M.E. Snel, Alessandra Cambi, Jan Greve, Bart G. De Grooth and Carl G. Figdor "Biomolecular Interactions Measured by Atomic Force Microscopy" Biophysical Journal, Volume 79, Issue 6, December 2000, Pages 3267-3281.
36. Koo-Hyun Chung and Dae-Eun Kim, "Wear characteristics of diamond-coated atomic force microscope probe". Ultramicroscopy, Volume 108, Issue 1, December 2007, Pages 1-10
37. Xu, Xin; Raman, Arvind (2007). "Comparative dynamics of magnetically, acoustically, and Brownian motion driven microcantilevers in liquids". J. Appl. Phys. 102: 034303. Bibcode:2007JAP...102a4303Y. doi:10.1063/1.2751415.
38. Hasselbach, K.; Ladam, C. (2008). "High resolution magnetic imaging : MicroSQUID Force Microscopy". Journal of Physics: Conference Series. 97: 012330. Bibcode:2008JPhCS..97a2330H. doi:10.1088/1742-6596/97/1/012330.
39. Giessibl, Franz J. (1 January 1998). "High-speed force sensor for force microscopy and profilometry utilizing a quartz tuning fork". Applied Physics Letters. 73 (26): 3956. Bibcode:1998ApPhL..73.3956G. doi:10.1063/1.122948.
40. Nishida, Shuhei; Kobayashi, Dai; Sakurada, Takeo; Nakazawa, Tomonori; Hoshi, Yasuo; Kawakatsu, Hideki (1 January 2008). "Photothermal excitation and laser Doppler velocimetry of higher cantilever vibration modes for dynamic atomic-force microscopy in liquid". Review of Scientific Instruments. 79 (12): 123703. Bibcode:2008RScI...79l3703N. doi:10.1063/1.3040500. PMID 19123565.
41. Rugar, D.; Mamin, H. J.; Guethner, P. (1 January 1989). "Improved fiber-optic interferometer for atomic-force microscopy". Applied Physics Letters. 55 (25): 2588. Bibcode:1989ApPhL..55.2588R. doi:10.1063/1.101987.
42. Göddenhenrich, T. "Force microscope with capacitive displacement detection". Journal of Vacuum Science and Technology A. 8 (1): 383. doi:10.1116/1.576401.
43. Giessibl, F. J.; Trafas, B. M. (1 January 1994). "Piezoresistive cantilevers utilized for scanning tunneling and scanning force microscope in ultrahigh vacuum". Review of Scientific Instruments. 65 (6): 1923. Bibcode:1994RScI...65.1923G. doi:10.1063/1.1145232.
44. Binnig, G.; Smith, D. P. E. (1986). "Single-tube three-dimensional scanner for scanning tunneling microscopy". Review of Scientific Instruments. 57 (8): 1688. Bibcode:1986RScI...57.1688B. doi:10.1063/1.1139196. ISSN 0034-6748.
45. R. V. Lapshin (1995). "Analytical model for the approximation of hysteresis loop and its application to the scanning tunneling microscope" (PDF). Review of Scientific Instruments. USA: AIP. 66 (9): 4718–4730. Bibcode:1995RScI...66.4718L. doi:10.1063/1.1145314. ISSN 0034-6748. (Russian translation is available).
46. R. V. Lapshin (2011). "Feature-oriented scanning probe microscopy". In H. S. Nalwa. Encyclopedia of Nanoscience and Nanotechnology (PDF). 14. USA: American Scientific Publishers. pp. 105–115. ISBN 1-58883-163-9.

47. R. V. Lapshin (1998). "Automatic lateral calibration of tunneling microscope scanners" (PDF). Review of Scientific Instruments. USA: AIP. 69 (9): 3268–3276. Bibcode:1998RScI...69.3268L. doi:10.1063/1.1149091. ISSN 0034-6748.

48. R. V. Lapshin (2004). "Feature-oriented scanning methodology for probe microscopy and nanotechnology" (PDF). Nanotechnology. UK: IOP. 15 (9): 1135–1151. Bibcode:2004Nanot..15.1135L. doi:10.1088/0957-4484/15/9/006. ISSN 0957-4484.

49. R. V. Lapshin (2007). "Automatic drift elimination in probe microscope images based on techniques of counter-scanning and topography feature recognition" (PDF). Measurement Science and Technology. UK: IOP. 18 (3): 907–927. Bibcode:2007MeScT..18..907L. doi:10.1088/0957-0233/18/3/046. ISSN 0957-0233.

50. V. Y. Yurov; A. N. Klimov (1994). "Scanning tunneling microscope calibration and reconstruction of real image: Drift and slope elimination" (PDF). Review of Scientific Instruments. USA: AIP. 65 (5): 1551–1557. Bibcode:1994RScI...65.1551Y. doi:10.1063/1.1144890. ISSN 0034-6748.

51. G. Schitter; M. J. Rost (2008). "Scanning probe microscopy at video-rate". Materials Today. UK: Elsevier. 11 (special issue): 40–48. doi:10.1016/S1369-7021(09)70006-9. ISSN 1369-7021. Archived from the original (PDF) on September 9, 2009.

52. R. V. Lapshin; O. V. Obyedkov (1993). "Fast-acting piezoactuator and digital feedback loop for scanning tunneling microscopes" (PDF). Review of Scientific Instruments. USA: AIP. 64 (10): 2883–2887. Bibcode:1993RScI...64.2883L. doi:10.1063/1.1144377. ISSN 0034-6748.

53. Jong, Wim H De; Borm, Paul JA (June 2008). "Drug Delivery and Nanoparticles: Applications and Hazards". Dovepress International Journal of Nanomedicine: 133–149.

54. Pyrgiotakis, Georgios; Blattmann, Christoph O.; Demokritou, Philip (10 June 2014). "Real-Time Nanoparticle-Cell Interactions in Physiological Media by Atomic Force Microscopy". ACS Sustainable Chemistry & Engineering (Sustainable Nanotechnology 2013): 1681–1690.

55. Evans, Evan A.; Calderwood, David A. (25 May 2007). "Forces and Bond Dynamics in Cell Adhesion". Science. 316 (5828): 1148–1153. Bibcode:2007Sci...316.1148E. doi:10.1126/science.1137592.

56. Scheuring, Simon; Lévy, Daniel; Rigaud, Jean-Louis (1 July 2005). "Watching the Components". Elsevier. 1712 (2): 109–127. doi:10.1016/j.bbamem.2005.04.005.

57. Alsteens, David; Verbelen, Claire; Dague, Etienne; Raze, Dominique; Baulard, Alain R.; Dufrêne, Yves F. (April 2008). "Organization of the Mycobacterial Cell Wall: A Nanoscale View". Pflügers Archive European Journal of Physiology. 456 (1): 117–125. doi:10.1007/s00424-007-0386-0.

Index

O

P

R

S

T